Oral Wound Healing

To my family

Oral Wound Healing

Cell Biology and Clinical Management

Edited by

Hannu Larjava
Professor and Chair,
Division of Periodontics
Faculty of Dentistry
University of British Columbia
Vancouver
BC, Canada

WILEY-BLACKWELL
A John Wiley & Sons, Ltd., Publication

This edition first published 2012 by John Wiley & Sons, Inc

Wiley-Blackwell is an imprint of John Wiley & Sons, Inc formed by the merger of Wiley's global Scientific, Technical and Medical business with Blackwell Publishing.

Registered Office
John Wiley & Sons, Ltd, The Atrium, Southern Gate, Chichester, West Sussex, PO19 8SQ, UK

Editorial Offices
2121 State Avenue, Ames, Iowa 50014-8300, USA
The Atrium, Southern Gate, Chichester, West Sussex, PO19 8SQ, UK
9600 Garsington Road, Oxford, OX4 2DQ, UK

For details of our global editorial offices, for customer services and for information about how to apply for permission to reuse the copyright material in this book please see our website at www.wiley.com/wiley-blackwell.

Library of Congress Cataloging-in-Publication Data

Oral wound healing : cell biology and clinical management / edited by Hannu Larjava.
p. ; cm.
Includes bibliographical references and index.
ISBN 978-0-8138-0481-1 (hardcover : alk. paper)
I. Larjava, Hannu.
[DNLM: 1. Periodontal Diseases–rehabilitation. 2. Mouth–injuries. 3. Oral Surgical Procedures–rehabilitation. 4. Wound Healing. WU 240]
617.6′32–dc23

2011042663

A catalogue record for this book is available from the British Library.

Wiley also publishes its books in a variety of electronic formats. Some content that appears in print may not be available in electronic books.

Set in 10/12pt Times by SPi Publisher Services, Pondicherry, India
Printed and bound in Singapore by Markono Print Media Pte Ltd

1 2012

Contents

Contributors

Editor

Hannu Larjava, DDS, PhD, Dip Perio
Professor and Chair, Division of Periodontics
Faculty of Dentistry
University of British Columbia
Vancouver, BC, Canada

Contributors

Ariane Berdal, DDS, MPhil, DSc
Centre de Recherche des Cordeliers
Physiologie Orale Moléculaire
Paris, France

Robert P. Carmichael, DMD, MSc, FRCDC
Chief of Dentistry, Bloorview Kids Rehab
Director, Ontario Cleft Lip and Palate Program
Co-ordinator of Prosthodontics, Hospital for Sick Children
Assistant Professor, University of Toronto
Toronto, Ontario, Canada

Cameron M.L. Clokie, DDS, PhD, FRCDC
Professor and Director of Graduate Program in Oral and Maxillofacial Surgery and Anaesthesia
University of Toronto
Toronto, Ontario, Canada

David L. Cochran, DDS, MS, PhD, MMSci
Chair and Professor
Department of Periodontics
University of Texas Health Science Center at San Antonio
San Antonio, TX, USA

Paul R. Cooper, BSc, PhD
Senior Lecturer in Molecular Biology
Oral Biology
School of Dentistry
University of Birmingham
St Chad's Queensway
Birmingham, UK

Douglas P. Dickinson, PhD
Associate Professor
Department of Oral Biology
Georgia Health Sciences University
College of Dental Medicine
Augusta, Georgia, USA

Luisa Ann DiPietro, DDS, PhD
Professor and Director
Center for Wound Healing and Tissue Regeneration
College of Dentistry
University of Illinois at Chicago
Chicago, IL, USA

Marc G. DuVal, DDS
Chief Resident, Graduate Program in Oral and Maxillofacial Surgery and Anaesthesia
University of Toronto
Toronto, Ontario, Canada

Roberto Farina, DDS, PhD, MSc
Research Assistant
Research Centre for the Study of Periodontal and Peri-implant Diseases
University of Ferrara
Ferrara, Italy

Gabrielle Fredman, PhD
Post Doctoral Fellow
Center for Experimental Therapeutics and Reperfusion Injury
Department of Anesthesiology, Perioperative, and Pain Medicine
Brigham and Women's Hospital/Harvard Medical School
Boston, Massachusetts, USA

Lari Häkkinen, DDS, PhD
Associate Professor
Laboratory of Periodontal Biology
Department of Oral Biological and Medical Sciences
Faculty of Dentistry
University of British Columbia
Vancouver, BC, Canada

Jyrki Heino, MD, PhD
Professor
Department of Biochemistry and Food Chemistry
University of Turku
Turku, Finland

Guy Huynh-Ba, DDS, Dr Med Dent, MS
Assistant Professor
Department of Periodontics
University of Texas Health Science Center at San Antonio
San Antonio, TX, USA

Ahmed Jan, DDS
Chief Resident in Oral and Maxillofacial Surgery and Anesthesia
University of Toronto
Toronto, Canada

Leeni Koivisto, PhD
Research Associate
Laboratory of Periodontal Biology
Department of Oral Biological and Medical Sciences
Faculty of Dentistry
University of British Columbia
Vancouver, BC, Canada

Jaebum Lee, DDS, MSD, PhD
Chief Clinical Scientist
Laboratory for Applied Periodontal and Craniofacial Regeneration
Departments of Periodontics and Oral Biology
Georgia Health Sciences University
College of Dental Medicine
Augusta, Georgia, USA

Philip J. Lumley, DDS, PhD
Director and Head
The School of Dentistry
University of Birmingham
Birmingham, UK

Michael P. Mills, DMD, MS
Clinical Associate Professor
Department of Periodontics
University of Texas Health Science Center at San Antonio
San Antonio, TX, USA

Carol Oakley, DDS, MSc, PhD
Clinical Associate Professor
Department of Oral Biological and Medical Sciences
Faculty of Dentistry
University of British Columbia
Vancouver, BC, Canada

Anthony Papp, MD, PhD, FRCSC
Medical Director BC Professional Firefighters' Burn, Plastic and Trauma Unit
Vancouver General Hospital
Vancouver, BC, Canada

Giuseppe Polimeni, DDS, MS
Clinical Associate Professor, Senior Clinical Scientist
Laboratory for Applied Periodontal and Craniofacial Regeneration
Departments of Periodontics and Oral Biology
Medical College of Georgia School of Dentistry
Augusta, Georgia, USA

Peter J. Polverini, DDS, DMSc
Professor and Dean
University of Michigan
School of Dentistry
Ann Arbor, Michigan, USA

Edward Putnins, PhD, DMD, Dip Perio, MSC, MRCD(C)
Associate Dean Research, Graduate and Post Graduate Studies
University of British Columbia
Faculty of Dentistry
Department of Oral Biological and Medical Sciences
Vancouver, BC, Canada

George K.B. Sándor, MD, DDS, PhD, Dr Habil, FRCDC, FRCSC, FACS
Professor of Tissue Engineering
Regea Institute for Regenerative Medicine
University of Tampere
Tampere, Finland
Professor of Oral and Maxillofacial Surgery
University of Oulu
Oulu, Finland

Charles N. Serhan, PhD
The Simon Gelman Professor of Anaesthesia (Biochemistry and Molecular Pharmacology) Harvard Medical School
Director, Center for Experimental Therapeutics and Reperfusion Injury
Department of Anesthesiology, Perioperative, and Pain Medicine
Brigham and Women's Hospital
Professor, Harvard School of Dental Medicine, Oral Medicine, Infection and Immunity
Boston, Massachusetts, USA

Stéphane Simon, DDS, PhD
Maitre de Conférence Hospitalo-Universitaire
Department of Oral Biology
University of Paris Diderot
Paris, France
Groupe Hospitalier Pitié Salpétrière
Paris, France
Associate Researcher
University of Birmingham
Birmingham, UK

Anthony J. Smith, PhD
Professor in Oral Biology
School of Dentistry
University of Birmingham
Birmingham, UK

Cristiano Susin, DDS, MSD, PhD
Associate Professor of Periodontics, Oral Biology and Graduate Studies
Associate Director, Laboratory for Applied Periodontal and Craniofacial Regeneration
Director, Clinical Research
Georgia Health Sciences University
College of Dental Medicine
Augusta, Georgia, USA

Leonardo Trombelli, DDS, PhD,
Professor and Director, Research Centre for the Study of Periodontal and Peri-implant Diseases
Director, Dental Clinic, University Hospital
University of Ferrara
Ferrara, Italy

Anna Turabelidze, BS
Center for Wound Healing and Tissue Regeneration
College of Dentistry
University of Illinois at Chicago
Chicago, IL, USA

Cristina Cunha Villar, DDS, MS, PhD
Assistant Professor
Department of Periodontics
University of Texas Health Science Center at San Antonio
San Antonio, TX, USA

Ulf M.E. Wikesjö, DDS, DMD, PhD, Diplomate ABP
Professor, Director
Laboratory for Applied Periodontal and Craniofacial Regeneration
Departments of Periodontics and Oral Biology
Georgia Health Sciences University
College of Dental Medicine
Medical College of Georgia School of Dentistry
Augusta, Georgia, USA

Yi Yang, DDS, MSD, MSC, PhD
University of British Columbia
Vancouver, BC, Canada

Leena P. Ylikontiola, MD, DDS, PhD
Assistant Professor, Institute of Dentistry
University of Oulu
Co-ordinator of Cleft Lip and Palate Surgery
Oulu University Hospital
Oulu, Finland

Preface

Our understanding about wound healing has vastly increased over the last decade. Currently, the PubMed search with the words 'wound healing' results in almost a hundred thousand citations. These publications range from basic science to clinical studies and cover multiple disciplines in biology and medicine. Explosion of new knowledge makes it difficult to process the information and condense it into meaningful concepts. The goal of this book was to filtrate the massive information to summaries of wound healing topics that were written by experts in the field. These experts covered not only their own endeavors but also the science at large in their topic area.

At the time of planning this book, there was no comprehensive book covering recent advancements in the field of oral wound care. Wound healing books covering healing of skin and other organs existed and had been extremely successful for dermatologists, wound healing researchers and other health professionals. Wounds are common in oral cavity, ranging from wounds on pulp tissue after tooth preparation to those caused by surgical procedures on soft tissue and bone. Oral wound care has several special features and covers unique processes such as soft tissue healing, healing of bone and extraction socket, regeneration of periodontal structures and healing around dental implants. Although many of these processes have been described in review articles over the years, there was no reference material (book) that covered the entire topic of oral wound healing. This book is the first one that focuses on wound healing in the oral cavity.

This book is intended for a diverse audience, from clinicians to wound healing students. The topics of the book can be useful especially for residents and graduate students who are in training programs aimed at surgical management of oral tissues (such as oral surgery, periodontics, endodontics and oral medicine) and for oral biology or other researchers who are investigating wound healing. In addition, undergraduate students and general practitioners who are advancing their training in surgical sciences would also benefit from the information presented in this book.

Oral Wound Healing is divided into 15 chapters. The first seven chapters cover the fundamentals of wound healing and they are organized to reflect the sequence of wound healing events, starting from blood clotting and ending with angiogenesis. The last eight chapters cover more clinical aspects of wound healing, ranging from healing of extraction sockets to large craniofacial defects.

I would like to express my deep gratitude to the contributors, without whom this book would have never seen completion. I would also like to thank Ms Melissa Wahl for patiently waiting for the final work and for John Wiley & Sons, Inc. for publishing the book.

1 Oral Wound Healing: An Overview

Hannu Larjava
Department of Oral Biological and Medical Sciences, Faculty of Dentistry, University of British Columbia, Vancouver, BC, Canada

In this Overview, I summarize the main content of each of the chapters in this book. Readers are encouraged to carefully read the chapters for more details and relevant literature.

CLOTTING AND INFLAMMATION (CHAPTERS 2, 3 AND 4)

Wounds are common in oral cavity, caused by either trauma or surgery. Soft tissue wound healing in oral cavity proceeds along the same principles as in other areas of the body such as the skin. Wound healing always starts with the blood clotting that initially seals the wound (Chapter 2). Platelet activation during the primary hemostasis releases a number of important cytokines that start the healing process via chemotactic signals to inflammatory and resident cells. In addition, the fibrin-fibronectin clot provides a provisional matrix that both epithelial cells and fibroblasts can use to migrate to the wound space. If a wound continues to bleed, healing is delayed because of the disturbed formation of granulation tissue. Cytokines released during the clotting phase initiate the inflammatory reaction that provides wound debridement, removing damaged tissue and microbes. During this innate immune response, inflammatory cells that have been recruited to the wound site release more cytokines and chemokines which critically modulate wound-healing outcome (Chapter 3). Macrophages appear to be especially critical cells for wound repair. Interestingly, recent evidence suggests that wound macrophage populations shift over time and cells with different phenotypes orchestrate different phases of wound healing (reviewed in Brancato and Albina 2011). Among the cytokines and other regulatory factors that they release, macrophages secrete vascular endothelial growth factor (VEGF), fibroblast growth factor (FGF) and transforming growth factor-beta1 (TGF-ß1) which appear to be the most significant regulators of tissue repair.

Persistent inflammation retards wound healing and can lead to the formation of chronic wounds and even to development of cancer (reviewed in Eming et al. 2007). In addition, inflammation seems to dictate the healing quality and outcome of the wound. Adult skin wounds heal with visible scars. Fetal skin wounds, however, heal without scars until late third trimester (Ferguson and O'Kane 2004). The most striking difference between fetal and adult healing is the lack of inflammation in fetal wound healing (Eming et al. 2007). It is

Oral Wound Healing: Cell Biology and Clinical Management, First Edition. Edited by Hannu Larjava.

crucial, therefore, to effectively down-regulate the inflammatory process to prevent wound fibrosis and chronic wounds. During the last decade, a number of chemical mediators have been found that regulate the resolution of inflammation (Chapter 4). During the early stage of the inflammatory reaction, pro-inflammatory mediators such as prostaglandins and leukotrienes dominate and they continue to dominate in 'unresolved' chronic inflammatory conditions (reviewed in Serhan 2011). In normal healing of acute inflammation, however, specialized pro-resolving lipid mediators are actively expressed to suppress inflammation (Chapter 4). These mediators include lipoxins, resolvins and protectins which have a variety of functions including suppression of influx of leucocytes, stimulation of uptake of apoptotic cells and activation of antimicrobial mechanisms (Serhan 2011). Resolvins are derived from the long-chain n-3 polyunsaturated fatty acids (PUFA) eicosapentaenoic acid (EPA), and docosahexaenoic acid (DHA). These compounds are found enriched in fish oils. The levels of resolvins increase in individuals consuming EPA. In addition, low-dose aspirin increases the resolving levels by a complex process involving acetylation of cyclooxygenase-2 by endothelial cells that converts EPA to a metabolite taken by the leukocytes which finally further convert it to resolvin (Chapter 4). Interestingly, preliminary studies suggest that oral supplementation of EPA and DHA together with low-dose aspirin may reduced inflammation and improve wound healing in acute human wounds (McDaniel et al. 2011).

Despite the enormous amount of data available about wound healing in general, molecular features of wound healing in different areas of oral cavity are still emerging. A common observation by clinicians is that oral wounds heal quickly and in some areas such as gingiva and palatal mucosa without significant scar formation. These observations are supported by experimental evidence showing that palatal wounds in humans and pigs heal with minimal scarring (Mak et al. 2009; Wong et al. 2009). Although the molecular mechanisms of the scar-free healing in oral cavity are still being dissected, the current evidence points to reduced or fast resolving inflammation that separates scar-free oral wounds from skin wounds that heal with scarring (Larjava et al. 2011a).

RE-EPITHELIALIZATION AND GRANULATION TISSUE FORMATION (CHAPTERS 5 AND 6)

Within 24 hours after wounding, epithelial cells at the margin of the wound dissolve their hemidesmosomal adhesions and show first signs of migration. In 48 hours, proliferation starts behind the leading edge, seeding more cells into the wound site. Epithelial cells migrate through fibrin-fibronectin provisional matrix until they contact the front of leading cells coming from the other side of the wound. This migration is a complex process that depends on cell surface integrin-type matrix receptors. Their expression is induced in the migratory cells to facilitate optimal adhesion strength to the extracellular matrix. This matrix is composed of proteins present in the provisional matrix and those synthesized by the cells, including laminin-332, fibronectin EDA and tenascin C. Too strong adhesion to the matrix would prevent migration and too weak adhesion would not provide sufficient force for migratory movement. When epithelial cells resume this optimal adhesion strength, their migration can be stimulated by a number of cytokines and growth factors such as epidermal growth factor (EGF), heparin-binding EGF (HB-EGF), TGF-ß1 and others. Furthermore, re-epithelialization is also critically dependent on proteolytic enzymes, including plasmin and matrix metalloproteinases. These enzymes support cell migration at multiple levels by breaking down the provisional matrix, loosening up the adhesions and also by activation of growth factors. The activity of these enzymes needs to be well balanced, as uncontrolled enzymatic activity is associated with chronic wounds that fail to re-epithelialize. Fortunately, most wounds re-epithelialize perfectly with complete regeneration of the epithelial structure and function.

The formation of granulation tissue starts simultaneously with re-epithelialization; however, its maturation to connective tissue takes much longer time and may in fact continue for months if not years. The purpose of granulation tissue is to replace the provisional wound matrix and provide scaffold for connective tissue formation. Small wounds with primary closure heal quickly with fast re-epithelialization and only a small amount of granulation tissue will form. Open wounds, however, heal with slower epithelial closure and more granulation tissue formation. Initially, fibrin-fibronectin provisional matrix contains neutrophil granulocytes that are subsequently replaced by macrophages, lymphocytes and mast cells. Inflammatory cells secrete a number of factors capable of activating and recruiting resident fibroblasts at the wound margin, mesenchymal progenitor cells (pericytes and other mesenchymal stem cells) and circulating fibroblast-like cells (fibrocytes) that migrate to the provisional matrix. These cells, along with cells forming the new blood vessels, form the granulation tissue and subsequently turn it to connective tissue. Analogous to epithelial cell migration, fibroblast migration also depends on induction of certain integrins, new matrix production (e.g. EDA- and EDB-fibronectins, tenascin-C, hyaluronan, type III collagen, matricellular proteins) and expression of several matrix-degrading enzymes. When sufficient amount of collagen is produced into the granulation tissue, wound contraction can start. This process pulls wound margins closer together, reducing surface area and increasing the speed of wound closure. Wound contraction is actively mediated by differentiated myofibroblasts that use integrin receptors to pull the matrix using their strong actin-rich cytoskeleton. Myofibroblasts differentiate from local resident fibroblasts or other progenitor cells in the presence of certain matrix molecules and growth factors including EDA-fibronectin and TGF-ß1. After wound contraction, granulation tissue remodeling takes place. During this process, fibroblasts degrade, remodel and re-organize the extracellular matrix. Altered mechanosensory signals from the remodeling tissue will reduce the cellular activity, and matrix production will cease and myofibroblasts undergo apoptosis. The end result of healing in the skin is often the formation of a connective tissue scar with reduced tensile strength, disoriented collagen fibers and other molecular alterations. In some parts of oral mucosa (gingiva, palatal mucosa), healing results in clinically scar-free healing with histological features of almost normal connective tissue (see above). The molecular differences of these two different healing responses are still not clear.

ANGIOGENESIS (CHAPTER 7)

Angiogenesis (formation of new blood vessels) is tightly associated with granulation tissue formation during wound healing. Injury to the tissue initiates the angiogenic process in the capillary network. Angiogenesis has many similarities to re-epithelialization (see above). Endothelial cells or their precursor cells in the pre-existing venules become activated by humoral factors (see below) and start to migrate to the wound provisional matrix within 24 hours after wounding. For migration, endothelial cells detach from the basement membrane and use their integrin receptors for cell movement. This process is similar to re-epithelialization but involves different integrins. Endothelial cells behind the leading edge start then to proliferate and feed more cells to the developing endothelial bud or sprout.

Finally, proximal to the proliferating and migrating cells, endothelial cells form a tube that is stabilized by surrounding basement membrane. At this stage, the new capillary is ready for blood flow that is necessary for maintenance of the new vessel.

Platelets, inflammatory cells (especially macrophages) and resident fibroblasts release many angiogenic factors, such as vascular endothelial growth factors (VEGFs) that play a crucial role in promotion of angiogenesis. Hypoxia in the wound site is a major inducer of VEGF expression in a variety of cells. The fully formed granulation tissue has a high number of new blood vessels. Some of these vessels need to regress during tissue maturation. This regression is linked to reduced or lack of angiogenic stimulus and also to active inhibition of angiogenesis by various factors, including thrombospondin-1. Balance between angiogenesis and its inhibition may be important for healing outcome. For example, skin wounds that form scars have more robust angiogenesis than palatal mucosal wounds that heal without scars (Mak et al. 2009). On the other hand, poor angiogenic response in wounds of diabetic patients contributes to wound healing morbidity in these patients.

HEALING OF EXTRACTION SOCKETS (CHAPTER 8)

One of the most common oral wounds is an extraction socket after tooth removal. Wound healing in the socket follows similar principles as the soft tissue healing except that it also involves healing of the bone, namely (1) clotting, (2) re-epithelialization, (3) granulation tissue formation and (4) bone formation. Within minutes after tooth extraction a blood clot forms into the extraction socket. Re-epithelialization starts as for any soft tissue wounds as described above. Granulation tissue also forms as explained above and within a week it has replaced the blood clot. What happens next differs from soft tissue healing. Osteogenic cells from the bottom and the walls of the socket are induced to migrate into the developing granulation tissue in which they differentiate and initiate bone deposition. It is likely that mesenchymal stem cells recruited locally together with bone marrow derived cells are induced for osteogenic differentiation by cytokines and growth factors released locally by platelets and inflammatory cells and bone cells. In addition, wounding stimulates osteoclastic activity and remodeling at the socket walls, which process releases growth factors and cytokines such as TGF-ß1 and BMPs that are stored in the bone matrix. Therefore, bony defect turns to bone rather than soft tissue. Most of the socket is filled with bone within 8 weeks after extraction. Bone remodeling continues, however, often for 6 months or more, with great individual variation. During this remodeling phase of socket healing, dimensions of socket walls change. A significant amount of bone height and width is lost due to resorption of the socket walls. The extent of this bone loss is again individual and dependent on several variables such as site, presence of adjacent teeth, treatment protocol and smoking. Grafting the socket with bone substitutes and covering them with membranes appears to show promising results in preventing some of the bone loss after extraction.

FLAP DESIGN FOR PERIODONTAL WOUND HEALING (CHAPTER 9)

Surgical maneuvering of the periodontal soft tissues plays a key role in optimal healing. It is well documented that large scalloped incisions cause significant tissue shrinkage during the healing period. In addition, anterior periodontal surgery with both labial and lingual opening of the flap frequently results in loss of papillary fill and creates so-called black holes. Furthermore, use of membranes and bone grafting materials makes it difficult to achieve primary closure, leading to membrane exposure and loss of bone grafting material. Different surgical techniques have been developed to optimize primary closure and therefore protect the fibrin-fibronectin clot that plays a crucial role in wound stability and healing outcome. Avoiding surgical incisions that compromise the integrity of the interdental supracrestal soft tissue seems to improve preservation of the interdental papilla. Various papilla preservation techniques have been designed and they seem to limit graft or membrane exposure as well as maintain the papilla. These techniques work well when adequate width of the interdental space is available. Since the interdental space is not often sufficiently wide for papilla preservation technique, a single flap approach could be considered. In this technique, only the buccal or lingual flap is elevated, allowing the flap to be repositioned to its original height with primary closure. Flap elevation from the bone is minimized. Specially designed micro surgical instruments can be used for these procedures. As for any surgical procedure, a key for success is a high level of oral hygiene before and after the surgical procedure to reduce the amount of microbial biofilm at the wound site, leading to reduced inflammatory reaction in the healing wound.

REGENERATION OF PERIODONTAL TISSUES (CHAPTERS 10 AND 11)

Conventional periodontal surgery aimed at reduction of periodontal pockets results in repair of periodontal structures that no longer mimic the normal architecture of the healthy periodontium. Periodontal regeneration is, however, a wound healing process that reproduces all the lost structures of the periodontium, namely alveolar bone, cementum, periodontal ligament and gingiva. Although wound healing at the tooth–gingiva interphase follows the same principles as in the skin or palatal mucosa, there are key differences that influence the healing outcome. In periodontal healing, the fibrin-fibronectin clot needs to be stabilized on a mechanically debrided root surface. This stabilization often fails leading to migration of the epithelium along the root surface, thus preventing connective tissue healing and regeneration. Periodontal ligament and bony walls of the tissue defect appear to serve as niches from which the progenitor cells migrate into the regenerating periodontium. Therefore, the defect configuration plays a critical role in periodontal regeneration. Stabilization of the wound and providing space are key elements for successful regeneration. Space can be provided by various barrier membranes or even bone grafting materials or other devices (see below). As indicated in the previous chapter, primary wound closure and appropriate control of microbial biofilm and thereby inflammation are crucial elements for successful regeneration.

Barrier membranes for space maintenance are cumbersome to use, make it difficult to achieve primary closure and often provide only partial regeneration. Therefore various biological agents have been developed to promote periodontal regeneration. At the present time, three different products are in clinical use and recommended for periodontal regenerative procedures. These are platelet-derived growth factor-BB (GEM 21S®; Osteohealth), type I collagen-derived synthetic peptide (PepGen P-15®; Dentsply) and enamel matrix protein mixture (Emdogain®, Straumann). Although the mechanisms explaining how these agents function when applied to the periodontal lesion are still unclear, they seem to produce positive clinical results. They do seem to share some common properties such as promotion of proliferation of fibroblasts and osteogenic cells. In addition, they all seem to positively promote stem cell recruitment. Other agents are also being tested for clincial use in humans, such as fibroblast growth factor-2 (FGF-2) and growth and differentiation factor-5 (GDF-5), with promising results. A common feature for all these agents is a large heterogeneity in treatment outcomes that could result from suboptimal release of the active ingredient (dose and time) from the scaffold. In addition, patient, site, type of defect and clinical application may critically influence the outcome. Since stem cell recruitment seems to be critical for the regenerative therapy, mesenchymal stem cells have been directly added into the periodontal defects in experimental setting. These studies have shown that this therapy may produce some regeneration of the periodontium. Future studies are needed to optimize these techniques and also to better explain the biological mechanisms that determine treatment outcomes and regeneration process.

OSTEOINTEGRATION AND SOFT TISSUE HEALING AROUND DENTAL IMPLANTS (CHAPTER 12)

Dental implants have become part of routine treatment in oral rehabilitation. Placing an implant into the alveolar bone initiates a wound healing response that typically involves healing of both soft tissues and bone. Implant fixtures can be placed at the level of the alveolar bone crest or left above it. They can also be either covered completely with the mucosal tissue or left exposed to oral cavity with a healing abutment. Wound healing response varies depending on the situation. In cases where an implant is placed at the level of bone with a cover screw and then completely covered with soft tissue with primary closure, the soft tissue will quickly heal following the principles described above with minimal granulation tissue formation. Wound healing reaction in the osteotomy site is initiated by clot formation at the inner parts of the treads. This clot is then infiltrated by inflammatory cells, namely polymorphonuclear leukocytes and macrophages. Fibroblastic progenitor cells then invade the provisional matrix and deposit granulation tissue that gets vascularized by migrating endothelial cells. These cells then differentiate to osteoblasts and start to deposit bone. Bone deposition can be seen as early as 4 days after implant placement, but complete osteointegration with maximum bone–implant contact takes 1–3 months. Implant stability can be tested during healing with various devices. Bone around the implant continues to remodel over the first year of implant placement and is dependent on the mechanical stress from occlusal forces. Osteointegration of dental implants is a very predictable procedure with success rates far above 90%, regardless of the implant loading protocol. Failure to osteointegrate or the development of peri-implant disease are often connected with patient-associated factors such as smoking, diabetes and history of periodontal disease, which can all affect various phases of the initial wound healing response (Mellado-Valero et al. 2007; Heitz-Mayfield and Huynh-Ba 2009).

When implants are immediately ‘restored’ with a healing abutment or a permanent abutment and restoration, the soft tissue healing response will differ from that associated with covered implants. In this case, a blood clot forms now between the abutment or the collar of the implant and the gingival soft tissue. During healing, epithelial cells from oral epithelium migrate towards the implant/abutment, flatten along the surface and create a peri-implant epithelium that mimics junctional epithelium. The adhesion of this epithelium may not fully recapitulate that of junctional epithelium (reviewed in Larjava et al. 2011b). During healing, fibroblasts apical to the peri-implant epithelium deposit collagen fibers that run parallel to the implant surface without insertion into the implant surface. This can be explained by the lack of cementum formation at the connective tissue–implant interphase. Several studies have shown that when the implant/abutment interphase is moved away from the bone crest, less crestal bone resorption will occur. It is probable, therefore, that soft tissue attachment to the abutment (or the implant) is not sufficiently strong to prevent biofilm penetration to the micro gap between the abutment and the implant. Future studies are needed to develop implant surface characteristics for better attachment of the soft tissue during the healing process. Improved therapy protocols are also needed to avoid multiple intrusive manipulations at the abutment/implant–soft tissue interphase that predispose the healing tissue to physical and microbiological insults.

THE PULP HEALING PROCESS (CHAPTER 13)

Wounding of the dental pulp happens commonly in a dental practice. Preparation of teeth for removal of caries and subsequent restoration or for bridge abutments often leads to traumatic injury or exposure of the pulp. If the injury is sufficiently weak and does not destroy the odontoblast layer, the cells are activated to produce tertiary dentin to protect the healing pulp from further injury. Bacterial products, cytokines released from the resident and inflammatory cells as well as growth factors of the TGF-ß family released from the dentin matrix are all able to stimulate this reactionary dentinogenesis. When the pulp is exposed with the damage to the odontoblast layer, healing process with a dentin bridge is possible but requires recruitment of progenitor cells that can differentiate to odontoblasts. Although reparative dentinogenesis can happen spontaneously in the absence of bacteria, many materials have been used to stimulate the reparative dentin formation. Traditionally, calcium hydroxide has been used for pulp capping after exposure. More recently, mineral trioxide aggregate (MTA) has been recommended for this purpose. Steps of wound healing in the pulp after calcium hydroxide application have been well characterized. Application of calcium hydroxide leads to superficial necrosis of the pulp followed by inflammatory reaction. Within a week the inflammatory layer is replaced by granulation tissue with numerous fibroblasts and blood vessels. Stem or progenitor cells are then induced to proliferate and migrate to the wound site where they differentiate into odontoblast-like cells that are able to synthesize proteins and vesicles involved in formation of reparative dentin. The origins of the stem/progenitor cells are still under investigation. If the inflammation persists in the pulp, the development of reparative dentin is inhibited and pulpal necrosis may follow. Future studies are likely to lead to new therapeutic approaches for pulp capping that further promote reparative dentin formation.

DERMAL WOUND HEALING AND BURN WOUNDS (CHAPTER 14)

As described in previous chapters, healing of relatively small traumatic or surgical soft tissue wounds usually results in fast repair with formation of a small scar, or in some cases in regeneration of the affected tissue. In contrast, thermal injuries in skin or mucosa may often cause more extensive damage, leading to severely compromised wound healing outcomes. The extent of thermal injury depends on temperature, contact time, thickness of the skin or mucosa and vascularity of the area. The central area of a burn wound shows necrosis often called the zone of coagulation. Necrotic area is surrounded by the heat-injured tissue that is still alive but has reduced tissue perfusion (zone of stasis). This area has potential for recovery if tissue perfusion can be re-established. The zone of hyperemia surrounds the zone of stasis and is characterized by viable cells and vasodilatation caused by inflammatory reaction. Burn injuries continue to progress into deeper structures for 48–72 hours after the initial insult. This is caused by vascular and inflammatory reactions. While the superficial wounds heal by re-epithelialization, the deeper wounds require surgical treatment for healing. To this end, all non-viable burn tissue will be removed and various skin grafts, artificial skins or flaps are used to reconstruct the area. The type of graft or whether flaps are utilized depends on the area and depth of the injury.

Superficial intraoral burn wounds are common and often caused by hot drinks. Fortunately, these wounds heal without complications and require no treatment. Deep intraoral wounds, however, are challenging to treat and numerous surgical procedures may be required to reduce the contractures that often develop to the commissural areas. Deep facial burns are also problematic as they often heal with visible scars that interfere with speech and expression of emotions. Such scars can have a detrimental effect on oral functions and also cause psychological trauma. Future burn therapies should focus on novel techniques for scar reduction, especially in the facial area.

HEALING OF LARGE DENTOFACIAL DEFECTS (CHAPTER 15)

Dentofacial defects are bone and soft tissue deficits in the jaws or other bones of the skull. They can result from congenital defects, trauma or tumors. Reconstruction of these defects can be challenging, as often a significant amount of new bone and soft tissue need to be engineered. Most bone defects require grafting with block or particulate grafts that can be harvested from the patient. Alternatively prepared cadaver bone graft materials or synthetic bone particles could be used. The bone graft is then completely covered with a resorbable or non-resorbable barrier membrane to prevent soft tissue invasion into the graft site. Graft site vascularity and wound stability are key factors for successful outcome. Lateral ridge augmentations and sinus elevation procedures are typical examples of bone grafting procedures aiming at augmentation of the alveolar ridge for implant placement. While sinus floor and lateral ridge augmentations are relatively predictable procedures, vertical augmentation of alveolar defects remains difficult and often unpredictable. Distraction osteogenesis has been used successfully to augment atrophic alveolar bone. This technique is, however, labor intensive and associated with significant morbidity and hardware costs.

Recently, synthetic bioimplants combined with growth factors have been considered for reconstruction of craniofacial defects. These implant materials contain bone morphogenic proteins (BMPs) that are known to support bone formation. Two products are currently in clinical use, namely BMP-7 (BMP-7, Stryker, Allendale, New Jersey, USA) and BMP-2 (BMP-2, Medtronic, Fridley, Minnesota, USA). BMP-2 has been approved by the US Food and Drug Administration (FDA) for anterior lumbar spinal fusion, sinus elevation and lateral ridge augmentation. BMP-7 device has been approved for posterolateral lumbar spine fusion and treatment of long bone non-union fractures. Both products use type I collagen as their carrier. Positive results with BMP-2 in sinus floor and lateral ridge augmentations have been reported (Jung et al. 2009; Triplett et al. 2009). In addition, positive results using BMP-7 in demineralized bone matrix for treatment of mandibular resection defects have been published (Clokie and Sándor 2008). Future studies should further evaluate the effectiveness of these products in the reconstruction of various defects in the craniofacial area when combined with autogenous mesenchymal stem cells (Sándor and Suuronen 2008).

REFERENCES

Brancato, S.K., Albina, J.E. (2011) Wound macrophages as key regulators of repair: origin, phenotype, and function. *Am J Pathol* **178**, 19–25.

Clokic, C.M., Sándor, G.K. (2008) Reconstruction of 10 major mandibular defects using bioimplants containing BMP-7. *J Canadian Dental Assoc* **74**, 67–72.

Eming, S.A., Krieg, T., Davidson, J.M. (2007) Inflammation in wound repair: molecular and cellular mechanisms. *J Invest Dermatol* **127**, 514–25.

Ferguson, M.W., O'Kane, S. (2004) Scar-free healing: from embryonic mechanisms to adult therapeutic intervention. *Phil Trans Royal Soc London. Series B, Biol Sci* **359**, 839–50.

Heitz-Mayfield, L.J., Huynh-Ba, G. (2009) History of treated periodontitis and smoking as risks for implant therapy. *Int J Oral Maxillofac Implants* **24** Suppl, 39–68.

Jung, R.E., Windisch, S.I., Eggenschwiler, A.M., et al. (2009) A randomized-controlled clinical trial evaluating clinical and radiological outcomes after 3 and 5 years of dental implants placed in bone regenerated by means of GBR techniques with or without the addition of BMP-2. *Clin Oral Implants Res* **20**, 660–66.

Larjava, H., Wiebe, C., Gallant-Behm, C., Hart, D.A., Heino, J., Häkkinen, L. (2011a) Exploring scarless healing of oral soft tissues. *J Can Dent Assoc* **77**, b18.

Larjava, H., Koivisto, L., Häkkinen, L., Heino, J. (2011b) Epithelial integrins with special reference to oral epithelia. *J Dent Res*, 25 March (Epub ahead of print).

Mak, K., Manji, A., Gallant-Behm, C., et al. (2009) Scarless healing of oral mucosa is characterized by faster resolution of inflammation and control of myofibroblast action compared to skin wounds in the red Duroc pig model. *J Dermatol Sci* **5**, 168–80.

McDaniel, J.C., Massey, K., Nicolaou, A. (2011) Fish oil supplementation alters levels of lipid mediators of inflammation in microenvironment of acute human wounds. *Wound Repair Regen* **19**, 189–200.

Mellado-Valero, A., Ferrer García, J.C., Herrera Ballester, A., et al. (2007) Effects of diabetes on the osteointegration of dental implants. *Med Oral Patol Oral Cir Bucal* **12**, E38–43.

Sándor, G.K., Suuronen, R. (2008) Combining adipose-derived stem cells, resorbable scaffolds and growth factors: an overview of tissue engineering. *J Can Dent Assoc* **74**, 167–70.

Serhan, C.N. (2011) The resolution of inflammation: the devil in the flask and in the details. *FASEB J* **25**, 1441–8.

Triplett, R.G., Nevins, M., Marx, R.E., et al. (2009) Pivotal, randomized, parallel evaluation of recombinant human bone morphogenetic protein 2/absorbable collagen sponge and autogenous bone graft for maxillary sinus floor augmentation. *J Oral Maxillofac Surg* **67**, 1947–60.

Wong, J.W., Gallant-Behm, C., Wiebe, C., et al. (2009) Wound healing in oral mucosa results in reduced scar formation as compared with skin: evidence from the red Duroc pig model and humans. *Wound Repair and Regen*, **17**, 717–29.

2 Hemostasis, Coagulation and Complications

Carol Oakley and Hannu Larjava

Department of Oral Biological and Medical Sciences, Faculty of Dentistry, University of British Columbia, Vancouver, BC, Canada

INTRODUCTION

One serious complication arising from wounding is the failure to control or stop bleeding. The point at which a clot is formed is known commonly as coagulation, yet coagulation is only one part of the complex hemostatic process. Hemostasis is the physiological process that maintains the fluidity of blood and, upon injury, limits blood loss yet preserves tissue perfusion and stimulates the local repair process. Hence, hemostasis is an intricate balance between clot formation and clot dissolution and any derangement of this balance leads to either hypercoagulation and thrombosis or hypocoagulation and hemorrhage. As minor injuries occur frequently, it is crucial that procoagulant reactions remain localized to the injured site and are not disseminated throughout the vascular system (Dahlback 2005).

Thrombosis occurs when an aggregation of platelets and fibrin forms within the vessel lumen. In either hemostasis or thrombosis, the coagulation process results in the conversion of prothrombin to thrombin that in turn converts circulating fibrinogen to insoluble fibrin.

Coagulation also triggers inflammatory reactions that are necessary for wound healing. In the converse direction, inflammation can trigger activation of the coagulation system (May et al. 2008). Even though the coagulation and immune systems are viewed as specialized systems, there is an extensive two-way interaction between the two systems both in health and disease (Delvaeye and Conway 2009; Rex et al. 2009; Verhamme and Hoylaerts 2009; Yeaman 2010).

The prevention of bleeding complications from a surgical procedure begins with a thorough review of the patient's health history and includes findings in the clinical examination so that patients with a potential bleeding problem can be identified. Bleeding disorders arise due to altered abilities of blood vessels, endothelial cells (ECs), platelets, coagulation and fibrinolytic factors to maintain hemostasis (Little et al. 2002). Some bleeding disorders are inherited, but the majority are acquired and occur secondarily to diseases and/or their management (Little et al. 2002) or are related to diet (e.g. Fugh-Berman 2000). Clinicians may rely upon various screening laboratory tests to provide an 'independent' assessment of specific coagulation deficiencies and hence the risk for clinical bleeding. However, clinicians may be misled by routine testing as these *in vitro* tests are often inadequate in explaining or predicting in vivo hemostasis and are inconsistent with clinical manifestations of several factor deficiencies.

Oral Wound Healing: Cell Biology and Clinical Management, First Edition. Edited by Hannu Larjava.

In this chapter, phases of hemostasis and models of coagulation are reviewed. In addition, laboratory testing and the prevention and management of bleeding complications in dental practice will be discussed.

PRIMARY HEMOSTASIS

The dynamics of the coagulation/hemostatic system are exceedingly complex and involve interrelationships between responses of endothelial cells (ECs), platelets, coagulation proteins and the fibrinolytic mechanism. Models have been developed to simplify the regulatory and biochemical mechanisms and many investigations into hemostasis and coagulation have been performed in cell-free static *in vitro* systems. However, advances in laboratory techniques, biochemistry and computerized mathematical models have provided paradigms that are more reliable and consistent with *in vivo* dynamics (Mann et al. 2006; 2009).

Blood flow differs between the venous and arterial systems and therefore their respective coagulation needs also differ. In the venous circulation, flow rates and bleeding are slower and hemostasis depends mostly on the rate of thrombin generation. In contrast, massive and rapid blood loss can result from even minor injury to pressurized arteries where platelets are essential to the rapid arrest of bleeding (Kriz et al. 2009). These differences are also reflected in thrombotic disorders and their therapeutic management. The predominant platelet aggregates in the arterial system are termed 'white thrombi' and antiplatelet agents such as aspirin, clopidogrel [Plavix™ (Bristol-Myers Squibb)], abciximab, epitifibatide and tirofiban are prescribed for the management of atherosclerotic disease. The 'red thrombus', rich in fibrin and trapped erythrocytes, forms in the venous system and cardiac atria and treatment and prophylaxis of venous thrombo-embolic disease includes heparin and warfarin (Bhatt and Francis 2003; Kriz et al. 2009; King 2010). Nevertheless, the soluble factors and cellular components are intertwined and the hemostatic system can be divided arbitrarily into primary, secondary and tertiary hemostasis (Stassen et al. 2004; Lippi et al. 2009).

In primary hemostasis, which includes the vascular phase and platelet phase, the vascular system and platelets respond to limit the loss of blood. The vascular system is a network of vessels comprised of muscular and elastic arteries which decrease in diameter and branch progressively into arterioles at the entrances to capillaries—the sites of nutrient, metabolite and blood gas exchange—and postcapillary venules and veins. Capillary ECs are surrounded by basal lamina and occasionally pericytes, which have a contractile function in regulating blood flow through the capillary. Following injury, pericytes can proliferate and differentiate into endothelial and smooth muscle cells. In general, veins conform to the three-layer anatomy of arteries, but veins have thinner walls and larger lumens than arteries and medium-sized veins contain valves to prevent blood backflow (Atkinson and White 1992). In healthy large arteries, the vessel size exceeds the size of blood cells and shear rates are sufficiently high enough so that interactions between particles and the vessel wall have a negligible effect on flow. Moreover, the high flow rate will preclude accumulation of activated coagulation factors. In narrower vessels, either healthy or diseased (e.g. atherosclerotic), the flow may be turbulent or transitional and resistance to flow changes significantly with respect to the radius of the vessel. Blood vessels quickly sense and adapt to changing rates of blood flow in order to maintain consistent blood pressure throughout the body. Blood vessels are active organs and their vascular functions are controlled by biochemical mediators (cytokines, hormones, neurotransmitters) as well as by biomechanical forces generated by blood flow and pressure (Esper et al. 2006).

The vascular phase of hemostasis begins immediately upon injury to blood vessels, which causes spasm of the smooth muscles in the vessel walls and results in retraction of severed arteries and vasoconstriction of arteries and veins, thus slowing the blood flow. As blood accumulates outside the vessel, increased extravascular pressure from the hematoma also slows bleeding by collapsing adjacent capillaries and veins, and blood flow is diverted around the site of the injury. The platelet phase includes platelet adhesion and platelet aggregation which results in formation of a soft platelet plug. Platelet adhesion (platelet contact to extracellular surfaces) and aggregation (contact between platelets) are usually considered distinct processes but are often mediated by the same receptors. The specific adhesion and aggregation interactions are regulated by the particular extracellular matrix (ECM) proteins exposed and the hydrodynamic conditions (shear stress and shear rate; see below) of blood flow at the lesion (Ruggeri and Mendolicchio 2007; Ruggeri 2009).

SECONDARY HEMOSTASIS AND THE COAGULATION SYSTEM

The Waterfall Cascade Model of clotting was developed independently by MacFarlane (1964) and Davie and Ratnoff (1964). The Waterfall Cascade Model (Fig. 2.1) comprises the distinct 'Y'-shaped pathways of the intrinsic and extrinsic pathways that both generate

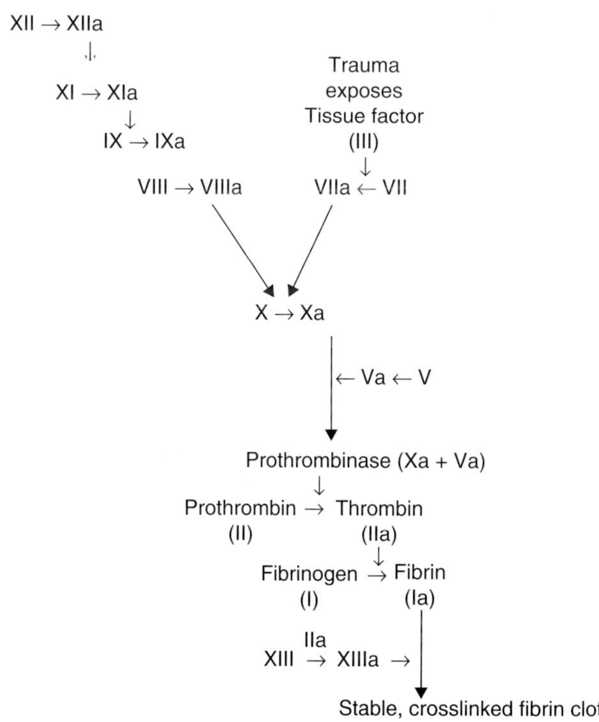

Fig. 2.1 The Waterfall Cascade Model of clotting. In the intrinsic pathway, a negatively charged surface initiates factor XII cleavage, while in the extrinsic pathway, tissue factor initiates factor VII cleavage. Both pathways lead to factor X activation and continue in a common pathway leading to fibrin clot formation.

Table 2.1 Coagulation factors and their functions.

Factor	Name	Pathways	Source	Function	Disorder
I	Fibrinogen	C	Liver	Forms fibrin	–
II*	Prothrombin (enzyme)	C	Liver	Active form activates I, V, VII, VIII, XI, XIII, protein C, platelets	–
III	Tissue factor (thromboplastin)	E, I	Damaged cells, platelets	Initiates the extrinsic pathway; cofactor of VIIa	–
IV	Calcium ions	N/A	Gut and bone	Required for coagulation factors to bind to membrane phospholipids	–
V	Labile cofactor, proaccelerin	E, I	Liver, MKS, α-granules		Factor V Leiden hypercoagulability disorder MCFD (FV and FVIII) multiple coagulation factor deficiency
(VI)	Activated factor V	N/A		Former name of FVa	–
VII*	Proconvertin	E	Liver	Activates IX, X	–
VIII	Antihemolytic cofactor	I	Endothelium, platelets	With IX forms the tenase complex	Hemophilia A MCFD (FV and FVIII) multiple coagulation factor deficiency
IX*	Christmas factor	I	Liver	Forms tenase with VIII	Hemophilia B
X*	Stuart Prower factor	E, I		Activates II, forms prothrombinase complex with FV	
XI	Plasma thromboplastin antecedent	I	Liver	Activates IX	Hemophilia C
XII	Hageman factor	I	Liver	Activates XI, VII and prekallikrein	–
XIII	Fibrin stabilizing factor	C	Liver	Cross-links fibrin	–

*Vitamin-K dependent factors.
E, extrinsic; I, intrinsic; C, common pathway.

activated factor X (FXa) and converge into the common pathway, resulting in generation of thrombin and the subsequent cleavage of fibrinogen to fibrin. Each pathway is a sequence of proteolytic reactions wherein enzymes cleave proenzymes or zymogen substrates to generate the next enzyme in the cascade (Table 2.1). In this model, coagulation is controlled primarily by the concentrations and kinetics of the coagulation proteins/cofactors, the presence of calcium, and anionic membrane phospholipids, which are required for the assembly and optimal function of the majority of the coagulation complexes. This model initially did not

Table 2.2 Coagulation cofactors and their functions.

Coagulation cofactor	Function
Alpha 2-antiplasmin	Inhibits plasmin
Antithrombin	Inhibits IIa, Xa and other proteases
Fibronectin	Mediates cell adhesion including platelets to the ECM
Heparin cofactor II	Inhibits IIa; cofactor for heparin
HMWK	High molecular weight kininogen; supports the activation of XI, XII
Plasminogen activator inhibitor-1 (PAI1)	Inactivates tPA and urokinase
Prekallikrein Fletcher factor	Activates XII, cleaves HMWK
Protein C	Inactivates Va, VIIIa
Protein S	Cofactor for activated protein C
Protein Z	Stimulates inhibition of FXa by ZPI (protein Z-related protease inhibitor)
Tissue plasminogen activator (tPA)	Activates plasminogen
Urokinase	Activates plasminogen
vWF (vonWillebrand factor)	Binds to VIII and mediates platelet adhesion
ZPI	Protein Z-related protease inhibitor; inhibits factor XIa; inhibits FXa in presence of protein Z

include any positive feedback loops or regulatory controls such as inhibitors of the clotting proteases or activation thresholds (Khanin and Semenov 1989) (Table 2.2). Nevertheless, this model is adequate enough to explain plasma-based *in vitro* coagulation.

In the 'extrinsic pathway', tissue factor (TF), formerly referred to as factor (F) III or tissue thromboplastin, was required in addition to circulating factors. Injury to ECs permits contact between FVII and TF which activates FVII to FVIIa. The TF/FVIIa complex then activates FX to FXa.

The 'intrinsic pathway' was so named because all components were present in the blood. The intrinsic pathway requires a negatively charged surface such as the membrane of an activated platelet. Cofactor high molecular weight kininogen (HMWK), attached to the platelet membrane and a likely product of platelets, aids in anchoring FXII to the platelet membrane and in its activation to FXIIa. This initial activation of FXII is limited in speed but once sufficient FXIIa accumulates, FXIIa converts prekallikrein to kallikrein, which forms a positive feedback loop accelerating activation of FXIIa. FXIIa/HMWK cleaves FXI to form FXIa/HMWK which cleaves FIX to FIXa. In turn, FIXa and downstream products, thrombin and FXa, in the presence of calcium, cleave FVIII to form FVIIIa. The complex of FIXa, FVIIIa and calcium form the tenase (FX cleaving) complex (Riddel et al. 2007).

The 'common pathway' begins with activation of FX to FXa from either or both of the extrinsic or intrinsic pathways. FXa, FVa and Ca^{2+} form the prothrombinase complex which, in the presence of membrane phospholipids, converts prothrombin to thrombin. In turn, thrombin catalyzes the proteolysis of soluble plasma protein fibrinogen to form fibrin monomers that polymerize into a fibrin gel. Thrombin also converts FXIII to FXIIIa which facilitates the covalent cross-linking of the fibrin polymers to a less-soluble mesh of stable fibrin. At the end of the coagulation phase, blood lost into the extravascular space has coagulated via the extrinsic and common pathways. Blood within vessels at the site of injury has coagulated via the intrinsic and common pathways.

TERTIARY HEMOSTASIS

The fibrinolytic system is initiated to disrupt clotting even as the clot is being formed. Fibrinolysis not only dissolves the clot once it has served its purpose in hemostasis but also prevents intravascular coagulation at sites distant from the site of the injury and protects against development of atherosclerotic vascular disease (for details, see below).

TISSUE FACTOR

Tissue factor (TF) is an integral transmembrane glycoprotein receptor with structural homology to class II cytokine receptors. TF is the principal *in vivo* initiator of the coagulation cascade and the only coagulation protein that is attached permanently to the membrane of the cell in which it was synthesized. Unlike other coagulation factors, TF does not require proteolytic activation. Under physiologic conditions, TF is expressed on several cell types outside the vasculature including fibroblasts, smooth muscle cells and keratinocytes. Within the walls of blood vessels, TF is localized to cells of the adventitia and media, especially pericytes, vascular smooth muscle cells (VSMCs) and adventitial fibroblasts. Cells that are in continuous contact with blood such as ECs and platelets express minimal TF or express an inactive or encrypted form of it (Bach 2006). This cell type-specific localized expression of TF forms a protective procoagulant envelope around the vascular system, whereas endothelium prevents contact between flowing blood and the TF-expressing cells and prevents intravascular clotting. However, upon vascular damage or activation of ECs, TF is exposed to blood and coagulation is rapidly triggered (Eilersten and Osterud 2004; Breitenstein et al. 2010). TF is essential for life as evidenced by it being the only coagulation factor for which a congenital disorder has not been described (Polgar et al. 2005).

However, the conventional view that TF serves as a hemostatic envelope surrounding the vascular bed has been challenged by a reservoir of blood-borne TF that is carried by cells in the blood (Mackman et al. 2007; Butenas et al. 2009; Mackman 2009; Mackman and Taubman 2009; Breitenstein et al. 2010). TF expression in ECs, circulating monocytes, eosinophils and neutrophils can be triggered by cytokines [e.g. TNF, interleukin-6 (IL6)] and bacterial endotoxin [lipopolysaccharide (LPS)], suggesting an important role of these cells in thrombosis. Although controversial, platelets appear to synthesize TF *de novo* and store it in α-granules and, upon activation, translocate TF to the cell surface. Platelets also have the capacity to bind TF-containing blood cells and transfer TF to monocytes via a mechanism involving P-selectin (P-sel) (Andre 2004; Mezzano et al. 2008).

Under physiologic conditions, most membrane TF exposed at cell surfaces is encrypted and does not trigger coagulation, although it is able to bind FVIIa. Intricate molecular interactions between ECs, platelets and phagocytes are considered essential for de-encryption of TF and TF-driven coagulation. The ability of TF to trigger coagulation is related to its phospholipid environment (see below), its association with membrane lipid rafts, loss of lipid symmetry and membrane shedding (Morel et al. 2008). The binding of TF to FVII/FVIIa enhances the catalytic activity of FVIIa by more than one-million-fold, thus rendering TF the prime initiator of coagulation (Polgar et al. 2005; Bach 2006).

VON WILLEBRAND FACTOR

von Willebrand factor (vWF) has two main functions in hemostasis. First, it binds FVIII, which stabilizes it from degradation, and second, it mediates platelet adhesion to the extracellular matrix (ECM) and to the injured vessel wall. Under conditions of very high shear stress, vWF also initiates platelet activation through interaction with platelet receptor GPIb-IX-V and participates in platelet aggregation by binding activated integrin $\alpha_{IIb}\beta_3$. vWF is synthesized in megakaryocytes (MKs) that partition into platelets which store vWF in α-granules, and in ECs which secrete vWF constitutively and secrete it from Weibel-Palade bodies (WPBs) upon stimulation by agonists including thrombin and histamine (Rondaij et al. 2006; Metcalf et al. 2007). vWF precursor protein forms dimers and then multimers which may be stored or secreted. Large vWF multimers enhance platelet aggregation via GPIb-IX-V complex. On the EC surface, P-selectin anchors the vWF multimers that become stretched in the flowing blood. Subsequently, stretching exposes vWF cleavage sites for ADAMST13, a plasma metalloprotease, which rapidly processes the multimers into less reactive fragments that are released into the circulation.

Plasma vWF is active only when immobilized onto a solid surface or when exposed to high fluid shear stress (Sadler 2002). vWF is the key component in initiating platelet adhesion and sustaining aggregation. Plasma vWF may reversibly self-associate with immobilized vWF multimers or bind to exposed ECM components such as collagen types I, III and VI. Platelets do not interact with soluble vWF in the circulation but they adhere quickly to immobilized vWF. Furthermore, platelet adhesion is more efficient under conditions of high shear such as in small arterioles as compared to veins because high shear unfolds vWF and exposes binding sites for the GPIb-IX-V complex (Ruggeri and Mendolicchio 2007). In contrast, large multimers of vWF bind to GPIbα under conditions in which plasma vWF fails to bind, causing platelets to adhere tightly. Deficiencies in ADAMTS13 favor platelet aggregation and thrombus formation which can occlude vessels locally or, if released, block small vessels downstream, leading to tissue infarction (Dong et al. 2002; Sadler 2002; Padilla et al. 2004).

OTHER COAGULATION FACTORS

Other coagulation factors contain glutamic acid (Gla) residues that, in the presence of Ca^{2+}, permit binding to negatively charged phospholipids in cell membranes. Factors VII, IX, X, prothrombin (FII) and proteins C, S, Z all require post-translational carboxylation of Gla via the vitamin K cycle in the liver, which facilitates binding to calcium (e.g. Dahlback 2005). Calcium (Ca^{2+}) binding produces a conformational change that permits interaction between Gla and membrane phospholipids of ECs and platelets. In the absence of carboxylation, the Gla proteins lack the ability to properly bind Ca^{2+} and hence cannot bind the activated membrane surface (Dahlback 2005; Smith 2009).

All coagulation factors except FVII circulate as inactive zymogens. Only a fraction (about 1%) of factor VII circulates as its active form under physiologic conditions (Morrisey 1996). Factors V and VIII are plasma cofactor proteins that circulate as inactive zymogens. FVIII circulates as a complex with vWF but it is liberated from vWF by a thrombin-mediated activation that enables free FVIIIa to bind to the activated platelet surface and participate in the tenase complex (FVIIIa, FIXa, Ca^{2+}). A portion of FV is localized within platelet α-granules and, upon activation of platelets, is released in a partially activated form. Both cofactors bind tightly to membranes containing acidic phospholipids allowing for their enzymatic action on the membrane surface (Mann et al. 1990; Dahlback 2005).

Coagulation proteins circulate in blood at different concentrations in relation to their role in coagulation. In general, early components circulate at lower concentrations than those involved at later stages and with amplification of clotting. The concentration of fibrinogen is about 50,000-fold higher than that of FVIII and, among vitamin K-dependent factors, prothrombin circulates at the highest concentration, FIX and FX at intermediate levels, and FVII at the lowest concentration (Dahlback 2005).

CELL-CENTRIC MODEL OF HEMOSTASIS: FROM INITIATION TO PROPAGATION

Hoffman and Monroe (2001, 2005, 2007; Monroe et al. 2002; Hoffman 2003; Roberts et al. 2006) proposed the cell-centric model which comprises three overlapping phases of hemostasis and in which the intrinsic and extrinsic pathways operate in parallel, but on different cell surfaces. In this model, clotting starts on TF-bearing cells ('the initiation phase;' Fig. 2.2A). The coagulation process is initiated only if the procoagulant stimulus is sufficiently strong and adequate quantities of FXa, IXa and thrombin are produced. If this threshold is met, then coagulation moves from the TF-bearing cell onto the platelets that adhere and become activated ('the amplification phase;' Fig. 2.2B). Cofactors with active proteases on the platelet surface then generate the burst of thrombin required for fibrin polymerization ('the propagation phase;' Fig. 2.2C). A stable clot is formed and blood loss stops. Fibrin formation and

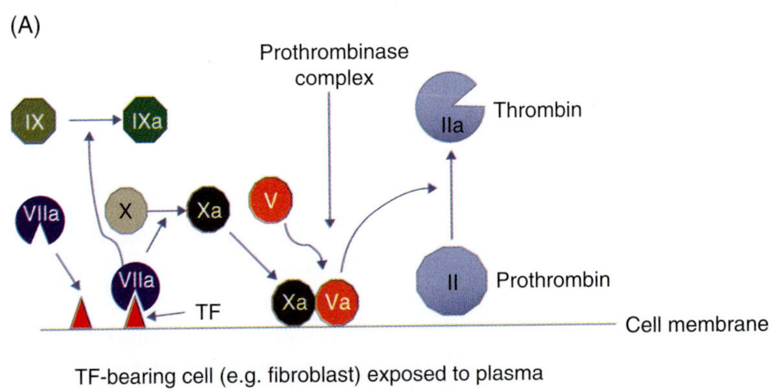

Fig. 2.2 (A) Simplified illustration of the cell-centric model of hemostasis.
Initiation Phase. The initiation phase occurs on the TF-bearing cell and results in the generation of small amounts of FIXa and thrombin that diffuse from the TF-bearing cell surface to the platelet. Injury permits contact between TF on a fibroblast and plasma which contains FVIIa to form the TF-FVIIa complex. The TF-FVIIa complex activates small amounts of FX and FIX. FXa that remains bound on the TF-cell surface binds plasma FV and generates FVa. FXa binding to its cofactor FVa forms the prothrombinase complex which rapidly cleaves prothrombin and generates small amounts of thrombin. If the procoagulant stimulus is strong enough, then enough FXa, FIXa and thrombin are generated for the coagulation process to progress to the amplification phase.

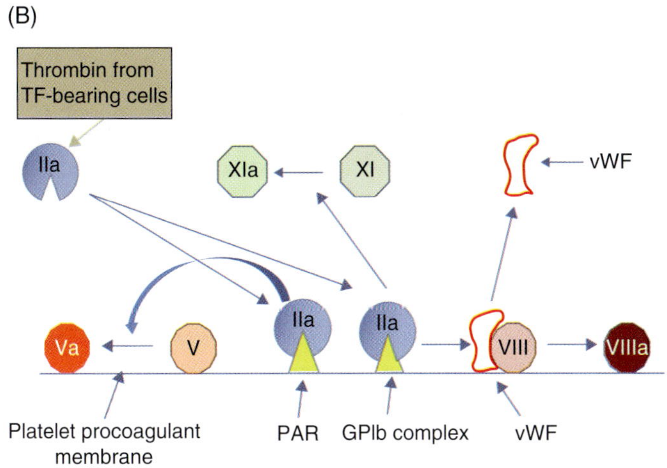

Fig. 2.2 (B) **Amplification Phase**. In the amplification phase, the coagulation response shifts from the TF-bearing cell to the platelet surface. Small amounts of thrombin generated by TF-bearing cells in the initiation phase activate platelets which release vWF and this leads to generation of FVa, FVIIIa and FXIa. Thrombin generated in the initiation phase diffuses away from the TF-bearing cell and is available to activate platelets. Thrombin enhances platelet adhesion, fully activates platelets and activates factors V, VIII and XI. Hence, thrombin primes the platelet surface for assembly of the procoagulant complex. Thrombin bound to protease-activated receptors (PARs) activates FV which is released from platelets. Thrombin bound to the GPIb complex cleaves FXI to FXIa. In addition, thrombin cleaves vWF from the vWF/FVIII complex leading to FVIII activation and the release of vWF.

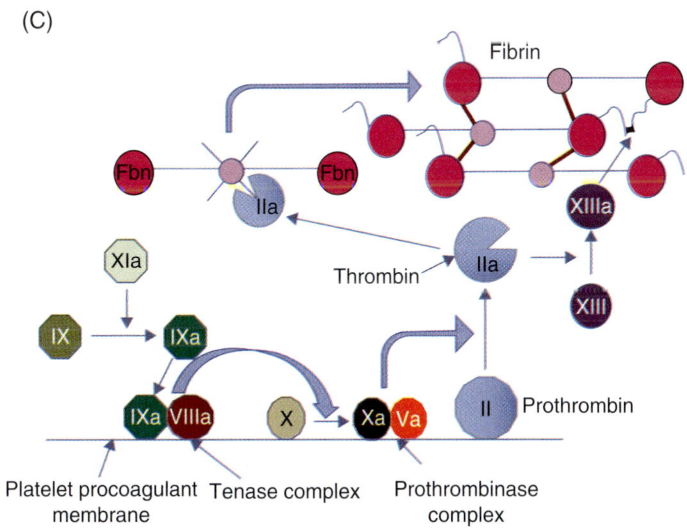

Fig. 2.2 (C) **Propagation Phase**. The activation of platelets in the amplification phase recruits additional platelets to the site of injury. Coagulation proteins, generated in the previous phases, assemble on the procoagulant membrane of recruited activated platelets, form tenase (FIXa-FVIIIa) and generate FXa on the platelet surface. Prothrombinase complex (FVa-FXa) forms and a burst of thrombin is generated directly on the platelet surface. Platelets possess high-affinity binding sites for FIXa, FXa and FXI and these receptors are essential for the coordinated assembly of the coagulation complexes. FIXa is generated by XIa (from the amplification phase) at the platelet surface and binds FVIIIa (from the amplification phase). A tenase complex of FVIIIa/IXa is formed. The tenase complex generates FXa which binds rapidly to FVa (generated by thrombin in the amplification phase) to form the prothrombinase complex (FXa-FVa). Thrombin removes the fibinopeptides from fibrinogen (Fbn) which then forms fibrin. Thrombin also activates FXIIIa (transglutaminase) which stabilizes the fibrin clot by cross-linking the fibrin oligomers.

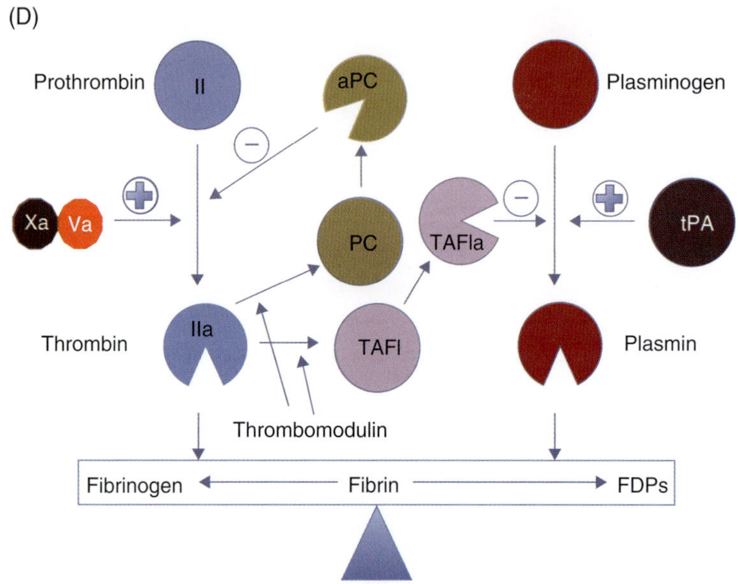

Fig. 2.2 (D) **Termination Phase**. Fibrin formation and fibrinolysis are regulated partially by the same enzymes in a delicate balance that can be shifted towards clotting or clot dissolution. The fibrinolytic system is initiated when plasminogen is converted to plasmin by tissue plasminogen activator (tPA) and plasmin degrades fibrin into soluble fibrin degradation products (FDPs). Fibrin itself is important for binding and activation of plasminogen. The limited cleavage of fibrin by plasmin exposes C-terminal lysine residues which bind both tPA and plasminogen. Fibrin now acts as a cofactor in the tPA-mediated catalysis of plasminogen, increasing its catalytic efficiency by 100- to 1,000-fold. Thrombin and thrombomodulin (TM) at the endothelial cell surface can activate both TAFI (thrombin-activable fibrinolysis inhibitor) and protein C (PC). TAFI is synthesized in the liver and circulates in plasma. Both thrombin and plasmin can activate TAFI but its activation is enhanced significantly by the thrombin/TM complex. TAFIa is a carboxypeptidase which cleaves the lysine residues from partially degraded fibrin and thereby eliminates fibrin as a cofactor in tPA conversion of plasminogen. The rate of plasmin formation is reduced and fibrinolysis is downregulated. PC is a circulating anticoagulant that is bound to endothelial cells where it is activated by the thrombin/TM complex. The PC pathway is an effective anticoagulant pathway as it inactivates FVIIIa and FVa, cofactors in tenase and prothrombinase complexes.

dissolution are regulated partially by the same enzymes. The thresholds and location regulate which process is promoted (see below and Fig. 2.2D, 'the termination phase').

In the cell-centric model, the intrinsic and extrinsic pathways are not redundant. The extrinsic pathway operates on the TF-bearing cell where the TF/FVIIa complex works with the FXa/Va complex to initiate and amplify coagulation. The intrinsic pathway, operating on the platelet surface, consists of FXIa working with the complexes of VIIIa/IXa and FXa/Va to generate the thrombin burst required for formation and stabilization of the fibrin clot.

THE PROCOAGULANT MEMBRANE

Eukaryotic cell membranes contain specialized functional microdomains called rafts, which modulate the lateral organization of the plasma membrane. External stimuli may elicit mobilization of rafts leading to signal transduction through the lipids (Hannun and Obeid

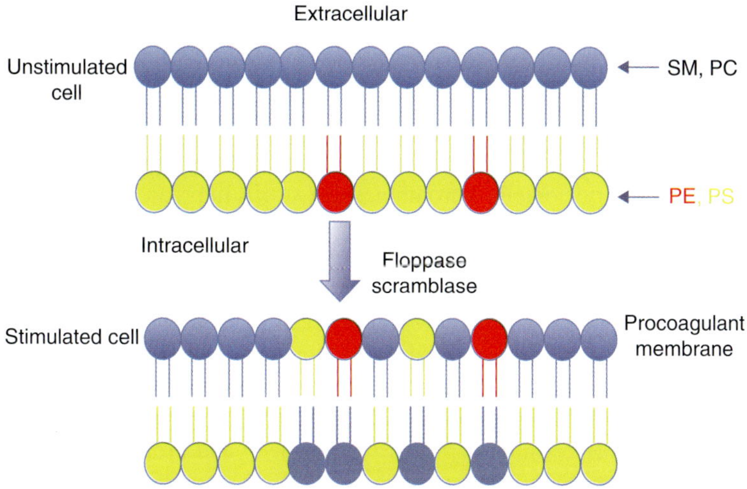

Fig. 2.3 Formation of procoagulant membrane. In a resting cell membrane, phosphatidylethanolamine (PE, red) and phosphatidylserine (PS, yellow) are concentrated on the cytoplasmic leaflet, whereas phosphotidylcholine (PC, blue) and sphingomyelin (SM, blue) are localized in the extra-cytosolic leaflet. The creation of lipid asymmetry is crucial for coagulation. Specialized protein transporters can either maintain or disrupt the lipid gradients. 'Flip-flop' is the ATP-dependent translocation of lipids from one leaflet to the other. Flippase transports from the outer leaflet towards the cytoplasmic leaflet and floppase transports from the inner leaflet to the extra-cytosolic leaflet. Scramblase is a third lipid transport system which functions to degrade the bilayer asymmetry. In stimulated cells, such as platelets, both floppase and scramblase activities are increased, resulting in exposure of PS and PE on the platelet surface. Hence, a procoagulant membrane is formed.

2008; van Meer et al. 2008; Spijkers et al. 2010). The main structural lipids are the glycerophospholipids including phosphatidylethanoloamine (PE), phosphadylserine (PS), phosphatidylinositol (PI), phosphatidic acid (PA), diacylglycerol (DAG) and phosphatidylcholine (PC), which comprises over 50% of the phospholipids in most membranes. Another class of structural membrane lipids forms the sphingophospholipids, namely sphingomyelin (SM), and the glycosphingolipids (GSLs). Significant functional consequences result from the asymmetric distribution of lipids. Under non-activated conditions, PS and PE are localized to the cytoplasmic surface but become shuffled to the outer membrane when cells are injured (Fig. 2.3). This shuffling is controlled by lipid transporters in either an inward (flippase) or outward (floppase) direction. In a resting membrane, flippase activity predominates. Upon cell stimulation, floppase activity predominates and scramblase (Ca^{2+}-dependent phospholipid transporter) is activated, leading to an alteration in membrane symmetry. Scramblase and floppase are essential for expression of PE and PS at the surface of activated cells (Yamaji-Hasegawa and Tsujimoto 2006; Morel et al. 2008). On the cell surface, PS functions as a propagation signal in blood coagulation through assembly of coagulation complexes and generation of soluble thrombin (Daleke 2003; Ikeda et al. 2006; Yamaji-Hasegawa and Tsujimoto 2006; Morel et al. 2008; van Meer et al. 2008). PS increases the speed of some coagulation reactions by thousands-fold, providing powerful local control of coagulation. In contrast, coagulation reactions occur very slowly on cells that do not express PS and therefore resting cells under normal physiologic conditions cannot support the coagulation cascade (Yamaji-Hasegawa and Tsujimoto 2006; Morel et al. 2008).

MEMBRANE PARTICLES

Membrane particles (MPs) are submicron membrane fragments or vesicles shed from activated or apototic cells. Specific stimuli may elicit a specific membrane response through raft mobilization and thereby promote the release of MPs with a specific membrane composition and specific content. Thrombin, shear stress, hypoxia, cytokines and ADP can all stimulate MP formation. Under physiologic conditions, MPs are shed from ECs, VSMCs, platelets and leukocytes. Platelets are probably the main source of MPs in the vascular compartment, but, in certain disease states, MPs are also shed from RBCs and neutrophils. The relative contribution of these different parent cell types to the pool of circulating MPs may depend upon the pathophysiological state (Morel et al. 2008).

MPs contain cell surface proteins that are similar to those of their parent cell. MPs may express PS rendering MPs procoagulant. Moreover, MPs may also express TF, vWF (if derived from ECs), P-selectin (if derived from platelets) and prothrombinase (complex of FXa, FVa). TF-positive MPs are the main reservoir of blood-borne TF. MPs shed from aggregating platelets may also participate in modification or amplification of platelet activity. Under shear stress, MPs are key players in promoting TF activity by vascular cells. TF-positive MPs shed from leukocytes can bind to activated platelets and promote recruitment of TF-positive MPs to a thrombus promoting its growth (Mackman et al. 2007). MPs also participate in anticoagulant activity as they may express thrombomodulin (TM), tissue factor pathway inhibitor (TFPI) (Crawley and Lane 2008), endothelial protein C receptor (EPCR) and protein S. However, in situations in which TF is upregulated, TF and prothrombinase activities overwhelm TM activity and coagulation prevails (Morel et al. 2008).

ENDOTHELIUM AND HEMOSTASIS

ECs are the primary contact between the blood and the vessels. Endothelium (E) functions as a receptor/effector organ that responds to both chemical and physical stimuli to regulate vasomotor tone, coagulation, SMC proliferation, leukocyte trafficking, inflammatory and immunological processes, ischemic and reperfusion injuries, and the development of atherosclerosis (Michiels 2003; Esper et al. 2006; Chien 2007). ECs are a heterogeneous population with different phenotypes reflected by a diversity of barrier functions and mechano-chemical responses (Chien 2007; Mitchell et al. 2007; Bogatcheva and Verin 2008; Vandenbroucke et al. 2008). Under physiologic conditions, the gaps between ECs are very small so that platelets and large proteins are sequestered within the intravascular space. Flow through capillaries is possible because both blood cells and ECs are flexible and deformable and because blood cells and ECs both carry a repelling negative electrostatic charge (Esper et al. 2006).

PRO- AND ANTICOAGULANT FUNCTIONS

Trauma, inflammation or exposure to thrombin, histamine and various cytokines can alter the phenotype of ECs to one that favors platelet aggregation, clot formation and suppression of anticoagulation (Fig. 2.4). Activated ECs synthesize and release two important mediators, namely vWF and platelet-activating factor (PAF). ECs secrete vWF into the subendothelium

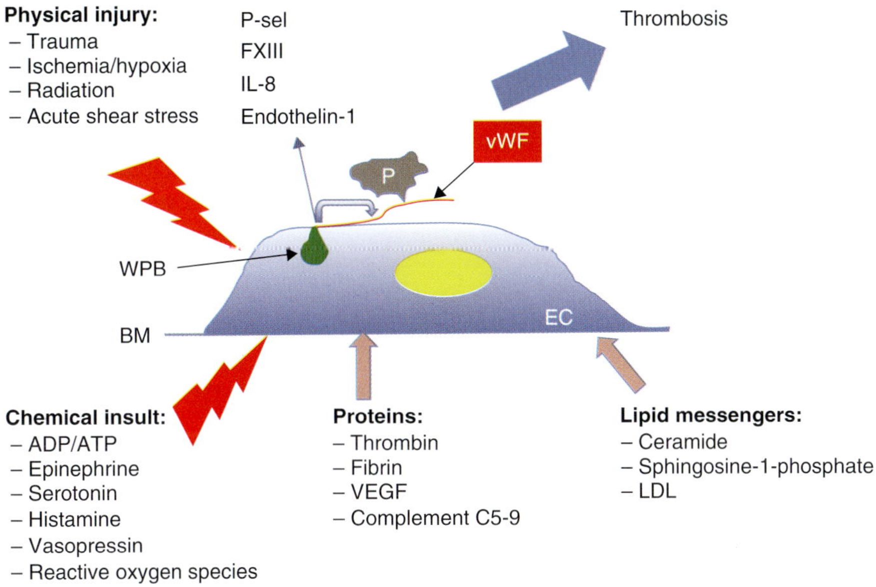

Fig. 2.4 Endothelial cell response to various stimuli. Endothelial cells contain specific storage vesicles called Weibel-Palade bodies (WPBs) which store proteins that regulate thrombosis and inflammation. vWF is the major component of WPBs but other contents include FXIIIa, P-selectin, IL-8 and endothelin-1. A large number of stimuli cause exocytosis of WPBs. Some stimuli, such as thrombin, trigger an immediate release of vWF. When released, vWF forms long fiber-like structures (red) on the endothelial cell surface which can attract platelets (P).

and ECM, which are sites that interact with platelets only if exposed by injury. vWF is a major adhesion protein for platelets, but fibronectin and collagen in the subendothelium also contribute to platelet adherence. Thrombin binding to an EC protease-activated receptor (PAR) causes ECs to produce and secrete PAF which promotes adhesion between platelets and ECs and subsequent platelet aggregation.

Activated ECs also release ADP and express TF. FVII binds with TF on the EC surface and remains active only when bound to TF. The TF-FVIIa complex can now activate FX directly on the EC membrane, allowing FX to form the prothrombinase complex. The TF-VIIa complex can also activate FX indirectly by activating FIX to form a complex with FVIII and phospholipids which activates FX. FXa activates thrombin which can diffuse into the interstitial fluid or plasma and cleave fibrinogen to fibrin (Shireman and Pearce 1996).

Under physiologic conditions, non-activated resting ECs constitute a non-thrombogenic surface through expression of a number of surface proteins with anticoagulant properties. Critical anticoagulant functions are provided by PE, TFPI, TM and heparin-sulfated proteoglycans (HSPGs). The luminal PE appears to be essential for binding protein C and maintaining its anticoagulant pathway. TFPI is an EC-bound plasma protein that interacts irreversibly with FXa leading to the formation of the TFPI-FXa complex, which further binds the TF-VIIa complex, thereby inactivating FXa and preventing thrombin formation.

TM is an EC thrombin receptor that binds thrombin, converting it to an anticoagulant protein through activation of protein C and thereby inhibiting thrombin formation (Fig. 2.2D). Expression of TM is a hundred-fold greater in capillary ECs as compared to

ECs in larger vessels; hence, any thrombin circulating in large vessels is rapidly extracted when the blood passes through a capillary. The TM–thrombin complex also activates circulating thrombin activable fibrinolysis inhibitor (TAFI) which stabilizes fibrin by decreasing plasminogen binding on the fibrin surface (Fig. 2.2D). Hence, fibrinolysis is decreased or inhibited (Antovic and Blomback 2002; Bouma and Mosnier 2006).

Luminal HSPGs expressed by ECs participate in the anticoagulation activity. HSPGs bind antithrombin (AT) and this complex promotes inactivation of thrombin. HSPGs provide the main site for inactivation of active thrombin and this mechanism is exploited clinically with the administration of heparin.

Endothelial cells also play an important role in the intravascular fibrinolysis that is initiated at the EC surface which binds plasminogen and tissue-type plasminogen activator (t-PA) and urokinase (uPA). Binding these molecules to EC greatly enhances the conversion of plasminogen to plasmin (Shireman and Pearce 1996; Bunte et al. 2008; Hoover-Plow 2010).

PLATELETS

Platelets are anuclear cytoplasmic fragments derived from MKs and hence they have limited biosynthetic function. However, platelets retain the capacity to synthesize proteins such as TF by translational pathways (Panes et al. 2007; Weyrich et al. 2007; Mezzano et al. 2008) and to generate functional progeny (Schwertz et al. 2009). The platelet lifespan averages 8–12 days in the circulation and about 30% of platelets are sequestered as a reserve in the spleen and microvasculature. Non-viable or aged platelets are removed primarily by the spleen but also by the liver (Camacho and Dimsdale 2000). Platelets are composed of membrane structures, the cytoskeleton and granules. Platelet cytoplasm contains three types of granules: lysosomal granules, dense granules and α-granules (Harrison and Cramer 1993; Camacho and Dimsdale 2000; Ren et al. 2008; Blair and Flaumenhaft 2009).

Under physiologic conditions, platelets are restricted to the intravascular space where they circulate freely in the blood without adhesion to each other or to the vessel walls. However, under conditions of activated ECs or exposure to ECM components, platelets adhere promptly and recruit additional platelets as well as different types of leukocytes to the site. Platelets provide a surface for binding adhesive proteins and for thrombin generation. Platelets express receptors for serotonin [5-hydroxytryptaimine (5-HT); Lopez-Vilechez et al. 2009], benzodiazepine and adenoreceptors (α-2, ß-2), protease-activated receptors (PARs) (Bilodeau and Hamm 2007), vWF, coagulation factors, collagen, thrombin and other agonists [ADP, epinephrine, thromboxane (TXA2)], TF-rich MPs and other platelets. Platelets are activated by several agonists including collagen, thrombin, Ca^{2+}, ADP, epinephrine, prostaglandin H2, TXA2, 5-HT and PAF. During activation and adhesion, platelets change from a discoid shape to a stellate form and shuffle their membrane phospholipids (see above), generating a procoagulant surface. However, only a fraction of platelets respond maximally. This differential platelet response may reflect differences in Ca^{2+} homeostasis or age of the platelets. Young platelets have increased capacity to form coated-platelets (formerly COAT-platelets, i.e. COllagen And Thrombin activated platelets). The simultaneous activation by both thrombin and collagen results in coated platelets that express surface PS and bind l α-granule proteins including FV, vWF, fibrinogen, fibronectin, thrombospondin and α-2 antiplasmin (Dale et al. 2002; Dale 2005).

During platelet activation, the granule secretions are released in a highly regulated fashion to establish a microenvironment at the wound site. Both inhibitors (endostatin, PF4, thrombospondin-1, α_2 macroglobulin, PAI-1, angiostatin) and promoters of angiogenesis [e.g. vascular endothelial growth factor (VEGF), platelet derived growth factor (PDGF), basic fibroblast growth factor (bFGF), EGF, MMPs] are sequestered in distinct populations of α-granules. Moreover, stimulated platelets do not release all of their granule contents during thrombogenesis. Similar differential packaging also exists for vWF and fibrinogen along with differential release in response to distinct agonists (Jurk and Kehrel 2005; Sehgal and Storrie 2007; Italiano et al. 2008). ECs exhibit a similar pattern of differential packaging and release of vWF and P-sel by WPBs (Lowenstein et al. 2005; Cleator et al. 2006).

Platelet adhesion and aggregation are influenced by the particular matrix proteins exposed during injury and by the local hydrodynamic conditions including shear stress and shear rate (Monroe et al. 2002; Aoki et al. 2007; Chien 2007; White and Frangos 2007; Ando and Yamamoto 2009; Chiu et al. 2009; Singh et al. 2009; Shibeko et al. 2010). Shear rate, related directly to flow velocity and velocity of cells within the fluid layer adjacent to the vessel wall, affects (1) how rapidly cells encounter the vessel wall or one another, (2) the duration of contact between components of the immobilized vessel wall and platelet receptors, (3) the forces on the adhesive bonds, and (4) how rapidly soluble mediators are delivered and removed from the site. Moreover, each reaction has its own threshold response caused by competition between activators and inhibitors and their respective concentrations and mobility at the site (Bach 2006; Runyon et al. 2007). Thus, shear rate limits the on-rate of the adhesive interactions and, with increasing shear rate, the efficiency of platelet recruitment onto the surface decreases. In contrast, shear stress affects the off-rate of the interaction or the lifetime of an adhesive bond. Under conditions of increasing shear stress, adherent cells detach (Ruggeri and Mendolicchio 2007; Diamond 2009). Moreover, the shear rate is variable as the flow field is unstable, first from the injury itself and then from vasoconstriction during the vascular phase of primary hemostasis and the shape and size of the forming clot (Ruggeri and Mendolicchio 2007; Diamond 2009).

The primary hemostatic response is contingent upon the nature of the lesion and the hydrodynamic threshold or critical threshold flow level that affects levels of circulating TF, active proteases and platelet capture, deformation, activation and arrest. First, the physical size of the injury determines the extent of TF-bearing cell membranes and ECM components exposed to the plasma (Beltrami and Jesty 2001; Jesty and Beltrami 2005). Flow determines the availability of coagulation proteases, TF and MPs. Depending on agonists, different platelet receptors (GPIbα in the GPIb-IX-V complex, GPVI, integrins $\alpha_2\beta_1$, $\alpha_{IIb}\beta_3$, $\alpha_5\beta_1$, GPVI, GPIV or CD-36) and ECM ligands (different collagen types I, III, VI, vWF, fibronectin, laminin, fibulin, thrombospondin), the platelet response to the injury varies. Dynamics of coagulation/hemostasis are further complicated by a changing platelet surface and changing concentrations in platelet numbers and coagulation factors (Stassen et al. 2004; Rivera et al. 2009).

Under conditions of elevated shear stress, vWF is primarily responsible for initiating platelet adhesion. vWF serves as a bridge between collagen (types I, III and IV) and the platelet receptor GPIα in the glycoprotein GPIb-IX-V receptor complex. However, the vWF-GPIα bond has a high dissociation rate and platelets tethered to the vessel wall solely through GPIα continue to move in the direction of flow. Nevertheless, this initial contact facilitates contact between activated platelets and stimulated ECs whose surface contains bound vWF and P-selectin, which mediates transient adhesion and rolling. Slowed motion of platelets further facilitates formation of additional bonds through integrins. Platelet activation is necessary to activate integrin function (e.g. $\alpha_{IIb}\beta_3$) and integrins are required for definitive arrest of platelets (Ruggeri and Mendolicchio 2007; Rivera et al. 2009).

COAGULATION AND WOUND HEALING

Platelet activation during primary hemostasis initiates the wound healing response via release of cytokines such as PDGF and TGFß1 (transforming growth factor beta 1) that serve as a chemotactic and stimulatory signal for many cell types essential for wound healing. Formation of a fibrin clot is also essential for the initiation of wound healing. During coagulation, fibrin is crosslinked to plasma fibronectin to create a plug for hemostasis. Although plasma fibronectin does not appear to be essential for hemostasis (Maurer et al. 2010), it can provide substratum for epithelial and fibroblast migration towards the clot (see Chapters 5 and 6). Fibrin itself in the wound provisional matrix provides adhesion for leukocytes, fibroblasts and endothelial cells (Laurens et al. 2006). In addition, fibrin provides a reservoir for many growth factors such as FGF-2 and VEGF that stimulate wound healing. As discussed previously, thrombin plays a critical role in the conversion of fibrinogen to fibrin. In addition, thrombin directly supports wound healing through its chemotactic and mitogenic activities towards macrophages, fibroblasts and endothelial cells (Hoffman and Monroe 2007). Coagulation and sustained thrombin production seem to be essential for wound healing. Mice deficient in FXIII or FIX have delayed wound healing because of continued bleeding into the granulation tissue and reduced thrombin production (Monroe et al. 2010).

LIMITATIONS OF THE WATERFALL CASCADE MODEL AND SCREENING LABORATORY TESTS

Screening laboratory tests for detection of potential bleeding problems are based upon the traditional Waterfall Cascade Model. The extrinsic/common pathways are assessed by PT (prothrombin time) and the intrinsic/common pathways by aPTT (activated partial thromboplastin time). These clot-based assays conclude with initial fibrin polymerization, before clot maturation which affects the quality of the fibrin clot that is formed (Mann et al. 2003, 2009). Hence, these assays fail to detect bleeding tendency in humans with factor XIII (FXIII) deficiency. As well, these *in vitro* tests show prolonged surface-activated coagulation (prolonged aPTT) with deficiencies of FXII, prekallikrein (PK) or high molecular weight kininogen (HMWK) yet clinical bleeding tendencies are not significant. It appears likely that PK, HMWK and FXII of the intrinsic pathway are not involved in physiologic hemostasis. However, FXII appears to be instrumental in pathological thrombosis formation as evidenced by the fact that FXII deficiency offers protection against pathological thrombosis (Kleinschnitz et al. 2006; Seligsohn 2007). In addition, deficiencies in each of the intrinsic pathway factors could have similarly prolonged aPTT values, yet the risks of hemorrhage vary greatly and FXI deficiency may or may not be associated with hemorrhage. The Waterfall Cascade Model also cannot explain why an intact 'extrinsic pathway' cannot activate adequate FX to compensate for the lack of FVIII (hemophilia A) or FIX (hemophilia B) (Hoffman and Monroe 2001, 2005, 2007; Hoffman 2003).

In general, the Waterfall Cascade Model assumed substrate specificity and fidelity of cofactors and enzymes with respect to components of the cascade. However, thrombin and FXa are multidirectional in that they can enhance their own formation rates by catalyzing activation of FV, FVII and FVIII. Thrombin also activates platelets. Furthermore, it has been identified as the physiologic activator of FXI and could thus bypass the initial contact-induced reactions (Gailani and Broze 1993; Vine 2009). In addition, membrane-bound FXa can cooperate in the FVIIa-TF activation of FIX (Lawson and Mann 1991). The FVIIa/TF complex (initiator of the extrinsic pathway) can also activate FX and FIX (of the intrinsic pathway); this observation has led to the conclusion that activity of the FVIIa/TF complex was the primary initiating event of hemostasis *in vivo* (Hoffman and Monroe 2001, 2005, 2007; Hoffman 2003; Roberts et al. 2006). Moreover, FVIIa can generate thrombin on the platelet surface independently of external TF (Monroe et al. 1998; Altman et al. 2006).

IMPLICATIONS FOR LABORATORY TESTS

All *in vitro* laboratory tests for defects of coagulation are severely restricted due to the absence of contributions to hemostasis by the vasculature and surrounding tissue. Moreover, there appears to be a circadian variation within hemostasis or a hemostatic clock that modulates EC and platelet functions and the concentration and activity of several coagulation and fibrinolytic proteins (Montagnana et al. 2009). As well, within the healthy population, there is wide variability in concentrations of pro- and anticoagulants. This heterogeneity is a consequence of genetic and environmental factors and because coagulation factors undergo a significant variety of posttranslational and proteolytic processing (Mann et al. 2009). Diet, including herbal supplements, alcohol and even glycemic spikes will modify coagulant activity (Brand-Miller et al. 2009).

PRE-SURGICAL EVALUATION TO PREVENT BLEEDING PROBLEMS

Medical history

The single best screening procedure to identify the patient with a possible bleeding disorder is the patient's history (Little et al. 2002). Presence of bleeding disorders in relatives is a strong indicator for a potential bleeding disorder. Hemophilia A (FVIII deficiency) and Christmas Disease (hemophilia B, FIX deficiency) are the two most common inherited coagulation disorders and they are transmitted in a sex-linked (X-chromosome) recessive mode. There is large variation in symptoms and severity. vWD is the most common inherited bleeding disorder and it is linked to an affected gene on chromosome 12. A history of spontaneous bleeding such as gingival bleeding, excessive bleeding after surgery, tooth extractions or trauma/injury, or bruising may suggest the need for laboratory testing to screen for a bleeding disorder (Little et al. 2002; Favaloro 2009). The patient should be asked about past or present illnesses such as alcoholism, liver disease, chronic pain such as arthritis, and heart disease. Liver diseases affect production of coagulation factors and may lead to an acquired bleeding disorder. Management of chronic pain and heart conditions may include regular use of medications that affect platelet functions or expression of coagulation factors (such as ASA/NSAIDs and coumadin). Coumadin inhibits the vitamin K-dependent carboxylation reaction required for the function of vitamin K-dependent clotting factors (II, VII, IX, X, proteins C, S). Coumadin is prescribed to prevent thrombosis and therefore bleeding is increased. The action of coumadin is increased by acetylsalicylic acid (ASA)/non-steroidal anti-inflammatory drugs (NSAIDs), acetaminophen in chronic high doses, metronidazole, erythromycin, tetracyclines, ciprofloxacin, antifungals (fluconazole, miconazole) and corticosteroids. In general, oral surgery requires prior consultation with the physician and INR (International Normalized Ratio) values ≤ 3.5 (Little et al. 2002). Stopping coumadin therapy for even a few days can increase the risk of a paralyzing stroke or death. Therefore, a moderate amount of bleeding may be the lesser risk and can often be managed with only local measures (Nematullah et al. 2009).

Heparin is a commonly used drug in anticoagulant prophylaxis and the treatment of thromboembolic disease. Heparin binds to and activates ATIII, which deactivates thrombin, hence preventing the conversion of fibrinogen to fibrin. ASA and NSAIDs will increase the anticoagulant effect of heparin. ASA irreversibly inhibits platelet cyclo-oxygenase which is required for the production of TXA_2 and subsequent platelet aggregation. The lifespan of a platelet is 8–12 days and the ASA effects will persist for this lifespan. Even a low dosage of ASA (81 mg daily or every second day), such as prescribed in prophylaxis for coronary thrombosis, is sufficient to inhibit platelet TXA_2 production, affect platelet aggregation and prolong the bleeding time. In ECs, cyclo-oxygenase is also inhibited by ASA but ECs can regenerate active cyclo-oxygenase. ASA also decreases EC production of prostacyclin (PGI_2) which is an inhibitor of platelet aggregation and a vasodilator. The overall net effect of ASA is that PGI_2 synthesis exceeds synthesis of TXA_2 so that EC-mediated inhibition of coagulation predominates (King 2010). Individual responses vary, however, and many patients can be treated without disrupting the prophylactic dose.

NSAIDs can also inhibit platelet cyclo-oxygenase, but the actions of NSAIDs are reversible. The duration of the NSAID effect depends upon the drug dose, serum level and half-life. The effects of ASA/NSAIDs are enhanced by the use of alcohol and in the presence of liver disease. NSAIDs should be avoided for patients taking selective serotonin reuptake inhibitors (SSRIs) as concurrent administration increases the risk of gastric bleeding (Horn and Hansten 2003; Wee et al. 2004). The SSRIs are compounds typically used as antidepressants in the treatment of depression, anxiety disorders and some personality disorders. SSRIs inhibit the reuptake of serotonin by platelets, resulting in a more than 80% decrease in intra-platelet serotonin. This reduction in intra-platelet serotonin leads to decreased exposure of activation proteins at the platelet surface, impaired platelet activation, aggregation and increased bleeding. The decreased volume of released serotonin also diminishes vasoconstriction of blood vessels. There are typically no abnormal test results of hemostatic function or even platelet aggregation in patients taking SSRIs, but patients may report occasional bruising or abnormal bleeding (McCloskey et al. 2008).

Clopidogrel (Plavix™; Bristol-Meyers Squibb) irreversibly and specifically blocks the ADP receptor on platelet membranes and thereby blocks activation of the GPIIb/IIIa receptor complex, which is involved in platelet aggregation and crosslinking by fibrin. Eptifibatide, abciximab and tirofiban target platelet receptor GPIIb-GPIIIa directly and therefore they are more effective at inhibiting platelet aggregation, regardless of agonist, than clopidogrel or ASA (King 2010). Dabigatran etexilate (Pradaxa TM, Boehringer Ingelheim) is a relatively new drug that acts as a direct thrombin inhibitor and may be prescribed as an anticoagulant alternative to warfarin. Dabigatran increases INR to some degree, but INR is not very sensitive to the effect of dabigatran and INR cannot be used to assess or adjust dosage.

Long-term antibiotic therapy may also affect the coagulation process. Long-term antibiotics disturb intestinal flora responsible for the vitamin K production required for production of factor II (prothrombin) and coagulation factors VII, IX and X, and proteins C and S. Beta-lactam antibiotics such as penicillin and cephalothins can also interfere with platelet function.

Table 2.3 List of herbal supplements with anticoagulant and antiplatelet effects.

Anticoagulants	Antiplatelets
	Danshen
	Dong quai
	Evening primrose
Fenugreek	Feverfew
	Garlic
	Ginger
	Gingko biloba
	Ginseng
	Grape seed
Horse chestnut	
Motherworth	
Omega-3 fatty acids	Omega-3 fatty acids
	Papaya
	Phenolic acids
Red clover	
	Turmeric
	Willow

Cohan and Jacobsen 2000; Fugh-Berman 2000; Abebe 2009.

Diet and herbal supplements

Many foods, medicinal herbs and pharmaceutical agents may be therapeutic at one dose but toxic at another. Furthermore, interactions between drugs, foods and supplements may affect the toxicological or pharmaceutical effects. Moreover, patients may not divulge the use of herbal medicines. In addition, labeling of herbal products may not be accurate and contamination, especially with heavy metals, is not uncommon. Many herbs may affect platelet function but not the coagulation cascade and hence their effects will not affect laboratory test values for PT, PPT or INR. However, the *in vivo* effects of certain herbs on platelet function and perioperative bleeding are in dispute (Cohan and Jacobsen 2000; Fugh-Berman 2000; Hu et al. 2005; Beckert et al. 2007; Abebe 2009; Table 2.3). The possibility of alcohol abuse cannot be ruled out on the basis of an individual's age, gender, socio-economic status, race/ethnicity or other groupings. Alcohol abuse is a potential contributing factor to bleeding problems due to liver disease, malabsorption problems and dietary insufficiencies. Alcohol also has a direct effect by interfering with platelet function (Salem and Laposata 2005). Even commonly consumed beverages such as coffee, tea, cocoa and wine, due to their content of phenolic acids, affect platelets (Natella et al. 2008). Omega-3 fatty acids may increase the risk of bleeding at higher doses (National Library of Medicine and the National Institutes of Health, http://www.nlm.nih.gov/medlineplus/druginfo/natural/patient-fishoil.html) and licorice and lavender contain low levels of coumarin which is found naturally in these plants (Ansell et al. 2004).

Clinical examination

Patients with a potential bleeding problem may present with clinical findings that include jaundice or pallor, extra- and/or intraoral spider angiomas, ecchymoses/petechia, oral ulcers, spontaneous oral or gingival bleeding, hyperplastic/enlarged gingival tissues and hemarthrosis (Little et al. 2002). These findings may indicate liver disease, chronic or heavy alcohol use or biliary tract obstruction. As the liver produces most coagulation factors, significant liver disease will compromise the coagulation phase, but up to 50% of patients with liver disease may be thrombocytopenic due to platelet sequestration in the spleen. These findings may also indicate other conditions such as malabsorption (vitamin K production affected), long-term antibiotic use, chronic renal disease, infectious diseases, autoimmune diseases, genetic coagulation disorders and leukemia (Little et al. 2002).

Presurgical planning

Consultation with the patient's physician is mandatory prior to proceeding with dental treatment for a patient with a serious bleeding disorder as they have an increased risk for spontaneous bleeding and for excessive bleeding from even minor trauma to the oral soft tissues. This topic is covered extensively by Little et al. (2002) and is beyond the scope of this chapter. Surgical incisions should be well planned and executed in a precise manner in order to avoid unnecessary trauma. Irregular, jagged incisions and tearing of the oral mucosa and/or periosteum will compromise hemostasis. In the raising of a mucoperiosteal flap, the incision should be directed to the crest of the underlying alveolar bone to sever the gingival attachment. The flap should be elevated with the periosteum preserved intact.

Local anesthetic (LA) with a vasoconstrictor is required for any oral surgery. One reason that LAs are formulated with vasoconstrictors (e.g. epinephrine) is in order to constrict blood vessels at the site of injection, decrease blood flow to the injection site and thereby minimize bleeding at the site of the injection. Vasoconstrictors also slow absorption of the anesthetic agent into the bloodstream and thereby produce lower blood levels of the anesthetic and reduce the risk of an anesthetic overdose reaction. Vasoconstrictors also maintain higher concentrations of the local anesthetic in/around the nerves for a longer time and thereby increase the duration of action of the local anesthetic. Epinephrine is the most useful vasoconstrictor. Epinephrine acts on both α adrenergic receptors and $\beta_{1,2}$ adrenergic receptors but the β_2 effects predominate. For the doses of epinephrine employed in dentistry, the epinephrine effects are usually limited to the direct action on α receptors causing vasoconstriction of smooth muscle in peripheral arterioles and results in increased systolic and diastolic blood pressure. However, after the α effects of vasoconstriction have worn off, epinephrine also produces a rebound vasodilation β_2 effect in arterioles. The rebound β effects can result in post-operative bleeding when epinephrine is used in either 1:50,000 or 1:100,000 concentrations. Epinephrine concentrations of 1:50,000 must never be used for block anaesthesia and must be used with caution during local infiltration. Due to profound vasoconstriction with epinephrine concentrations of 1:50,000, tissue ischemia and necrosis are a risk. In order to prevent or minimize bleeding, epinephrine-containing LA may be infiltrated locally into the site of operation. However, minimal amounts of LA must be used as excessive vasoconstriction at the surgical site will compromise healing and complicate post-operative hemostasis due to the rebound β effects (Malamed 1986; Little et al. 2002).

Control of intra-operative/primary bleeding

Intra-operative bleeding must be controlled as soon as possible. Uncontrolled bleeding places the patient at risk, obscures the surgical field and delays the completion of surgery. However, intra-operative sites of bleeding from the bone and/or mucoperiosteal flap may be obscured during the time of surgery due to the use of LA with a vasoconstrictor. When the vasoconstrictor effects have worn off and rebound vasodilation occurs, the bleeding will become apparent. In typical fashion, this secondary/post-operative bleeding will become apparent several hours after the patient has been dismissed from the clinic.

Common sources of intra-operative bleeding include granulation tissue within periodontal defects, vessels in the periosteum, nutrient vessels or marrow spaces in bone. Pressure packs/ gauze applied to the granulation tissue will usually not stop the bleeding from granulation tissue. Once the pressure packs are removed, blood will usually diffuse back into the surgical field. Therefore, to control the bleeding, the osseous defects should be quickly and thoroughly debrided of granulation tissue. Adequate flap reflection, careful suctioning and good lighting should identify bleeding vessels in the periosteum. Clamping of the vessels with a small hemostat and/or placement of a resorbable suture should control the bleeding. Nutrient vessels/marrow spaces may be encountered during debridement or performance of ostectomy/ plasty. Crushing or burnishing the surrounding bone will usually control the bleeding from these sites. If bleeding from marrow spaces cannot be controlled with application of pressure or compression of the bone, then bone wax may be applied into the space.

After performance of tooth extractions, ostectomy and/or osteoplasty, all loose bone spicules and sharp osseous protrusions should be removed. All debris must be removed from the site by thorough irrigation with sterile saline. Primary closure is preferred for the establishment and maintenance of hemostasis. After placement of sutures, gentle pressure may be placed at the surgical site with a damp gauze sponge. Maintaining pressure at the surgical for at least 5 minutes should establish hemostasis. Some pressure may also be applied via placement of periodontal dressing.

Topical agents may be applied to residual sites of bleeding and include tissue cyanoacrylate adhesives (e.g. Histoacryl®, B. Braun), microfibrillar collagen (e.g. Oxycel, Surgicel; Surgicel fibrillar, Johnson & Johnson), topical thrombin or Gelfoam (gelatin sponge; Gelfoam, Pharmacia & Upjohn) and chitin-based polymers (e.g. HemCon Dental Dressing, HDD; HemCon Medical Technologies, Inc, Beaverton, Oregon). If absorbable agents must be used on/near a bony or neural space, use the minimal amount of material necessary, ensure that hemostasis is achieved before closing the wound, and remove as much as possible (preferably all) of the agent as soon as possible after hemostasis is achieved (FDA Bulletin, Health Canada Bulletin, www.hc-sc.gc.ca/dhp-mps/medeff/advisories-avis/ prof/_2004/hemostat_agents)

Lasers and electrocautery may also be used to establish hemostasis as both methods coagulate the soft tissues and hence occlude the vessels. A CO_2 or Nd:YAG laser may be used to establish hemostasis at sites of soft-tissue wounds such as graft donor sites. However, CO_2, Nd:YAG (or argon) lasers or the use of electrocautery are not indicated for contact with bone or other hard tissues and therefore the use of these techniques to establish hemostasis from a bleeding extraction socket is not indicated.

Post-operative/secondary bleeding

When a patient is concerned about bleeding following an oral surgical procedure, the patient's emotional/mental state will probably include anxiety, stress and fear. These emotions promote the release of endogenous catecholamines, which increase the sympathetic tone. The resulting increased blood pressure and heart rate may promote bleeding from the wound sites. Moreover, the patient's mental state may not allow the patient to clearly focus and follow post-operative instructions; therefore, the assistance and reassurance of a family member can be helpful. It may be necessary to recall the patient to the clinic. Upon arrival, the patient's vital signs (blood pressure, pulse and breathing rate) should be recorded and the source of bleeding determined. Integrity of the periodontal dressing (if placed) should be assessed and removed if necessary to examine the bleeding site. Pooled blood, saliva and soft clots should be evacuated. Firm pressure should be applied to reduce bleeding before other means are initiated. Active sites of bleeding can arise in the bone and/or mucoperiosteal flap. These sites may not have been evident during the surgery due to the use of LA with a vasoconstrictor. The surgical site (and source of bleeding) may be painful if the LA effect has worn off. Injection of LA with a vasoconstrictor for pain relief is indicated to permit further local measures for the control of bleeding. Local infiltration of LA with a vasoconstrictor will aid in establishing hemostasis. The source of the bleeding should be identified prior to administration of LA with a vasoconstrictor.

Measures that may be used alone or in combination include additional sutures, obtaining primary closure, placing blind sutures (e.g. at the palatal graft donor site) to exert mechanical tension onto the underlying vasculature and thereby promote hemostasis, application of tissue adhesive and topical hemostatic agents, use of lasers and electrocautery.

CONCLUSIONS

This chapter reviews hemostasis and coagulation models as well as protocols for predicting, preventing and managing bleeding complications. It is easy for clinicians to take for granted the complex reactions that establish hemostasis after wounding until challenged with a bleeding complication. Whereas the intrinsic and extrinsic pathways of the Waterfall Cascade Model are easy to understand, no such division exists *in vivo*: tissue factor VIIa complex is a potent activator of FX, FIX and FVIIa and can generate thrombin on the platelet surface independently of external TF. Coagulation reactions are finely regulated by stimulatory and inhibitory mechanisms that maintain the fluid phase of blood but can respond rapidly to injury with clot formation. Under physiologic conditions, there is a minor predominance of anticoagulant processes and the healthy endothelium is an integral component. Derangements in the complex interactions between cellular (endothelium, platelets) and protein components of the hemostatic system can quickly lead to pathological conditions. Although *in vitro* laboratory testing cannot accurately replicate the *in vivo* processes, it remains a useful guideline for predicting and managing bleeding complications as long as the limitations are recognized. Clinicians are well aware of the importance of a patient's health history, including bleeding history and drug history. However, it is easy for clinicians to overlook the significance of nutritional history including daily supplements from the health food store in regards to the potential for bleeding tendencies, especially in combination with prescribed or over-the-counter drugs.

REFERENCES

Abebe, W. (2009) Herbal supplements may require modifications of dental treatment. *Dentistry Today.com*, accessed 1/15/2009.

Altman, R., Alejandra, S.S., de Lourdes Herrera, M., Gonzalez, C. (2006) Thrombin generation by activated factor VII on platelet activated by different agonists. Extending the cell-based model of hemostasis. *Thrombosis Journal* **4**, 5; http://www.thrombosisjournal.com/content/4/1/5.

Ando, J., Yamamoto, K. (2009) Vascular mechanobiology – endodothelial cell responses to fluid shear stress. *Circulation Journal* **73**, 1983–92.

Andre, P. (2004) P-selectin in haemostasis. *British Journal of Hematology* **126**, 298–306.

Ansell, J., Hirsh, J., Poller, L., et al. (2004) The pharmacology and management of vitamin K antagonists: the seventh ACCP conference on antithrombotic and thrombolytic therapy. *Chest* **126** (3 Suppl), 204S–33S.

Antovic, J.P., Blomback, M. (2002) Thrombin-activatable fibrinolysis inhibitor antigen and TADI activity in patients with APC resistance caused by factor V Leiden mutation. *Thrombosis Research* **106**(1), 59–62.

Aoki, A.S., Osada, M., Kaneko, M., et al. (2007) Fluid shear stress enhances the sphingosine 1-phosphate responses in cell–cell interactions between platelets and endothelial cells. *Biochemical and Biophysical Research Communications* **358**, 1054–7.

Atkinson, M.E., White, F.H. (1992) *Principles of Anatomy and Oral Anatomy for Dental Students*. Chapter 26, The Vascular System. Churchill Livingstone, Edinburgh, London.

Bach, R.R. (2006) Tissue factor encryption. *Arteriosclerosis, Thrombosis, and Vascular Biology* **26**, 456–61.

Beckert, B.W., Concannon, J., Henry, S.L., et al. (2007) The effect of herbal medicines on platelet function: an *in vivo* experiment and review of the literature. *Plastic and Reconstructive Surgery* **120**(7), 2044–50.

Beltrami, E., Jesty, J. (2001) The role of membrane patch size and flow in regulating a proteolytic feedback threshold on a membrane: possible application in blood coagulation. *Mathematical Biosciences* **172**, 1–13.

Bhatt, D.L., Francis, G.S. (2003) Red vs white thrombi: treating the right clot is crucial. *Archives Internal Medicine* **163**(20), 2535.

Bilodeau, M.L., Hamm, H.E. (2007) Regulation of protease-activated receptor (PAR) 1 and PAR4 signaling in human platelets by compartmentalized cyclic nucleotide actions. *Journal of Pharmacology and Experimental Therapeutics* **322**, 778–88.

Blair, P., Flaumenhaft, R. (2009) Platelet alpha-granules: basic biology and clinical correlates. *Blood Reviews* **23**(4), 177–89.

Bogatcheva, N.V., Verin, A.D. (2008) The role of cytoskeleton in the regulation of vascular endothelial barrier function. *Microvascular Research* **76**, 202–207.

Bouma, B.N., Mosnier, L.O. (2006) Thrombin activatable fibrinolysis inhibitor (TAFI) – how does thrombin regulate fibrinolysis? *Annals of Medicine* **38**, 378–88.

Brand-Miller, J., Dickinson, S., Barclay, A., et al. (2009) Glycemic index, glycemic load, and thrombogenesis. *Seminars in Thrombosis and Hemostasis* **35**(1), 111–18.

Breitenstein, A., Camici, G.G., Tanner, F.C. (2010) Tissue factor: beyond coagulation in the cardiovascular system. *Clinical Science* **118**, 159–72.

Bunte, M.C., Patnaik, M.M., Pritzker, M.R., et al. (2008) Pulmonary veno-occlusive disease following hematopoietic stem cell transplantation: a rare model of endothelial dysfunction. *Bone Marrow Transplantation* **41**, 677–86.

Butenas, S., Orfeo, T., Mann, K.G. (2009) Tissue factor in coagulation. Which? Where? When? *Arteriosclerosis, Thrombosis and Vascular Biology* **29**, 1989–96.

Camacho, A., Dimsdale, J.E. (2000) Platelets and psychiatry: lessons learned from old and new studies. *Pysochomatic Medicine* **62**, 326–36.

Chien, S. (2007) Mechanotransduction and endothelial cell homeostasis: the wisdom of the cell. *American Journal of Physiology – Heart and Circulatory Physiology* **292**, H1209–24.

Chiu, J., Usami, S., Chien, S. (2009) Vascular endothelial responses to altered shear stress: pathologic implications for atherosclerosis. *Annals of Medicine* **41**, 19–28.

Cleator, J.H., Zhu, W.Q., Vaughan, D.E., et al. (2006) Differential regulation of endothelial exocytosis of P-selectin and von Willebrand factor by protease-activated receptors and cAMP. *Blood* **107**(7), 2736–44.

Cohan, R.P., Jacobsen, P.L. (2000) Herbal supplements: considerations in dental practice. *Journal of the California Dental Association*, **28**(8), 600–610; http://www.cda.org/library/cda_member/pubs/journal/jour0800/index.html.

Crawley, J.T.B., Lane, D.A. (2008) The haemostatic role of tissue factor pathway inhibitor. *Arteriosclerosis, Thrombosis and Vascular Biology* **28**, 233–42.

Dahlback, B. (2005) Blood coagulation and its regulation by anticoagulant pathways: genetic pathogenesis of bleeding and thrombotic diseases. *Journal of Internal Medicine* **257**, 209–23.

Dale, G.L. (2005) Coated platelets: an emerging component of the procoagulant response. *Journal of Thrombosis and Haemostasis* **3**(10), 2185–92.

Dale, G.L., Friese, P., Batar, P., et al. (2002) Stimulated platelets use serotonin to enhance their retention of procoagulant proteins on the cell surface. *Nature* **415**(6868), 175–9.

Daleke, D.L. (2003) Regulation of transbilayer plasma membrane phospholipid asymmetry. *Journal of Lipid Research* **44**, 233–42.

Davie, E.W., Ratnoff, O.D. (1964) Waterfall sequence for intrinsic blood clotting. *Science* **145**, 1310–12.

Delvaeye, M., Conway, E.M. (2009) Coagulation and innate immune responses: can we view them separately? *Blood* **114**, 2367–74.

Diamond, D.L. (2009) Systems biology to predict blood function. *Journal of Thrombosis and Haemostasis* **7** (Suppl 1), 177–80.

Dong, J., Moake, J.L., Nolasco, L., et al. (2002) ADAMTS-13 rapidly cleaves newly secreted ultralarge von Willebrand factor multimers on the endothelial surface under flowing conditions. *Hemostatis, Thrombosis, and Vascular Biology* **100**, 4033–9.

Eilersten, K.E., Osterud, B. (2004) Tissue factor: (patho)physiology and cellular biology. *Blood Coagulation and Fibrinolysis* **15**(7), 521–38.

Esper, R.J., Nordaby, R.A., Vilarino, J.O., et al. (2006) Endothelial dysfunction: a comprehensive appraisal. *Cardiovascular Diabetology* **5**, 4; http://www.cardiab.com/content/5/1/4.

Favaloro, E.J. (2009) Toward a new paradigm for the identification and functional characterization of von Willebrand disease. *Seminars in Thrombosis and Hemostasis* **35**(1), 60–75.

Fugh-Berman, A. (2000) Herb–drug interactions. *Lancet* **355**, 134–8.

Gailani, D., Broze Jr., G.J. (1993) Factor XI activation by thrombin and factor XIa. *Seminars in Thrombosis and Hemostasis* **19**(4), 396–404.

Hannun, Y.A., Obeid, L.M. (2008) Principles of bioactive lipid signaling: lessons from sphingolipids. *Nature Reviews Molecular Cell Biology* **9**(2), 139–50.

Harrison, P., Cramer, E.M. (1993) Platelet alpha-granules. *Blood Reviews* **7**(1), 52–62.

Hoffman, M. (2003) Remodeling the blood coagulation cascade. *Journal of Thrombosis and Thombolysis* **16**(1–2), 17–20.

Hoffman, M., Monroe, D.M. (2001) A cell-based model of hemostasis. *Journal of Thrombosis and Haemostasis* **85**(6), 958–65.

Hoffman, M., Monroe, D.M. (2005) Rethinking the coagulation cascade. *Current Hemotology Reports* **4**(5), 391–6.

Hoffman, H., Monroe, D.M. (2007) Coagulation 2006: a modern view of hemostasis. *Hematology/Oncology Clinics of North America* **21**, 1–11.

Hoover-Plow, J. (2010) Does plasmin have anticoagulant activity? *Vascular Health and Risk Management* **6**, 199–205.

Horn, J.R., Hansten, P.D. (2003) SSRIs and NSAIDs: increasing the risk of upper gastrointestinal bleeding? *Drug Interactions and Insights* **December**, 68–9.

Hu, A., Yang, X., Ho., P.C., et al. (2005) Herb–drug interactions: a literature review. *Drugs* **65**(9), 1239–82.

Ikeda, M., Kihara, A., Igarashi, Y. (2006) Lipid asymmetry of the eukaryotic plasma membrane: functions and related enzymes. *Biological and Pharmaceutical Bulletin* **29**(8), 1542–6.

Italiano, J.E., Richardson, J.L., Patel-Hett, S., et al. (2008) Angiogenesis is regulated by a novel mechanism: pro- and antiangiogenic proteins are organized into separate platelet alpha granules and differentially released. *Hemostasis, Thrombosis, and Vascular Biology* **111**, 1227–33.

Jesty, J., Beltrami, E. (2005) Positive feedbacks of coagulation; their role in threshold regulation. *Arteriosclerosis, Thrombosis and Vascular Biology* **25**, 2463–9.

Jurk, K., Kehrel, B.E. (2005) Platelets: physiology and biochemistry. *Seminars in Thrombosis and Hemostasis* **31**(4), 381–92.

Khanin, M.A., Semenov, V.V. (1989) A mathematical model of the kinetics of blood coagulation. *Journal of Theoretical Biology* **136**(2), 127–34.

King, M. (2010). Blood coagulation. *The Medical Biochemistry Page*; http://themedicalbiochemistrypage.org/ blood-coagulation.html.

Kleinschnitz, C., Stoll, G., Bendszus, M., et al. (2006) Targeting coagulation factor XII provides protection from pathological thrombosis in cerebral ischemia without interfering with hemostasis. *Journal Experimental Medicine* **203**(3), 513–18.

Kriz, N., Rinder, C.S., Rinder, H.M. (2009) Physiology of hemostasis: with relevance to current and future laboratory testing. *Clinical Laboratory Medicine* **29**, 159–74.

Laurens, N., Koolwijk, P., De Maat, M.P.M. (2006) Fibrin structure and wound healing. *Journal of Thrombosis and Haemostasis* **4**, 932–9.

Lawson, J.H., Mann, K.G. (1991) Cooperative activation of human factor IX by the human extrinsic pathway of blood coagulation. *Journal of Biological Chemistry* **266**(17), 11317–27.

Lippi, G., Favaloro, E.J., Franchini, M., et al. (2009) Milestones and perspectives in coagulation and hemostasis. *Seminars in Thrombosis and Hemostasis* **35**(1), 009–022.

Little, J.W., Falace, D.A., Miller, C.S., Rhodus, N.L. (2002) *Dental Management of the Medically Compromised Patient*, 6th edn. Chapter 4, Hypertension, and Chapter 19, Bleeding Disorders. Mosby, St Louis, Missouri.

Lopez-Vilechez, I., Diaz-Ricart, M., White, J. B., et al. (2009) Serotonin enhances platelet procoagulant properties and their activation induced during platelet tissue factor uptake. *Cardiovascular Research* **84**(2), 309–16.

Lowenstein, C.J., Morrell, C.N., Yamakuchi, M. (2005) Regulation of Weibel-Palade body exocytosis. *Trends in Cardiovascular Medicine* **15**, 302–308.

MacFarlane, R.G. (1964) An enzyme cascade in the blood clotting mechanism, and its function as a biochemical amplifier. *Nature* **202**, 498–9.

Mackman, N. (2009) The role of tissue factor and factor VIIa in hemostasis. *Anesthesia Analgesia* **108**(5), 1447–52.

Mackman, N., Taubman, M. (2009) Tissue factor past, present and future. *Arteriosclerosis, Thrombosis and Vascular Biology* **29**(12), 1986–8.

Mackman, N., Tilley, R.E., Key, N.S. (2007) Role of the extrinsic pathway of blood coagulation in hemostasis and thrombosis. *Arteriosclerosis, Thrombosis and Vascular Biology* **27,** 1687–93.

Malamed, S.F. (1986) *Handbook of Local Anaesthesia*. Chapter 3, Pharmacology of Vasoconstrictors. CV Mosby, St Louis, Toronto, London.

Mann, K.G., Nesheim, M.E., Church, W.R., et al. (1990) Surface-dependent reactions of the vitamin K-dependent enzyme complexes. *Journal of the American Society of Hematology* **76**, 1–16.

Mann, K.G., Brummel, K., Butenas, S. (2003) What is all that thrombin for? *Journal of Thrombosis and Haemostasis* **1**(7), 1504–14.

Mann, K.G., Brummel-Ziedins, K., Orfeo, T., et al. (2006) Models of blood coagulation. *Blood Cells, Molecules, and Diseases* **36**, 108–117.

Mann, K.G., Orfeo, T., Butenas, S., et al. (2009) Blood coagulation dynamics in haemostasis. *Hamostaseologie* **29**(1), 7–16.

Maurer, L.M., Tomasini-Johansson, B.R., Mosher, D.F. (2010) Emerging roles of fibronectin in thrombosis. *Thrombosis Research* **125,** 287–91.

May, A.E., Seizer, P., Gawaz, M. (2008) Platelets: inflammatory firebugs of vascular walls. *Arteriosclerosis, Thrombosis and Vascular Biology* **28**, s5–10.

McCloskey, D.J., Postolache, T.T., Vittone, B.J., et al. (2008) Selective serotonin reuptake inhibitors (SSRIs): measurement of effect on platelet function. *Translational Research* **151**(3), 168–72.

Metcalf, D.J., Nightingale, T.D., Zenner, H.L., et al. (2007) Formation and function of Weibel-Palade bodies. *Journal of Cell Science* **121**, 19–27.

Mezzano, D., Matus, V., Saez, C.G., et al. (2008) Tissue factor storage, synthesis and function in normal and activated human platelets. *Thrombosis Research* **122** (Suppl1), S31–6.

Michiels, C. (2003) Endothelial cell functions. *Journal of Cellular Physiology* **196**, 430–43.

Mitchell, J.A., Ali, F., Bailey, L. et al. (2007) Role of nitric oxide and prostacyclin as vasoactive hormones released by endothelium. *Experimental Physiololgy* **93**(1), 141–7.

Monroe, D.M., Hoffman, N.M., Oliver, J.A., et al. (1998) A possible mechanism of action of activated factor VII independent of tissue factor. *Blood Coagulation and Fibrinolysis*, **9** (S1), S15–20.

Monroe, D.M., Hoffman, M., Roberts, H.R. (2002) Platelets and thrombin generation. *Arteriosclerosis, Thrombosis and Vascular Biology* **22**, 1381–9.

Monroe, D.M., Mackman, N., Hoffman, M. (2010) Wound healing in hemophilia B mice and low tissue factor mice. *Thrombosis Research* **125**, S74–7.

Montagnana, M., Salvagno, G.L., Lippi, G. (2009) Circadian variation within hemostasis: an underrecognized link between biology and disease. *Seminars in Thrombosis and Hemostasis* **35**(1), 23–33.

Morel, O., Morel, N., Freyssinet, J.M., et al. (2008) Platelet microparticles and vascular cell interactions: a checkpoint between haemostatic and thrombotic response. *Platelets* **19**(1), 9–23.

Morrisey, J.J. (1996) Plasma factor VIIa: measurement and potential clinical significance. *Haemostasis* **26**(S1), 66–71.

Natella, F., Nardini, M., Bellili, F., et al. (2008) Effect of coffee drinking on platelets: inhibition of aggregation and phenols incorporation. *British Journal of Nutrition* **100**, 1276–82.

Nematullah, A., Alabousi, A., Blanas, N., et al. (2009) Dental surgery for patients on anticoagulant therapy with warfarin: a systematic review and meta-analysis. *Journal of the Canadian Dental Association* **75**(1), 41–50.

Padilla, A., Moake, J.L., Bernardo, A., et al. (2004) P-selectin anchors newly released ultralarge von Willebrand factor multimers to the endothelial cell surface. *Blood* **103**, 2150–56.

Panes, O., Matus, V., Saez, C., et al. (2007) Human platelets synthesize and express functional tissue factor. *Blood* **109**, 5242–50.

Polgar, J., Matuskova, J., Wagner, D.D. (2005) The P-selectin, tissue factor, coagulation triad. *Journal of Thrombosis and Haemostasis* **3**(8), 1590–96.

Ren, Q., Ye, S., Whiteheard, S.W. (2008) The platelet release reaction: just when you thought platelet secretion was simple. *Current Opinion in Hematology* **15**(5), 537–41.

Rex, S., Beaulieu, L.M., Perlman, D.H., et al. (2009) Immune versus thrombotic stimulation of platelets differentially regulates signalling pathways, intracellular protein–protein interactions, and alpha-granule release. *Journal of Thrombosis and Haemostasis* **102**(1), 97–110.

Riddel, J.P., Aouizerat, B.E., Miaskowski, C., et al. (2007) Theories of blood coagulation. *Journal of Pediatric Oncology Nursing* **24**, 123–31.

Rivera, J., Lozano, M.L., Navarro-Nunez, L., et al. (2009) Platelet receptors and signalling in the dynamics of thrombus formation. *Haematologica* **94**, 700–711.

Roberts, H.R., Hoffman, M., Monroe, D.M. (2006) A cell-based model of thrombin generation. *Seminars in Thrombosis and Hemostasis* **32**(S1), 32–8.

Rondaij, M.G., Bierings, R., Kragt, A., et al. (2006) Dynamics and plasticity of Weibel-Palade bodies in endothelial cells. *Arteriosclerosis, Thrombosis and Vascular Biology* **26**, 1002–7.

Ruggeri, Z.M. (2009) Platelet adhesion under flow. *Microcirculation* **16**(1), 58–83.

Ruggeri, Z.M., Mendolicchio, G.L. (2007) Adhesion mechanisms in platelet function. *Circulation Research* **100**, 1673–85.

Runyon, M.K., Johnson-Kerner, B.L., Kastrup, C.J., et al. (2007) Propagation of blood clotting in complex biochemical network of hemostasis is described by a simple mechanism. *Journal of the American Chemical Society* **129**, 7014–15.

Sadler, J.E. (2002) A new name in thrombosis, ADAMTS13. *Proceedings of the National Academy of Sciences, USA* **99**, 11552–4.

Salem, R.O., Laposata, M. (2005) Effects of alcohol on hemostasis. *American Journal of Clinical Pathology* **123**, S96–105.

Schwertz, H., Koster, S., Kahr, W.H.A., et al. (2009) Anucleate platelets generage progeny. *Blood* **115**(18), 3801–9; http://bloodjournal.hematologylibrary.org /cgi /content /abstract/ blood-2009-08-239558v1.

Sehgal, S., Storrie, B. (2007) Evidence that differential packaging of the major platelet granule proteins von Willebrand factor and fibrinogen can support their differential release. *Journal of Thrombosis and Haemostasis* **5**, 2009–16.

Seligsohn, U. (2007) Factor XI in haemostasis and thrombosis: past, present and future. *Journal of Thrombosis and Haemostasis* **98**, 84–9.

Shibeko, A.M., Lobanova, E.S., Panteleev, M.A., et al. (2010) Blood flow controls coagulation onset via the positive feedback of factor VII activation by factor Xa. *BioMed Central Systems Biology* **4**, 5.

Shireman, P.K., Pearce, W.H. (1996) Endothelial cell function: biologic and physiologic functions in health and disease. *American Journal of Roentgenology* **166**, 7–13.

Singh, I., Temistou, E., Porcar, K., et al. (2009) Fluid shear induces conformation change in human blood protein von Willebrand factor in solution. *Biophysical Journal* **96**, 1312–20.

Smith, S. (2009) The cell-based model of coagulation. *Journal of Veterinary Emergency and Critical Care* **19**(1), 3–10.

Spijkers, L.J.A., Alewijnse, A.E., Peters, S.L.M. (2010) Sphingolipids and the orchestration of endothelium-derived vasoactive factors: when endothelial function demands greasing. *Molecules and Cells* **29**, 105–11.

Stassen, J.M., Arnout, J., Deckmyn, H. (2004) The hemostatic system. *Current Medicinal Chemistry* **11**(17), 2245–60.

Vandenbroucke, E., Mehta, D., Minshall, R., et al. (2008) Regulation of endothelial junctional permeability. *Annals of the New York Academy of Sciences* **1123**, 134–45.

van Meer, G., Voelker, D.R., Feigenson, G.W. (2008) Membrane lipids: where they are and how they behave. *Nature Reviews Molecular and Cellular Biology* **9**(2), 112–24.

Verhamme, P., Hoylaerts, M.F. (2009) Hemostasis and inflammation: two of a kind? *Thrombosis Journal* **5**, 15–17.

Vine, A.K. (2009) Recent advanced in haemostasis and thrombosis. *Retina* **29**, 1–7.

Wee, M., Heerdink, E.R., Nolen, W.A., et al. (2004) Do serotonin reuptake inhibitors increase the risk of bleeding? *American Psychosocial Onclogy Society,* clinical e-mail update #14; http://www.apos-society.org/professionals/clincal/updates/2004/ClinUPdate14.122304.htm.

Weyrich, A.S., Schwertz, H., Mackman, N. (2007) Platelet tissue factor comes of age. *Blood* **109**, 5069–70.

White, C.R., Frangos, J.A. (2007) The shear stress of it all: the cell membrane and mechanochemical transduction. *Philosophical Transactions of the Royal Society B: Biological Sciences* **362**, 1459–67.

Yamaji-Hasegawa, A., Tsujimoto, M. (2006) Asymmetric disbribution of phospholipids in biomembranes. *Biological and Pharmaceutical Bulletin* **29**(8), 1547–53.

Yeaman, M.R. (2010) Platelets in defence against bacterial pathogens. *Cellular and Molecular Life Sciences* **67,** 525–44.

3 Inflammation and Wound Healing

Anna Turabelidze and Luisa Ann DiPietro

Center for Wound Healing and Tissue Regeneration, University of Illinois at Chicago, Chicago, IL, USA

INTRODUCTION

With few exceptions, a vigorous inflammatory response is a hallmark of the initial response to injury. Beginning with studies performed in the early 20th century by Dr Alexis Carrel, mounting evidence suggests that the appropriate function of inflammatory cells is important to successful wound healing (Carrel 1922). The study of wound inflammation continues to receive intense attention, with more than 1,000 articles on the topic published within the past 5 years. Inflammatory cells can assist the repair process by performing microbial decontamination, and via the production of multiple growth factors and cytokines. Indeed, studies in a variety of model systems suggest that key inflammatory cytokines are critical to wound healing (Gillitzer and Goebeler 2001). However, it should be noted that reduced or absent wound inflammation has been associated with improved tissue repair in specific settings, such as fetal wounds and oral mucosal wounds (Wetzler et al. 2000; Szpaderska et al. 2003). This chapter reviews the current information on the mechanisms that dictate the inflammatory response in wounds, and examines the emerging concepts concerning the role of inflammation in modulating reparative outcomes.

THE INNATE IMMUNE RESPONSE IN WOUNDS

Immediately following injury, innate immune cells at the site of injury initiate an inflammatory response (Shaw and Martin 2009). Cells of the innate immune system stand at the ready, acting as sentinels to respond quickly to tissue damage or microbes (Fig. 3.1). The innate immune cells within the skin are of several types, and include mast cells (Noli and Miolo 2001), dendritic cells, fixed macrophages (Cumberbatch et al. 2000), and some specialized gamma-delta T-cell populations (Jameson et al. 2004). In the skin, keratinocytes are often considered a part of the immune sentinel system as well, as this cell type can quickly respond to stimuli and produces several pro-inflammatory mediators (Kupper and Fuhlbrigge 2004). The response of the innate immune cells to injury is rapid, with cells such as keratinocytes and macrophages able to produce inflammatory mediators within the first hour following insult. Resident mast cells respond even more rapidly. Mast cells can be activated by numerous stimuli, including trauma, antigen, superoxides, complement, neuropeptides and lipoproteins (Marshall 2004). Once activated, mast cells immediately degranulate, releasing

Oral Wound Healing: Cell Biology and Clinical Management, First Edition. Edited by Hannu Larjava.

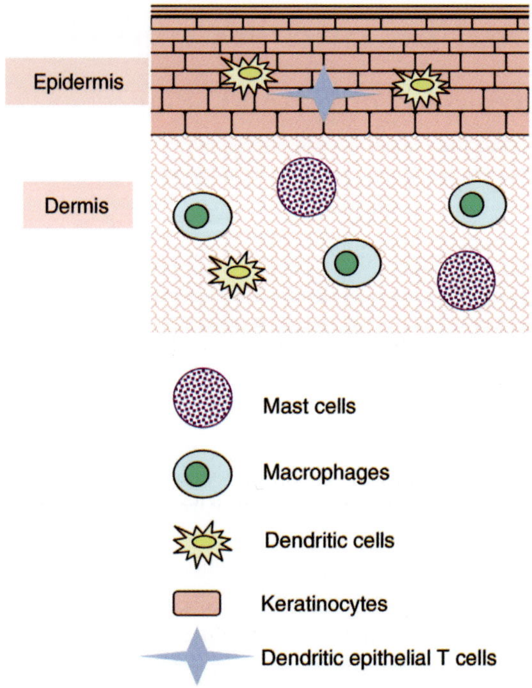

Fig. 3.1 Resident innate immune cells that contribute to wound inflammation in skin. Many types of innate immune cells stand at the ready, acting as sentinels to respond quickly to tissue damage or microbes.

preformed proinflammatory mediators, including histamine, leukotrienes, prostanoids and cytokines. The mediators produced by resident innate immune cells in response to injury or insult trigger vascular responses, including vasodilation, endothelial cell activation and increased vascular permeability. Further, early mediators from resident innate immune cells assist in recruiting the first wave of circulating leukocytes from the bloodstream into the injured tissue. Thus the resident innate immune cells trip the inflammatory switch, initiating the robust cellular inflammatory response that is observed in wounds.

INFLAMMATORY CELL INFILTRATION INTO WOUNDS

Following tissue injury and innate immune cell activation, the early inflammatory phase is marked by neutrophil infiltration (Fig. 3.2). Neutrophils, a cell type that is rarely found in normal tissue, begin to accumulate in the wound within minutes and continue to increase in number for several days after injury. Similar to all immune cells, the recruitment of neutrophils into wounds is mediated by chemotactic factors generated at the site. As mentioned above, there are many sources of chemotactic factors in the wound, including innate immune cells. Additional chemoattractants can be released by platelets, are produced during complement activation and may also derive from microorganisms (Robson et al. 2001; Szpaderska and DiPietro 2005).

Sometime after neutrophil infiltration is well underway, the macrophage population within the wound begins to increase. Resident macrophages become activated, and their

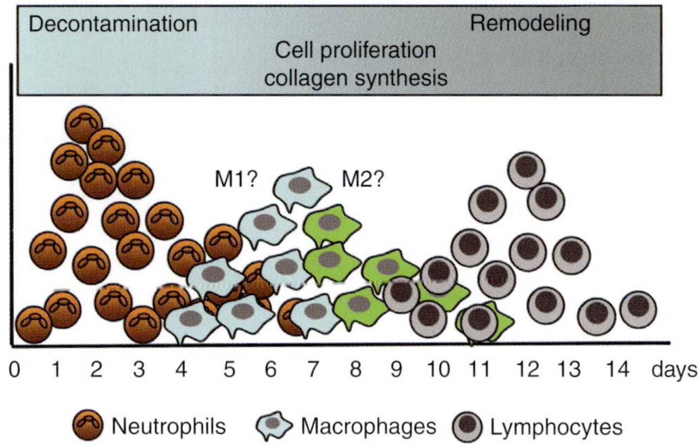

Fig. 3.2 Inflammatory cell infiltration and function in wounds. Following injury and activation of the innate immune system, successive waves of neutrophils, macrophages (both M1 and M2 types) and lymphocytes move into the wound. The presumed functions of these cell types are shown in the box above the cells.

numbers increase as circulating monocytes move into the extravascular space and differentiate into mature tissue macrophages (Martinez et al. 2006). Although it has been commonly thought that activated macrophages behave uniformly, more recent studies have shown that macrophages are capable of developing diverse phenotypes. *In vitro* studies suggest that macrophages readily acquire two different phenotypes that are dependent upon the method of activation. Classically activated macrophages, or the M1 phenotype, are pro-inflammatory cells that produce an array of pro-inflammatory cytokines. Alternatively activated macrophages, or the M2 phenotype, are anti-inflammatory and support proliferation by producing growth factors (Shaw and Martin 2009). While these dichotomous phenotypes are well described in some systems, the situation with wound macrophages themselves seems much more complex. Within acute skin wounds, multiple and perhaps intermediate phenotypes are found within the macrophage population (Daley et al. 2010).

Another cell type that also increases in density in the wound bed is mast cells, with most of the infiltrating mast cells originating in the adjacent tissue (Artuc et al. 1999). As the leukocyte density within the wound increases, the leukocytes that have been recruited into the wound produce large amounts of cytokines and chemoattractants, amplifying the inflammatory response.

In the late inflammatory phase of wound repair, T lymphocytes appear in the wound bed, and may support the resolution and remodeling of the wound (Barbul et al. 1989a, 1989b). T-cells may be attracted by interleukin-1 (IL-1), complement components and immunoglobulin G (IgG) breakdown products (Hunt et al. 2000; Hart 2002; Broughton et al. 2006a).

INFLAMMATORY CELL FUNCTION IN WOUNDS

Neutrophils

Inflammatory cells have multiple functions in both early and late phases of inflammation (Velnari et al. 2009). The first inflammatory cells to arrive at the site of injury are neutrophils. In the early response, the main function of neutrophils is considered to be prevention of infection by the killing of microbes (Broughton et al. 2006b). Neutrophils are highly phagocytic, and are important for decontamination of the wound. However, in the absence of microbial insult, neutrophils are not essential for proper wound healing in the skin (Simpson and Ross 1972). In a classic study by Simpson and Ross, no discernable differences in fibrin content or distribution were observed in wounds of neutropenic and control guinea pigs. More contemporary studies suggest that in the absence of microbial contamination, neutrophils may be detrimental to repair. The depletion of neutrophils has been shown to accelerate wound closure in both normal and diabetic mice (Dovi et al. 2004). This depletion had no significant effect on collagen deposition, wound disruption strength or macrophage infiltration in wounds of neutropenic mice in comparison to control.

The negative role for neutrophils in wound healing is thought to derive from the bystander damage caused by these cells as they attempt to clear microbes and debris. Neutrophils achieve the clearance of bacteria, foreign materials and damaged cells in the wound by phagocytosis (Robson et al. 2001; Hart 2002). Neutrophils may also attack microbes by trapping them in extruded nets of histones and DNA (Brinkmann et al. 2004). To perform this function, neutrophils move through intact capillary walls into surrounding body tissue and to the bacteria. However, this fight against infectious organisms does not come without casualties. Activated neutrophils release a set of microbicidal substances that are essential in the fighting of invading pathogens. Many of these factors, such as reactive oxygen species, cationic peptides, eicosanoids and proteases, not only kill microbes but also affect healthy host cells (Dovi et al. 2004; Richardson 2004; Martin and Leibovich 2005; Broughton et al. 2006a). Neutrophil elastase, for instance, can degrade virtually every component of the extracellular matrix, as well as proteins as diverse as clotting factors, complement, immunoglobulins and cytokines (Weiss 1989).

Once the bacteria and foreign material have been cleared from the wound site, neutrophils are no longer needed and the task of the host is then to eliminate them from the wound site. However, clearing of neutrophils from the wound must neither initiate an inflammatory response nor damage the tissue. This is achieved by their extrusion to the wound surface as slough and by apoptosis (Hunt et al. 2000; Hart 2002; Velnari et al. 2009). Apoptotic neutrophils are recognized by wound macrophages and are thought to stimulate the macrophages to adopt the M2, or alternative, phenotype.

Mast cells

Mast cells are part of the resident innate immune population. They are thought to be critical for the maintenance of tissue integrity and function (Maurer et al. 2003). Once an injury occurs, mast cells degranulate and release a variety of pre-stored mediators from their granules (Puxeddu et al. 2003). Mast cell-deficient mice have been described as exhibiting impaired wound healing of large sized wounds, although smaller wounds heal equally well in these mice (Egozi et al. 2003; Weller et al. 2006). The depletion of mast cells also leads to a decrease in neutrophils in wounds (Egozi et al. 2003; Weller et al. 2006; Wilgus 2008). However, the number of macrophages and CD-3-positive T-cells in wounds is similar to those in wild-type wounds (Egozi et al. 2003; Wilgus 2008). In addition to the resident population, mast cells are recruited to wounds, albeit in a slower time-course than neutrophils. Martin and Leibovich (2005) suggested that the small numbers of resident mast cells in tissues of injury play a surprisingly important role in the immediate–early activation events, especially to draw in neutrophils. What happens to mast cells in wounds after their job is complete is not well understood. Some studies suggest that they might disperse into the surrounding tissues by the lymphatic drainage (Burman et al. 2005).

Macrophages

Macrophages have been quoted as 'essential', 'indispensable' and 'most important to a successful outcome of wound healing', as these cells have been shown to produce growth factors that stimulate angiogenesis and fibrogenesis (Leibovich and Ross 1975; Hunt et al. 1984; Danon et al. 1989). Meszaros et al. (2000) demonstrated that macrophages, which arrive in the wound bed just after the neutrophils and just prior to neutrophil disappearance, are capable of inducing neutrophil apoptosis *in vitro*. Further, neutrophil-derived fragments have been found in phagosomes inside of macrophages (Meszaros et al. 1999). It seems that one of the most important functions of macrophages in wound healing is to assist in the regression of the inflammatory response via the elimination of neutrophils.

Macrophages also appear to be an important source of proliferative factors in wounds. Macrophage depletion was first shown to lead to delayed wound healing by Leibovich and Ross, who performed such a depletion study in guinea pigs in 1975 (Leibovich and Ross 1975). More recent studies have used sophisticated genetic manipulations to very specifically deplete macrophage populations in wounds. These studies reinforce the concept that macrophages play an integral role in a successful outcome of wound healing through the generation of growth factors that promote not only cell proliferation but also protein synthesis (Goren et al. 2009; Mirza et al. 2009).

Macrophages release many growth factors within wounds (Rappolee et al. 1988). Growth factors that are important to wound healing, including transforming growth factor-alpha (TGFα), transforming growth factor-beta (TGFβ) and platelet-derived growth factor are expressed by wound macrophages. Wound macrophages can also stimulate re-epithelialization and angiogenesis by secreting growth factors such as fibroblast growth factor-2 (FGF-2) and vascular endothelial growth factor (VEGF) (Kovacs and DiPietro 1994; Bingle et al. 2002). The fate of macrophages in the wound is not completely known. A study by Bellingan et al. (1996) suggests that the inflammatory macrophages do not die in the wounds but emigrate to the draining lymph node.

The balance of neutrophils and macrophages is also critical to wound healing outcomes. If the inflammatory process is altered such that the recruitment of neutrophils is increased, this may stimulate increased recruitment of macrophages to remove them. The end result of excessive inflammation is local tissue damage and hypoxia, and, ultimately, delayed healing.

T lymphocytes

T lymphocytes arrive in the wound after neutrophils and macrophages at about day 7 after injury. Their presence is at its peak during the late proliferative/early remodeling phase.

While the function of T lymphocytes in wounds is not well understood, a reduced level of T-cells has been shown to impair healing outcomes. The specific type of T-cell appears to be critical to function, as CD4+ cells (T-helper cells) have been suggested to accelerate wound healing while CD8+ cells (T-suppressor-cytotoxic cells) inhibit wound healing (Barbul et al. 1989a, 1989b; Park and Barbul 2004). Studies in mice deficient in both T- and

B-cells have shown that scar formation is diminished in the absence of lymphocytes (Gawronska-Kozak et al. 2006).

Gamma delta T-cells or dentritic epidermal T-cells (DETCs)

The resident gamma delta T-cell populations found in epithelial tissues are different from anywhere else in the body (Allison and Havran 1991) due to their differences in expression of tissue-restricted T-cell receptors (TCRs) (Jameson and Havran 2007). These cells are also called dendritic epidermal T-cells (DETC) due to their unique dendritic morphology. DETCs are activated by stressed, damaged or transformed keratinocytes.

The role of DETCs in wound healing was shown by Jameson et al. (2002). Full-thickness wounds of TCR delta -/- knockout mice exhibited delayed wound closure that could be rescued by the addition of either activated DETCs or recombinant KGF-1 (Jameson et al. 2002; Jameson and Havran 2007).

A role for DETCs in wound inflammation has also been demonstrated. The inflammatory cell content of full-thickness wounds in TCR delta -/- knockout mice is normal as far as neutrophils are concerned, yet exhibits delayed infiltration of macrophages in comparison to wild-type mice (Jameson et al. 2005; Jameson and Havran 2007). The difference in the level of macrophage infiltration was seen in the upper dermal compartment, where wild-type mice exhibit large numbers of macrophages by day 2 after injury (Jameson et al. 2005). This absence of macrophages was not believed to be from a defect in extravasation of macrophages from the bloodstream but from a defect in macrophage migration within the damaged dermis (Jameson et al. 2005).

In mice there are different subsets of gamma/delta T-cells, depending on such factors as time of appearance in ontogeny, anatomical location, TCR repertoires and thymus dependence (Haas et al. 1993). Each subset expresses unique adhesion proteins that are responsible for the differences in their migration capacity (Haas et al. 1993). Two different subsets are concentrated in skin epithelia and in the mucosal surfaces of the tongue (Itohara et al. 1990); however, they are both derived from the gamma delta T-cells which appear first in the fetal thymus (Haas et al. 1993).

CYTOKINES AND CHEMOKINES IN WOUNDS

Pro-inflammatory cytokines play a critical role in wound healing. Neutrophils and macrophages are major producers of pro-inflammatory cytokines. These include: interleukin-lα (IL-1α), IL-1β, IL-6, IL-8 and tumor necrosis factor-α (TNF-α). IL-1, IL-6 and TNF- α are upregulated during the inflammatory phase of wound healing (Singer and Clark 1999). Together, cytokines prevent infection, stimulate cellular recruitment and activate immune cells. In addition, cytokines regulate the ability of fibroblasts and epithelial cells to remodel damaged tissue.

Chemokines (chemotactic cytokines) are small heparin-binding proteins that direct the movement of circulating leukocytes to sites of inflammation or injury. They are active participants in the wound healing process because they stimulate the migration of multiple cell types in the wound site, especially inflammatory cells (Barrientos et al. 2008). The CXC, CC and C families of ligands act by binding to G protein-coupled surface receptors, CXC receptors and the CC receptor.

Here we review some of the chemokines and cytokines that are known to be critical to wound inflammation.

Interleukin-1 (IL-1)

IL-1 is highly upregulated during the inflammatory phase of wound healing (Singer and Clark 1999). This cytokine is produced by diverse groups of cells: keratinocytes, neutrophils, monocytes and macrophages. IL-1 plays a role in the proliferation of keratinocytes and endothelial cells, and in the activation of neutrophils, natural killer cells, T-cells, B-cells and macrophages at the wound site (Barrientos et al. 2008).

Upon injury, pre-stored IL-1 is immediately released by keratinocytes, acting as the initial signaling for barrier damage and calling for neutrophils to the damaged site (Barrientos et al. 2008). In addition, neutrophils further stimulate the inflammatory response by secreting IL-1α and IL-1β (Werner and Grose 2003). This is achieved by recruiting monocytes, inducing adhesion molecule expression in blood vessels to promote diapedesis, and supporting macrophage survival and retention at the wound site.

IL-1 has both paracrine and autocrine effects on migration and proliferation of keratinocytes. It induces the expression of K6 and K16 keratins in migrating keratinocytes (Komine et al. 2000), activates fibroblasts and increases secretion of fibroblast growth factor 7(FGF-7) (Tang and Gilchrest 1996).

Interleukin-6 (IL-6)

IL-6 is another pro-inflammatory cytokine and has been shown to be crucial in initiating the healing response. Studies have shown that IL-6 expression increases and remains high after wounding (Grellner et al. 2000; Di Vita et al. 2006). Sources of IL-6 in the wound include neutrophils, monocytes, fibroblasts and activated mature macrophages

IL-6 has a proliferative effect on keratinocytes and is chemoattractive to neutrophils (Gallucci et al. 2004). IL-6 can also act as an endogenous pyrogen and augments immunoglobulin production by B-cells and enhances B-cell growth and differentiation.

The importance of IL-6 in healing has been shown by studies in mouse model systems. Mice genetically deficient for IL-6 exhibit a healing time that is three times that of wild-type controls. In these knockouts, re-epithelialization was delayed and the granulation tissue formation was also impaired (Gallucci et al. 2000). However, this impaired healing would be rescued through administering recombinant murine IL-6 protein 1 hour prior to wounding. Therefore, IL-6 may be more crucial at the beginning of the healing process, which is in accordance with its chemoattractive effect on neutrophils and mitogenic effects upon wound-edge keratinocytes.

Interestingly, IL-6 is also associated with severe scar formation, such as that seen in keloid formation. A study by Xue et al. (2000) showed that there is increased IL-6 expression at both gene and protein levels in keloids. This is suggested to occur through interferon-gamma (IFN-gamma) regulation of IL-6 secretion from fibroblasts (Maruyama et al. 1995; Yellin et al. 1995).

Interleukin-8 (IL-8 or CXCL8)

IL-8 is a member of the CXC family (Raja et al. 2007) and its expression is increased in acute wounds (Engelhardt et al. 1998). IL-8 is a strong chemoattractant for neutrophils, thus participating in the inflammatory response (Rennekampff et al. 2000). A direct homolog of IL-8 is not present in mice, creating some confusion as to its function in rodent systems.

Tumor necrosis factor (TNF alpha)

TNF-alpha is produced in the early wound at relatively high concentrations, suggesting that this factor is important to healing outcomes. However, when TNF-alpha is applied to wounds, its impact depends on concentration and duration of exposure. At low levels, TNF-alpha can promote wound healing by indirectly stimulating inflammation and increasing macrophage-produced growth factors. However, at higher levels, especially for prolonged periods of time, TNF-alpha has a detrimental effect on healing. It suppresses synthesis of extracellular matrix (ECM) proteins and tissue inhibitors of metalloproteinases (TIMPs) while increasing synthesis of matrix metalloproteinases (MMPs) (Barrientos et al. 2008).

Macrophage chemoattractant protein (MCP-1 or CCL2)

MCP-1 is a CC family chemokine. It is provided by in keratinocytes and macraphages upon wounding. It is a chemoattractant for monocytes, macrophages, T-cells and mast cells (DiPietro et al. 1995).

In MCP-1 knockout mice, wound healing is delayed, including re-epithelialization, angiogenesis and collagen synthesis (Low et al. 2001); This phenotype is also suggested in humans (Engelhardt et al. 1998). When exogenous MCP-1 is applied to wounds in animals, there is only moderate improvement in wound healing (DiPietro et al. 2001).

Interferon inducible protein 10 (IP-10 or CXCL10)

IP-10 is a member of the alpha or cysteine-X amino acid-cysteine (CXC) chemokine family of chemotactic cytokines. It is produced late in wound healing, becoming evident 4 days after wounding (Engelhardt et al. 1998). IP-10 is a chemoattractant for monocytes and T lymphocytes. It can inhibit the proliferation of endothelial cells and inhibit the growth of tumors *in vivo* (Luster et al. 1998). An IP-10 transgenic mouse, which constitutively expresses IP-10, demonstrates an abnormal wound healing response. It displays an intense inflammatory phase and a prolonged and disorganized granulation phase with impaired blood vessel formation (Luster et al. 1998).

In vitro studies show that IP-10 delays re-epithelialization and prolongs the granulation phase (Shiraha et al. 1999). It inhibits the migration of dermal fibroblasts by blocking their release from the substratum regulated by IP-10 inhibition of EGF and heparin-binding EGF-like growth factor receptor-mediated calpain activity (Shiraha et al. 1999). Studies have also shown that IP-10 inhibits angiogenesis (Barrientos et al. 2008).

Stromal cell-derived factor (SDF-1 or CXCL12)

The chemokine SDF-1 is a member of the CXC family and is angiogenic (Salcedo et al. 1999). It binds to CXCR4 receptors on endothelial cells and induces endothelial cell chemotaxis and formation of blood vessels (Salcedo et al. 1999). SDF-1 is constitutively abundant in many tissues (Shirozu et al. 1995). Mice lacking SDF-1 or its receptor CXCR4 present with severe developmental defects in the immune, circulatory and central nervous systems (Ma et al. 1998; Tachibana et al. 1998; Zou et al. 1998).

SDF-1 plays a role in the inflammatory response by recruiting lymphocytes to the wound and promoting angiogenesis. Endothelial cells, myofibroblasts and keratinocytes express SDF-1. When homeostasis is disturbed in an acute wound, SDF-1 expression increases at the wound margin in humans (Toksoy et al. 2007). However, starting from day 10 after wounding, SDF-1 is almost completely suppressed in the fibrous neostroma that replaces the provisional matrix covering the initial wound defect, whereas endothelial cells, major producers of SDF-1, are abundant at this site (Toksoy et al. 2007). However, in a mouse wound healing model, there is downregulation of SDF-1 (Fedyk et al. 2001). Further, in incisional wounding there is no expression of SDF-1 mRNA expression during the first 5 days (Florin et al. 2005). However, there is an increase in the expression of SDF-1 in diabetic db/db at the wound margin (Asai et al. 2006). In addition, during the initial phase of skin recovery following burns, an increase of SDF-1 protein is observed in rats (Avniel et al. 2006).

Transforming growth factor-beta (TGF-β)

One particular factor that seems critically involved in the wound healing process is TGF-β. TGF-β is chemotactic for fibroblasts, keratinocytes and inflammatory cells (Roberts and Sporn 1996).The TGF-β family of proteins consists of several structurally related but functionally distinct isoforms. In mammals, three isoforms, TGF-β1, -β2 and -β3, are identified (Massague et al. 1990). Studies have suggested specific roles for each of the TGF-β isoforms in the inflammation, proliferation and the remodeling stages of wound healing (Wahl et al. 1987; Roberts et al. 1988). TGF-β1 promotes inflammatory cell recruitment. Inflammatory cells recruited to the wound produce additional TGF- β1, increasing the inflammatory cell response (Moses et al. 1990). TGF- β1 is also believed to be a regulator in the development of hypertrophic scarring and keloid formation (Shal et al. 1995; Russell et al. 1988; Ghahary et al. 1993), while increased levels of TGF-β3 are associated with improved healing and reduced scar formation.

INFLAMMATION IN ORAL MUCOSAL WOUNDS

The healing of oral mucosal wounds proceeds through similar stages to that of dermal wounds. Yet wound healing in the oral mucosa is clinically distinguished from skin healing in terms of both its rapidity and relatively minimal scar formation. Studies in at least three different models of oral mucosal wound healing demonstrate that reduced inflammation and reduced scar formation are universal features of the superior healing phenotype that is observed in the oral cavity (Szpaderska et al. 2003; Mak et al. 2009; Wong et al. 2009). The one exception that has been seen are excisional wounds placed on the hard palate of the mouse. In this model, the underlying connective tissue is extremely thin, so the wound depth reaches the periosteal bony surface and healing slows (Graves et al. 2001). Nearly all other oral mucosal wounds, including palatal wounds in humans and pigs, heal more quickly than skin. At these oral sites, wounds exhibit less inflammation than skin wounds, with lower neutrophil, macrophage and T-cell infiltration (Szpaderska et al. 2003). Cytokine production is also decreased in oral wounds, including diminished production of IL-6, TNFα and keratinocyte-derived chemokine (KC) (Szpaderska et al. 2003). In a study performed by Mak et al. (2009) oral mucosal wounds showed significantly fewer mast cells than did skin wounds at 60 days post-wounding in the red Duroc pig model. T lymphocyte cell content in wounds is also significantly decreased in oral mucosal wounds on day 7 post injury in comparison to skin wounds in mice (Szpaderska et al. 2003). In equivalent sized excisional oral and dermal wounds of murine model tissues, reduced levels of TGF-β1 are associated with minimal oral mucosal scarring (Schrementi et al. 2008). Further, in the oral mucosa, there is a threefold increase in TGF-β3 production compared with unwounded tissue by 24 hours post wounding. Schrementi et al. suggest that the altered levels of TGF-β1 and -β3 play a key role in the privileged healing of the oral mucosa. Together, these studies contribute to the conclusion that inflammation in oral mucosal wounds is far less than in dermal wounds.

The reduced inflammation seen at sites of oral mucosal injury may derive partially from faster repair processes, such as accelerated cellular proliferation, and faster migration. Yet, an innate decrease in the inflammatory response in the oral mucosal wound seems to be involved. The abridged inflammatory response in oral mucosal wounds is reminiscent of findings in fetal wound healing models. Wounds produced in the early to mid-gestation fetus exhibit very little, if any, inflammatory response while healing in a scarless fashion (Adzick 1985; Cowin et al. 1998; Liechty et al. 1998).

INFLAMMATION IN FETAL WOUNDS

Scarless healing has been shown to occur in the early stages of development, and this outcome seems to be specifically confined to approximately the first two trimesters of gestation. Inflammatory cells such as neutrophils, macrophages, T-cells and B-cells are all absent in scarless fetal wounds (Adolph et al. 1993; Hopkinson-Woolley et al. 1994; Armstrong and Ferguson 1995; Cowin et al. 1998). This reduced inflammatory cell infiltration may begin with platelets. Fetal platelets produce less platelet-derived growth factor (PDGF), TGF-β1 and -β2, thus impairing their effectiveness in neutrophil and macrophage recruitment (Olutoye et al. 1996). The introduction of inflammation into normally scarless wounds produces a dose-dependent increase in wound macrophages, neutrophils, collagen deposition and scarring (Frantz et al. 1993). Overall, then, the switch to healing with scar formation is marked by the presence of inflammatory cells (Cass et al. 1997; Beanes et al. 2002).

Several studies suggest that fetal scarless healing is dependent upon the absence of acute inflammation and a lack of immune cell infiltration and not on the intrauterine environment (Block 1960; Dixon 1960; Somasundaramand and Prathap 1970; Burrington 1971; Goss 1977; Rowlatt 1979). For example, a study by Armstrong and Ferguson (1995) demonstrated that fetal marsupials heal cutaneous wounds without scar formation even though they develop outside the uterus in a maternal pouch. More evidence to support the hypothesis that fetal scarless wound healing is intrinsic comes from investigations in which adult sheep skin was transplanted onto the back of a fetal sheep bathed in the amniotic fluid of the intrauterine environment (Longaker et al. 1994). The transplanted adult skin healed incisional wounds with scar while adjacent incisional wounds in fetal skin healed without scar formation.

Non-scarring fetal wounds demonstrate a reduced level of TGF-β1 expression when compared with adult skin wounds (Krummel et al. 1988; Cowin et al. 2001). When an exogenous TGF-β1 is added to the non-scarring fetal wound, the outcome is scar formation (Lanning et al. 1999). Further, the addition of TGF-β1 neutralizing antibodies to adult wounds reduces scarring (Nath et al. 1994; Shah et al. 1995).

Several other factors are different in fetal non-scarring wounds when compared to scar-forming sites. A decrease in platelet derived growth factor (PDGF) occurs between the 16th and 18th gestational day, the transition period between scarless and scarring repair in rats (Peled et al. 2001). The expression of interleukins is also interesting in fetal wounds. IL-6 and IL-8 expression are greatly attenuated in fetal wounds (Liechty et al. 1998, 2000a). In contrast, the production of IL-10, an anti-inflammatory cytokine that deactivates macrophages, is critical for scarless fetal repair, since wounds of fetal mice lacking IL-10 heal with marked inflammation and scarring (Liechty et al. 2000b). When adult mouse wounds are treated with an IL-10 adenoviral vector, inflammation is reduced and scarless healing results (Gordon et al. 2001).

ROLE OF INFLAMMATION IN KELOIDS

Keloids are a result of abnormal wound healing and are benign dermal fibroproliferative tumors. They are unique to humans, with the highest frequency of occurrence in the African-American population. Keloids occur at areas of cutaneous injury, grow continuously beyond the original margins of the scar (Seifert and Mrowietz 2009) and tend to recur after excision.

Several cytokines are upregulated in patients with keloids. Notably, the overproduction of IL-6 is implicated in the formation of keloids. Studies of both peripheral blood monocyte and fibroblasts demonstrate an increased production of IL-6 in patients with keloids (McCauley et al. 1992; Xue et al. 2000; Tosa et al. 2005). The inhibition of IL-6 or its receptor IL-6Ra by their corresponding antibodies in keloid fibroblasts significantly and dose-dependently reduces collagen and fibronectin mRNA expression (Ghazizadeh et al. 2007). These findings suggest that altered levels of immunoregulatory cytokines may play a significant role in the proliferation of fibroblasts and net increase in collagen synthesis, which characterizes keloid formation (Ghazizadeh et al. 2007). TGF-β has also been implicated in playing a role in keloid formation. TGF- β1 and -β2 proteins are produced at higher levels in keloid fibroblast cultures compared with normal human dermal fibroblast cultures. The expression of TGF- β3 has been reported to be comparable or higher in normal versus keloid cell lines (Lee et al. 1999; Bran et al. 2010).

Even though keloids are frequent in the general population, the mechanisms underlying keloid formation are not completely understood. Further, no single treatment has proven to be widely effective. Additional studies are needed to understand the complexity of keloid pathogenesis and help in the development of an effective therapeutic strategy.

INFLAMMATION AND DIABETIC WOUNDS

Abnormal wound healing is a major complication in diabetic patients, and non-healing ulcers, particularly on the lower extremities, remain a critical clinical issue. In addition to chronic wounds, healing following acute injury proceeds more slowly and with an increased incidence of complications such as infection and wound dehiscence in diabetic persons. The mechanisms that underlie the altered healing outcomes seen in diabetic individuals are many (Falanga 2005; Eming et al. 2009). To begin with, several common complications of diabetes, such as neuropathy and poor tissue perfusion, exert an obvious negative influence on repair processes. Of particular relevance to this chapter is that the wounds of diabetics display a distinctly modified inflammatory response which includes an increased inflammatory reaction, altered protease balance and aberrant angiogenesis. Wounds of diabetic persons contain an abundance of neutrophils, yet exhibit a significant impairment in bacterial decontamination (Acosta et al. 2008). The exaggerated yet ineffective inflammatory response creates additional tissue destruction, and the resolution of repair is delayed. Along with the increased inflammatory cell content, cytokines and chemokines are abundant in the wounds of diabetic persons. These inflammatory mediators, as well as advanced glycation end-products, create a circumstance of excessive cellular apoptosis. A link between pro-inflammatory pathways and insulin resistance has also been suggested, as adipose tissue itself appears to be an important modifier of the inflammatory response (Balistreri et al. 2010). These many factors combine to yield a highly dysfunctional repair process.

Given the central role of aberrant inflammation in diabetic wound healing outcomes, therapies aimed at modifying the local inflammatory response have been suggested as possible methods to improve healing in this population. Such approaches might be beneficial to wound healing outcomes in both skin and other tissues, such as oral mucosa. Interestingly, the diminished repair capacity of diabetics has been suggested to play a role in the increased prevalence of periodontal disease in this population (Iacopino 2001).

CONCLUSIONS

Inflammation in wounds is a highly ordered process that significantly impacts wound healing outcomes. Several pieces of evidence point to a positive role for leukocytes in the stimulation of the proliferative phase of healing. In particular, macrophages appear to support healing through the generation of growth factors that promote cell proliferation and protein synthesis. While much remains to be learned, the accumulated information suggests that a carefully balanced inflammatory response is needed to provide maximal support for both infection prevention and optimal healing outcomes following injury. Wounds in the oral mucosa seem to benefit from a minimized inflammatory response that is supportive of repair.

REFERENCES

Acosta J.B., del Barco D.G., Vera D.C., et al. (2008) The pro-inflammatory environment in recalcitrant diabetic foot wounds. *International Wound Journal* **5**, 530–39.

Adolph V.R., DiSanto S.K., Bleacher J.C., Dillon P.W., Krummel T.M. (1993) The potential role of the lymphocyte in fetal wound healing. *Journal of Pediatric Surgery* **28**, 1316–20.

Adzick N.S., Harrison M.R., Glick P.L., et al. (1985) Comparison of fetal, newborn, and adult wound healing by histologic, enzyme-histochemical, and hydroxyproline determinations. *Journal of Pediatric Surgery* **20**, 315–19.

Allison J.P., Havran W.L. (1991) The immunobiology of T cells with invariant gd antigen receptors. *Annual Reviews in Immunology* **9**, 679–705.

Armstrong J.R., Ferguson M.W. (1995) Ontogeny of the skin and the transition from scar-free to scarring phenotype during wound healing in the pouch young of a marsupial, *Monodelphis domestica. Developmental Biology* **169**, 242–60.

Artuc M., Hermes B., Steckelings U. M., Grutzkau A., Henz B.M. (1999) Mast cells and their mediators in cutaneous wound healing – active participants or innocent bystanders? *Experimental Dermatololgy* **8**, 1–16.

Asai J., Takenaka H., Katoh N., et al. (2006) Dibutyryl cAMP influences endothelial progenitor cell recruitment during wound neovascularization. *Journal of Investigative Dermatology* **126**,1159–67.

Avniel S., Arik Z., Maly A., et al. (2006) Involvement of the CXCL12/CXCR4 pathway in the recovery of skin following burns. *Journal of Investigative Dermatology* **126**, 468–76.

Balistreri C.R., Caruso C., Candore G. (2010) The role of adipose tissue and adipokines in obesity-related inflammatory diseases. *Mediators of Inflammation* 802078 (Epub).

Barbul A., Breslin R.J., Woodyard J.P., Wasserkrug H.L., Efrom G. (1989a) The effect of in vivo T helper and T suppressor lymphocyte depletion on wound healing. *Annals of Surgery* **209**, 479–83.

Barbul A., Shawe T., Rotter S.M., Efrom J.E., Wasserkrug H.L., Badawy S.B. (1989b) Wound healing in nude mice: a study on the regulatory role of lymphocytes in fibroplasia. *Surgery* **105**, 764–9.

Barrientos S., Stojadinovic O., Golinko M.S., Brem H., Tomic-Canic M. (2008). Growth factors and cytokines in wound healing. *Wound Repair and Regeneration* **16**, 585–601.

Beanes S.R., Hu F.Y., Soo C., et al. (2002) Confocal microscopic analysis of scarless repair in the fetal rat: defining the transition. *Plastic and Reconstructive Surgery* **109**, 160–70.

Bellingan G.J., Caldwell H., Howie S.E., Dransfield I., Haslett C. (1996) In vivo fate of the inflammatory macrophage during the resolution of inflammation: inflammatory macrophages do not die locally, but emigrate to the draining lymph nodes. *Journal of Immunology* **157**, 2577–85.

Bingle L., Brown N.J., Lewis C.E. (2002) The role of tumour-associated macrophages in tumour progression: implications for new anticancer therapies. *Journal of Pathology* **196** (3), 254–65.

Block M. (1960) Wound healing in the new-born opossum (*Didelphis virginianam*). *Nature* **187**, 340–41.

Bran G.M., Goessler U.R., Schardt C., Hormann K., Riedel F., Sadick H. (2010) Effect of the abrogation of TGF-beta1 by antisense oligonucleotides on the expression of TGF-beta isoforms and their receptors I and II in isolated fibroblasts from keloid scars. *International Journal of Molecular Medicine* **25** (6), 915–21.

Brinkmann V., Reichard U., Goosmann C., et al. (2004) Neutrophil extracellular traps kill bacteria. *Science* **303**, 1532–5.

Broughton G., Janis J.E., Attinger C.E. (2006a) The basic science of wound healing. *Plastic and Reconstructive Surgery* **117** (Suppl 7), 12S–34S.

Broughton G., Janis J.E., Attinger C.E. (2006b) Wound healing: an overview. *Plastic and Reconstructive Surgery* **117**(Suppl 7), 1e-S–32e-S.

Burman A., Haworth O., Bradfield P., et al. (2005) The role of leukocyte–stromal interactions in chronic inflammatory joint disease. *Joint Bone Spine* **72**, 10–16.

Burrington J.D. (1971) Wound healing in the fetal lamb. *Journal of Pediatric Surgery* **6**, 523–8.

Carrel A. (1922) Growth-promoting function of leucocytes. *Journal of Experimental Medicine* **36**, 385–91.

Cass D.L., Bullard K.M., Sylvester K.G., Yang E.Y., Longaker M.T., Adzick N.S. (1997) Wound size and gestational age modulate scar formation in fetal wound repair. *Journal of Pediatric Surgery* **32**, 411–15.

Cowin A.J., Brosnan M.P., Holmes T.M., Ferguson M.W. (1998) Endogenous inflammatory response to dermal wound healing in the fetal and adult mouse. *Developmental Dynamics* **212**, 385–93.

Cowin A.J., Holmes T.M., Brosnan P., Ferguson M.W. (2001) Expression of TGF-beta and its receptors in murine fetal and adult dermal wounds. *European Journal of Dermatology* **11**, 424–31.

Cumberbatch M., Dearman R.J., Griffiths C.E., Kimber I. (2000) Langerhans cell migration. *Clinical and Experimental Dermatology* **25**, 413–18.

Daley J.M., Brancato S.K., Thomay A.A., Reichner J.S., Albina J.E. (2010) The phenotype of wound macrophages. *Journal of Leukocyte Biology* **87**, 59–67.

Danon D., Kowatch M.A., Roth G.S. (1989) Promotion of wound repair in old mice by local injection of macrophages. *Proceedings of National Academy of Sciences USA* **86**, 2018–20.

DiPietro L.A., Polverini P.J., Rahbe S.M., Kovacs E.J. (1995) Modulation of JE/MCP-1 expression in dermal wound repair. *American Journal of Pathology* **146**, 868–75.

DiPietro L.A., Reintjes M.G., Low Q.E., Levi B., Gamelli R.L. (2001) Modulation of macrophage recruitment into wounds by monocyte chemoattractant protein-1. *Wound Repair and Regeneration* **9**, 28–33.

Di Vita G., Patti R., D'Agostino P., et al. (2006) Cytokines and growth factors in wound drainage fluid from patients undergoing incisional hernia repair. *Wound Repair and Regen*eration **14**, 259–64.

Dixon J.B. (1960) Inflammation in the foetal and neonatal rat: the local reactions to skin burns. *Journal of Pathology Bacteriology* **80**, 73–82.

Dovi J.V, Szpaderska A.M., DiPietro L.A. (2004) Neutrophil function in the healing wound: Adding insult to injury? *Thrombosis and Haemostasis* **92**, 275–80.

Egozi E.I., Ferreira A.M., Burns A.L., Gamelli R.L., Dipietro L.A. (2003) Mast cells modulate the inflammatory but not the proliferative response in healing wounds. *Wound Repair and Regeneration* **11**, 46–54.

Eming S.A., Hammerschmidt M., Krieg T., Roers A. (2009) Interrelation of immunity and tissue repair or regeneration. *Seminars in Cell and Developmental Biology* **20**, 517–27.

Engelhardt E., Toksoy A., Goebeler M., Debus S., Brocker E.B., Gillitzer R. (1998) Chemokines IL-8, GROalpha, MCP- 1, IP-10, and Mig are sequentially and differentially expressed during phase-specific infiltration of leukocyte subsets in human wound healing. *American Journal Pathology* **153**, 1849–60.

Falanga V. (2005) Wound healing and its impairment in the diabetic foot, *Lancet* **366**, 1736–43.

Fedyk E.R., Jones D., Critchley H.O., et al. (2001) Expression of stromal-derived factor-1 is decreased by IL-1 and TNF and in dermal wound healing. *Journal of Immunology* **166**, 5749–54.

Florin L., Maas-Szabowski N., Werner S., et al. (2005) Increased keratinocyte proliferation by JUN-dependent expression of PTN and SDF-1 in fibroblasts. *Journal of Cell Science* **118**, 1981–9.

Frantz F.W., Bettinger D.A., Haynes J.H., et al. (1993) Biology of fetal repair: the presence of bacteria in fetal wounds induces an adult-like healing response. *Journal of Pediatric Surgery* **28**, 428–34.

Gallucci R.M., Simeonova P.P., Matheson J.M., et al. (2000) Impaired cutaneous wound healing in interleukin-6-deficient and immunosuppressed mice. *FASEB Journal* **14**, 2525–31.

Gallucci R.M., Sloan D.K., Heck J.M., Murray A.R., O'Dell S.J. (2004) Interleukin 6 indirectly induces keratinocytes migration. *Journal of Investigative Dermatology* **122**, 764–72.

Gawronska-Kozak B., Bogacki M., Rim J.S., Monroe W.T., Manuel J.A. (2006) Scarless skin repair in immunodeficient mice. *Wound Repair and Regeneration* **14**, 265–76.

Ghahary A., Shen Y.J., Scott P.G., Gong Y., Tredget E.E. (1993) Enhanced expression of mRNA for transforming growth factor-beta, type I and type III procollagen in human postburn hypertrophic scar tissues. *Journal of Laboratory and Clinical Medicine* **122**, 465–73.

Ghazizadeh M., Tosa M., Shimizu H., Hyakusoku H., Kawanami O. (2007) Functional implications of the IL-6 signaling pathway in keloid pathogenesis. *Journal of Investigative Dermatology* **127**, 98–105.

Gillitzer R, Goebeler M. (2001) Chemokines in cutaneous wound healing. *Journal of Leukocyte Biology* **69**, 513–21.

Gordon A.D., Karmacharya J., Herlyn M., Crombleholme T.M. (2001) Scarless wound healing induced by adenoviral-mediated over expression of interleukin-10. *Surgery Forum* **52**, 568–9.

Goren I., Allmann N., Yogev N., et al. (2009) A transgenic mouse model of inducible macrophage depletion: effects of diphtheria toxin-driven lysozyme M-specific cell lineage ablation on wound inflammatory, angiogenic, and contractive processes. *American Journal of Pathology* **175**, 132–47.

Goss A.N. (1977) Intra-uterine healing of fetal rat oral mucosal, skin and cartilage wounds. *Journal of Oral Pathology* **6**, 35–43.

Graves D.T., Nooh N., Gillen T., et al. (2001) IL-1 plays a critical role in oral, but not dermal, wound healing. *Journal of Immunology* **167** (9): 5316–20.

Grellner W., Georg T., Wilske J. (2000) Quantitative analysis of proinflammatory cytokines (IL-1 beta, IL-6, TNF-alpha) in human skin wounds. *Forensic Sciences International* **113**, 251–64.

Haas W., Pereira P., Tonegawa S. (1993) Gamma/delta cells. *Annual Reviews Immulogy* **11**, 637–85.

Hart J. (2002) Inflammation. 1: Its role in the healing of acute wounds. *Journal of Wound Care* **11**, 205–209.

Hopkinson-Woolley J., Hughes D., Gordon S., Martin P. (1994) Macrophage recruitment during limb development and wound healing in the embryonic and foetal mouse. *Journal of Cell Science* **107**, 1159–67.

Hunt T.K., Knighton D.R., Thakral K.K., Goodson W.H., Andrews W.S. (1984) Studies on inflammation and wound healing: angiogenesis and collagen synthesis stimulated in vivo by resident and activated wound macrophages. *Surgery* **96**, 48–54.

Hunt T.K., Hopf H., Hussain Z. (2000) Physiology of wound healing. *Advances in Skin and Wound Care* **13**, 6–11.

Iacopino A.M. (2001) Periodontitis and diabetes interrelationships: role of inflammation. *Annals of Periodontology* **6**, 125–37.

Itohara S., Farr A.G., Lafaille J.J., et al. (1990) Homing of a 1′/15 thymocyte subset with homogenous T-cell receptors to mucosal epithelial. *Nature* **343,** 754–7.

Jameson J., Ugarte K., Chen N., et al. (2002) A role for skin gd T cells in wound repair. *Science* **296,** 747–9.

Jameson J., Havran W.L. (2007) Skin gamma delta T-cell functions in homeostasis and wound healing. *Immunological Reviews* **215,** 114–22.

Jameson J.M., Sharp L.L., Witherden D.A., Havran W.L. (2004) Regulation of skin cell homeostasis by gamma delta T-cells. *Frontiers in Bioscience* **9,** 2640–51.

Jameson J.M., Cauvi G., Sharp L.L., Witherden D.A., Havran W.L. (2005) gd T cell-induced hyaluronan production by epithelial cells regulates inflammation. *Journal of Experimental Medicine* **201**, 1269–79.

Komine M., Rao L.S., Kaneko T., et al. (2000) Inflammatory versus proliferative processes in epidermis. Tumor necrosis factor alpha induces K6b keratin synthesis through a transcriptional complex containing NFkappa B and C/EBPbeta. *Journal of Biological Chemistry* **275**, 32077–88.

Kovacs E.J., DiPietro L.A. (1994) Fibrogenic cytokines and connective tissue production. *FASEB Journal* **8**, 854–61.

Krummel T.M., Michna B.A., Thomas B.L. et al. (1988) Transforming growth factor beta (TGFβ) induces fibrosis in a fetal wound model. *Journal of Pediatric Surgery* **23**, 647–52.

Kupper T.S., Fuhlbrigge R.C. (2004) Immune surveillance in the skin: mechanisms and clinical consequences. *Nature Reviews in Immunology* **4**, 211–22.

Lanning D.A., Nwomeh B.C., Montante S.J., Yager D.R. Diegelmann R.F., Haynes J.H. (1999) TGF-beta 1 alters the healing of cutaneous fetal excisional wounds. *Journal of Pediatric Surgery* **34**, 695–700.

Lee T.Y., Chin G.S., Kim W.J., Chau D., Gittes G.K., Longaker M.T. (1999) Expression of transforming growth factor 1, 2, and 3 proteins in keloids. *Annal of Plastic Surgery* **43** (2), 179–84.

Leibovich S.J., Ross R. (1975) The role of the macrophage in wound repair. A study with hydrocortisone and antimacrophage serum. *American Journal of Pathology* **78**, 71–100.

Liechty K.W., Crombleholme T.M., Cass D.L., Martin B., Adzick N.S. (1998) Diminished interleukin-8 (IL-8) production in the fetal wound healing response. *Journal of Surgery Research* **77**, 80–84.

Liechty K.W., Adzick N.S., Crombleholme T.M. (2000a) Diminished interleukin 6 (IL-6) production during scarless human fetal wound repair. *Cytokine* **12**, 671–6.

Liechty K.W., Kim H.B., Adzick N.S., Crombleholme T.M. (2000b) Fetal wound repair results in scar formation in interleukin-10 deficient mice in a syngeneic murine model of scarless fetal wound repair. *Journal of Pediatric Surgery* **35**, 866–72.

Longaker M.T., Whitby D.J., Ferguson M.W.J., Lorenz H.P., Harrison M.R., Adzick N.S. (1994) Adult skin wounds in the fetal environment heal with scar formation. *Annals Surgery* **219**, 65–72.

Low Q.E., Drugea I.A., Duffner L.A., et al. (2001) Wound healing in MIP-1alpha(-/-) and MCP-1(-/-) mice. *American Journal of Pathology* **159**, 457–63.

Luster A.D., Cardiff R.D., MacLean J.A., Crowe K., Granstein R.D. (1998) Delayed wound healing and disorganized neo-vascularization in transgenic mice expressing the IP-10 chemokine. *Proceedings of the Association of American Physicians* **110**, 183–96.

Ma Q., Jones D., Borghesani P.R., et al.(1998). Impaired B-lymphopoiesis, myelopoiesis, and derailed cerebellar neuron migration in CXCR4- and SDF-1-deficient mice. *Proceedings of Natlional Academy of Sciences USA*. **95**, 9448–53.

Mak K., Manji A., Gallant-Behm C., et al. (2009) Scarless healing of oral mucosa is characterized by faster resolution of inflammation and control of myofibroblast action compared to skin wounds in the red Duroc pig model. *Journal of Dermatological Sciences* **56**, 68–80.

Marshall J.S. (2004) Mast-cell response to pathogens. *Nature Reviews Immunology* **4**, 787–99.

Martin P., Leibovich S.J. (2005) Inflammatory cells during wound repair: the good, the bad and the ugly. *Trends in Cell Biology* **15**, 599–607.

Martinez F.O., Gordon S., Locati M., Mantovani A. (2006) Transcriptional profiling of the human monocyte-to-macrophage differentiation and polarization: new molecules and patterns of gene expression. *Journal of Immunology***177**, 7303–11.

Maruyama K., Zhang J.Z., Nihei Y., Ono I., Kaneko F. (1995) Regulatory effects of gamma-interferon on IL-6 and IL-8 secretion by cultured human keratinocytes and dermal fibroblasts. *Journal of Dermatology* **22**, 901–906.

Massague J., Cheifetz S., Boyd F.T., Andres J.L. (1990) TGF-beta receptors and TGF-beta binding proteoglycans: recent progress in identifying their functional properties. *Annals of the New York Academy of Sciences* **593**, 59–72.

Maurer M., Theoharides T., Granstein R.D., et al. (2003) What is the physiological function of mast cells? *Experimental Dermatology* **12**, 886–910.

McCauley R.L., Chopra V., Li Y.Y., Herndon D.N., Robson M.C. (1992) Altered cytokine production in black patients with keloids. *Journal of Clinical Immunology* **12**, 300–308.

Meszaros A.J., Reichner J.S., Albina J.E. (1999) Macrophage phagocytosis of wound neutrophils. *Journal of Leukocyte Biology* **65**, 35–42.

Meszaros A.J., Reichner J.S., Albina J.E. (2000) Macrophage induced neutrophil apoptosis. *Journal of Immunology* **165**, 435–41.

Mirza R., DiPietro L.A., Koh T.J. (2009) Selective and specific macrophage ablation is detrimental to wound healing in mice. *American Journal of Pathology* **175**, 2454–62.

Moses H.L., Yang E.Y., Pietenpol J.A. (1990) TGF-beta stimulation and inhibition of cell proliferation: new mechanistic insights. *Cell* **63**, 245–7.

Nath R.K., LaRegina M., Markham H., Ksander G.A., Weeks P.M. (1994) The expression of transforming growth factor type beta in fetal and adult rabbit skin wounds. *Journal of Pediatric Surgery* **29**, 416–21.

Noli C, Miolo A. (2001) The mast cell in wound healing. *Veterinary Dermatology* **12**, 303–313.

Olutoye O.O., Yager D.R., Cohen I.K., Deigelmann R.F. (1996) Lower cytokine release by fetal porcine platelets: a possible explanation for reduced inflammation after fetal wounding. *Journal of Pediatric Surgery* **31**, 91–5.

Park J.E., Barbul A. (2004) Understanding the role of immune regulation in wound healing. *American Journal of Surgery* **187**, 11S–16S.

Peled Z., Rhee S., Hsu M., Chang J., Krummell T., Longaker M. (2001) The ontogeny of scarless healing II: EGF and PDGF-B gene expression in fetal rat skin and fibroblasts as a function of gestational age. *Annuals of Plastic Surgery* **47**, 417–24.

Puxeddu I., Piliponsky A.M., Bachelet I., Levi-Schaffer F.(2003) Mast cells in allergy and beyond. *International Journal of Biochemistry and Cell Biology* **35**, 1601–7.

Raja, Sivamani K., Garcia M.S., Isseroff R.R. (2007) Wound re-epithelialization: modulating keratinocyte migration in wound healing. *Frontiers in Bioscience* **12**, 2849–68.

Rappolee D.A., Mark D., Banda M.J., Werb Z. (1988) Wound macrophages express TGF alpha and other growth factors in vivo: analysis by mRNA phenotyping. *Science* **241**, 708–712.

Rennekampff H.O., Hansbrough J.F., Kiessig V., Dore C., Sticherling M., Schroder J.M. (2000) Bioactive interleukin-8 is expressed in wounds and enhances wound healing. *Journal of Surgical Research* **93**, 41–54.

Richardson M. (2004) Acute wounds: an overview of the physiological healing process. *Nursing Times* **100**, 50–53.

Roberts A.B., Sporn M.B. (1996) Transforming growth factor-β. In: Clark R.A.F. (ed.) *The Molecular and Cellular Biology of Wound Repair*, Vol xxiii. Plenum Press, New York, pp. 275–308.

Roberts A.B., Thompson N.L., Heine U., Flanders C., Sporn M.B. (1988) Transforming growth factor-beta: possible roles in carcinogenesis. *British Journal of Cancer* **57**, 594–600.

Robson M.C., Steed D.L., Franz M.G. (2001) Wound healing: biologic features and approaches to maximize healing trajectories. *Current Problems in Surgery* **38**, 72–140.

Rowlatt U. (1979) Intrauterine wound healing in a 20 week human fetus. *Virchows Archiv. Pathological Anatomy and Histology* **381**, 353–61.

Russell W.E., Coffey R.J. Jr, Ouellette A.J., Moses H.L. (1988) Type beta transforming growth factor reversibly inhibits the early proliferative response to partial hepatectomy in the rat. *Proceedings National Academy of Sciences USA* **85**, 5126–30.

Salcedo R., Wasserman K., Young H. A., et al. (1999) Vascular endothelial growth factor and basic fibroblast growth factor induce expression of CXCR4 on human endothelial cells. In vivo neovascularization induced by stromal-derived factor-1a. *American Journal of Pathology* **154**, 1125–35.

Schrementi M.E., Ferreira A.M., Zender C., DiPietro L.A. (2008) Site-specific production of TGF-beta in oral mucosal and cutaneous wounds. *Wound Repair and Regeneration* **16**, 80–86.

Seifert O., Mrowietz U. (2009) Keloid scarring: bench and bedside. *Archives of Dermatological Research* **301**, 259–72.

Shah M., Foreman D.M., Ferguson M.W. (1995) Neutralisation of TGF-beta 1 and TGF-beta2 or exogenous addition of TGF beta 3 to cutaneous rat wounds reduces scarring. *Journal of Cell Science* **108**, 985–1002.

Shaw T.J., Martin P. (2009) Wound repair at a glance. *Journal of Cell Science* **15**(122), 3209–13.

Shiraha H., Glading A., Gupta K., Wells A. (1999) IP-10 inhibits epidermal growth factor-induced motility by decreasing epidermal growth factor receptor-mediated calpain activity. *Journal of Cell Biology* **146**, 243–54.

Shirozu M., Nakano T., Inazawa J., et al. (1995) Structure and chromosomal localization of the human stromal cell-derived factor 1 (SDF1) gene. *Genomics* **28**, 495–500.

Simpson D.M., Ross R. (1972) The neutrophilic leukocyte in wound repair: a study with antineutrophil serum. *Journal of Clinical Investigation* **51**, 2009–23.

Singer A.J., Clark R.A. (1999) Cutaneous wound healing. *New England Journal of Medicine* **341**, 738–46.

Somasundaramand K., Prathap K. (1970) Intra-uterine healing of skin wounds in rabbit foetuses. *Journal of Pathology* **100**, 81–6.

Szpaderska A.M., DiPietro L.A. (2005) Inflammation in surgical wound healing: friend or foe? *Surgery* **137**, 571–3.

Szpaderska A.M., Zuckerman Z.D., DiPietro L.A. (2003) Differential injury responses in oral mucosal and cutaneous wounds. *Journal of Dental Research* **82**, 621–6.

Tachibana K., Hirota S., Iizasa H., et al. (1998) The chemokine receptor CXCR4 is essential for vascularization of the gastrointestinal tract. *Nature* **393**, 591–4.

Tang A., Gilchrest B.A. (1996) Regulation of keratinocytes growth factor gene expression in human skin fibroblasts. *Journal of Dermatological Sciences* **11**, 41–50.

Toksoy A., Muller V., Gillitzer R., Goebeler M. (2007) Biphasic expression of stromal cell-derived factor-1 during human wound healing. *British Journal of Dermatology* **157**, 1148–54.

Tosa M., Ghazizadeh M., Shimizu H., Hirai T., Hyakusoku H., Kawanami O. (2005) Global gene expression analysis of keloid fibroblasts in response to electron beam irradiation reveals the involvement of interleukin-6 pathway. *Journal of Investigative Dermatology* **124**, 704–13.

Velnari T, Bailey T, Smroklj V. (2009) The wound healing process: an overview of the cellular and molecular mechanisms. *Journal of International Medical Research* **37** (5), 1528–42.

Wahl S.M., Hunt D.A., Wakefield L.M., et al. (1987) Transforming growth factor type beta induces monocyte chemotaxis and growth factor production. *Proceedings National Academy of Sciences USA* **84**, 5788–92.

Weiss S.J. (1989) Tissue destruction by neutrophils. *New England Journal of Medicine* **320**, 365–76.

Weller K., Foitzik K., Paus R., Syska W., Maurer M. (2006) Mast cells are required for normal healing of skin wounds in mice. *FASEB Journal* **20**, 2366–8.

Werner S., Grose R. (2003) Regulation of wound healing by growth factors and cytokines. *Physiology Reviews* **83**, 835–70.

Wetzler C., Kampfer H., Stallmeyer B., Pfeilschifter J., Frank S. (2000) Large and sustained induction of chemokines during impaired wound healing in the genetically diabetic mouse: prolonged persistence of neutrophils and macrophages during the late phase of repair. *Journal of Investigative Dermatology* **115**, 245–53.

Wilgus T.A. (2008) Immune cells in the healing skin wound: influential players at each stage of repair. *Pharmacological Research* **58**, 112–16.

Wong J. W., Gallant-Behm C., Wiebe C., et al. (2009) Wound healing in oral mucosa results in reduced scar formation as compared with skin: evidence from the red Duroc pig model and humans. *Wound Repair and Regeneration* **17**, 717–29.

Xue H., McCauley R.L., Zhang W. (2000) Elevated IL-6 expression in keloid fibroblasts. *Journal of Surgical Research* **89**, 74–7.

Yellin M.J., Winikott S., Fortune S.M., et al. (1995) Ligation of CD40 on fibroblasts induces CD54 (ICAM-1) and CD 106 (VCAM-1) up-regulation and IL-6 production and proliferation. *Journal of Leukocyte Biology* **58**, 209–16.

Zou Y.R., Kottmann A.H., Kuroda M., et al. (1998) Function of the chemokine receptor CXCR4 in haematopoiesis and in cerebellar development. *Nature* **393**, 595–9.

4 Specialized Pro-resolving Lipid Derived Fatty Acid Mediators: Wiring the Circuitry of Effector Immune Homeostasis

Gabrielle Fredman and Charles N. Serhan

Center for Experimental Therapeutics and Reperfusion Injury, Department of Anesthesiology, Perioperative, and Pain Medicine, Brigham and Women's Hospital and Harvard Medical School, Boston, MA, USA

INFLAMMATION: THE CARDINAL SIGNS

Mesopotamian writings, Egyptian hieroglyphics and texts from ancient Greece and China all describe the flame of inflammation (Majno 1991), but only insofar as its observable signs, such as redness, heat, swelling and pain (initially noted by Celsus in AD 30). These accounts, however, mistakenly concluded that inflammation is a disease unto itself (Majno 1991; Majno and Joris 2004). Centuries later (1794), John Hunter, a Scottish surgeon who was noted for his contributions to the fields of anatomy and dentistry, posited that inflammation was actually a consequence of injury or disease (Majno 1991). Since this important clarification, many endeavors were undertaken to decipher the cellular and molecular mediators of inflammation. During the late 1800s and early 1900s, some notable contributors to our understanding of the mechanisms of tissue injury were Julius Cohnheim and Samuel Gross, who reported on leukocyte emigration and vascular permeability. Additionally, Elie Metchnikoff discovered that cells play a central role in inflammation and he was the first to characterize host defense processes of phagocytosis (Tauber and Chernyak 1991). In the mid-20th century, the chemical mediators of inflammation were beginning to unfold. Seminal work from Bengt Samuelsson (Samuelsson 1979), John Vane (Vane 1976) and Sune Bergstrom (Bergstroem et al. 1964) led to the elucidation of prostaglandins, thromboxanes and prostacyclins (collectively termed the eicosanoid family) associated with hemodynamic, reproductive and inflammatory processes. Still, little was known about the mechanisms that might turn off or self-limit the acute inflammatory response. Inflammation was initially thought to cease by the passive catabolism of pro-inflammatory mediators. Recently, work from this laboratory revealed a class of novel lipid mediators that are generated during inflammation to *actively* resolve injury or infection. This chapter will overview and highlight our current understanding of the cellular and

Oral Wound Healing: Cell Biology and Clinical Management, First Edition. Edited by Hannu Larjava.

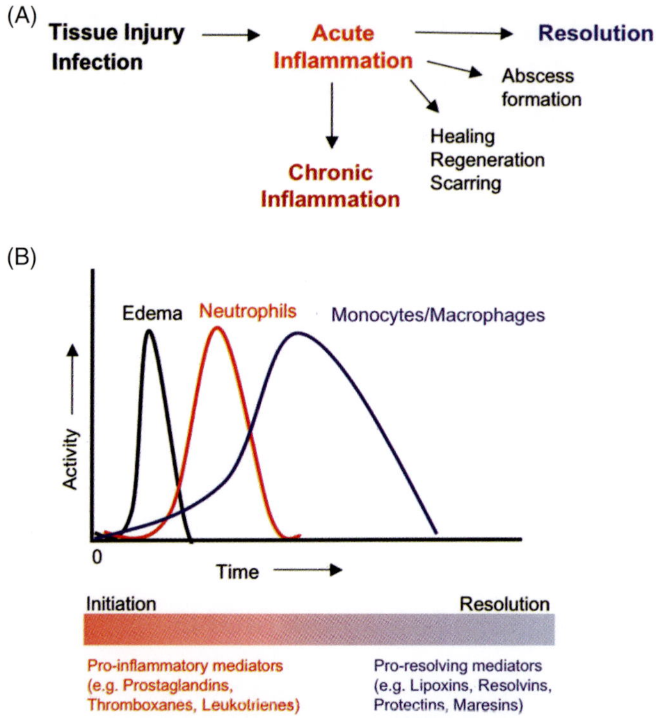

Fig. 4.1 Outcomes and cellular mediators of acute inflammation. (A) Acute inflammation is initiated by injury or infection and has several outcomes that include progression to chronic inflammation, healing by connective tissue replacement, abscess formation (particularly in infections) or complete resolution. (B) Acute inflammation is a highly coordinated process and is characterized by specific cellular mediators. At the onset of acute inflammation, vascular leakage (edema) occurs. Neutrophils are among the first responders during an acute inflammatory response, followed by monocytes and macrophages. The first cellular hallmark of tissue resolution is defined by a decrease in neutrophil infiltration. Classically, eicosanoids such as PGE_2, TXA_2 and LTB_4 are known to exert pro-inflammatory actions such as vasodilation, platelet activation and chemotaxis, respectively. Pro-resolving molecules are generated during inflammation that block vasodilation/edema formation and limit further chemotaxis of neutrophils, thus allowing for the return to homeostasis. (Adapted from Kumar et al. 2005.).

chemical mediators in the resolution of acute inflammation and the implications of this for novel treatments for inflammatory diseases including periodontal disease. For further details on these topics, readers are directed to recent reviews covering the original research in this area (Serhan 2005, 2007; Serhan et al. 2008a, 2008b).

COMPLETE RESOLUTION AND TISSUE HOMEOSTASIS IS THE IDEAL OUTCOME OF ACUTE INFLAMMATION

Acute inflammatory responses have several possible outcomes that include progression to chronic inflammation, scarring and fibrosis or ideally complete resolution (Fig. 4.1A); see Kumar et al. (2005) for further details. Acute inflammation is a response that eliminates or neutralizes foreign bodies or organisms and is protective against injury or infection (Majno

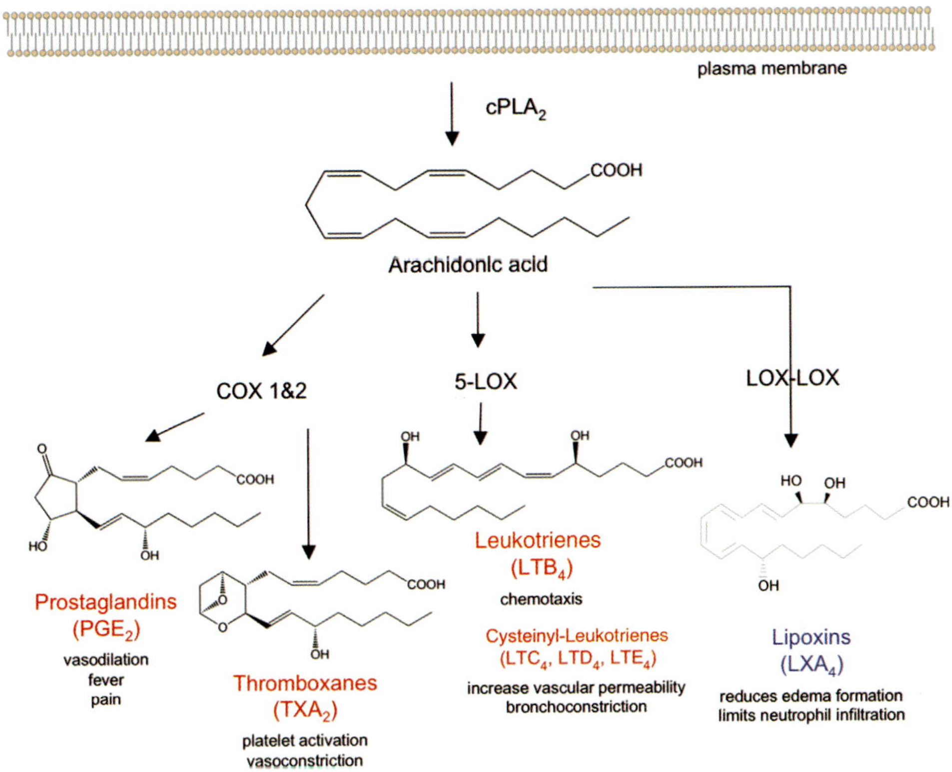

Fig. 4.2 Eicosanoid biosynthesis. The activation of PLA_2 leads to the liberation of arachidonic acid (AA). AA can be further metabolized by (left) cyclo-oxygenase (COX) 1 and 2 to generate prostaglandins (i.e. PGE_2) via isomerases or thromboxanes (i.e. TXA_2) via thromboxane synthase in platelets. AA can be further metabolized via lipoxygenase (LOX) to generate leukotrienes, such as LTB_4 (middle). Lipoxins are generated during transcellular biosynthesis, a mechanism that requires a donor cell to synthesize and release one component of the biosynthetic cascade and a second accessory cell to take up that intermediate to process each into the final biologically active product.

and Joris 2004; Kumar et al. 2005). This process is characterized by vascular dilation, enhanced permeability of capillaries, increased blood flow and the production of fibrin-rich inflammatory exudates (Majno and Joris 2004). Vascular permeability and increased blood flow give rise to leukocyte recruitment from the circulation (Ryan and Majno 1977).

Leukocyte recruitment is classically defined by the initial trafficking of polymorphonuclear (PMN) granulocytes followed by monocytes that differentiate locally into macrophages (Fig. 4.1B). These events in pro-resolving responses are coupled with release of factors that prevent further or excessive trafficking of leukocytes in self-limited inflammation allowing for resolution (Serhan et al. 2000, 2002). Early in the inflammatory response, pro-inflammatory mediators such as prostaglandins and leukotrienes play an important role (Borgeat and Samuelsson 1979a; Samuelsson 1983; Samuelsson et al. 1987) (Fig. 4.2). The progression from acute to chronic inflammation as in many occurring human diseases, such as arthritis, periodontal disease and cardiovascular disease, is widely viewed as an excess of pro-inflammatory mediators (Van Dyke and Serhan 2006; Serhan et al. 2007). Although mononuclear cells can in many settings contribute to pro-inflammatory responses, they are also critical in wound healing, tissue repair and remodeling in a non-inflammatory, non-phlogistic manner (Kumar et al. 2005). Most successful inflammatory processes are self-limiting (Majno and Joris 2004), which implies the existence of endogenous anti-inflammation pathways (Serhan et al. 2004b, Serhan and Savill 2005). In this regard, it is possible that defects in mounting endogenous pro-resolving circuits and compounds *de novo* could underlie some of the aberrant mechanisms in chronic inflammation (Serhan et al. 2007).

Complete or successful resolution of an acute inflammatory response and the local return to homeostasis is necessary for ongoing health. Hence, the ideal outcome is the removal of leukocytes from infected or inflamed tissues without leaving remnants of the host's combat between leukocytes, invading microbes and/or other initiators of inflammation. This laboratory has focused on the question 'How is the acute inflammatory response regulated and are these specialized mediators involved in the successful resolution process?' It was widely believed and argued that simple dilution of pro-inflammatory mediators was enough to turn off or 'burn out' inflammation, with the subsequent responses ending naturally or passively (Kumar et al. 2005). Along these lines, recent evidence demonstrates that resolution of inflammation and the return to homeostasis is not passive but an active and highly regulated process that can be considered programmed resolution at the tissue level (Serhan 2007).

LIPOXINS, RESOLVINS, PROTECTINS AND MARESINS: SEMPER VIGILANTES OF ANTI-INFLAMMATION AND PRO-RESOLUTION

Specialized pro-resolving lipid mediators (SPMs) comprise a genus (chemically distinct families) of endogenous mediators, including lipoxins, resolvins, protectins (Serhan 2007) and maresins (Serhan et al. 2009; Table 4.1). They are actively biosynthesized during the resolution phase of acute inflammation and are potent agonists that control the magnitude and duration of inflammation (Fig. 4.3). They are also potent chemoattractants, but via a non-inflammatory mechanism: for example, lipoxins activate mononuclear cell infiltration without stimulating release of pro-inflammatory chemokines or activation of pro-inflammatory gene pathways and

Table 4.1 List of important acronyms for lipoxins, resolvins, protectins and maresins.

ATLa	Aspirin-triggered lipoxin analog (15-epi-16-(para-fluoro)-phenoxy-lipoxin A_4)
LTB_4	Leukotriene B_4, 5*S*,12*R*-dihydroxy-eicosa-6*Z*,8*E*,10*E*,14*Z*-tetraenoic acid
LXA_4	Lipoxin A_4 (5S, 6R, 15S-trihydroxy-eicosa-7E, 9E, 11Z, 13E-tetraenoic acid)
LXB_4	Lipoxin B_4 (5S, 14R, 15S-trihydroxy-eicosa-6E, 8Z, 10E, 12E-tetraenoic acid)
RvE1	Resolvin E1 (5S, 12R, 18R-trihydroxy-eicosa-6*Z*, 8*E*, 10*E*, 14*Z*, 16*E*-pentaenoic acid)
RvE2	Resolvin E2 (5*S*,18*R*-dihydroxy-eicosapentaenoic acid)
PD1/NPD1	Protectin D1/neuroprotectin D1 (10*R*, 17*S*-dihydroxy-docosa-4*Z*, 7*Z*, 11*E*, 13*E*, 15*Z*, 19*Z*-hexaenoic acid)
PGE_2	Prostaglandin E_2, 9-oxo-11α,15*S*-dihydroxy-prosta-5*Z*,13*E*-dien-1-oic acid
RvD1	Resolvin D1 (7*S*, 8*R*, 17*S*-trihydroxy-4*Z*, 9*E*, 11*E*, 13*Z*, 15*E*, 19*Z*-docosahexaenoic acid)
RvD2	Resolvin D2 (7*S*,16*R*,17*S*-trihydroxydocosa-4*Z*,8*E*,10*Z*,12*E*,14*E*,19*Z*-hexaenoic acid)
RvD3	Resolvin D3 (4*S*,11,17*S*-trihydroxydocosa-5,7*E*,9*E*,13*Z*,15*E*,19*Z*-hexaenoic acid)
RvD4	Resolvin D4 (4*S*,5,17*S*-trihydroxydocosa-6*E*,8*E*,10*Z*,13*Z*,15*E*,19*Z*-hexaenoic acid)
RvD5	Resolvin D5 (7*S*,17*S*-dihydroxy-docosa-5*Z*,8*E*,10*Z*,13*Z*,15*E*,19*Z*-hexaenoic acid)
MaR1	Maresin 1 (7,14-dihydroxy-docosa-4Z,8,10,12,16Z,19Z-hexaenoic acid)

products (Maddox and Serhan 1996; Maddox et al. 1997; Qiu et al. 2001). Lipoxins also stimulate the uptake of apoptotic PMNs (Godson et al. 2000) and activate endogenous antimicrobial defense mechanisms stimulating the mucosa to release bactericidal/permeability-increasing protein (BPI) (Canny et al. 2002). Importantly, resolvin E1 (RvE1) stimulates clearance on mucosal surfaces (Campbell et al. 2007). Lipoxins, resolvins, protectins and maresins are unique chemical mediator families; they each have different chemical structures that bind distinct receptors and exert actions on selective cellular targets (Serhan and Chiang 2008). In this regard, SPMs are agonists that stimulate the resolution of inflammation.

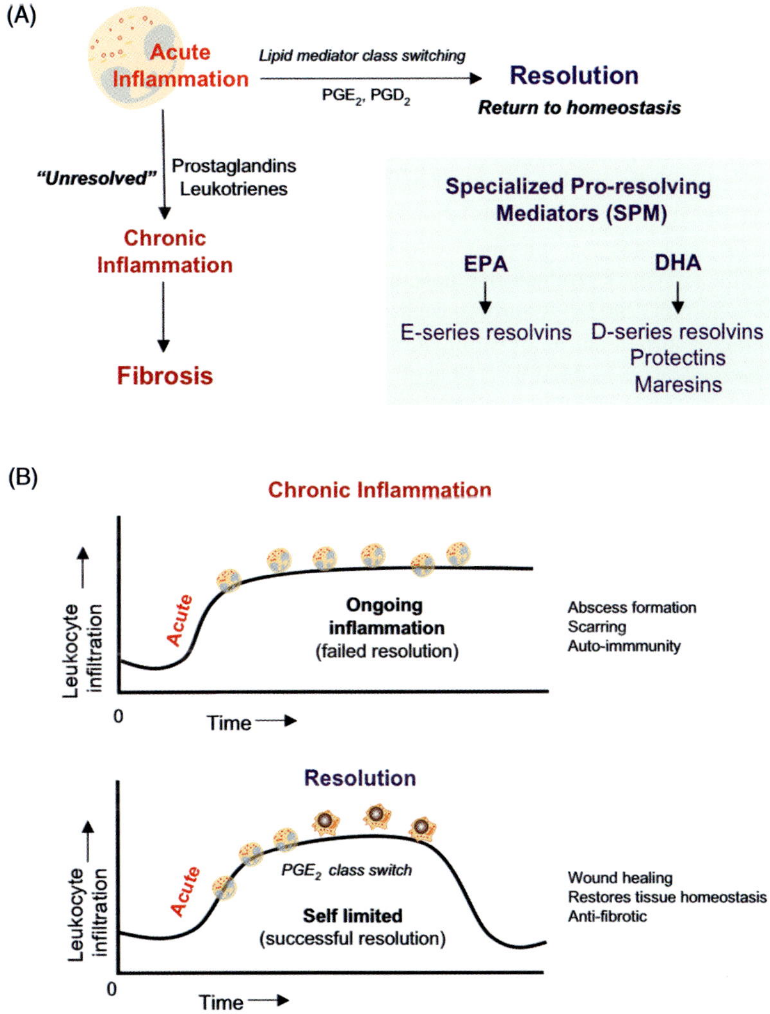

Fig. 4.3 Specialized pro-resolving mediators in resolution of acute inflammation. In response to injury or infection, acute inflammation is a protective mechanism, initiated by neutrophils summoned to the site to engulf and destroy invading microbes. In this process, neutrophil-derived pro-inflammatory mediators, such as leukotrienes and prostaglandins, and the unintentional release of hydrolytic enzymes and reactive oxygen species can be detrimental to this process, potentially leading to chronic inflammation and potential tissue fibrosis. The ideal outcome is complete resolution that is actively turned on by specialized pro-resolving mediators (SPMs), including resolvins derived from omega-3 PUFAs eicosapentaenoic acid (EPA; E-series resolvins), docosahexaenoic acid (DHA; D-series resolvins) and protectins and maresins enzymatically derived from DHA. (Adapted from Serhan et al. 2007.).

Lipoxins

Lipoxins, such as lipoxin A_4 (LXA_4) and LXB_4, were the first lipid mediators of endogenous anti-inflammation and pro-resolution (Serhan 2005). Lipoxins (Fig. 4.2) are lipoxygenase-derived eicosanoids, derived enzymatically from arachidonic acid (AA), an omega-6 fatty acid that is released and mobilized during inflammation (Samuelsson et al. 1987). Lipoxins are made in humans via cell–cell interactions involving mucosa, i.e. epithelial cells of the gastrointestinal tract, bronchial tissue interactions with leukocytes, or platelet–leukocyte interactions within the vasculature (Serhan 2007). Single cells, such as trout macrophages (Rowley et al. 1994) and murine macrophages (Schwab et al. 2007), also generate lipoxins. Aspirin has an unexpected impact within resolution. In humans, aspirin 'jump-starts' this process via its ability to trigger the endogenous biosynthesis of lipid mediators (Serhan et al. 2000, 2002; Chiang et al. 2004). For example, aspirin-triggered epimeric lipoxin generation leads to the production of mediators known as aspirin-triggered lipoxins (ATLs). These are biosynthesized initially by the actions of the cyclo-oxygenase-2 (COX-2) pathway (Claria and Serhan 1995). Aspirin, via acetylation of COX-2, does not inhibit the activity of the enzyme in the same way as a selective COX-2 inhibitor. Instead, the acetylation changes the chirality of the enzyme's products and generates 15*R*-HETE, a precursor to 15-epi-lipoxins [reviewed in Serhan (2007)]. Aspirin thus has the unique mode of action and ability to initiate resolution of inflammation by stimulating the early formation of mediators that would normally be made later in the time course of an inflammatory response.

During local contained inflammation, the first line of host defense, namely the neutrophils, can undergo apoptosis as well as necrotic cell death. As part of resolution, lipoxins signal macrophages to enhance their uptake of the remains of these cells (Godson et al. 2000; Mitchell et al. 2002). Lipoxins are potent anti-inflammatory mediators that act in picogram to nanogram amounts with human tissues and in animal disease models. They have the specific actions of limiting PMN recruitment, chemotaxis and adhesion to the site of insult. Essentially they are breaking signals for PMN-mediated tissue injury. The 5-lipoxygenase (5-LO) pathway, for example, generates leukotrienes (Fig. 4.2) that are primarily pro-inflammatory mediators (Borgeat and Samuelsson 1979b; Samuelsson 1983). Topical application of leukotriene B_4, a potent pro-inflammatory mediator and neutrophil chemoattractant, on the skin of mice ears stimulates rapid and significant PMN infiltration that is enhanced with PGE_2 (Serhan and Drazen 1997; Takano et al. 1998). Neutrophils rapidly (within minutes) infiltrate the ear tissue and when in high flux excessive PMN infiltration can lead to local tissue damage and increased vascular permeability causing leakage. When metabolically stable LXA_4 (aspirin-triggered) analogs were applied topically to ear skin, they rapidly 'stopped' PMN infiltration as well as reduced vascular permeability (Takano et al. 1998). To date, at least four generations of stable lipoxin analogs have now been introduced that show promise in a number of different *in vivo* settings and for large-scale manufacturing (Serhan et al. 1995; O'Sullivan et al. 2007; Petasis et al. 2008). Thus, the lipoxin analogs were the first anti-inflammatory and pro-resolving biotemplates that may lead to a new avenue of therapeutics (Serhan and Chiang 2008).

Resolvins

Resolvins are a family of endogenous compounds generated during resolution of inflammation. Using an unbiased systems approach, resolvins were identified via LC-MS-MS, and complete structural elucidation of the bioactive mediators and related compounds was

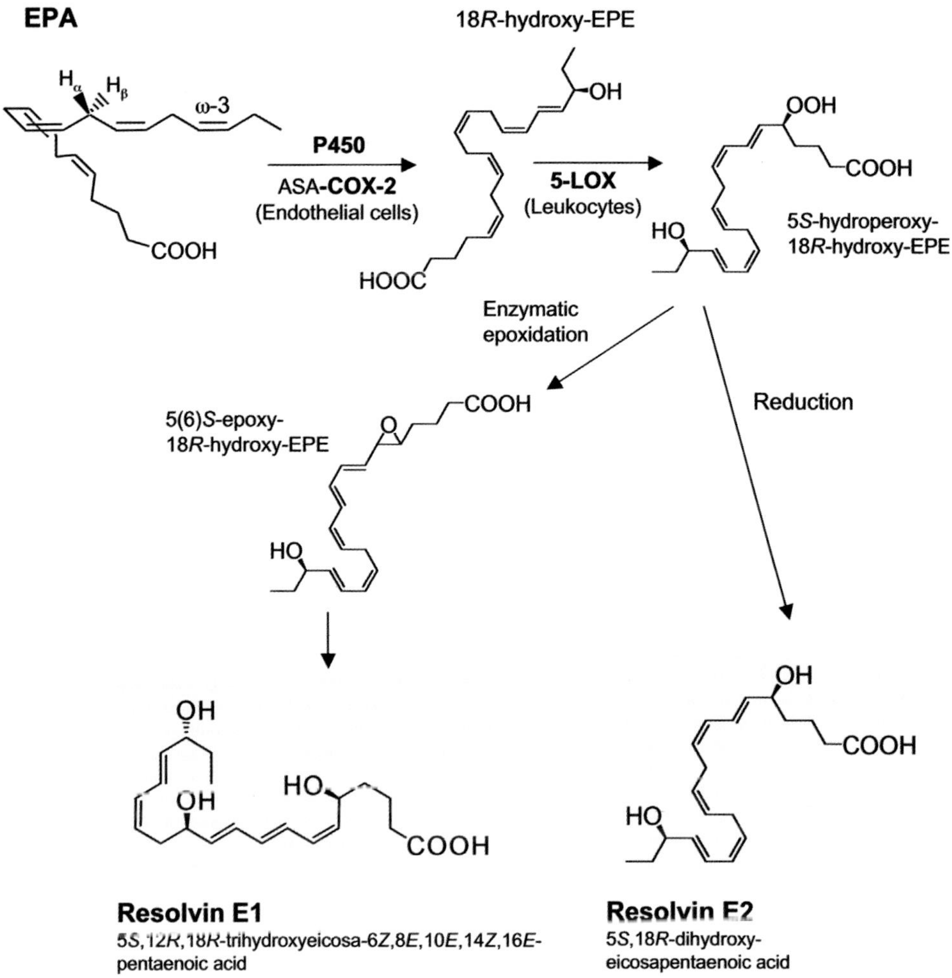

Fig. 4.4 Biosynthesis of E-series resolvins. Aspirin acetylated COX-2 in vascular endothelial cells stereoselectively generates 18*R*-hydroperoxy-EPE (18*R*-H(p)EPE). 18*R*-HEPE is further converted via sequential actions of leukocyte 5-LOX, leading to formation of RvE1. The complete stereochemistry of RvE1 was recently established as 5*S*,12*R*,18*R*-trihydroxyeicosa-6*Z*,8*E*,10*E*,14*Z*,16*E*-pentaenoic acid (Arita et al. 2005a). Microbial P-450s can also contribute to RvE biosynthesis via converting eicosapentaenoic acid (EPA) to 18-HEPE. Human recombinant 5-LOX also generates resolvin E2 (RvE2) from 18-HEPE (Tjonahen et al. 2006).

performed (Serhan et al. 2000, 2002, 2006; Hong et al. 2003). Resolvins or *resolution-phase interaction products* are endogenous compounds biosynthesized from the omega-3 fatty acid eicosapentaenoic acid (EPA) (Serhan et al. 2000), docosahexaenoic acid (DHA) (Serhan et al. 2002) and docosapentaenoic acid (DPA) (Dangi et al. 2009). E series resolvins (RvEs) such as RvE1 and RvE2 (Tjonahen et al. 2006) are biosynthesized from EPA (Fig. 4.4) and the D series (RvDs) resolvins are generated from DHA (Fig. 4.5) (Serhan et al. 2002).

Resolvins are also produced by COX-2-initiated routes. For example, in the presence of aspirin, the 17*R* series of resolvins can be generated from DHA (Serhan et al. 2004a).

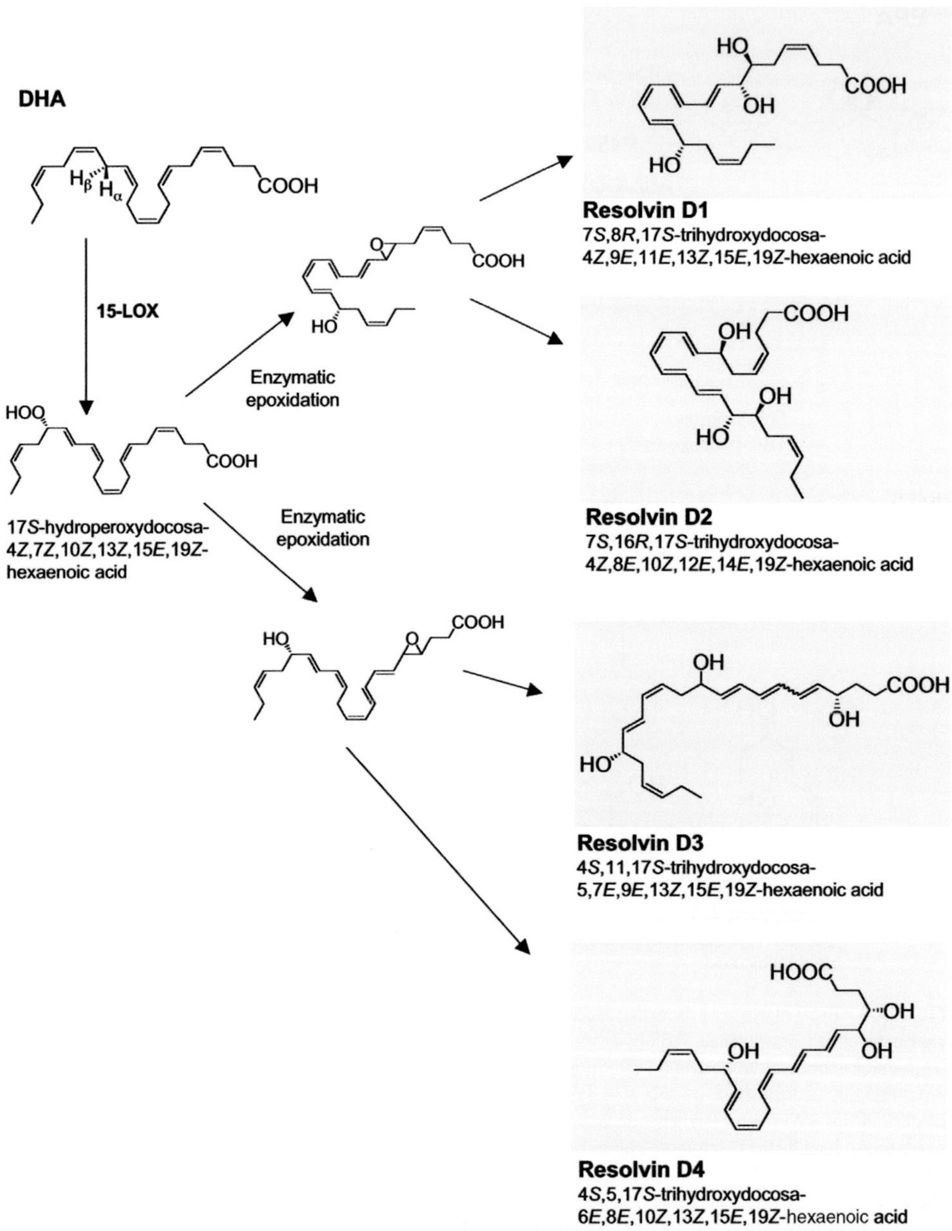

Fig. 4.5 D-series resolvins. These are formed from docosahexaenoic acid (DHA). The biosynthetic pathways reconstructed *in vitro* involve the lipoxygenase (LOX) product 17*S*-H(p)DHA, which is rapidly transformed by the LOX activity in human polymorphonuclear leukocyte (PMN) into two epoxide intermediates. These two novel epoxide intermediates open to form bioactive products denoted 17*S*- D series resolvins (RvD1—7*S*,8*R*,17*S*-trihydroxy-4*Z*,9*E*,11*E*,13*Z*,15*E*,19*Z*-docosahexaenoic acid; RvD2—7*S*,16*R*,17*S*-trihydroxydocosa-4*Z*,8*E*,10*Z*,12*E*,14*E*,19*Z*-hexaenoic acid; RvD3—4*S*,11, 17*S*-trihydroxydocosa-5,7*E*,9*E*,13*Z*,15*E*,19*Z*-hexaenoic acid; and RvD4—4*S*,5,17*S*-trihydroxydocosa-6*E*,8*E*,10*Z*,13*Z*,15*E*,19*Z*-hexaenoic acid are shown).

A growing body of evidence indicates that resolvins possess potent anti-inflammatory and immunoregulatory actions that include blocking the production of pro-inflammatory mediators and regulating the trafficking of leukocytes to sites of inflammation (Serhan et al. 2008a). Specifically, resolvins limit further PMN infiltration *in vivo* and transmigration (Serhan et al. 2002; Sun et al. 2007). They also reduce cytokine expression by isolated microglia cells (Hong et al. 2003). Moreover, we recently established the stereochemistry and actions of RvD1 (Fig. 4.5) and AT-RvD1 (aspirin-triggered-RvD1). RvE1 and PD1 (*vide infra*) also demonstrated the stereoselective basis for their potent actions as well as their enzymatic inactivation (Arita et al. 2005a, Serhan et al. 2006; Sun et al. 2007). In a recent set of experiments, we compared the actions of RvD1 and the 17R-aspirin triggered (AT)-RvD1 (0–1,000 nM) on human PMN transendothelial migration (Sun et al. 2007). Both RvD1 and AT-RvD1 stopped PMN transmigration in a concentration-dependent manner ($P < 0.001$), with a similar efficacy. The potency of these compounds is noteworthy, with an approximately 50% reduction in PMN transmigration observed with concentrations as low as 10 nM. RvD1 has been studied in several inflammatory disease models displaying potent and stereoselective activity.

Protectins

Protectins, another family of pro-resolving mediators, are biosynthesized from the precursor DHA but via a separate enzymatic pathway to the DHA-derived resolvins. Protectins are distinguished by the presence of their conjugated triene-containing structure (Fig. 4.6) (Serhan et al. 2006). The name 'protectins' was coined from the observed anti-inflammatory (Hong et al. 2003) and protective actions in neural tissues and systems. The prefix *neuro*protectin gives the tissue address to the production and local actions of these, such as neuroprotectin D1 (NPD1) (Mukherjee et al. 2004; Serhan et al. 2006). Like resolvins, the protectins stop PMN infiltration (Hong et al. 2003; Serhan et al. 2006). They are biosynthesized by and act on glial cells by reducing cytokine expression (Hong et al. 2003). NPD1 reduces retinal and corneal injury (Mukherjee et al. 2004) and stroke damage (Marcheselli et al. 2003), and improves corneal wound healing in mouse models (Gronert et al. 2005).

Maresins

Using self-resolving inflammatory exudates and lipidomics, we identified a new pathway involving biosynthesis of potent anti-inflammatory and pro-resolving mediators from the essential fatty acid, DHA (Serhan et al. 2009). During the resolution of murine peritonitis, exudates accumulated both 17-HDHA, a known marker of 17S-D-series resolvin and protectin biosynthesis, and 14S-HDHA from endogenous DHA. Addition of either DHA or 14S-hydroperoxydocosa-4Z,7Z,10Z,12E,16Z,19Z-hexaenoic acid (14S-HpDHA) to activated macrophages converted these substrates to novel dihydroxy-containing products that possessed potent anti-inflammatory and pro-resolving activity with a potency similar to resolvin E1 and protectin D1. Stable isotope incorporation, intermediate trapping and characterization of physical and biological properties of the products demonstrated a novel 14-lipoxygenase pathway, generating bioactive 7,14-dihydroxy-docosa-4Z,8,10,12,16Z,19Z-hexaenoic acid (Fig. 4.6), coined maresin (macrophage mediator in resolving inflammation, or MaR1). Thus, maresins are the first to define this new macrophage metabolome and therefore may be involved in some of the beneficial actions of DHA when utilized by resolving macrophages during inflammation-resolution, host defense and wound healing.

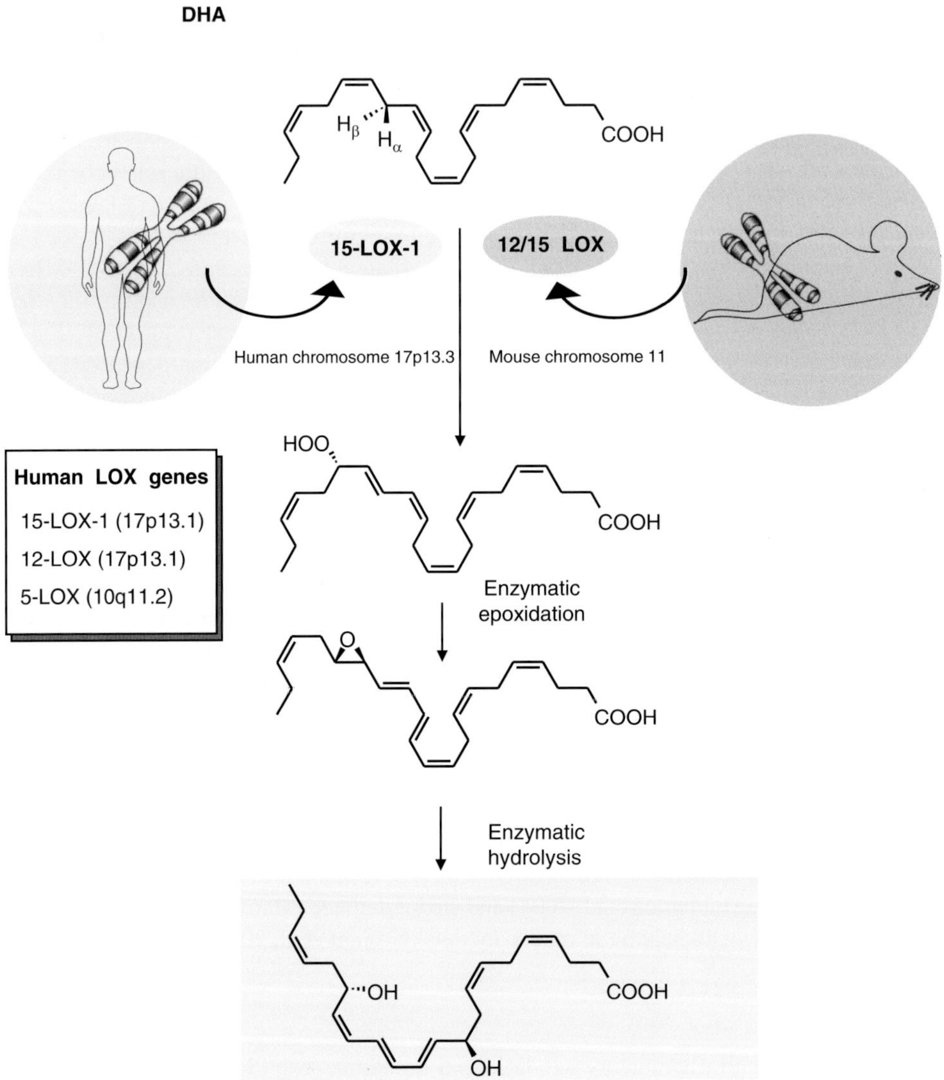

Protectin D1

10*R*, 17S-dihydroxydocosa-4Z,7Z,11E,13E,15Z,19Z-hexaenoic acid

Fig. 4.6 Biosynthesis of protectins. Protectins are generated from DHA; the initial enzymatic product 17*S*-H(p)DHA is enzymatically converted to an epoxide intermediate, which is then enzymatically hydrolyzed to bioactive protectin D1 (PD1). The complete stereochemistry of PD1 is established as 10*R*,17*S*-dihydroxydocosa-4Z,7Z,11E,13E,15Z,19Z-hexaenoic acid.

RESOLUTION OF INFLAMMATION IS AN ACTIVELY REGULATED PROCESS *IN VIVO*

In order to study resolution via a systems biology approach, the murine dorsal air pouch system was particularly helpful in yielding contained exudates (Serhan et al. 2000, 2002). This system permitted direct analysis of exudate, in terms of lipidomics (bioaction products, as well as metabolites), proteomics and cellular composition, by monitoring leukocyte trafficking. Importantly, this system allowed for the direct comparison of the timing and location of different mediators that are produced and activated during resolution, namely temporal and spatial differential analyses (Bannenberg et al. 2005; Serhan 2007). In this context, we used the murine dorsal air pouch to determine the formation and roles of endogenous LXA_4 in the resolution of acute inflammation (Levy et al. 2001). Upon initiation of inflammation with TNF-α, there was a typical acute-phase response denoted by rapid PMN infiltration preceded by both local prostaglandins and leukotrienes. Unexpectedly, the eicosanoids then underwent what we've termed a 'class switch'. As the exudate evolved, the eicosanoid profiles switched and the lipid mediators made within that milieu changed with time (Levy et al. 2001). Leukotrienes (potent chemoattractants) were deactivated and the transcriptional regulation of enzymes needed for production of lipoxins was activated. This in turn attracted mononuclear cells and stimulated macrophages to ingest apoptotic neutrophils within the contained inflammatory exudate site. These results suggested a dual action in that specific eicosanoids, namely lipoxins, actively reduced the entry of neutrophils into the site of inflammation while accelerating uptake of apoptotic neutrophils (Serhan 2007).

Within the inflammatory exudate, arachidonate-derived eicosanoids changed from initial production of prostaglandins and leukotrienes to lipoxins, which halted further recruitment of neutrophils. This class switch was driven in part by COX-derived prostaglandins E_2 and D_2, which regulate transcription of enzymes involved in lipoxin biosynthesis (Levy et al. 2001). Along with Sir John Savill, we coined the phrase 'alpha signals omega', the beginning signals the end (Serhan and Savill 2005), because the appearance of lipoxins within inflammatory exudates was concomitant with spontaneous resolution of inflammation (Levy et al. 2001). Generally, lipoxins stimulated non-phlogistic monocyte recruitment and enhanced macrophage phagocytosis of apoptotic PMNs, demonstrating pro-resolving actions (Maddox and Serhan 1996; Godson et al. 2000).

RESOLVINS AND PROTECTINS ARE PROTECTIVE IN EXPERIMENTAL MODELS OF INFLAMMATORY DISEASES

Pro-resolving mediators are protective in various animal models of disease, including peritonitis (Bannenberg et al. 2004, 2005; Serhan et al. 2006; Sun et al. 2007) (Table 4.2). PD1, as an example, was protective in microbial peritonitis initiated by intraperitoneal administration of zymosan A (Serhan et al. 2006). To assess whether PD1 could reduce leukocyte infiltration, doses as low as 1 ng were injected. At 4 hours, peritoneal lavages were collected and analyzed. PD1 had a potent action, blocking > 90% of further leukocyte infiltration, specifically stopping PMN migration and infiltration into the peritoneum (Serhan et al. 2006). RvE1 (10 ng) significantly reduced PMN infiltration, although the response was less than that obtained with PD1 (10 ng). When both PD1 and RvE1 were injected together to determine whether their actions were synergistic or additive, the reduction in PMN number was even greater, which suggests that there was an additive effect of protectin D1 and resolvin E1 *in vivo* in murine peritonitis.

Inflammatory bowel disorders, like colitis, are characterized by a relapsing inflammatory process due to mucosal damage and abnormal mucosal responses (Blumberg and Strober 2001). We found that RvE1 protects against bowel inflammation using the well-studied

Table 4.2 *In vivo* actions of lipoxins, resolvins and protectins in complex disease models.

Mediators	Species/Disease model	Action(s)
LXA_4/ATL	Rabbit/Periodontitis	Reduces PMN infiltration; prevents connective tissue and bone loss (Serhan et al. 2003a)
	Mouse/Peritonitis	Inhibits neutrophil recruitment and lymphatic removal of phagocytes (Bannenberg et al. 2005) (Schwab et al. 2007)
	Mouse/Dorsal air pouch	Inhibits neutrophil recruitment (Clish et al. 1999)
	Mouse/Dermal inflammation	Inhibits neutrophil recruitment and vascular leakage (Takano et al. 1998)
	Mouse/Colitis	Attenuates pro-inflammatory gene expression and reduces severity of colitis. Inhibits weight loss, inflammation and immune dysfunction (Gewirtz et al. 2002)
	Mouse/Asthma	Inhibits airway hyper-responsiveness and pulmonary inflammation (Levy et al. 2002)
	Mouse/Cystic fibrosis	Decreases neutrophilic inflammation, pulmonary bacterial burden and disease severity (Karp et al. 2004)
	Mouse/Ischemia-reperfusion	Attenuates hind-limb I/R-induced lung injury (Chiang et al. 1999). Detachment of adherent leukocytes in mesenteric I/R (Scalia et al. 1997) Reduces myocardial infarct size and area at risk in myocardial I/R (infarction)
	Mouse/Cornea	Accelerates cornea re-epithelialization, limits sequelae of thermal injury (i.e. neovascularization, opacity) and promotes host defense (Gronert et al. 2005)
	Mouse/Angiogenesis	Reduces angiogenic phenotype, endothelial cell proliferation and migration (Fierro et al. 2002)
	Mouse/Bone marrow transplant (BMT)	Protects against BMT-induced graft-vs.-host diseases (GvHD) (Devchand et al. 2005)
	Rat/Glomerulonephritis	Reduces leukocyte rolling and adherence. Decreases neutrophil recruitment (Papayianni et al. 1995)
	Rat/Hyperalgesia	Prolongs paw withdraw latency, reducing hyperalgesic index. Reduces paw edema (Svensson et al. 2007)
	Rat/Pleuritis	Shortens the duration of pleural exudation (Bandeira-Melo et al. 2000)
RvE1	Rabbit/Periodontitis	Reduces PMN infiltration; prevents connective tissue and bone loss; promotes healing of diseased tissues and regeneration of lost soft tissue and bone (Hasturk et al. 2006, 2007)
	Mouse/Peritonitis	Inhibits neutrophil recruitment; regulates chemokine/cytokine production (Arita et al. 2005a; Bannenberg et al. 2005). Promotes lymphatic removal of phagocytes (Schwab et al. 2007)
	Mouse/Dorsal air pouch	Inhibits neutrophil recruitment (Serhan et al. 2000)
	Mouse/Retinopathy	Protects against neovascularization (Connor et al. 2007)
	Mouse/Colitis	Decreases PMN recruitment and pro-inflammatory gene expression; improves survival; reduces weight loss (Arita et al. 2005b)
	Mouse/Obesity	Regulates adipokines and protects against liver steatosis (Gonzalez-Periz et al. 2009)
RvD1	Mouse/Peritonitis	Inhibits neutrophil recruitment (Hong et al. 2003; Sun et al. 2007)

Table 4.2 (*Continued*).

Mediators	Species/Disease model	Action(s)
	Mouse/Dorsal air pouch	Inhibits neutrophil recruitment (Serhan et al. 2002; Hong et al. 2003)
	Mouse/Kidney ischemia-reperfusion	Protects from ischemia-reperfusion-induced kidney damage and loss of function; regulates macrophages (Duffield et al. 2006)
	Mouse/Retinopathy	Protects against neovascularization (Connor et al. 2007)
PD1	Mouse/Peritonitis	Inhibits neutrophil recruitment; regulates chemokine/cytokine production (Arita et al., 2005a; Bannenberg et al. 2005). Promotes lymphatic removal of phagocytes (Schwab et al. 2007). Regulates T-cell migration (Ariel et al. 2005)
	Mouse/Asthma	Protects from lung damage, airway inflammation and hyperresponsiveness (Levy et al. 2007)
	Human/Asthma	PD1 is generated in human asthma (Levy et al. 2007)
	Mouse/Kidney ischemia-reperfusion	Protects from ischemia-reperfusion-induced kidney damage and loss of function; regulates macrophages (Duffield et al. 2006)
	Mouse/Retinopathy	Protects against neovascularization (Connor et al. 2007)
	Rat/Ischemic stroke	Inhibits leukocyte infiltration, NFkB and cyclo-oxygenase-2 induction (Marcheselli et al. 2003)
	Human/Alzheimer's disease	Diminished PD1 production in human Alzheimer's disease (Lukiw and Bazan 2008)
	Mouse/Liver injury	Protects from necro-inflammatory liver injury (Gonzalez-Periz et al. 2009)
RvD2	Mouse/Sepsis	Prevents hypothermia, decreases bacterial load in the blood and peritoneum, and promotes survival (Spite et al. 2009)
	Mouse/Peritonitis	Potently blocks PMN infiltration into the peritoneum (Spite et al. 2009)

experimental colitis model where mice were challenged with an intrarectal antigenic hapten, 2,4,6-trinitrobenzene sulfonic acid (TNBS) (Arita et al. 2005b). RvE1 was administered prior to the induction of colitis in one group, which was compared with mice that received TNBS alone. With treatment of as little as 1 μg of RvE1 per mouse, there was dramatic reduction in mortality, weight loss and less severe histologic display of colitis, namely reduction in the associated inflammatory cells, such as PMN, and lymphocytes compared with mice with TNBS-induced colitis. In addition, RvE1 is protective in periodontal disease in rabbits, where it appears to stimulate alveolar bone regeneration (Hasturk et al. 2006, 2007), which will be discussed; *vide infra*.

Recently, work from our laboratory also demonstrated that RvD2 is protective in a murine model for sepsis, cecal ligation and puncture (or CLP) (Spite et al. 2009). RvD2 in amounts as low as 100 ng prevented hypothermia, and reduced neutrophilic infiltration into the peritoneum and systemic and local bacterial burden as compared to vehicle treated mice. Of note, RvD2-treated mice also exhibited significantly higher survival rates than the CLP-control mice. These new findings expand our knowledge regarding the scope and breadth of resolvins as not only protective mediators in various self-limited inflammatory diseases but also potent regulators of complex infection. Thus, pro-resolving mediators display anti-inflammatory, antifibrotic and anti-infectious actions in several widely used laboratory models of inflammation.

SPECIALIZED PRO-RESOLVING LIPID MEDIATORS IN ORAL MEDICINE: RESTORATION OF TISSUE HOMEOSTASIS IN EXPERIMENTAL PERIODONTITIS

In order to underscore the importance of the critical enzymatic machinery involved in the generation of SPM, a 15-lipoxygenase (15-LO) transgenic rabbit was engineered (Serhan et al. 2003). The overexpression of 15-LO leads to a rise in the product 15-HETE, which is rapidly utilized by myeloid 5-LO to generate lipoxin A_4. The resulting phenotype is a rabbit with increased circulating LXA_4. In addition, when fed with a high fat diet accompanied by ligature-induced periodontitis, the transgenic animals were resistant to induction of cardiovascular disease (CVD) and were protected against development of periodontitis (Serhan et al. 2003). From these results we were able to conclude that resolution agonists such as LXA_4 play a pivotal role in restoring homeostasis. In addition, our results underscore that inflammation is an aggressor in the pathogenesis of both periodontitis and cardiovascular diseases and regulating inflammatory processes and prevents both periodontitis and early vascular changes in this rabbit model.

Additionally, resolvin E1 has potent and protective actions *in vivo* by reducing inflammation and tissue destruction in rabbit models of periodontitis (Hasturk et al. 2006, 2007). RvE1 treatment appeared to stimulate the resolution of inflammation by restoring *P.g.*-induced bone loss (Hasturk et al. 2006, 2007). RvE1 treatment resulted in a significant reduction in viable counts of oral microflora (Hasturk et al. 2006). These results were not anticipated, based on previous studies that failed to demonstrate direct antibacterial action of RvE1 alone over vehicle (ethanol) treatment (Hasturk et al. 2006). The reasons for a reduction in the complexity of biofilm composition with RvE1 treatment remain of interest (Van Dyke 2008). One possibility is that resolvins promote the release of antimicrobial peptides, such as defensins and bactericidal/permeability-increasing protein, resulting in the destruction of select micro-organisms (Levy et al. 2003). A second possibility is that *P.g.*, being an asaccharolytic organism that requires essential amino acids as its food source, survives on peptides formed by the degradation of collagen fragments, such as those produced during an inflammatory response (Van Dyke 2007). As such, an inflammatory state is a more hospitable environment for pathogenic bacteria, with formation of deep pockets favoring the survival of certain species. This explanation would suggest that the magnitude of inflammation generated by the host determines the composition of flora within the biofilm (Van Dyke 2008).

Recently, we also found that RvE1 topical treatment allowed for regeneration of hard and soft tissues of the periodontium lost to inflammatory disease (Fig. 4.7) (Hasturk et al. 2007). Overall, RvE1 acts as a modulator of the inflammatory response by shifting the response to more rapid resolution, effectively preventing the chronic phase. Elimination of inflammation in the healing lesion promotes tissue regeneration. These principles may be applicable to other inflammatory diseases including arthritis and CVD due to the similarities between these diseases, such as the neutrophil-induced panus formation in arthritis (Abramson et al. 1983) and the inflammatory damage to blood vessels stimulating atherogenesis (Libby et al. 2002).

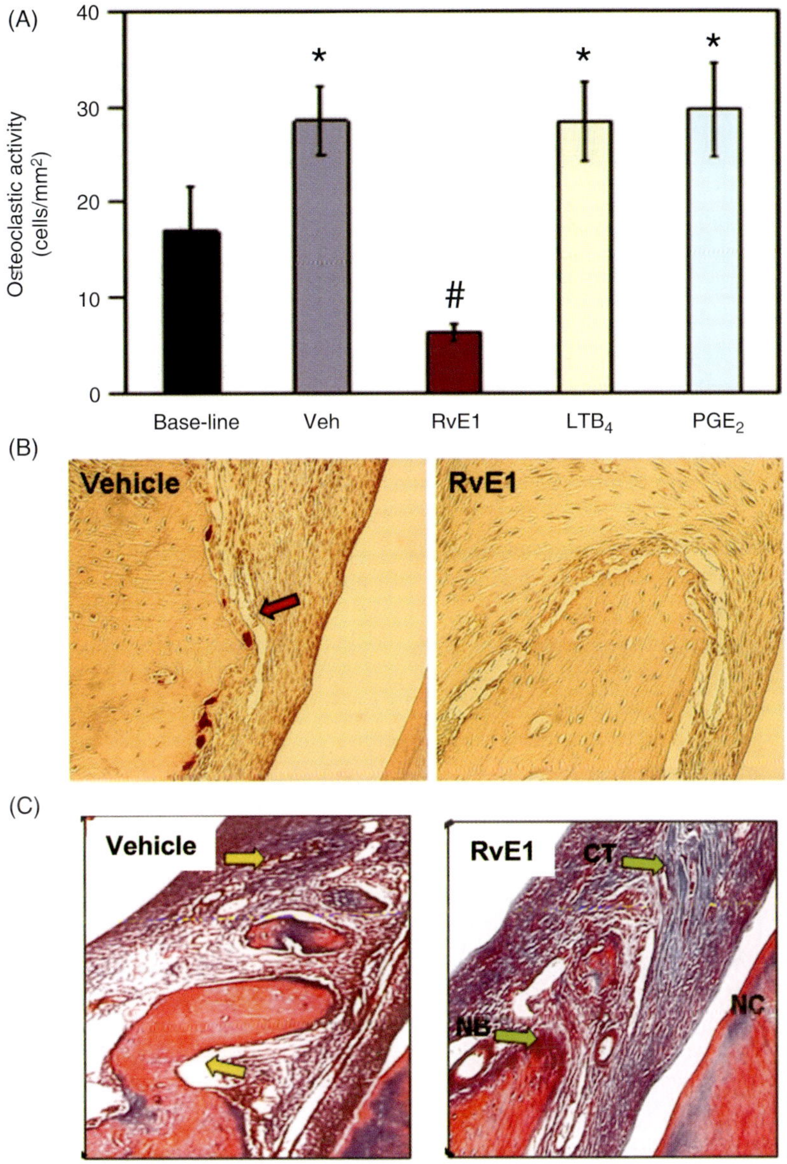

Fig. 4.7 Resolvin E1 restores tissue homeostasis in experimental periodontitis. (A) Resolvin E1 (4 μg) significantly blocks osteoclast activity as assessed by TRAP (tartrate resistant acid phosphatase) staining of rabbit alveolar bone sections. (B) Representative tissue sections clearly demonstrate decreased TRAP staining in RvE1-treated rabbits. (C) RvE1 also restored new bone and connective tissue (evaluated by Masson's trichrome staining). Experimental periodontitis resulted in soft tissue degradation (loss of interdental papillae) and bone loss as indicated by yellow arrows (×100 magnification). Green arrows indicate RvE1 stimulated new bone (NB), connective tissue (CT) formation and new cementum (NC). (Adapted from Hasturk et al. 2006, 2007. Copyright 2007. The American Association of Immunologists, Inc.).

RESOLUTION AND WOUND HEALING

When uncontrolled, inflammation can lead to fibrosis and potential tissue damage. Lipoxins demonstrate antifibrotic actions in murine models of acute renal failure (ARF). Administration of the stable lipoxin analog [ATLa; 15-epi-16-(para-fluoro)-phenoxy-lipoxin A_4] prior to ischemia resulted in significant functional and morphologic protection and attenuated cytokine and chemokine responses (Leonard et al. 2002). In addition, treatment with ATLa prior to injury modified the expression of many differentially expressed pathogenic mediators, including cytokines, growth factors, adhesion molecules and proteases (Kieran et al. 2003). Also, resolvins of the D-series limit interstitial fibrosis that persist from ischemia-reperfusion injury of the kidney (Duffield et al. 2006).

DHA-derived resolvins also have direct action on corneal wound healing. DHA is important in neural function and is one of the major polyunsaturated fatty acids (PUFA) found in the retina along with AA (Bazan et al. 1992). In addition, EPA is found in the retinal vascular endothelium (SanGiovanni and Chew 2005). In order to determine whether EPA, DHA and AA regulate retinal vaso-obliteration and neovascularization *in vivo*, an oxygen-induced retinopathy murine model to compare the effects of omega-3 and -6 PUFAs on retinal angiogenesis in wild-type mice with mice that overexpress the *C. elegans fat-1* gene was studied (Kang et al. 2004). This gene converts omega-6 PUFA into omega-3 resulting in elevated tissue levels of omega-3 PUFA within the *fat-1* overexpressing mice. A protective effect against pathological angiogenesis was found in the retina when there was a lower ratio of omega-6:omega-3 PUFA (Connor et al. 2007). Wild-type mice lacking the *fat-1* transgene had more extensive vaso-obliteration and more severe retinal neovascularization compared with *fat-1* mice (Connor et al. 2007). Of interest, in mice fed omega-3 PUFA, there were markers of biosynthesis of neuroprotectin D1 (NPD1) and RvE1 in the retinal tissues. In mice without omega-3 PUFA supplementation, administration of RvD1, RvE1 or NPD1 each gave protection from vaso-obliteration and neovascularization. Interestingly, these *fat-1* mice are also protected from colitis (Hudert et al. 2006).

Corneal injury by partial thermal cauterization stimulates inflammatory responses including temporally defined wound closure and PMN infiltration (Gronert 2005). Topical treatment (1 µg/cornea/t.i.d.) with LXA_4 reduces all parameters of corneal injury, such as accelerating wound closure, as well as attenuating corneal opacity and neovascularization. LXA_4 actions on wound healing precede PMN infiltration, suggesting that attenuation of neovascularization and corneal opacity are a consequence of accelerated epithelial wound healing. The role of LXA_4 in epithelial wound healing has been investigated by selective de-epithelialization of the mouse cornea and quantitating re-epithelialization by biomicroscopy and fluorescent image analysis (Gronert et al. 2005). These experiments have identified novel actions for both native LXA_4 and ATLa because they increase the rate (~ 2×) of re-epithelialization within the first 48 hours of injury and reduce the time for complete wound closure (Gronert et al. 2005). Thus, pro-resolving mediators display anti-inflammatory and antifibrotic actions in several widely used laboratory models of inflammation.

ANTI-INFLAMMATION VS. PRO-RESOLUTION

An emerging body of evidence now indicates that anti-inflammation, i.e. inhibiting the cardinal signs of inflammation (Kumar et al. 2005) and pro-resolution (namely activating endogenous resolution programs) are distinct mechanisms in the control of inflammation

(Serhan 2007). In addition to serving as agonists to reduce neutrophil infiltration to inflamed tissues, pro-resolution molecules promote the uptake and clearance of apoptotic cells and micro-organisms by macrophages in inflamed sites (Schwab et al. 2007), and stimulate the antimicrobial activities of mucosal epithelial cells (Canny et al. 2002; Campbell et al. 2007). The resolution of inflammation is accompanied by an active switch in the mediators that predominate in exudates (Levy et al. 2001). Initially, classic prostaglandins and leukotrienes, which activate and amplify the cardinal signs of inflammation, are generated. Next, prostaglandin E_2 and prostaglandin D_2, by inducing the production of key enzymes, promote the synthesis of mediators (Levy et al. 2001) that have both anti-inflammatory and pro-resolution activities, such as the lipoxins, resolvins and protectins. These SPMs are not immunosuppressive but instead function in the resolution of inflammation by activating specific mechanisms to promote homeostasis (Serhan et al. 2008a). In general, SPMs stimulate and accelerate resolution via mechanisms at the tissue level. Specific SPMs provide potent signals that selectively stop neutrophil (Bannenberg et al. 2005) and eosinophil infiltration (Haworth et al. 2008); stimulate non-phlogistic recruitment of monocytes; activate macrophage phagocytosis of micro-organisms and apoptotic cells (Schwab et al. 2007); increase the exit of phagocytes from the inflamed site through the lymphatics; and stimulate the expression of molecules involved in antimicrobial defense (Canny et al. 2002; Campbell et al. 2007). Additionally, RvD2 stimulates human PMN to enhance phagocytosis and the killing of *E. coli* (Spite et al. 2009), a novel pro-resolution and anti-infection action of resolvins.

Resolution toxicity

The conceptual difference between anti-inflammation and pro-resolution is underscored by certain anti-inflammatory therapies. It is becoming increasingly apparent that certain widely used drugs are 'resolution toxic' in that they impair the timely return to homeostasis. Most of the anti-inflammatories in use inhibit key biochemical pathways and/or block the signaling of key pro-inflammatory mechanisms (Serhan et al. 2007). For example, this is most notable in the case of the inhibition of COX-2 with selective COX-2 inhibitors, where these inhibitors block the production of PGE_2 and PGD_2 and thus block the switch to resolution (Gilroy et al. 1999; Levy et al. 2001). These researchers' findings also highlight the pivotal role of COX-2-derived mediators in both the initiation of acute inflammatory response and its resolution. Thus, temporal and spatial positioning of these biochemical pathways can dictate the actions of their local mediators (Serhan et al. 2007).

In addition to blocking COX, LO inhibition is considered to be 'resolution toxic'. LO inhibition by baicalein at 100 μg/mouse significantly increased the number of PMNs in exudates at 24 hours and reduced zymosan clearance to lymph nodes, indicating a 'resolution deficit', characterized by an impaired phagocyte removal (Schwab et al. 2007). In contrast, when 300 ng of either ATL analog, RvE1 or PD1 was administered together with the enzyme inhibitor, resolution of inflammation was 'rescued', as evidenced by a marked reduction of exudate PMNs and an increase of zymosan in the lymphatic samples. It now seems apparent that attempting to control inflammation via inhibition of key enzymes causes a pharmacological defect, reducing the ability to resolve inflammation, potentially resulting in exacerbating chronic inflammation. Hence, it is important to develop drugs that spare the resolution process. Besides COX-2 inhibitors, another example may be antiTNF therapy. It has been proposed that the poor clinical outcome observed in systemic inflammatory response syndrome (SIRS) patients is related to the derailment of a proper temporal anti-inflammatory pro-resolving response (Serhan et al. 2007).

In addition to anti-inflammatories, commonly used anesthetics (e.g. lidocaine) have been reported to have various side effects such as delayed wound healing (Drucker et al. 1998; Lee et al. 2004). Thus, we recently investigated the impact of lidocaine on resolution of inflammation using a self-limited microbial peritonitis model of inflammation-resolution (Chiang et al. 2008). We found that lidocaine increased PMN infiltration during zymosan stimulation and delayed resolution. Also, lidocaine reduced PMN apoptosis and clearance by macrophages. Interestingly, ATLa (300 ng), when added concomitantly with lidocaine and zymosan, rescued the delayed resolution (Chiang et al. 2008).

In contrast, there are some drugs that are considered 'resolution friendly'. As mentioned *vide supra*, the commonly used drug aspirin jump-starts resolution by generating epimeric pro-resolving lipid mediators such as the aspirin-triggered lipoxins (e.g. ATL) and resolvins (e.g. AT-RvD1). In addition, it was reported that statins (e.g. pioglitazone and atorvastatin) augment myocardial production of ATL, which may underlie some of the protective actions of statins (Birnbaum et al. 2006).

CLINICAL IMPLICATIONS AND THE DEVELOPMENT OF STABLE ANALOGS

Current anti-inflammatory therapy arises from the need to control the cardinal signs of inflammation. Most of the anti-inflammatories studied to date block/antagonize key pro-inflammatory mediator pathways that are elicited on the initiation of an acute inflammatory response (Serhan et al. 2007). SPMs offer a novel strategy toward curtailing the cardinal signs of inflammation since they are agonists that actively stimulate resolution circuitry within cells and more broadly within systems.

Endogenous SPMs are autacoids, by definition molecules that are locally generated and rapidly utilized. Thus, the development of stable lipoxin, resolvin, protectin or maresin analogs for clinical uses that harness the inherent structural features to withstand enzymatic degradation may prove to be useful therapeutic tools for the treatment of a wide range of inflammatory diseases. The systemic administration of PD1 and the RvE1 analog RX-10008 (Bannenberg 2009) or the topical administration of an isopropyl ester RvE1 analog RX-10045 reduced choroidal neovascularization after laser-induced injury of the retina (Sheets et al. 2009). A phase 2, 28-day randomized placebo-controlled clinical trial was carried out to assess the potential protective actions of RX-10045 in the ocular surface of 232 patients with chronic dry eye syndrome (Clinicaltrials.gov identifier: NCT00799552). The trial produced a dose-dependent, statistically significant improvement in symptoms and signs of dry eye. This is the first demonstration of clinical efficacy for this novel class of SPM.

CONCLUSIONS

Table 4.3 summarizes the key points covered in this chapter. The acute inflammatory response is a self-limited protective mechanism. In response to injury or infection, excessive or uncontrolled inflammatory responses can lead to chronic disorders. Neutrophil-derived pro-inflammatory mediators, including leukotrienes and prostaglandins, are produced from arachidonic acid. They are made in the initial phase of contained acute inflammatory responses that they can amplify. Within contained inflammatory exudates, we found that neutrophils can change phenotypes with time to generate protective mediators, derived from

Table 4.3 Summary of key points.

1. The resolution of acute inflammation is an active, highly regulated process.
2. PMN change their phenotype in resolving exudates, initially biosynthesizing prostaglandin and leukotrienes to temporally generate anti-inflammatory and pro-resolving lipid mediators.
3. Lipoxins, resolvins, protectins and maresins (SPMs) are enzymatically generated families of local acting chemical mediators that coordinate resolution.
4. SPMs are potent in the picogram to nanogram range *in vivo;* they regulate cytokines and chemokines and thus are antifibrotic and pro wound healing.
5. SPMs are anti-inflammatory, pro-resolving mediators that are not immunosuppressive.

essential polyunsaturated fatty acids, to promote resolution. There is an active catabasis to return tissues to a homeostatic health state from the inflammatory battle (Bannenberg et al. 2005). These protective mediators include the arachidonic acid-derived lipoxins as well as omega-3 EPA-derived resolvin E-series, DHA-derived resolvin-D series, protectins and maresins. These findings provide evidence that the resolution of acute inflammation is not a passive burning out of chemotactic signals, but rather an active, regulated process that orchestrates the clearance of inflammatory exudates. Thus, the production of pro-resolving lipid mediators, such as lipoxins, protectins and resolvins, when administered *in vivo* can accelerate the resolution of acute inflammation and the return to tissue homeostasis.

ACKNOWLEDGMENTS

We thank M. Halm Small for chapter preparation. This study was supported, in part, by National Institutes of Health grant nos GM38765, DK074448, DE019938 and RC2AT005909 (C.N. Serhan). CNS is an inventor on patents [resolvins] assigned to BWH and licensed to Resolvyx Pharmaceuticals. CNS is a scientific founder of Resolvyx Pharmaceuticals and owns equity in the company. CNS' interests were reviewed and are managed by the Brigham and Women's Hospital and Partners HealthCare in accordance with their conflict of interest policies.

REFERENCES

Abramson, S., Edelson, H., Kaplan, H., Given, W., Weissmann, G. (1983) The neutrophil in rheumatoid arthritis: its role and the inhibition of its activation by nonsteroidal antiinflammatory drugs. *Seminars in Arthritis and Rheumatism,* **13**, 148–53.

Ariel, A., Li, P.L., Wang, W., et al. (2005) The docosatriene protectin D1 is produced by TH2 skewing and promotes human T cell apoptosis via lipid raft clustering. *J Biol Chem,* **280,** 43079–86.

Arita, M., Bianchini, F., Aliberti, J., et al. (2005a) Stereochemical assignment, antiinflammatory properties, and receptor for the omega-3 lipid mediator resolvin E1. *Journal of Experimental Medicine,* **201**, 713–22.

Arita, M., Yoshida, M., Hong, S., et al. (2005b) Resolvin E1, an endogenous lipid mediator derived from omega-3 eicosapentaenoic acid, protects against 2,4,6-trinitrobenzene sulfonic acid-induced colitis. *Proceedings of the National Academy of Sciences USA,* **102**, 7671–6.

Bandeira-Melo, C., Serra, M.F., Diaz, B.L., et al. (2000) Cyclooxygenase-2-derived prostaglandin E2 and lipoxin A4 accelerate resolution of allergic edema in *Angiostrongylus costaricensis*-infected rats: relationship with concurrent eosinophilia. *J Immunol,* **164,** 1029–36.

Bannenberg, G.L. (2009) Resolvins: current understanding and future potential in the control of inflammation. *Current Opinion in Drug Discovery and Development*, **12**, 644–58.

Bannenberg, G., Moussignac, R.L., Gronert, K., et al. (2004) Lipoxins and novel 15-epi-lipoxin analogs display potent anti-inflammatory actions after oral administration. *British Journal of Pharmacology*, **143**, 43–52.

Bannenberg, G.L., Chiang, N., Ariel, A., et al. (2005) Molecular circuits of resolution: formation and actions of resolvins and protectins. *Journal of Immunology*, **174**, 4345–55.

Bazan, N.G., Gordon, W.C., Rodriguez de Turco, E.B. (1992) Docosahexaenoic acid uptake and metabolism in photoreceptors: retinal conservation by an efficient retinal pigment epithelial cell-mediated recycling process. *Advances in Experimental Medicine and Biology*, **318**, 295–306.

Bergstroem, S., Danielsson, H., Samuelsson, B. (1964) The enzymatic formation of prostaglandin E2 from arachidonic acid prostaglandins and related factors 32. *Biochim Biophysica Acta*, **90**, 207–10.

Birnbaum, Y., Ye, Y., Lin, Y., et al. (2006) Augmentation of myocardial production of 15-epi-lipoxin-a4 by pioglitazone and atorvastatin in the rat. *Circulation*, **114**, 929–35.

Blumberg, R.S., Strober, W. (2001) Prospects for research in inflammatory bowel disease. JAMA, 285, 643–7.

Borgeat, P., Samuelsson, B. (1979a) Arachidonic acid metabolism in polymorphonuclear leukocytes: effects of ionophore A23187. *Proceedings of the National Academy of Sciences USA*, **76**, 2148–52.

Borgeat, P., Samuelsson, B. (1979b) Transformation of arachidonic acid by rabbit polymorphonuclear leukocytes. Formation of a novel dihydroxyeicosatetraenoic acid. *Journal of Biological Chemistry*, **254**, 2643–6.

Campbell, E.L., Louis, N.A., Tomassetti, S.E., et al. (2007) Resolvin E1 promotes mucosal surface clearance of neutrophils: a new paradigm for inflammatory resolution. *FASEB Journal*, 21, 3162–70.

Canny, G., Levy, O., Furuta, G.T., et al. (2002) Lipid mediator-induced expression of bactericidal/ permeability-increasing protein (BPI) in human mucosal epithelia. *Proceedings of the National Academy of Sciences USA*, **99**, 3902–7.

Chiang, N., Bermudez, E.A., Ridker, P.M., Hurwitz, S., Serhan, C.N. (2004) Aspirin triggers antiinflammatory 15-epi-lipoxin A4 and inhibits thromboxane in a randomized human trial. *Proceedings of the National Academy of Sciences USA*, **101**, 15178–83.

Chiang, N., Gronert, K., Clish, C.B., O'Brien, J.A., Freeman, M.W., Serhan, C.N. (1999) Leukotriene B4 receptor transgenic mice reveal novel protective roles for lipoxins and aspirin-triggered lipoxins in reperfusion. *J Clin Invest,* **104,** 309–316.

Chiang, N., Schwab, J.M., Fredman, G., Kasuga, K., Gelman, S., Serhan, C.N. (2008) Anesthetics impact the resolution of inflammation. *PLoS ONE*, **3**, e1879.

Claria, J., Serhan, C.N. (1995) Aspirin triggers previously undescribed bioactive eicosanoids by human endothelial cell-leukocyte interactions. *Proceedings of the National Academy of Sciences USA,* **92**, 9475–9.

Clish, C.B., O'Brien, J.A., Gronert, K., Stahl, G.L., Petasis, N.A., Serhan, C.N. (1999) Local and systemic delivery of a stable aspirin-triggered lipoxin prevents neutrophil recruitment in vivo. *Proc Natl Acad SciUSA,* **96,** 8247–52.

Connor, K.M., Sangiovanni, J.P., Lofqvist, C., et al. (2007) Increased dietary intake of omega-3-polyunsaturated fatty acids reduces pathological retinal angiogenesis. *Nature Medicine,* **13**, 868–73.

Dangi, B., Obeng, M., Nauroth, J.M., et al. (2009) Biogenic synthesis, purification, and chemical characterization of anti-inflammatory resolvins derived from docosapentaenoic acid (DPAn-6). *Journal of Biological Chemistry,* **284**, 14744–59.

Devchand, P.R., Schmidt, B.A., Primo, V.C., et al. (2005) A synthetic eicosanoid LX-mimetic unravels host–donor interactions in allogeneic BMT-induced GvHD to reveal an early protective role for host neutrophils. *FASEB J,* **19,** 203–210.

Drucker, M., Cardenas, E., Arizti, P., Valenzuela, A., Gamboa, A. (1998) Experimental studies on the effect of lidocaine on wound healing. *World Journal of Surgery,* **22**, 394–7; discussion 397–8.

Duffield, J.S., Hong, S., Vaidya, V.S., et al. (2006) Resolvin D series and protectin D1 mitigate acute kidney injury. *Journal of Immunology,* **177**, 5902–11.

Fierro, I.M., Kutok, J.L., Serhan, C.N. (2002) Novel lipid mediator regulators of endothelial cell proliferation and migration: aspirin-triggered-15R-lipoxin A(4) and lipoxin A(4). *J Pharmacol Exp Ther,* **300,** 385–92.

Gewirtz, A.T., Neish, A.S., Madara, J.L. (2002) Mechanisms of active intestinal inflammation and potential down-regulation via lipoxins. *Adv Exper Med Biol,* **507,** 229–36.

Gilroy, D.W., Colville-Nash, P.R., Willis, D., Chivers, J., Paul-Clark, M.J., Willoughby, D. A. (1999) Inducible cyclooxygenase may have anti-inflammatory properties. *Nature Medicine,* **5**, 698–701.

Godson, C., Mitchell, S., Harvey, K., Petasis, N.A., Hogg, N., Brady, H.R. (2000) Cutting edge: lipoxins rapidly stimulate nonphlogistic phagocytosis of apoptotic neutrophils by monocyte-derived macrophages. *Journal of Immunology,* **164**, 1663–7.

Gonzalez-Periz, A., Horrillo, R., Ferre, N., et al. (2009) Obesity-induced insulin resistance and hepatic steatosis are alleviated by ω-3 fatty acids: a role for resolvins and protectins. *FASEB J,* **23**, 1946–57.

Gronert, K. (2005) Lipoxins in the eye and their role in wound healing. *Prostaglandins, Leukotrienes and Essential Fatty Acids,* **73**, 221–9.

Gronert, K., Maheshwari, N., Khan, N., Hassan, I.R., Dunn, M., Laniado Schwartzman, M. (2005) A role for the mouse 12/15-lipoxygenase pathway in promoting epithelial wound healing and host defense. *Journal of Biological Chemistry,* **280**, 15267–78.

Hasturk, H., Kantarci, A., Ohira, T., et al. (2006) RvE1 protects from local inflammation and osteoclast-mediated bone destruction in periodontitis. *FASEB Journal, 20*, 401–403.

Hasturk, H., Kantarci, A., Goguet-Surmenian, E., et al. (2007) Resolvin E1 regulates inflammation at the cellular and tissue level and restores tissue homeostasis in vivo. *Journal of Immunology,* **179**, 7021–9.

Haworth, O., Cernadas, M., Yang, R., Serhan, C.N., Levy, B.D. (2008) Resolvin E1 regulates interleukin 23, interferon-gamma and lipoxin A4 to promote the resolution of allergic airway inflammation. *Nature Immunology,* **9**, 873–9.

Hong, S., Gronert, K., Devchand, P.R., Moussignac, R.L., Serhan, C.N. (2003) Novel docosatrienes and 17S-resolvins generated from docosahexaenoic acid in murine brain, human blood, and glial cells. Autacoids in anti-inflammation. *Journal of Biological Chemistry,* **278**, 14677–87.

Hudert, C.A., Weylandt, K.H., Lu, Y., et al. (2006) Transgenic mice rich in endogenous omega-3 fatty acids are protected from colitis. *Proceedings of the National Academy of Sciences USA,* **103**, 11276–81.

Kang, J.X., Wang, J., Wu, L., Kang, Z.B. (2004) Transgenic mice: fat-1 mice convert n-6 to n-3 fatty acids. *Nature,* **427**, 504.

Karp, C.L., Flick, L.M., Park, K.W., et al. (2004) Defective lipoxin-mediated anti-inflammatory activity in the cystic fibrosis airway. *Nat Immunol,* **5,** 388–92.

Kieran, N.E., Doran, P.P., Connolly, S.B., et al. (2003) Modification of the transcriptomic response to renal ischemia/reperfusion injury by lipoxin analog. *Kidney International,* **64**, 480–92.

Kumar, V., Abbas, A.K., Fausto, N., Robbins, S.L., Cotran, R.S. (2005) *Robbins and Cotran Pathologic Basis of Disease*. Philadelphia, Elsevier/Saunders.

Lee, H.T., Krichevsky, I.E., Xu, H., Ota-Setlik, A., D'agati, V.D., Emala, C.W. (2004) Local anesthetics worsen renal function after ischemia-reperfusion injury in rats. *American Journal of Physiology. Renal Physiology,* **286**, F111–19.

Leonard, M.O., Hannan, K., Burne, M.J., et al. (2002) 15-Epi-16-(para-fluorophenoxy)-lipoxin A(4)-methyl ester, a synthetic analogue of 15-epi-lipoxin A(4), is protective in experimental ischemic acute renal failure. *Journal of the American Society of Nephrology,* **13**, 1657–62.

Levy, B.D., Clish, C.B., Schmidt, B., Gronert, K., Serhan, C.N. (2001) Lipid mediator class switching during acute inflammation: signals in resolution. *Nature Immunology,* **2**, 612–19.

Levy, B.D., De Sanctis, G.T., Devchand, P.R., et al. (2002) Multi-pronged inhibition of airway hyper-responsiveness and inflammation by lipoxin A(4). *Nat Med,* **8,** 1018–23.

Levy, B.D., Kohli, P., Gotlinger, K., et al. (2007a) Protectin D1 is generated in asthma and dampens airway inflammation and hyperresponsiveness. *J Immunol,* **178,** 496–502.

Levy, O., Canny, G., Serhan, C.N., Colgan, S.P. (2003) Expression of BPI (bactericidal/permeability-increasing protein) in human mucosal epithelia. *Biochemical Society Transactions,* **31**, 795–800.

Libby, P., Ridker, P.M., Maseri, A. (2002) Inflammation and atherosclerosis. *Circulation,* **105**, 1135–43.

Lukiw, W.J., Bazan, N.G. (2008) Docosahexaenoic acid and the aging brain. *J Nutr,* **138,** 2510–14.

Maddox, J.F., Serhan, C.N. (1996) Lipoxin A4 and B4 are potent stimuli for human monocyte migration and adhesion: selective inactivation by dehydrogenation and reduction. *Journal of Experimental Medicine,* **183**, 137–46.

Maddox, J.F., Hachicha, M., Takano, T., Petasis, N.A., Fokin, V.V., Serhan, C.N. (1997) Lipoxin A4 stable analogs are potent mimetics that stimulate human monocytes and THP-1 cells via a G-protein-linked lipoxin A4 receptor. *Journal of Biological Chemistry,* **272**, 6972–8.

Majno, G. (1991) *The Healing Hand: Man and Wound in the Ancient World.* Cambridge, Massachusetts, Harvard University Press.

Majno, G., Joris, I. (2004) *Cells, Tissues, and Disease: Principles of General Pathology.* New York, Oxford University Press.

Marcheselli, V.L., Hong, S., Lukiw, W.J., et al. (2003) Novel docosanoids inhibit brain ischemia-reperfusion-mediated leukocyte infiltration and pro-inflammatory gene expression. *Journal of Biological Chemistry,* **278**, 43807–17.

Mitchell, S., Thomas, G., Harvey, K., et al. (2002) Lipoxins, aspirin-triggered epi-lipoxins, lipoxin stable analogues, and the resolution of inflammation: stimulation of macrophage phagocytosis of apoptotic neutrophils in vivo. *Journal of the American Society of Nephrology,* **13**, 2497–507.

Mukherjee, P.K., Marcheselli, V.L., Serhan, C.N., Bazan, N.G. (2004) Neuroprotectin D1: a docosahexaenoic acid-derived docosatriene protects human retinal pigment epithelial cells from oxidative stress. *Proceedings of the National Academy of Sciences USA,* **101**, 8491–6.

O'Sullivan, T.P., Vallin, K.S., Shah, S.T., et al. (2007) Aromatic lipoxin A4 and lipoxin B4 analogues display potent biological activities. *Journal of Medicinal Chemistry,* **50**, 5894–902.

Papayianni, A., Serhan, C.N., Phillips, M.L., Rennke, H.G., Brady, H.R. (1995) Transcellular biosynthesis of lipoxin A4 during adhesion of platelets and neutrophils in experimental immune complex glomerulonephritis. *Kidney Int,* **47,** 1295–302.

Petasis, N.A., Keledjian, R., Sun, Y.P., et al. (2008) Design and synthesis of benzo-lipoxin A4 analogs with enhanced stability and potent anti-inflammatory properties. *Bioorganic and Medicinal Chemistry Letters,* **18**, 1382–7.

Qiu, F.H., Devchand, P.R., Wada, K., Serhan, C.N. (2001) Aspirin-triggered lipoxin A4 and lipoxin A4 up-regulate transcriptional corepressor NAB1 in human neutrophils. *FASEB Journal,* **15**, 2736–8.

Rowley, A.F., Lloyd-Evans, P., Barrow, S.E., Serhan, C.N. (1994) Lipoxin biosynthesis by trout macrophages involves the formation of epoxide intermediates. *Biochemistry,* **33**, 856–63.

Ryan, G.B., Majno, G. (1977) Acute inflammation. A review. *American Journal of Pathology,* **86**, 183–276.

Samuelsson, B. (1979) Prostaglandins, thromboxanes, and leukotrienes: formation and biological roles. *Harvey Lecture,* **75**, 1–40.

Samuelsson, B. (1983). Leukotrienes: mediators of immediate hypersensitivity reactions and inflammation. *Science,* **220**, 568–75.

Samuelsson, B., Dahlen, S.E., Lindgren, J.A., Rouzer, C.A., Serhan, C.N. (1987) Leukotrienes and lipoxins: structures, biosynthesis, and biological effects. *Science,* **237**, 1171–6.

Sangiovanni, J.P., Chew, E.Y. (2005) The role of omega-3 long-chain polyunsaturated fatty acids in health and disease of the retina. *Progress in Retinal and Eye Research,* **24**, 87–138.

Scalia, R., Gefen, J., Petasis, N.A., Serhan, C.N., Lefer, A.M. (1997) Lipoxin A4 stable analogs inhibit leukocyte rolling and adherence in the rat mesenteric microvasculature: role of P-selectin. *Proc Natl Acad Sci USA,* **94,** 9967–72.

Schwab, J.M., Chiang, N., Arita, M., Serhan, C.N. (2007) Resolvin E1 and protectin D1 activate inflammation-resolution programmes. *Nature,* **447**, 869–74.

Serhan, C.N. (2007) Resolution phase of inflammation: novel endogenous anti-inflammatory and proresolving lipid mediators and pathways. *Annual Review of Immunology,* **25**, 101–37.

Serhan, C.N., Chiang, N. (2008) Endogenous pro-resolving and anti-inflammatory lipid mediators: a new pharmacologic genus. *British Journal of Pharmacology,* **153** (Suppl 1), S200–215.

Serhan, C.N., Drazen, J.M. (1997) Antiinflammatory potential of lipoxygenase-derived eicosanoids: a molecular switch at 5 and 15 positions? *Journal of Clinical Investigation,* **99**, 1147–8.

Serhan, C.N., Guest Ed. (2005) Special issue on lipoxins and aspirin-triggered lipoxins. *Prostaglandins, Leukotrienes and Essential Fatty Acids,* **73**(3–4), 139–321.

Serhan, C.N., Savill, J. (2005) Resolution of inflammation: the beginning programs the end. *Nature Immunology,* **6**, 1191–7.

Serhan, C.N., Maddox, J.F., Petasis, N.A., et al. (1995) Design of lipoxin A4 stable analogs that block transmigration and adhesion of human neutrophils. *Biochemistry,* **34**, 14609–15.

Serhan, C.N., Clish, C.B., Brannon, J., Colgan, S.P., Chiang, N., Gronert, K. (2000) Novel functional sets of lipid-derived mediators with antiinflammatory actions generated from omega-3 fatty acids via cyclooxygenase 2-nonsteroidal antiinflammatory drugs and transcellular processing. *Journal of Experimental Medicine,* **192**, 1197–204.

Serhan, C.N., Hong, S., Gronert, K., et al. (2002) Resolvins: a family of bioactive products of omega-3 fatty acid transformation circuits initiated by aspirin treatment that counter proinflammation signals. *Journal of Experimental Medicine,* **196**, 1025–37.

Serhan, C.N., Jain, A., Marleau, S., et al. (2003) Reduced inflammation and tissue damage in transgenic rabbits overexpressing 15-lipoxygenase and endogenous anti-inflammatory lipid mediators. *Journal of Immunology,* **171**, 6856–65.

Serhan, C.N., Jain, A., Marleau, S., et al. (2003a) Reduced inflammation and tissue damage in transgenic rabbits overexpressing 15-lipoxygenase and endogenous anti-inflammatory lipid mediators. *J Immunol,* **171,** 6856–65.

Serhan, C.N., Arita, M., Hong, S., Gotlinger, K. (2004a) Resolvins, docosatrienes, and neuroprotectins, novel omega-3-derived mediators, and their endogenous aspirin-triggered epimers. *Lipids,* **39**, 1125–32.

Serhan, C.N., Gotlinger, K., Hong, S., Arita, M. (2004b) Resolvins, docosatrienes, and neuroprotectins, novel omega-3-derived mediators, and their aspirin-triggered endogenous epimers: an overview of their protective roles in catabasis. *Prostaglandins Other Lipid Mediators,* **73**, 155–72.

Serhan, C.N., Gotlinger, K., Hong, S., et al. (2006) Anti-inflammatory actions of neuroprotectin D1/protectin D1 and its natural stereoisomers: assignments of dihydroxy-containing docosatrienes. *Journal of Immunology,* **176**, 1848–59.

Serhan, C.N., Brain, S.D., Buckley, C.D., et al. (2007) Resolution of inflammation: state of the art, definitions and terms. *FASEB Journal,* **21**, 325–32.

Serhan, C.N., Chiang, N., Van Dyke, T.E. (2008a) Resolving inflammation: dual anti-inflammatory and pro-resolution lipid mediators. *Nature Review Immunology,* **8**, 349–61.

Serhan, C.N., Yacoubian, S., Yang, R. (2008b) Anti-inflammatory and proresolving lipid mediators. *Annual Review of Pathology,* **3**, 279–312.

Serhan, C.N., Yang, R., Martinod, K., et al. (2009) Maresins: novel macrophage mediators with potent antiinflammatory and proresolving actions. *Journal of Experimental Medicine,* **206**, 15–23.

Sheets, K.G., Elison, Z.Y. Jr, Gjörstrup, P., Gordon, W.C., Bergsma, D.R., Bazan, N.G. (2009) An analog of resolvin E1 inhibits endothelial cell growth in retina following laser-induced choroidal neovascularization (CNV). In: *Association for Research in Vision and Ophthalmology Annual Meeting*, Fort Lauderdale, Florida, USA.

Spite, M., Norling, L.V., Summers, L., et al. (2009) Resolvin D2 is a potent regulator of leukocytes and controls microbial sepsis. *Nature,* **461**, 1287–91.

Sun, Y.P., Oh, S.F., Uddin, J., et al. (2007) Resolvin D1 and its aspirin-triggered 17R epimer. Stereochemical assignments, anti-inflammatory properties, and enzymatic inactivation. *Journal of Biology and Chemistry,* **282**, 9323–34.

Svensson, C.I., Zattoni, M., Serhan, C.N. (2007) Lipoxins and aspirin-triggered lipoxin inhibit inflammatory pain processing. *J Exp Med,* **204,** 245–52.

Takano, T., Clish, C.B., Gronert, K., Petasis, N., Serhan, C.N. (1998) Neutrophil-mediated changes in vascular permeability are inhibited by topical application of aspirin-triggered 15-epi-lipoxin A4 and novel lipoxin B4 stable analogues. *Journal of Clinical Investigation,* **101**, 819–26.

Tauber, A.I., Chernyak, L. (1991) *Metchnikoff and the Origins of Immunology: From Metaphor to Theory*. Oxford, Oxford University Press.

Tjonahen, E., Oh, S.F., Siegelman, J., et al. (2006) Resolvin E2: identification and anti-inflammatory actions: pivotal role of human 5-lipoxygenase in resolvin E series biosynthesis. *Chemistry and Biology,* **13**, 1193–202.

Van Dyke, T.E. (2007) Control of inflammation and periodontitis. *Periodontol 2000,* **45**, 158–66.

Van Dyke, T.E. (2008) The management of inflammation in periodontal disease. *Journal of Periodontology,* **79**, 1601–8.

Van Dyke, T.E., Serhan, C.N. (2006) A novel approach to resolving inflammation. *Scientific American Oral and Whole Body Health*, 2006, 42–45.

Vane, J.R. (1976) The mode of action of aspirin and similar compounds. *Journal of Allergy and Clinical Immunology,* **58**, 691–712.

5 Re-epithelialization of Wounds

Leeni Koivisto, Lari Häkkinen and Hannu Larjava
Laboratory of Periodontal Biology, Department of Oral Biological and Medical Sciences, Faculty of Dentistry, University of British Columbia, Vancouver, BC, Canada

INTRODUCTION

Stratified squamous epithelium of mucosa and skin, the epidermis, serves as an important barrier between an organism and its environment, protecting the host from physical, chemical and microbial damage (Kirfel and Herzog 2004). It also regulates the function and integrity of the underlying connective tissue. Therefore, re-epithelialization after trauma or wounding has to be a robust process to restore the barrier function. Only a few studies directly explore the mechanisms of re-epithelialization that are specific for human oral mucosal epithelium. Therefore, much of the data presented below draw from wound re-epithelialization in general and come from reports on human skin wound healing, from experiments with cultured keratinocytes or organotypic epithelial cell cultures, or from research conducted in different mouse skin wound healing models. Since the process of wound healing is highly evolutionally and mechanistically conserved, one can assume that oral wound re-epithelialization occurs mostly by a similar mechanism.

KERATINOCYTES FORM A PROTECTIVE BARRIER BETWEEN AN ORGANISM AND ITS ENVIRONMENT

The epithelium is separated from the underlying connective tissue by a basement membrane (Figs. 5.1 and 5.2). Keratinocytes of the basal layer attach to it via hemidesmosomes. In the epithelium, keratinocytes form a tight sheet by connecting to neighboring cells by specialized cell–cell adhesions, including desmosomes, adherens junctions and gap junctions. During tissue homeostasis, the daughter cells of the proliferating basal cells that lose their contact with the basement membrane are slowly pushed to the outer layers of the epithelium and undergo gradual terminal differentiation until they become anucleated and flattened, eventually shedding away from the epithelial surface (Blanpain and Fuchs 2009). This process is tightly controlled and is crucial to maintaining epithelial integrity and appropriate barrier function during tissue homeostasis. A significant portion of the epithelial stem cells appear to reside in the basal cell layer. It has been long assumed that in epidermal homeostasis of skin, a subpopulation of interfollicular basal keratinocytes which are slowly cycling contain epidermal stem cells that give rise to transit-amplifying cells that can themselves

Oral Wound Healing: Cell Biology and Clinical Management, First Edition. Edited by Hannu Larjava.

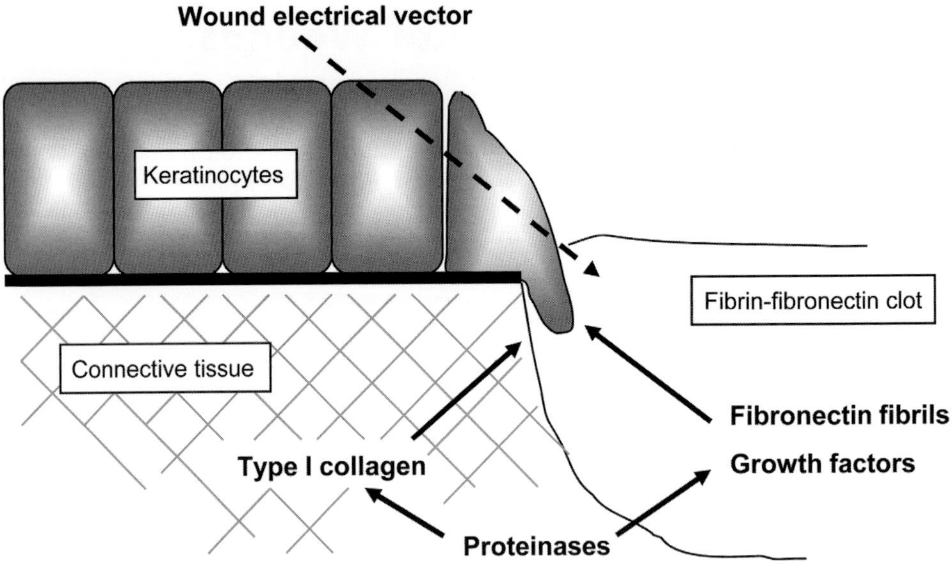

Fig. 5.1 Schematic presentation of factors that contribute to initiation of keratinocyte migration after wounding. Upon wounding, the basement membrane is disrupted and keratinocytes become exposed to wound-induced electrical fields, to pro-migratory matrix molecules, including type I collagen in the connective tissue and fibronectin fibrils in the clot, and to pro-migratory growth factors secreted by the wound cells. Proteinases synthesized by keratinocytes themselves and by other wound cells contribute to collagen denaturation, to growth factor release and activation and to modulation of the molecular structure of the fibrin-fibronectin clot. Wounding also disrupts the endogenous intra-epithelial electrical field and creates a new, laterally oriented one.

divide a small number of times (Potten 1981; Jensen et al. 1999; Watt 2002; Morasso and Tomic-Canic 2005). This model has been recently challenged with a new model of homeostasis in which tissue maintenance depends on a single population of proliferating cells (Clayton et al. 2007). In addition to interfollicular basal cells, stem cells residing in hair follicles and sepaceous glands in skin may participate in maintaining the epithelial intergrity (Morasso and Tomic-Canic 2005; Nowak et al. 2008). In oral mucosa that lacks adnexae typical to skin, a putative stem cell population has been recently linked to a subpopulation of basal cells facing the connective tissue papilla area (Hosoya et al. 2008). Since epithelial stem cells are difficult to identify, the true hierarchies of these stem cell populations remain under investigation (Jones et al. 2007; Fuchs 2009).

KERATINOCYTES ARE ACTIVATED RAPIDLY TO RESTORE THE EPITHELIAL BARRIER AFTER WOUNDING

Considering the important barrier function of epithelium, it is necessary to re-establish tissue integrity as fast and as efficiently as possible after injury (Schaffer and Nanney 1996; Martin 1997). Shortly after wounding, epithelial keratinocytes become activated through the combined effects of the exposure to (1) pro-migratory matrix molecules within the wound site, (2) growth factors and cytokines that are released by inflammatory and other wound cells and from the blood clot and surrounding extracellular matrix, and (3) wound-generated electrical fields (Fig. 5.1; Schultz and Wysocki 2009; Zhao 2009; see below).

Upon activation, keratinocytes dissolve their hemidesmosomal contacts with the basement membrane, and the lateral desmosomal connections between the wound edge keratinocytes also decrease. Some desmosomal cell–cell connections are required for optimal re-epithelialization nonetheless (Beaudry et al. 2010). Intercellular communication between keratinocytes adjacent to the wound through gap junctions is also reduced via increased phosphorylation of connexin43, the main structural protein of epithelial gap junctions (Richards et al. 2004). The downregulation of connexin43 at the wound edge appears to be a prerequisite for keratinocyte mobilization during wound healing (Kretz et al. 2003; Richards et al. 2004). The morphology of keratinocytes changes from polarized basal keratinocytes to flattened and elongated when they assume the migratory phenotype (Odland and Ross 1968). Long actin-rich lamellipodia that extend to the wound bed are observed in migrating keratinocytes in the provisional matrix. This lamellipodia extension requires the activities of intracellular signaling molecules Rac1 GTPase and glycogen synthase kinase-3 (Fenteany et al. 2000; Koivisto et al. 2004, 2006). Many cytokines, including keratinocyte growth factor (KGF), epidermal growth factor (EGF) and insulin-like growth factor (IGF), which promote keratinocyte migration (see below) are able to cause alterations in the organization of the cytoskeleton and cell shape (Putnins et al. 1999; Haase et al. 2003).

The morphological changes caused by initial keratinocyte activation occur within hours after wounding and appear to be a prerequisite for keratinocyte migration. Histological studies have shown that keratinocytes start to migrate from the wound edge to the provisional matrix during the first 24 hours, initiating the re-epithelialization of the wound defect. In skin, epidermal stem cells or their progeny residing in hair follicle bulges as well as sebaceous and sweat glands are also recruited to the pool of migrating cells. Although most of these cells are short-lived and eliminated from the epidermis over several weeks, some persist long term (Ito et al. 2005; Levy et al. 2007; Nowak et al. 2008). As oral mucosa lacks hair follicles and sweat glands, the major source for wound keratinocytes lies most likely in the basal layer of the oral mucosal epithelium. Once the keratinocyte migration is well underway, basal keratinocytes adjacent to the migrating epithelial front start proliferating 48–72 hours after the injury, seeding more migratory, non-proliferating cells to the wound (Odland and Ross 1968; Patel et al. 2006; Fig. 5.2). Also some bone marrow-derived cells may engraft at the wound site as transit-amplifying keratinocytes to assist wound re-epithelialization, although they may not play a significant role in the process (Badiavas et al. 2003; Borue et al. 2004; Fan et al. 2006).

Different models of keratinocyte migration during re-epithelialization have been proposed. In the first model, the basal keratinocytes migrate on the wound matrix and actively pull along the suprabasal cell layers (Stenn and Malhotra 1992). In the second proposed mechanism, the epithelial cells behind the wound margin also actively crawl and slide as a sheet together with the cells located at the wound margin. This mechanism of cell motility has been observed in wounded epithelial cell cultures and in corneal wounds *in vivo* (Zhao et al. 2003; Farooqui and Fenteany 2004). Evidence for the third mechanism (the so-called leap-frog model), in which the cells at the wound margin do not in fact migrate, but the suprabasal keratinocytes leap over the basal keratinocytes and attach to the wound matrix forming a new leading front, comes from an organotypic model of wound healing (Garlick and Taichman 1994; Laplante et al. 2001). This model also involves intra-epithelial migration. It is possible that all of these different mechanisms of keratinocyte movement contribute to re-epithelialization of multilayered epithelia *in vivo* (Usui et al. 2005; Hosoya et al. 2008).

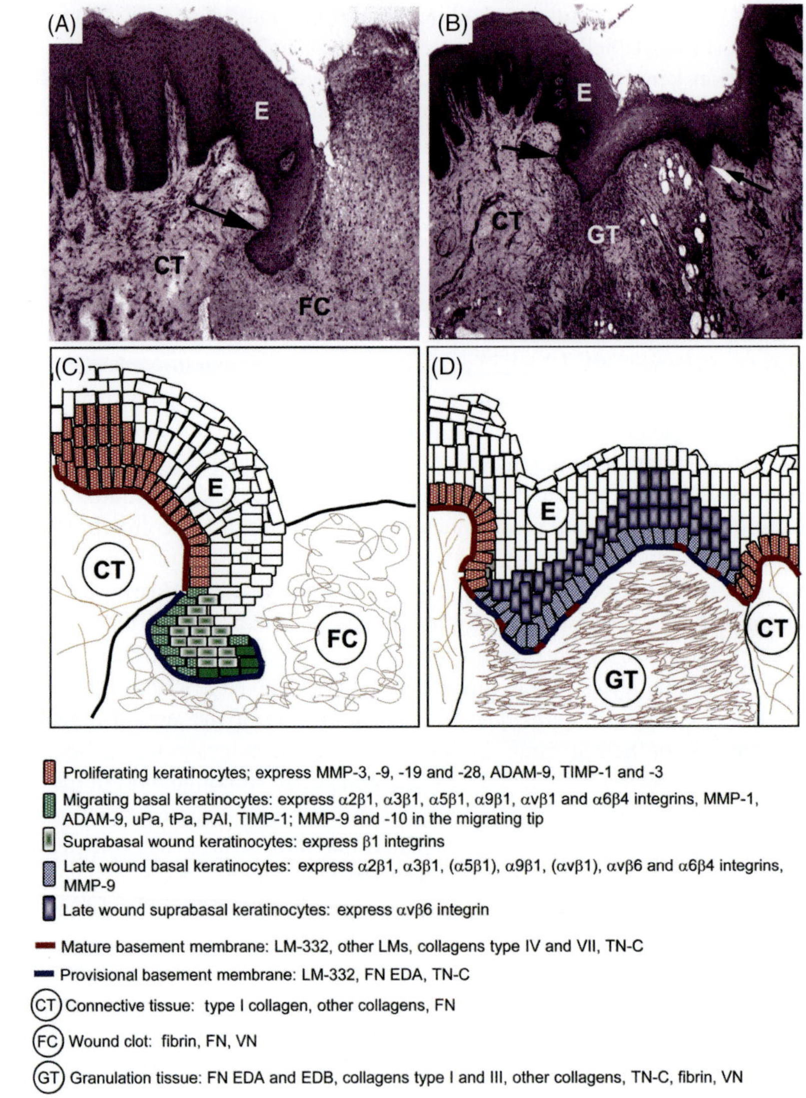

Fig. 5.2 Structural organization [hematoxylin-eosin staining (A, B) and schematic presentation (C, D)] of wounded human gingival mucosa, including integrin, proteinase and extracellular matrix molecule expression patterns. Three-day wound (early wound; A, C) and 7-day wound (migrating epithelial fronts have just joined; B, D). E, epithelium; CT, connective tissue; FC, fibrin clot; GT, granulation tissue; FN, fibronectin; LM, laminin; TN, tenascin; VN, vitronectin. Arrows mark the wound margin. Red cells, proliferating wound edge keratinocytes; blue cells, activated wound keratinocytes.

MANY DIFFERENT FACTORS CONTRIBUTE TO RE-EPITHELIALIZATION

Wound healing involves coordinated expression of several new extracellular matrix molecules, their receptors (integrins) and proteinases, which cleave matrix molecules to reveal functionally active domains within these molecules and release matrix-bound growth factors (Davis et al. 2000; Kirfel and Herzog 2004; Fig. 5.1). The contact of keratinocyte integrins with these pro-migratory wound matrix molecules and binding of soluble motogenic cytokines and growth factors to their receptors on the cell surface of the wound edge keratinocytes then collaboratively promote wound closure (Streuli and Akhtar 2009). In addition, loss of neighboring cells, disruption of cell–cell contacts by decreased extracellular Ca^{2+} concentration and changes in the intra-epithelial electrical field contribute to the re-epithelialization process (Kirfel and Herzog 2004; Song et al. 2004; Zhao 2009; Fig. 5.1).

Keratinocytes become exposed to novel extracellular matrix molecules in wounds

In unwounded tissue, basal epithelial cells are in close proximity with the extracellular matrix components of the intact basement membrane, including laminin-111 (formerly known as laminin-1), laminin-332 (formerly laminin-5) and type IV collagen. Rapidly after formation of a full-thickness epithelial wound that penetrates the basement membrane, keratinocytes come into contact with a new pericellular environment, consisting of the type I collagen- and fibronectin-rich connective tissue and the plasma-derived proteins, including fibronectin, fibrinogen and vitronectin, which are recruited to the wound site by the injury-induced vascular permeability (Davis et al. 2000). In the blood clot, plasma fibronectin is cross-linked to fibrin and assembled into a polymerized matrix (Figs. 5.1 and 5.2), which acts as a scaffold for further accumulation of other molecules, such as denatured collagen released from the wound margin connective tissue by proteolysis (see below) and heparin released by activated mast cells during tissue injury (Johansson and Hook 1980; Ruoslahti et al. 1982; Noli and Miolo 2001; Pankov and Yamada 2002). Wound matrix also contains matricellular molecules, such as osteopontin, thrombospondins, SPARC (secreted protein acidic and rich in cysteine), tenascins and alternatively spliced forms of fibronectin that are released or synthesized by cells in the injury site (e.g. mesenchymal cells and macrophages) and modulate tissue repair (Brown et al. 1993; Reed et al. 1993; Davis et al. 2000; Häkkinen et al. 2000a).

Wound keratinocytes also deposit and process their own matrix. For example, the migrating keratinocytes assemble alternatively spliced EDA (extra domain A) fibronectin underneath themselves against the wound bed matrix in the leading epithelial front during re-epithelialization (ffrench-Constant et al. 1989; Larjava et al. 2002). They also deposit the unprocessed form of laminin-332 as well as tenascin-C and its large molecular weight splicing variant (Larjava et al. 1993; Kainulainen et al. 1998; Goldfinger et al. 1999; Häkkinen et al. 2000a; Fig 5.2). Notably, the unprocessed form of the $\alpha3$ chain in the heterotrimeric laminin-332 ($\alpha3\beta3\gamma2$) promotes keratinocyte migration, whereas its proteolytically processed form inhibits motility (O'Toole et al. 1997; Goldfinger et al. 1998). Epidermal hyaluronan, a secreted large, non-sulphated glycosaminoglycan, is also expressed in the wound margin where it may promote keratinocyte proliferation and migration (Oksala et al. 1995; Kaya et al. 1997). In addition, migrating keratinocytes appear to recognize the tracks of other keratinocytes and to migrate along them (Kirfel and Herzog 2004). This is supported by findings that, at least *in vitro*, migrating keratinocytes leave behind tracks of ripped-off membrane proteins and matrix molecules that provide multiple adhesion sites for other cells migrating behind them.

At present, it is not completely clear how the connective tissue, wound cell and blood clot-derived pericellular matrix regulates wound re-epithelialization. Studies in knockout

Table 5.1 Effect of knockout or overexpression of extracellular matrix molecules on re-epithelialization in mice.

ECM molecule	Method	Effect on re-epithelialization	Refs
Fibrinogen	Knockout	Re-epithelialization speed normal although migration pattern altered; increased epithelial hyperplasia. (Somewhat increased initial bleeding, defects in granulation tissue formation and reduced wound tensile strength)	1, 2
Fibronectin	Knockout	Not tested (embryonic lethal phenotype)	3
Plasma fibronectin	Hepatocyte-targeted knockout	No abnormalities	4
Fibronectin EDA	Exclusion of EDA domain	Keratinocyte migration normal; blurred border between the new epidermis and granulation tissue; ulceration in the newly formed epidermis; influx of inflammatory cells to ulcerated area	5
Laminin-332	Knockout of $\alpha 3$ or $\gamma 2$ subunit of laminin-332	Not tested (neonatal lethal phenotype). (Epidermal/dermal blistering; apoptosis in the basal cells of the blistered skin; abnormal hemidesmosomes in intact epithelium)	6, 7
Tenascin-C	Knockout	Skin wound re-epithelialization normal; defects in corneal wound re-epithelialization; reduced fibronectin expression in wounds	8, 9
Tenascin-X	Knockout	Re-epithelialization normal. (Defects in granulation tissue remodeling and maturation)	10
Vitronectin	Knockout	Keratinocyte migration normal. (Slightly delayed dermal wound healing)	11
Thrombospondin-1	Overexpression (K14-promoter)	Keratinocyte migration normal. (Delayed wound closure; reduced granulation tissue formation and diminished wound angiogenesis)	12
Thrombospondin-2	Knockout	Keratinocyte migration normal; thickened epithelium. (Accelerated wound healing with reduced inflammation and scarring; altered granulation tissue organization and vascularization)	13
Osteopontin	Knockout	Re-epithelialization normal. (Defects in granulation tissue organization)	14
SPARC	Knockout	Re-epithelialization normal. (Accelerated wound closure due to enhanced granulation tissue contractibility)	15
Hevin (SPARC-like 1)	Knockout	Re-epithelialization normal. (Accelerated wound closure due to enhanced granulation tissue formation)	16

Effects on the other aspects of wound healing mentioned in brackets. References: [1] Bugge et al. 1996; [2] Drew et al. 2001; [3] George et al. 1993; [4] Sakai et al. 2001; [5] Muro et al. 2003; [6] Ryan et al. 1999; [7] Meng et al. 2003; [8] Forsberg et al. 1996; [9] Mackie and Tucker 1999; [10] Egging et al. 2007; [11] Jang et al. 2000; [12] Streit et al. 2000; [13] Kyriakides et al. 1999; [14] Liaw et al. 1998; [15] Bradshaw et al. 2002; [16] Sullivan et al. 2008 mice have provided some insight into the importance of the various extracellular matrix molecules for wound re-epithelialization *in vivo* (details and references in Table 5.1). Wound re-epithelialization in most of the knockout mouse models appears normal, although many exhibit changes in other aspects of wound healing (e.g. in granulation tissue formation and vascularization). Fibrin matrix assembly in the wound clot and re-epithelialization also proceed normally in the absence of plasma fibronectin. However, transgenic mice that are unable to express EDA fibronectin exhibit impaired skin wound re-epithelialization. While knocking out laminin-332 produces a neonatal lethal phenotype in mice, other evidence points to its importance for wound re-epithelialization. Importantly, people with laminin-332 mutations suffer from profoundly compromised epithelial healing of wounds (Schneider et al. 2007). Also cell culture experiments point to its essential role in keratinocyte migration (Hartwig et al. 2007). Thus, the matrix molecules that the migrating keratinocytes assemble underneath themselves in the leading epithelial front during re-epithelialization (e.g. EDA fibronectin and laminin-332) appear, indeed, more fundamental for wound closure than the proteins derived from the connective tissue or blood clot.

Integrins are signaling molecules that mediate cell adhesion to extracellular matrix and cell migration

The interaction of cells with extracellular matrix molecules is mainly mediated by integrins, a family of cell-surface glycoproteins consisting of two subunits, α and β, that are noncovalently associated with each other. In addition to attaching the cell to its surrounding matrix, integrins convey two-way signaling across the plasma membrane, influencing cell growth, differentiation, survival, morphology and migration (Häkkinen et al. 2000b; Hynes 2002; Stupack 2005; Legate et al. 2009; Fig. 5.3). Integrin affinity (the binding of an integrin to a single ligand motif) and avidity (combined affinity of integrins to multiple ligand binding sites that can be modified by integrin clustering by the ligands) can induce different signaling events (Defilippi et al. 1999; Giancotti and Ruoslahti 1999; Krissansen 2001; DeMali et al. 2003; Fig. 5.3). One integrin can typically bind several different matrix molecules and, additionally, many matrix molecules are recognized by several different integrin heterodimers (Table 5.2).

The maximum cell migration speed is achieved at an intermediate ratio of cell-substrate adhesiveness (DiMilla et al. 1991; Palecek et al. 1997; Greenwood and Murphy-Ullrich 1998). Substratum ligand level, the level of integrin expression in cells and integrin–ligand binding affinity all contribute to the strength of cell adhesion. Strong adhesion of cells to matrix molecules prevents the cells from detaching, whereas weak adhesion does not generate the contractile force that is necessary for directional cell movement. Controlled de-adhesion has been proposed as an initial step in the induction of cell motility (Greenwood and Murphy-Ullrich 1998). It may thus be beneficial for keratinocyte migration on the wound composite matrix to utilize several intermediate strength integrin–matrix interactions in cooperation.

Integrin-mediated signaling pathways show heterodimer-specific variations that can be modified further by integrin association with transmembrane adaptor proteins and membrane lipids, such as caveolin-1, members of the transmembrane-4 superfamily (also called tetraspanins or tetraspans), growth factor receptors and urokinase-type plasminogen activator receptor (uPAR) (Hemler 1998; Porter and Hogg 1998; Giancotti and Ruoslahti 1999; Berditchevski 2001; Krissansen 2001; Kugler et al. 2003; Ivaska and Heino 2010; Table 5.3). Several types of these molecules can accumulate in the same complexes and

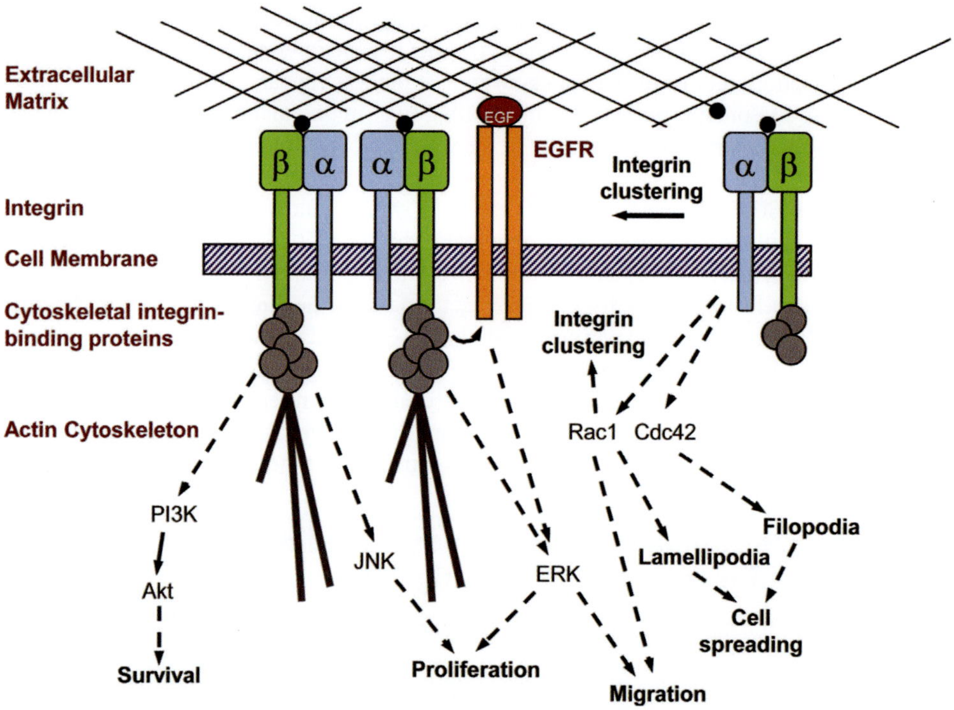

Fig. 5.3 Schematic presentation of common integrin-mediated signaling pathways that regulate cell spreading, proliferation, migration and survival. Integrin engagement leads to cytoplasmic accumulation of several different cytoskeletal proteins such as paxillin, talin, vinculin and α-actinin, and the subsequent integrin clustering triggers the β subunit cytoplasmic domain-mediated activation and autophosphorylation of focal adhesion kinase (FAK), creating a binding site for protein tyrosine kinases of the Src family. Subsequently, adaptor proteins, including Grb2, Ras, Sos, Fyn, phosphatidylinositol 3-kinase (PI3K) and p130Cas, are recruited and assembled to these cytoplasmic complexes, linking the integrin β subunit cytoplasmic tails to cellular signaling pathways and to the actin cytoskeleton. (The cytoplasmic tail of β4 integrin is an exception as it associates with the keratin intermediate filaments instead of actin.) Main pathways that are activated by integrin complexes include the activation of mitogen-activated protein kinase (MAPK) cascades, leading to the activation of extracellular signal-regulated kinases (ERK) and c-Jun amino terminal kinase (JNK), which regulate cell growth and/or motility. Interaction of EGFR with activated integrins results in EGFR transactivation and further activation of MAPK signaling that is synergistically enhanced by ligand binding to EGFR. PI3K activation by integrin complexes and the subsequent activation of protein kinase B/Akt (PKB/Akt) promote cell survival and protect adherent epithelial cells from apoptosis. Epithelial cell survival also requires FAK activation and paxillin tyrosine phosphorylation. Via organization of the cytoskeleton, integrin binding to the ligand can activate Rac and Cdc42, two small GTPases of the Rho family that regulate actin polymerization to form lamellipodia and filopodia, respectively. Rac1 also promotes integrin clustering, which may cause further Rac1 activation, establishing a positive feedback loop. The picture is by necessity simplified and excludes many important signaling molecules that are associated with integrin-mediated cellular signaling pathways. In addition, much of the data concerning these pathways have been obtained by using fibroblasts and other non-keratinocytic cell lines and may not directly apply to keratinocytes in all aspects. [References: Khwaja et al. 1997; D'Souza-Schorey et al. 1998; Price et al. 1998; Giancotti and Ruoslahti 1999; Huang et al. 2004; Legate and Fässler 2009; Moser et al. 2009; Zouq et al. 2009.]

affect each other's functions (e.g. Toledo et al. 2005). These binding partners may alter integrin conformation and affinity directly, modulate the avidity of integrins by regulating their clustering, assist in recruiting signaling molecules to cell adhesion sites, regulate receptor endocytosis or facilitate cell migration through tissues. The importance of cellular

Table 5.2 Keratinocyte integrins in re-epithelialization.

Integrin	Epithelial ligands	Expression in wounds	Functions	Involvement in re-epithelialization in animal models	Refs
$\alpha 2\beta 1$	Collagens (types I and III with high avidity), LM-332, MMP-1	Expressed: leading edge of migrating front, basal and lateral surfaces	Regulates expression and localization of MMP-1; mediates keratinocyte migration on fibrillar collagen and LM-332; may support the innate epithelial immune system	Re-epthelialization normal in $\alpha 2$ integrin knockout mice; increased neoangiogenesis	1–6
$\alpha 3\beta 1$	LM-332, other LMs, (collagens, FN)	Expressed: leading edge of migrating front, basal and lateral surfaces	Binds to newly deposited LM-332; regulates maintenance of basement membrane; maintains keratinocyte adhesion during migration; promotes keratinocyte survival; regulates cell polarization; delays keratinocyte migration; controls wound angiogenesis and TGF-β1-mediated responses	Keratinocyte migration is slightly accelercted or not affected with normal proliferation in keratinocyte-targeted $\alpha 3$ integrin knockout mice; re-epithelialization is retarded in $\alpha 3$ integrin null mouse skin grafts	7–15
$\alpha 5\beta 1$	FN	Expressed: leading edge of migrating front	Promotes keratinocyte migration, mediates cell growth signaling and suppresses apoptosis	Not tested (embryonic lethal phenotype)	16–20
$\alpha 9\beta 1$	TN-C, FN EDA	Upregulated: leading edge of migrating front	May regulate cell migration on TN-C and FN EDA; controls keratinocyte proliferation	Reduced keratinocyte proliferation, thinner migrating epithelium and delayed wound closure in keratinocyte-targeted $\alpha 9$ integrin knockout mice	21–27
$\alpha 6\beta 4$	LM-332, other LMs	Expressed: lateral localization at the leading edge, basal localization distally	Promotes keratinocyte adhesion, motility and proliferation; may regulate HGF signaling	Deletion of $\beta 4$ integrin intracellular signaling domain causes decelerated wound re-epithelialization and reduced keratinocyte migration	17, 28, 29

(*Continued*)

Table 5.2 (*Continued*).

Integrin	Epithelial ligands	Expression in wounds	Functions	Involvement in re-epithelialization in animal models	Refs
$\alpha v\beta 1$	FN, VN, latent TGF-β1	Expressed: leading edge of migrating front	Mediates cell adhesion to FN; may help to sequester a pool of inactive TGF-β1 into close proximity of the cells		24, 30, 31
$\alpha v\beta 5$	VN, latent TGF-β1	Upregulated in skin wounds: leading edge of migrating front. Not detected in oral mucosal wounds	May mediate keratinocyte migration on VN	Re-epithelialization is normal in β5 integrin knockout mice	30, 32–34
$\alpha v\beta 6$	FN, TN-C, VN, latent TGF-β1	Expressed: basal and suprabasal keratinocyte layers; strongest when migrating fronts joined	Regulates inflammation and keratinocyte proliferation; contributes to basement membrane reorganization and granulation tissue remodeling; activator of TGF-β1 and TGF-β3; downregulates uPAR expression and function; induces the expression of MMP-9	Re-epithelialization is normal in β6 integrin knockout mice if not challenged; faster epithelial advancement and more robust keratinocyte proliferation in knockouts after glucocorticoid treatment; mice with keratinocyte-targeted β6 integrin overexpression are susceptible to chronic, non-healing wounds	24, 31, 33, 35–42
$\alpha v\beta 8$	LM-111, type IV collagen, FN, latent TGF-β1	Not reported (expressed in suprabasal keratinocytes in intact epithelium)	–		43, 44

FN, fibronectin; LM, laminin; MMP, matrix metalloproteinase; TGF, transforming growth factor; TN, tenascin; VN, vitronectin.

References: [1] Pilcher et al. 1997; [2] Décline and Rousselle 2001; [3] Chen et al. 2002; [4] Grenache et al. 2007; [5] Parks 2007; [6] Zweers et al. 2007; [7] Carter et al. 1991; [8] DiPersio et al. 1997; [9] Oh et al. 2002; [10] Choma et al. 2004; [11] Frank and Carter 2004; [12] Manohar et al. 2004; [13] Reynolds et al. 2008; [14] Margadant et al. 2009; [15] Mitchell et al. 2009; [16] Cavani et al. 1993; [17] Larjava et al. 1993; [18] Yang et al. 1993; [19] Zhang et al. 1995; [20] Bata-Csorgo et al. 1998; [21] Palmer et al. 1993; [22] Yokosaki et al. 1994; [23] Häkkinen et al. 2000a; [24] Larjava et al. 2002; [25] Liao et al. 2002; [26] Singh et al. 2004; [27] Singh et al. 2009; [28] Trusolino et al. 2001; [29] Nikolopoulos et al. 2005; [30] Munger et al. 1998; [31] Munger et al. 1999; [32] Juhasz et al. 1993; [33] Haapasalmi et al. 1996; [34] Huang et al 2000; [35] Breuss et al. 1995; [36] Huang et al. 1996; [37] Niu et al. 1998; [38] Annes et al. 2002; [39] Dalvi et al. 2004; [40] Häkkinen et al. 2004; [41] AlDahlawi et al. 2006; [42] Xie et al. 2009; [43] Stepp 1999; [44] Cambier et al. 2000.

Table 5.3 Some examples of transmembrane proteins and membrane lipids that form complexes with integrins and modulate their function and cellular signaling.

Adaptor molecule	Partner	Mechanism of action	Effect on keratinocytes	Refs
Caveolin-1	α5β1 integrin	Integrin cluster formation; organization of specialized plasma membrane rafts enriched in Src kinases; MAPK pathway activation	Cell survival	1, 2
CD9 tetraspanin	α3β1 integrin	Recruitment of signaling molecules (e.g. PKC)	Cell motility	3–5
CD9 tetraspanin	α6β4 integrin	Recruitment of signaling molecules	Cell motility	6
CD81 tetraspanin	α3β1 integrin	Recruitment of signaling molecules (e.g. PI4K and PKC)	Cell motility	4, 5, 7
CD151 tetraspanin	α3β1 integrin	Recruitment of signaling molecules; modulation of the integrin ligand-binding activity through stabilizing its activated conformation	Cell motility, adhesion and proliferation on LM-332; basement membrane organization	8–10
CD151 tetraspanin	α6β4 integrin	Recruitment of signaling molecules	Hemidesmosome organization; cell motility, adhesion and proliferation on LM-332; basement membrane organization; re-epithelialization and basement membrane organization are impaired in CD151-null mouse skin wounds	9–11
EGFR	α5β1 integrin	Receptor clustering; synergistically enhanced MAPK signaling	Cell proliferation and motility	12–15
EGFR	α6β4 integrin	Activation of integrin-associated tyrosine kinase Fyn, phosphorylation of β4 integrin cytoplasmic domain	Disruption of hemidesmosomes; cell motility and proliferation	16–17
uPAR	α3β1 integrin	Focalized activation of plasmin; plasmin-mediated digestion of LM-332	Invasion to the fibrin clot during wound healing	18, 19
Ganglioside GT1b	α5β1 integrin	Abrogation of α5β1 integrin–fibronectin interaction	Inhibition of cell adhesion and migration on fibronectin	20–22
Ganglioside GM3	β1 integrins	Disruption of β1 integrin–EGFR association; abrogation of integrin-mediated, ligand-independent EGFR signaling	Inhibition of cell proliferation	23, 24

EGFR, epidermal growth factor receptor; LM, laminin; MAPK, mitogen-activated protein kinase; PI4K, phosphatidylinositol 4-kinase; PKC, protein kinase C; uPAR, urokinase-type plasminogen activator receptor.

References: [1] Wary et al. 1996; [2] Wary et al. 1998; [3] Jones et al. 1996; [4] Peñas et al. 2000; [5] Zhang et al. 2001; [6] Baudoux et al. 2000; [7] Berditchevski et al. 1997; [8] Nishiuchi et al. 2005; [9] Cowin et al. 2006; [10] Geary et al. 2008; [11] Sterk et al. 2000; [12] Miyamoto et al. 1996; [13] Moro et al. 1998; [14] Kuwada and Li 2000; [15] ffrench-Constant and Colognato 2004; [16] Mainiero et al. 1996; [17] Mariotti et al. 2001; [18] Ghosh et al. 2000; [19] Steffensen et al. 2001; [20] Paller et al. 1995; [21] Sung et al. 1998; [22] Wang et al. 2001; [23] Paller et al. 1993; [24] Wang et al. 2003.

signaling pathways jointly mediated by integrins and growth factors for wound closure has been evidenced in recent animal studies, in which deficiencies in extracellular signal-regulated kinase-2 (ERK2), signal tranducer and activation of transcription 3 (Stat3) or Rac1 signaling impairs re-epithelialization (DiPersio 2007; Tscharntke et al. 2007; Sano et al. 2008; Satoh et al. 2009; Castilho et al. 2010).

Epithelial keratinocytes need to readjust their cell adhesion receptors to interact with the wound matrix and to modulate cellular signaling

Basal keratinocytes in healthy epithelium express mainly α3β1, α2β1, α9β1 and α6β4 integrins which serve to anchor the cells to the underlying basement membrane as well as to maintain normal epithelial proliferation and differentiation patterns and the innate epithelial immune system (Häkkinen et al. 2000a; Watt 2002; Parks 2007; Margadant et al. 2010). During wound healing, keratinocytes have to adjust their integrin receptors to be able to adhere and migrate on the wound matrix proteins (see above) that resting keratinocytes do not normally encounter. Thus, an exposure to these novel matrix molecules and the influence of growth factors and cytokines in the wound environment causes a change in the expression levels and/or distribution of the existing keratinocyte integrins and induces novel matrix receptors, most notably the three fibronectin receptor integrins, α5β1, αvβ1 and αvβ6 (Larjava et al. 1993, 1996; Table 5.2).

Expression and localization of α2β1, α3β1 and α9β1 integrins are altered to mediate novel functions during wound closure

The expression of β1 integrins is strongly upregulated after wounding and expands to several suprabasal keratinocyte layers (Cavani et al. 1993; Juhasz et al. 1993; Larjava et al. 1993; Fig. 5.2). Their expression is critical for proper re-epithelialization, and mice with keratinocyte-specific knockout of the β1 integrin subunit display severely impaired wound keratinocyte migration (Raghavan et al. 2000; Grose et al. 2002). However, the importance of the individual α subunit partners of the β1 subunit in mediating re-epithelialization is not yet clearly understood.

In early skin wounds, keratinocytes come into contact with fibrillar dermal collagens (mainly type I collagen) that become exposed at the wound edge. The major keratinocyte collagen receptor, α2β1 integrin, binds collagen with high affinity and, therefore, this interaction is unlikely to support cell migration. Instead, it induces the expression of matrix metalloproteinase-1 (MMP-1) in keratinocytes (Pilcher et al. 1997), producing a focalized denaturation of the collagen matrix. Integrin α2β1 shows minimal binding to denatured collagen (Davis 1992). Since keratinocytes do not express any other known receptors for denatured collagen, they cannot directly migrate on it. However, denatured collagen may aid wound matrix assembly by binding other matrix proteins that support cell migration (see above). This process may help to regulate the directionality of keratinocyte migration in wounds (Pilcher et al. 1997). In addition to collagen, α2β1 integrin may recognize another ligand during re-epithelialization. In wounds, most of the laminin-332 γ2 chains produced by migrating keratinocytes are present in an unprocessed form that can serve as ligands for α2β1 integrin to mediate keratinocyte migration (Décline and Rousselle 2001). While knockout mouse studies have shown that these functions of α2β1 integrin can be compensated by other mechanisms in the mouse skin wound healing, it is indispensable for human skin re-epithelialization with dense dermis consisting of thick fibrillar collagens (Parks 2007; Table 5.2). It is not yet known whether α2β1 integrin is also required for the re-epithelialization of human oral mucosal wounds where the keratinocytes migrate through the wound clot and not beneath it on the connective tissue as in the skin (Larjava et al. 1993; Woodley 1996).

The role of the other major keratinocyte β1 integrin, the laminin-332 receptor α3β1, in re-epithelialization is complex. Depending on the experimental setup, it can either advance or inhibit migration of cultured keratinocytes (Kim et al. 1992; Zhang and Kramer 1996; Goldfinger et al. 1999; Décline and Rousselle 2001; deHart et al. 2003). Animal studies indicate that α3β1 integrin either does not affect keratinocyte migration during skin wound re-epithelialization or delays it by binding to the laminin-332 that is newly deposited on the wound bed at the rear of the cell, thus regulating cell polarization and maintaining adhesion during migration (Frank and Carter 2004; Margadant et al. 2009; Mitchell et al. 2009; Table 5.2). On the other hand, this integrin may also augment re-epithelialization by controlling transforming growth factor-β1 (TGF-β1)-mediated responses in the wound or by functioning as a trans-dominant inhibitor of other β1 integrins, including α2β1 and α5β1 (Hodivala-Dilke et al. 1998; Reynolds et al. 2008), providing yet another mechanism for the migrating keratinocytes to reduce the strength of their attachment during re-epithelialization. Keratinocyte α3β1 integrin also regulates wound angiogenesis by promoting the expression of pro-angiogenic factor mitogen-regulated protein 3 (MRP3) in epidermis (Mitchell et al. 2009).

The expression of α9β1 integrin is upregulated in the migrating basal epithelial cells at the leading edge during early wound repair of human oral mucosal wounds and rat skin wounds, coinciding with the deposition of its ligands tenascin-C and fibronectin EDA (Häkkinen et al. 2000a; Larjava et al. 2002; Singh et al. 2004; Table 5.2). While integrin α9β1 may also participate in the regulation of cell migration, it seems to be crucial for keratinocyte proliferation at the wound edge. Mice with conditional α9 integrin knockout in keratinocytes display poor skin wound re-epithelialization due to significantly reduced number of proliferating keratinocytes (Singh et al. 2009; Table 5.2).

Integrin α6β4 signaling is necessary for re-epithelialization and EGF signaling

After basement membrane disruption by wounding, the wound edge keratinocytes detach from the basement membrane and dissolve their hemidesmosomes. Integrin α6β4, which is a receptor for laminin-332 and a part of the hemidesmosome, loses its basal localization and its distribution around basal keratinocytes becomes diffuse (Larjava et al. 1993, 1996; Borradori and Sonnenberg 1999). Chemotactic factors (e.g. EGF; see below) promote the mobilization of α6β4 integrin from hemidesmosomes, leading to its localization to wound edge actin protrusions in migrating keratinocytes and other epithelial cells *in vitro*; this is associated with increased phosphorylation of the β4 integrin cytoplasmic domain (Gipson et al. 1993; Mainiero et al. 1996; Lotz et al. 2000; Santoro et al. 2003; Margadant et al. 2008). The expression of α6β4 integrin seems to be necessary for EGF-induced keratinocyte migration, and abolition of α6β4 integrin signaling leads to delayed re-epithelialization and reduced keratinocyte migration in mouse skin wounds (Russell et al. 2003; Nikolopoulos et al. 2005; Table 5.2). In a later phase of wound healing, α6β4 integrin relocates back to the basal surface of keratinocytes that are away from the wound edge and binds to the proteolytically cleaved α3 subunit of laminin-332, stabilizing epithelial attachment to the reforming basement membrane.

Fibronectin receptor integrins regulate multiple aspects of re-epithelialization

In normal resting adult epithelium, keratinocytes do not interact with fibronectin and thus do not typically express fibronectin receptors (Larjava et al. 1993; Haapasalmi et al. 1996; Häkkinen et al. 2000b). Upon wounding, keratinocytes come into contact with the fibronectin-rich provisional matrix and start expressing three different new fibronectin receptor integrins, α5β1, αvβ1 and αvβ6 (Larjava et al. 1993; Häkkinen et al. 2000a; Fig. 5.2; Table 5.2).

Induction of α5β1 fibronectin receptor expression occurs at early stages of wound healing when the epithelium starts to migrate across the wound provisional matrix (Cavani et al. 1993; Larjava et al. 1993, 2002; Fig. 5.2; Table 5.2). It promotes keratinocyte adhesion and motility and its interaction with EDA fibronectin may also contribute to the increased proliferation of the non-migratory keratinocytes behind the leading edge during wound healing (Zhang et al. 1995; Bata-Csorgo et al. 1998; Table 5.2). Tenascin-C present underneath the migrating keratinocytes reduces the strength of high affinity fibronectin binding to α5β1 integrin and may thereby transform this interaction to more conducive for cell motility (Lightner and Erickson 1990; Hauzenberger et al. 1999; Ingham et al. 2004). While no obvious defects in re-epithelialization were detected in the tenascin-C-deficient mice, the loss of its expression was associated with significantly reduced deposition of fibronectin underneath the migrating epithelium in both skin and corneal wounds (Forsberg et al. 1996; Mackie and Tucker 1999).

Integrin αvβ1 is strongly expressed by basal epithelial cells located against the fibrin-fibronectin clot and at the tip of the migrating front in re-epithelializing human oral mucosal wounds (Larjava et al. 2002; Fig. 5.2; Table 5.2). It is a low affinity fibronectin receptor that can mediate cell adhesion to fibronectin but only weakly supports keratinocyte migration (Vogel et al. 1990; Zhang et al. 1993; Koivisto et al. 1999). It may thus facilitate keratinocyte migration on the underlying fibronectin EDA during re-epithelialization by supporting cell attachment without decelerating the migration speed. While αvβ1 integrin interacts with the latency-associated peptide of the TGF-β1 complex, unlike αvβ6 integrin (see below), it is not capable of activating it (Munger et al. 1998, 1999). It may, however, help to sequester a pool of inactive TGF-β1 into close proximity of the cells where it can be activated, for example, by proteolytic cleavage when necessary (Yu and Stamenkovic 2000; Maeda et al. 2001).

In early healing of oral mucosal and skin wounds, migrating keratinocytes occasionally weakly express αvβ6 integrin that localizes against the fibrin-fibronectin clot and to the tip of the migrating cell sheet together with its substrates fibronectin EDA and tenascin-C (Breuss et al. 1995; Haapasalmi et al. 1996; Huang et al. 1998; Häkkinen et al. 2000a; Larjava et al. 2002). The expression of αvβ6 integrin is, however, most prominently upregulated in basal and several suprabasal keratinocyte layers after the epithelial sheets have joined, coinciding with basement membrane reorganization and granulation tissue formation (Haapasalmi et al. 1996; Fig. 5.2; Table 5.2). It regulates keratinocyte proliferation, inflammation and deposition of extracellular matrix in the granulation tissue by locally activating matrix-bound TGF-β1 and presenting it to the neighboring epithelial cells and/or fibroblasts (Wipff and Hinz 2008; Xie et al. 2009; Margadant and Sonnenberg 2010; Table 5.2). In addition, αvβ6 integrin-mediated signaling downregulates the expression and function of uPAR (see below) and induces the expression of MMP-9, which is required for remodeling of the basement membrane zone and for removal of the fibrin provisional matrix during late wound healing (Mohan et al. 2002; Dalvi et al. 2004).

Several types of cell adhesion molecules in different wound cells jointly contribute to wound healing

Integrin expression in cells other than keratinocytes in the wound environment can also influence re-epithelialization, highlighting the cross-talk between the different cell types within the wound. For example, knocking out neutrophil and monocyte integrin Mac-1 delays skin wound re-epithelialization in mice, whereas elimination of $\alpha v\beta 3$ integrin that is expressed in wounds by platelets, endothelial cells, macrophages and dermal fibroblast accelerates it (Reynolds et al. 2005; Sisco et al. 2007).

While integrins are the major mediators of cell–extracellular matrix interactions, other types of keratinocyte cell surface adhesion receptors collaborate with them and may thus contribute to re-epithelialization (Morgan et al. 2007). Keratinocytes in human oral mucosal wounds express transmembrane heparan sulfate proteoglycans syndecan-1 and -4 which can mediate keratinocyte attachment to the unprocessed laminin-332 (Oksala et al. 1995; Gallo et al. 1996; Okamoto et al. 2003). It is not currently known whether this interaction promotes cell motility, as neither syndecan-1 nor syndecan-4 knockout mice exhibited defects in keratinocyte migration during re-epithelialization of skin wounds, although in the wounds of syndecan-1 null mice, keratinocyte proliferation was reduced (Echtermeyer et al. 2001; Stepp et al. 2002). Oral keratinocytes also express heparan sulfate proteoglycan CD44, a receptor for hyaluronan, which regulates their proliferation in wounds (Oksala et al. 1995; Kaya et al. 1997).

Growth factor receptors, including EGF receptor (EGFR), may interact with extracellular matrix molecules to promote keratinocyte migration by binding to their matrikine domains (Swindle et al. 2001; Tran et al. 2004). The individual EGF-like repeats of tenascin-C and laminin-332 bind to EGFR with very low affinity, but the presence of multiple repeats in these matrix proteins contributes to high-avidity interactions to favor migratory pathways over proliferative pathways (Swindle et al. 2001; Haugh 2002). In agreement with this principle, EGFR binding to these repeats initiates EGFR-dependent downstream signaling cascades, inducing motility rather than proliferation (Tran et al. 2004). EGF-like domains in matrix molecules may also serve to bring integrins into a close proximity with EGFR to potentiate their signaling.

Re-epithelialization also involves regulated de-adhesion. For example, the large variant of tenascin-C has been shown to decrease cell adhesiveness by binding to annexin II on the cell surface and to alter integrin–matrix interactions through modulation of intracellular signaling pathways (Chung and Erickson 1994; Chung et al. 1996). Since the expression of annexin II is induced in keratinocytes during early wound healing (Munz et al. 1997), this mechanism for modulating the dynamics of cell adhesiveness may also have an effect on re-epithelialization.

Cytokines and growth factors are important mediators of wound healing

Although they are apparently only able to stimulate cell migration when the cells are in contact with pro-migratory matrix molecules through integrins (Li et al. 2004), the cytokines and growth factors that are released by wound platelets in the clot and appended by inflammatory cells, fibroblasts and keratinocytes themselves are vital for the initiation and sustenance of re-epithelialization. Many growth factors bind to heparin, fibronectin or denatured collagen, which leads to their accumulation in the proximity of migrating keratinocytes (Davis et al. 2000). The major growth factors that regulate re-epithelialization include members of the EGF-family, TGF-β1 and KGFs, but also other growth factors and cytokines are involved (Table 5.4).

Table 5.4 The role of growth factors, cytokines and other secreted factors and their receptors in re-epithelialization.

Growth factor	Expression in wounds	Effects on keratinocytes	Involvement in re-epithelialization as evidenced by *in vivo* studies	Refs
EGF	Expressed by platelets, fibroblasts and mast cells	Promotes motility and proliferation; induces expression of $\alpha2\beta1$ integrin, uPA, MMP-1, MMP-9, fibronectin and LM-332; promotes hemidesmosome disassembly	Promotive: topical application of EGF enhances re-epithelialization	1–5
TGF-α	Expressed by platelets, macrophages, keratinocytes and fibroblasts; upregulated in keratinocytes 1–5 days after injury	Promotes motility and proliferation; induces expression of $\alpha2\beta1$ integrin	Promotive: topical application of TGF-α enhances re-epithelialization; delayed closure of ear wounds in TGF-α knockout mouse healing mainly by re-epithelialization but no significant differences in full thickness wound repair	2, 4, 6, 7
HB-EGF	Expressed by macrophages and keratinocytes; a major component in the wound fluid after injury in porcine skin and in human burn wounds	Promotes motility and proliferation; induces expression of MMP-1, HB-EGF; its expression and shedding are critical events for keratinocyte migration	Promotive: delayed re-epithelialization and reduced epithelial migration in keratinocyte-targeted HB-EGF knockout mice, keratinocyte proliferation normal	2, 4, 8–12
Amphiregulin	Expressed at the leading edge of migrating wound keratinocytes	Promotes proliferation		2, 13
Epiregulin	Expressed by keratinocytes and macrophages	Promotes proliferation	Redundant: normal wound repair in epiregulin knockout mice	2, 14, 15
EGF receptor (EGFR, ErbB1)	Strongly and transiently upregulated in keratinocytes at the wound edge localizing in the migrating tip of the advancing epithelium; also present in the hypertrophic proliferating area of epithelium	Binds to and is activated by EGF, TGF-α, HB-EGF, amphiregulin, betacellulin and epiregulin; collaboration with $\alpha5\beta1$ integrin induces both keratinocyte migration and proliferation during wound repair; blocking induces apoptosis; activation upregulates expression of $\alpha2\beta1$ integrin, uPA, MMP-1	Promotive: decreased proliferation and epithelial migration into the wound during the first 3 days after injury in EGFR null mouse skin grafts	2, 4, 13, 16–23
Heregulin-α	Expressed by keratinocytes; present in wound fluids	Promotes motility		13

NDF-α2	Expressed by fibroblasts (its receptor ErbB3 is strongly upregulated in keratinocytes at the wound edge)	Promotes motility and proliferation; induces expression of $\alpha5\beta1$, $\alpha6\beta4$ integrins	Promotive: topical application of NDF-α2 enhances re-epithelialization, epidermal migration and epidermal thickness	13, 16, 24
TGF-β1	An early surge of cytokine released by the degranulating platelets in the fibrin clot and by the infiltrating macrophages and fibroblasts; also expressed in wound edge keratinocytes; a second peak of expression when re-epithelialization is complete	Promotes motility; inhibits proliferation; induces expression of $\alpha5\beta1$, $\alpha v\beta5$ and $\alpha v\beta6$ integrins, FN EDA and uPA; prevents the proteolytic processing of both the $\alpha3$ and $\gamma2$ chains of LM-332; downregulates the expression of $\alpha3\beta1$ and $\alpha6\beta4$ integrins	Either promotive or restrictive depending on the study model: re-epithelialization normal in TGF-β1 knockout mice with increased rate, delayed wound repair at the later stages of healing due to severe inflammation; TGF-β1 overexpression stimulates re-epithelialization of partial thickness mouse ear wounds but delays it in full-thickness skin wounds with profound inflammation present; keratinocyte-targeted overexpression of dominant-negative TGF-β receptor accelerates re-epithelialization of full-thickness skin wounds, increased keratinocyte proliferation at the wound edge and reduced apoptosis in the re-epithelialized wounds; re-epithelialization is accelerated and keratinocyte proliferation increased in Smad3 (a signal mediator of TGF-β1) knockout mice	1, 4, 25–41
BMP-6	Upregulated in suprabasal keratinocyte layers distal to the wound edge; not in keratinocytes directly bordering the wound	Counteracts and controls hyperproliferation	Restrictive: keratinocyte-targeted overexpression of BMP-6 delays re-epithelialization; repression of keratinocyte proliferation during later stages of wound healing	42
Activin A	Expressed by mesenchymal cells in early wound healing	Inhibits the growth of cultured keratinocytes and induces their differentiation	Possibly promotive: keratinocyte-targeted overexpression of activin A may slightly accelerate re-epithelialization, increased keratinocyte proliferation, enhanced wound closure due to increased deposition of granulation tissue; keratinocyte-targeted overexpression of activin A antagonist follistatin resulted in thinner epithelium but re-epithelialization was not significantly altered; keratinocyte-targeted expression of dominant-negative activin A receptor slightly delayed re-epithelialization	43–47

(*Continued*)

Table 5.4 *(Continued)*.

Growth factor	Expression in wounds	Effects on keratinocytes	Involvement in re-epithelialization as evidenced by *in vivo* studies	Refs
KGF-1 (FGF-7)	Upregulated rapidly in dermal fibroblasts beneath the wound and at the wound after injury; remains elevated for several days	Promotes motility and proliferation; protects from apoptosis; increases attachment and migration on FN and Coll I by inducing $\beta 1$ integrin clustering and increasing integrin avidity; stimulates uPA, MMP-10 and TGF-α synthesis	Promotive but redundant: topical delivery of KGF-1 or its cDNA accelerates re-epithelialization, increases keratinocyte proliferation and decreases apoptosis; no defects in re-epithelialization in KGF-1-deficient mice	48–59
KGF-2 (FGF-10)	Expressed by fibroblasts; highly induced 1 day after injury, decreasing rapidly by 3 days in mouse skin wounds	Promotes motility and proliferation	Promotive: topical application of KGF-2 accelerates re-epithelialization	54, 57, 60
FGF-22	Expressed by keratinocytes; high expression in late stages of wound healing			61
KGF receptor; FGFR2-IIIb	Expressed by keratinocytes		Promotive: decreased keratinocyte proliferation at the wound edge by more than 90% and severely delayed resurfacing of wounds in mice with keratinocyte-targeted overexpression of defective KGF receptor	54, 57, 62
FGF-1			Promotive but redundant: topical application of FGF-1 stimulates re-epithelialization; wound healing normal in FGF-1 knockout mice	57, 63
FGF-2			Promotive: topical application of FGF-2 accelerates re-epithelialization; reduced re-epithelialization in FGF-2 knockout mice	57, 64
HGF/SF	Expressed by fibroblasts; increased transiently in early wounds together with its receptor c-Met	Promotes motility and proliferation; induces expression of FN EDA and MMP-9	Promotive: topical delivery of HGF/SF or its cDNA accelerates re-epithelialization; its neutralization with antibodies delays it	3, 65–70

IGF-1	Increased after wounding (fibroblasts, macrophages)	Promotes motility and proliferation; induces activation of PI3K and Rac1 GTPase	Promotive: topical delivery of IGF cDNA stimulates re-epithelialization and increases epithelial cell proliferation and KGF expression	71–75
sAPP	Expressed by platelets and keratinocytes; biphasic increase in mice: the first peak 1 day after injury and the second after 5 days (in the hyperproliferative epithelium at the wound margin)	Promotes motility and proliferation; operates synergistically with FN; motogenic action involves Rac1 activation		76–79
MSP	From blood plasma	Promotes motility and proliferation		80
GM-CSF	Secreted by keratinocytes shortly after injury	Promotes motility; modulates the release of cytokines (e.g. IL-1, IL-6, TNF-α, TGF-β1, IFN-γ)	Promotive: accelerated re-epithelialization; and increased proliferation of wound keratinocytes in mice with keratinocyte-targeted GM-CSF overexpression	81
IL-1	Increased within 24 hours of injury (keratinocytes, leucocytes, monocytes, macrophages)	Promotes proliferation; induces KGF and IL-6 expression in human and mouse dermal and gingival fibroblasts; promotes sAPP expression in keratinocytes	Promotive: topical application of IL-1α enhances re-epithelialization and increases keratinocyte proliferation	54, 77, 82–89
IL-6	Expressed by keratinocytes at the leading wound edge and by neutrophils	Promotes proliferation; decreases AP-1 transcription factor activation	Promotive: delayed re-epithelialization in IL-6-deficient mice and in mice wounds treated with a neutralizing IL-6 antibody	90–92
TNF-α	Increased transiently with maximal expression levels 6 hours after injury (keratinocytes, neutrophils, macrophages)	Promotes proliferation; downregulates TGF-β1 expression	Restrictive: enhanced re-epithelialization in TNF receptor knockout mice	87, 93
Angiotensin II	Expression increased in wounds (also its receptor)	Promotes motility and proliferation; induces HB-EGF expression and EGFR transactivation	Promotive: angiotensin II receptor knockout delays re-epithelialization	94

(*Continued*)

Table 5.4 (*Continued*).

Growth factor	Expression in wounds	Effects on keratinocytes	Involvement in re-epithelialization as evidenced by *in vivo* studies	Refs
ANGPTL4	Expressed by keratinocytes; increased after injury	Promotes motility; interacts with FN and VN in the wound bed delaying their proteolytic degradation by MMPs; regulates cell-matrix communications; binds to β1 and β5 integrins and modulates their signaling	Promotive: delayed re-epithelialization with reduced keratinocyte migration in ANGPTL4-deficient mice and in wounds with topically applied anti-ANGPTL4 antibody	95, 96
Acetylcholine		Promotes motility; regulates keratinocyte adhesion	Promotive: acetylcholine receptor α9 knockout delays re-epithelialization	97

ANGPTL4, angiopoietin-like 4; BMP, bone morphogenic protein; Coll, collagen; EGF, epidermal growth factor; FGF, fibroblast growth factor; FN, fibronectin; GM-CSF, granulocyte-macrophage colony-stimulating factor; HB-EGF, heparin-binding EGF-like growth factor; HGF/SF, hepatocyte growth factor/scatter factor; IFN, interferon; IGF, insulin-like growth factor; IL, interleukin; KGF, keratinocyte growth factor; LM, laminin; MSP, macrophage stimulating protein; NDF, neu differentiation factor; sAPP, secretory form of Alzheimer amyloid precursor protein; TGF, transforming growth factor; TNF, tumor necrosis factor; VN, vitronectin.

References: [1] Nickoloff et al. 1988; [2] Hudson and McCawley 1998; [3] McCawley et al. 1998; [4] Hashimoto 2000; [5] D'Alessio et al. 2008; [6] Antoniades et al. 1993; [7] Kim et al. 2001; [8] Marikovsky et al. 1993; [9] McCarthy et al. 1996; [10] Tokumaru et al. 2000; [11] Ellis et al. 2001; [12] Shirakata et al. 2005; [13] Schelfhout et al. 2002; [14] Shirakata et al. 2000; [15] Shirasawa et al. 2004; [16] Stoscheck et al. 1992; [17] Wenczak et al. 1992; [18] Chen et al. 1993; [19] Jensen and Rodeck 1993; [20] Nanney and King 1996; [21] Rodeck et al. 1997; [22] Pilcher et al. 1999; [23] Repertinger et al. 2004; [24] Danilenko et al. 1995; [25] Wikner et al. 1988; [26] Kane et al. 1991; [27] Levine et al. 1993; [28] Brown et al. 1995; [29] Zambruno et al. 1995; [30] Ashcroft et al. 1999; [31] Yang et al. 1999; [32] Koch et al. 2000; [33] Décline and Rousselle 2001; [34] Yang et al. 2001; [35] Amendt et al. 2002; [36] Chan et al. 2002; [37] Larjava et al. 2002; [38] Décline et al. 2003; [39] Falanga et al. 2004; [40] Tredget et al. 2005; [41] Wang et al. 2006; [42] Kaiser et al. 1998; [43] Hübner et al. 1996a; [44] Munz et al. 1999; [45] Seishima et al. 1999; [46] Wankell et al. 2001; [47] Bamberger et al. 2005; [48] Werner et al. 1992; [49] Tsuboi et al. 1993; [50] Dlugosz et al. 1994; [51] Marchese et al. 1995; [52] Guo et al. 1996; [53] Madlener et al. 1996; [54] Werner 1998; [55] Putnins et al. 1999; [56] Jeschke et al. 2002; [57] Steiling and Werner 2003; [58] Firth and Putnins 2004; [59] Marti et al. 2004; [60] Tagashira et al. 1997; [61] Beyer et al. 2003; [62] Werner et al. 1994; [63] Miller et al. 2000; [64] Ortega et al. 1998; [65] Matsumoto et al. 1991; [66] Inoue et al. 1999; [67] Nakanishi et al. 2002; [68] Yoshida et al. 2003; [69] Yoshida et al. 2004; [70] Bevan et al. 2004; [71] Rappolee et al. 1988; [72] Barreca et al. 1992; [73] Hodak et al. 1996; [74] Haase et al. 2003; [75] Jeschke et al. 2004; [76] Hoffman et al. 2000; [77] Kummer et al. 2002; [78] Kirfel et al. 2002; [79] Schmitz et al. 2002; [80] Wang et al. 1996; [81] Mann et al. 2001; [82] Sauder et al. 1990; [83] Waelti et al. 1992; [84] Brauchle et al. 1994; [85] Boxman et al. 1996; [86] Goretsky et al. 1996; [87] Hübner et al. 1996b; [88] Sanaie et al. 2002; [89] Efron and Moldawer 2004; [90] Grossman et al. 1989; [91] Gallucci et al. 2000; [92] Lin et al. 2003; [93] Mori et al. 2002; [94] Yahata et al. 2006; [95] Goh et al. 2010a; [96] Goh et al. 2010b; [97] Chernyavsky et al. 2007.

EGF family of growth factors promote keratinocyte migration and proliferation

Of the EGF family of growth factors, EGF, TGF-α, heparin-binding EGF-like growth factor (HB-EGF), amphiregulin, betacellulin and epiregulin bind to and activate homo- or heterodimers of EGFR (ErbB1), a receptor with intrinsic tyrosine kinase activity, and thereby promote mitogenesis and/or motility of keratinocytes (Hudson and McCawley 1998; Hashimoto 2000; Table 5.4). Activation of the EGFR by any EGFR ligand induces autocrine expression of other EGFR ligands in keratinocytes (cross-induction). EGFR ligands are synthesized as membrane-bound precursors and activated by ADAM (a disintegrin and matrix metalloproteinase)-mediated shedding to produce bioactive soluble growth factors (Higashiyama and Nanba 2005). After tissue injury, EGFR is strongly upregulated in keratinocytes at the wound edge, and it remains present in the hypertrophic proliferating area of epithelium until the proliferative phase ceases (Stoscheck et al. 1992; Wenczak et al. 1992; Schelfhout et al. 2002). Among the EGFR ligands, HB-EGF is a major component in the wound fluid (Marikovsky et al. 1993; McCarthy et al. 1996). Its autocrine expression and shedding are critical events for keratinocyte migration *in vivo* and also *in vitro* regardless of the type of the initial stimulus (Tokumaru et al. 2000; Ellis et al. 2001; Koivisto et al. 2006). Studies with cultured keratinocytes as well as results obtained from animal wound healing models indicate that EGFR signaling may promote re-epithelialization by at least three distinct mechanisms. First, in collaboration with integrin signaling, it can activate pro-migratory and pro-mitogenic cellular signaling pathways, especially the mitogen-activated protein kinase pathway. Second, it can induce disruption of hemidesmosomes and intercellular attachments to release keratinocytes for migration. Third, it can induce expression of integrins, proteases and matrix molecules that facilitate re-epithelialization (details and references in Table 5.4).

TGF-β1 promotes keratinocyte migration but inhibits their proliferation

The TGF-β superfamily consists of isoforms TGF-β1–5, of which TGF-β1–3 are expressed in humans, and related molecules, including bone morphogenic proteins (BMP) and activins. They bind to receptors with protein-serine/threonine kinase activity initiating signaling pathways that involve Smad proteins as cytoplasmic mediators (Hashimoto 2000). The degranulating platelets in the fibrin clot and infiltrating macrophages and fibroblasts release an early surge of active TGF-β1, while a second peak of TGF-β1 expression occurs when re-epithelialization is complete (Levine et al. 1993; Yang et al. 1999; Table 5.4). TGF-β1 inhibits the growth of keratinocytes but stimulates their motility by switching the cells from a differentiating to a regenerative phenotype (Hashimoto 2000). The role of TGF-β1 in the re-epithelialization is complex, and its proper spatio-temporal regulation is necessary for effective wound closure. Studies with transgenic animals and organotypic epithelial cell cultures have produced variable results with TGF-β1 either enhancing re-epithelialization due to increased keratinocyte migration or delaying it because of decreased keratinocyte proliferation, depending on the experimental model (Garlick and Taichman 1994; Reynolds et al. 2005; details and references in Table 5.4). TGF-β1 also seems to have a major function in regulation of inflammation and granulation tissue formation, as TGF-β1 null mice show delayed wound repair at the later stages of healing due to severe inflammation (Brown et al. 1995). On the other hand, its overexpresson has also been associated with profound inflammation in wounds (Wang et al. 2006), highlighting the importance of proper control of TGF-β1 activity for successful wound healing. Other members of the TGF-β superfamily are also involved in the re-epithelialization process (Table 5.4).

KGFs promote keratinocyte proliferation

In human and mouse skin wounds, KGF-1 (FGF-7) expression is upregulated rapidly after injury in dermal fibroblasts beneath the wound and at the wound edge, and it remains elevated for several days (Werner et al. 1992; Marchese et al. 1995). KGF-2 (FGF-10) expression is also highly induced (Tagashira et al. 1997). Both forms of KGF act on keratinocytes in a paracrine manner by binding to keratinocyte growth factor receptor (FGFR2-IIIb; KGFR) that is exclusively expressed in epithelial cells. Wound keratinocytes themselves also express a related growth factor, FGF-22, which acts via the same receptor in an autocrine manner (Beyer et al. 2003; Zhang et al. 2006). The activity of these KGFR ligands may be enhanced by the FGF-binding protein, which is also upregulated during wound healing (Beer et al. 2005). Results from studies using cultured keratinocytes, topical application of KGF-1 or KGF-2 to wounds and animal models with overexpression or knock down of the KGFs or their receptors show that KGFR signaling improves re-epithelialization by increasing keratinocyte proliferation, by protecting epithelial cells from apoptosis, and possibly also by enhancing keratinocyte migration (details and references in Table 5.4).

Keratinocytes express cytokines and growth factors that modulate wound healing beyond re-epithelialization

Cytokines and growth factors provide one mechanism for cross-talk between different cell types in the wound environment. In addition to the growth factors that regulate keratinocyte behavior during re-epithelialization, keratinocytes themselves express cytokines that affect other aspects of wound healing (Werner et al. 2007). For example, keratinocytes produce vascular endothelial growth factor, which mediates the ingrowth of new blood vessels into the wound bed, and platelet-derived growth factor-AA, which promotes growth and vascularization of the underlying dermal tissue (Brown et al. 1992; Eming et al. 1995). In addition, TGF-β1 produced by keratinocytes regulates fibroblast behavior, dermal remodeling, angiogenesis and inflammation in wounds and, when excessive, may even contribute to fibrosis, emphasizing the importance of keratinocytes in the whole process of wound healing (Häkkinen et al. 2004; Koskela et al. 2010; Owens et al. 2010).

Serine proteases and matrix metalloproteinases modulate extracellular matrix and generate biologically active molecules

An essential feature of wound healing is the controlled proteolytic degradation and substantial remodeling of the extracellular matrix that involves serine proteases, especially plasmin, as well as matrixins (MMPs) and transmembrane protease adamalysins (a disintegrin and metalloproteinase domain or ADAMs) (Steffensen et al. 2001; Higashiyama and Nanba 2005; Gill and Parks 2008). Their roles in re-epithelialization include removal of the provisional matrix, clearing paths for keratinocyte migration, pericellular proteolysis to loosen keratinocyte attachment and cell–cell contacts to allow migration, creation of biologically active matrix fragments (matricryptins) and the release and activation of growth factors from the extracellular matrix or cell surface (e.g. TGF-β1 and HB-EGF, respectively). Keratinocyte MMPs also regulate inflammation in wounds by controlling, for example, chemokine activity, establishment of chemotactic gradients and transepithelial migration of leukocytes (Parks et al. 2004; Gill and Parks 2008). Their activities need to be precisely controlled, as dysregulated proteolysis may contribute to the inability of wounds to heal (Pilcher et al. 1999; Philipp et al. 2004; see below).

Plasmin is required for keratinocyte invasion into the fibrin-fibronectin clot

To re-epithelialize a wound, the leading keratinocytes have to first proteolytically dissolve and remodel the fibrin barrier ahead of them to create a path for migration (Steffensen et al. 2001; Kirfel and Herzog 2004). Migrating keratinocytes are highly phagocytic, allowing them to penetrate into the clot (Woodley 1996). In skin, wound edge keratinocytes start migrating along the underlying exposed type I collagen-containing connective tissue underneath the fibrin-fibronectin clot. In oral mucosal wounds, however, the keratinocytes cut their path directly through the clot and may not directly interact with the connective tissue matrix (Larjava et al. 1993; Woodley 1996). The main enzyme for fibrinolysis is plasmin derived from plasminogen in the clot and activated either by urokinase-type plasminogen activator (uPA) or tissue-type plasminogen activator (tPA) on the cell surface. Both uPA and tPA as well as their receptor uPAR are upregulated at the migratory edge of the epithelium (Vaalamo et al. 1996). Association of uPAR with integrins on the keratinocyte cell surface leads to focalized activation of plasmin that is crucial for localized fibrin digestion at the leading edge and for the advancement of the epithelial front (Ghosh et al. 2000; Steffensen et al. 2001). Consequently, wound re-epithelialization is almost completely blocked in plasminogen-deficient as well as in uPA/tPA double knockout mice (Carmeliet et al. 1994; Rømer et al. 1996; Table 5.5). Since plasmin activity needs to be focalized and well controlled, the expression of plasminogen activator inhibitors (PAI) is also upregulated in the leading epithelial front. Plasmin may also serve other functions in re-epithelialization (details and references in Table 5.5).

Several MMPs are expressed during re-epithelialization

MMPs can cleave several components of the extracellular matrix as well as other types of molecules in wounds (Steffensen et al. 2001; Illman et al. 2008). Topical or systemic administration of broad-spectrum MMP inhibitors retards wound re-epithelialization without affecting the proliferation of wound keratinocytes, indicating that MMPs are involved in keratinocyte migration during wound healing *in vivo* (Lund et al. 1999; Ågren 1999 Ågren et al. 2001; Mirastschijski et al. 2004). Rather than exerting their activities freely in tissue fluid compartments, MMPs function in close proximity to cells and may be positioned, activated and released as needed from cell surfaces by several mechanisms (Basbaum and Werb 1996; Steffensen et al. 2001). In early wounds, the migrating wound keratinocytes express at least MMP-1 (interstitial collagenase), MMP-9 (92-kDa gelatinase, gelatinase B) and MMP-10 (stromelysin-2), while the proliferating, non-migrating keratinocytes at the wound margin express MMP-3 (stromelysin-1), MMP-9, MMP-19 (RASI) and MMP-28 (epilysin; references and details in Table 5.5). After re-epithelialization is complete, MMP-9 expression continues, whereas the expression of the other MMPs is downregulated (Parks 1999; Steffensen et al. 2001). Of these keratinocyte MMPs, at least MMP-9 appears essential for proper re-epithelialization, since wound keratinocyte migration is delayed and clearance of the fibrin clot is reduced in skin wounds of MMP-9-deficient mice (Kyriakides et al. 2009). In addition to keratinocytes, other cell types in the wound environment, including fibroblasts and macrophages, secrete MMPs into

Table 5.5 Proteinases in re-epithelialization.

Proteinase	Expression in wounds	Roles in re-epithelialization	Transgenic animal studies	Refs
Plasmin	Derived from plasminogen in the wound clot	Crucial for fibrin digestion and for the advancement of the epithelial front; cleaves fibronectin; cleaves the $\alpha3$ chain of LM-332 to render its structure conducive for hemidesmosome formation	Wound re-epithelialization almost completely blocked in plasminogen-deficient and in uPA/tPA double knockout mice	1–5
MMP-1	Expressed by migrating human keratinocytes in early wounds	Guides directional movement of the migrating keratinocytes by cleaving type I collagen; lessens the affinity of collagen–$\alpha2\beta1$ integrin contacts	Transgenic mice expressing mutated type I collagen resistant to collagenase cleavage display severely delayed re-epithelialization; transgenic mice overexpressing human MMP-1 in the epidermis show retarded re-epithelialization	6–11
MMP-3	Expressed by proliferating keratinocytes at the wound margin		Re-epithelialization normal in MMP-3-deficient mice, but wound contraction decreased	12
MMP-9	Expressed by both migrating and proliferating keratinocytes; expression continues after re-epithelialization is complete	Required for normal progression of wound closure; cleaves basement membrane collagens IV and VII; clears fibrin clots; regulates matrix deposition	MMP-9-deficient mice display compromised re-epithelialization and reduced clearance of fibrin clots; also exhibit abnormal matrix deposition, as evidenced by the irregular alignment of immature collagen fibers	13, 14
MMP-10	Expressed by migrating keratinocytes	May control keratinocyte migration in wounds by cleaving the $\gamma2$ chain of LM-332	Wound re-epithelialization rate normal but the migrating epidermal front is scattered and the deposition of LM-332 impaired in mouse skin overexpressing active MMP-10 in the basal keratinocytes	15, 16
MMP-19	Expressed by proliferating keratinocytes at the wound margin			17
MMP-28	Expressed by proliferating keratinocytes at the wound margin	Possibly associated with wound keratinocyte proliferation, basement membrane restructuring and intercellular adhesion cleavage		18
ADAM-9	Expressed by migrating and proliferating wound keratinocytes	ADAMs are sheddases for the EGF family of growth factors, APP, CXC chemokine ligand 16 and end E-cadherin; cleave extracellular matrix proteins; regulate keratinocyte cell–cell contacts, migration, proliferation and MMP-9 expression	Accelerated re-epithelialization in ADAM-9 knockout mice due to increased keratinocyte migration	19–24

References: [1] Carmeliet et al. 1994; [2] Rømer et al. 1996; [3] Goldfinger et al. 1998; [4] Ghosh et al. 2000; [5] Pankov and Yamada 2002; [6] Saarialho-Kere et al. 1992; [7] Stricklin et al. 1993; [8] Inoue et al. 1995; [9] Pilcher et al. 1997; [10] Di Colandrea et al. 1998; [11] Beare et al. 2003; [12] Bullard et al. 1999; [13] Salo et al. 1994; [14] Kyriakides et al. 2009; [15] Tran et al. 2004; [16] Krampert et al. 2004; [17] Impola et al. 2003 [18] Saarialho-Kere et al. 2002; [19] Asai et al. 2003; [20] White 2003; [21] Maretzky et al. 2005; [22] Scholz et al. 2007; [23] Zigrino et al. 2007; [24] Mauch et al. 2010.

wound fluids, which can affect keratinocyte behavior. For example, active MMP-2 has been detected in wound fluids (Moses et al. 1996).

Proper control of MMP activity is required for successful wound closure

MMP activity is tightly controlled in tissues. Tissue inhibitors of metalloproteinases (TIMPs) are the main regulators of MMP activity (Gill and Parks 2008). They are secreted proteins widely distributed in tissues and serve as specific inhibitors for MMPs. In wounds, the expression of TIMPs is upregulated in parallel with MMPs (Schaffer and Nanney 1996; Steffensen et al. 2001). In early wounds, TIMP-1 is expressed at the migratory front, whereas non-migrating keratinocytes at the wound margin express TIMP-1 and TIMP-3. Disturbance in the balance between MMPs and TIMPs results in poor wound healing: TIMP-1 expression is missing from chronic wounds, but TIMP-1 overexpression in wound keratinocytes also significantly retards the advancement of the epithelial front in mice (Vaalamo et al. 1996; Salonurmi et al. 2004). Similarly, transgenic mice expressing mutated type I collagen, which is resistant to collagenase cleavage, display severely delayed re-epithelialization (Beare et al. 2003), whereas also increased levels of MMP-1 activity are linked to retarded epithelial migration in wounds (Saarialho-Kere et al. 1992; Vaalamo et al. 1996; Di Colandrea et al. 1998).

Levels of divalent cations in the wound fluid affect re-epithelialization

Wound fluids collected throughout the early stages of cutaneous wound healing show elevations in Mg^{2+} and decreases in Ca^{2+} that correlate with the period of epithelial migration (Grzesiak and Pierschbacher 1995a). When re-epithelialization is complete, the concentrations of these cations return to normal plasma levels. Keratinocytes lose their migratory phenotype when exposed to dialyzed wound fluid, and migration resumes with the restoration of post-injury concentrations of Mg^{2+} and Ca^{2+} in the wound fluid (Grzesiak and Pierschbacher 1995a). Extracellular Mg^{2+} and Ca^{2+} levels may have an impact on several aspects of keratinocyte migration during re-epithelialization: Mg^{2+} enhances the ligand-binding ability of several integrins, including $\alpha2\beta1$, $\alpha5\beta1$ and $\alpha v\beta1$, whereas a high concentration of Ca^{2+} is inhibitory (Kirchhofer et al. 1991; Grzesiak and Pierschbacher 1995b; Mould et al. 1995). In addition, high extracellular Ca^{2+} concentration depresses the mRNA expression of the critical autocrine wound-healing growth factor HB-EGF in keratinocytes, whereas it is upregulated in low Ca^{2+} (Varani et al. 2001). In the presence of Ca^{2+}, E-cadherins that form the transmembrane core of adherens junctions interact in a homophilic manner with E-cadherins on the surface of adjacent keratinocytes (Kirfel and Herzog 2004). Wounding *in vivo* and exposure of keratinocytes to low extracellular Ca^{2+} concentration *in vitro* lead to the disruption of E-cadherin-mediated keratinocyte cell–cell contacts (Grzesiak and Pierschbacher 1995b). In addition, a high extracellular Ca^{2+} concentration induces keratinocyte stratification and terminal differentiation and reduces their proliferation, whereas low extracellular Ca^{2+} concentration promotes keratinocyte mitogenesis (Hennings et al. 1980). Thus, the increased concentration of Mg^{2+} in wound fluids may enhance integrin function, whereas the reduced concentration of Ca^{2+} may promote re-epithelialization by inducing the synthesis of pro-migratory growth factors, by disrupting intercellular contacts in wound edge keratinocytes and by promoting keratinocyte proliferation.

Wound-induced electrical field directs re-epithelialization

It has been demonstrated in cornea and skin that intact mammalian epithelia have established transepithelial voltage differences with apical to basal orientations that are introduced by actively pumping Na^+ and K^+ inwards and Cl^- outwards across the epithelial layers and that are maintained by epithelial tight junctions (Barker et al. 1982; Song et al. 2004; Zhao 2009). Wounding of epithelial sheets collapses this potential difference at the wound edge, leading to formation of a wound-induced, laterally oriented electrical field that is directed towards the wound. This electric field will persist until the migrating epithelial edges join and re-establish their cellular connections. Remarkably, epithelial cell migration and cell division are directed by the wound-induced electrical field, making it a fundamentally important factor for guiding directional keratinocyte migration in wounds (Song et al. 2002, 2004; Zhao 2009). Enhancing or suppressing the electric field pharmacologically increases or decreases wound re-epithelialization, respectively. The effect of the wound electrical field may be conveyed to the cell by the association of integrins with voltage-gated potassium channels, resulting in polarized integrin activation and asymmetrical lamellipodia extension, a process that also involves activities of EGFR, ERK, phosphatidylinositol 3-kinase and Rac1 GTPase, to promote keratinocyte directional migration (Zhao et al. 2002, 2006; Pullar et al. 2006; Brown and Dransfield 2008). Interestingly, electrical stimulation therapy that is believed to imitate the natural electrical currents in wounded skin significantly improves re-epithelialization of human chronic and diabetic ulcers (Baker et al. 1997; Gardner et al. 1999).

FINAL STAGES OF RE-EPITHELIALIZATION

Once the migrating epithelial fronts have joined and the denuded wound surface is covered, epithelial migration ceases due to contact inhibition, and a new stratified epithelium with the underlying basement membrane is re-established from the margins of the wound inward in skin (Uitto et al. 1996; Martin 1997). In small gingival wounds, the nucleation of the basement membrane appears to occur at multiple sites at the same time (Larjava et al. 1993). Both keratinocytes and connective tissue cells contribute to the basement membrane regeneration, and this process requires CXC chemokine signaling (El Ghalbzouri and Ponec 2004; Werner et al. 2007; Paquet-Fifield et al. 2009; Yates et al. 2009). Concurrently with basement membrane regeneration, keratinocytes start undergoing their normal differentiation program and new hemidesmosomal adhesions to basal lamina reassemble. Granulation tissue deposition and remodeling will still continue long after re-epithelialization is complete (Schaffer and Nanney 1996).

The proteolytic processing of the laminin-332 $\alpha3$ chain by focalized action of plasmin supports $\alpha6\beta4$ integrin-mediated hemidesmosome formation and retards migration (Goldfinger et al. 1998). Hemidesmosomes appear to function as nucleation sites for the reformation of the basement membrane (Jones et al. 1994). Once the cells have become stationary, they start to deposit basement membrane proteins, including laminin-111 and type IV and VII collagens that have been missing from underneath the migrating keratinocytes (Larjava et al. 1993). Laminin-111 may signal keratinocytes that they are in stable unwounded normal skin, do not need to migrate and can resume their normal proliferation pattern (Woodley et al. 1993).

FAILURE TO RE-EPITHELIALIZE: CHRONIC WOUNDS

Healing of acute wounds progresses smoothly, transitioning from one phase to another and resulting in stable wound closure. However, sometimes, often due to systemic conditions such as diabetes or venous insufficiency, re-epithelialization fails to complete, leading to the development of chronic, non-healing ulcers, mostly in the skin, that compromise the quality of life of the affected individuals and expose them to potentially life-threatening infections. Contrary to acute, normally healing wounds, wound edge keratinocytes in chronic ulcers are highly proliferative, are unable to migrate and do not display markers for epidermal differentiation (Morasso and Tomic-Canic 2005; Usui et al. 2008). Persistent inflammation, biochemical abnormalities of the extracellular matrix, increased levels of proteases and abnormalities of growth factor expression are all characteristics of chronic wounds. Overexpression and increased activity of MMPs, including MMP-1, -2, -3, -8 and -9, as well as ADAM-9 and -12, and reduced expression of TIMPs are common findings in non-healing chronic human wounds (Vaalamo et al. 1996; Nwomeh et al. 1999; Pilcher et al. 1999; Trengove et al. 1999; Philipp et al. 2004; Harsha et al. 2008; Mauch et al. 2010). Also plasmin activity may be impaired in chronic wounds, since tPA expression is strongly increased relative to PAI-1 in chronic, non-healing ulcers (Weckroth et al. 2004). This excessive and dysregulated protease activity may cause degradation of adhesion proteins, preventing the cell adhesion necessary for normal wound healing (Grinnell et al. 1992; Reiss et al. 2010). For example, wound fluids from normally healing skin wounds contain mainly intact fibronectin, but in chronic ulcers part or all of the fibronectin in the wound fluid becomes fragmented, and fibronectin supplementation into these non-healing ulcers seems to improve re-epithelialization (Wysocki and Grinnell 1990; Woodley 1996). Degradation of vitronectin and tenascin-C is also increased, whereas the presence of the uncleaved form of laminin-332 is reduced (Grinnell et al. 1992; Latijnhouwers et al. 1998; Usui et al. 2008). Increased MMP activity may also cause degradation of growth factors important for re-epithelialization (e.g. EGF; Trengove et al. 1999). Changes in growth factor expression are also detected in chronic wounds, for example diminished expression of IGF and increased expression of BMP-6 (Kaiser et al. 1998; Blakytny et al. 2000).

CONCLUSIONS

To date, great progress has been made in understanding the biological processes involved in wound healing. At the same time, it has become increasingly clear that wound healing is a very complex process that requires spatially and temporally regulated expression, downregulation or cleavage of various matrix molecules, their receptors and proteinases, as well as coordinated interplay between many different types of cells, including platelets, leukocytes, fibroblasts and keratinocytes, all of them influenced by the multiple growth factors and cytokines present in the wound environment. Many of the molecules have diverse functions during the different phases of wound healing and the cells also express several molecules with obviously overlapping activities. Considering the critical importance of timely re-epithelialization for the survival of an organism, the mechanism of wound healing clearly needs to be evolutionally well protected. Thus, targeted knock down of molecules that are shown to be essential for wound closure *in vitro* often results in mild effects in animal models where all the different interacting molecules and cell types are present. It is fundamental to our understanding of wound-healing biology to learn about the signals that trigger the different cell types at wound margins to proliferate, become invasive, lay down new matrix and finally reconstruct the tissue. Recent advances in understanding of micro-RNA (miRNA), epigenetic regulation of cell function and detoxification of reactive oxygen species by small proline-rich (SPRR) proteins suggest that these mechanisms are also involved in wound healing and may provide novel insights to the re-epithelialization process (Shaw and Martin 2009; Banerjee et al. 2010; Vermeij and Backendorf 2010). To date, as also evidenced by this chapter, most of the functional studies on wound healing have been carried out in rodents, in which the skin wound closure occurs largely by contraction. In contrast, re-epithelialization and granulation tissue formation are the major mechanisms of human wound healing. Recently, new experimental models that more closely parallel human wound healing have been developed that utilize grafting of human tissue-engineered skin onto the backs of nude mice or splinting to prevent the contraction of mouse wounds (Escámez et al. 2004; Galiano et al. 2004; Geer et al. 2004). Wound healing studies in porcine models may also provide results that are more applicable for human wound repair, including oral healing (Eslami et al. 2009; Mak et al. 2009; Wong et al. 2009). The developing knowledge of mechanisms of normal human wound healing may aid in solving the problems associated with excessive scarring, chronic non-healing ulcers and even invasion of epithelial cancers.

REFERENCES

Ågren, M.S. (1999) Matrix metalloproteinases (MMPs) are required for re-epithelialization of cutaneous wounds. *Archives of Dermatological Research*, **291**, 583–590.

Ågren, M.S., Mirastschijski, U., Karlsmark, T., et al. (2001) Topical synthetic inhibitor of matrix metalloproteinases delays epidermal regeneration of human wounds. *Experimental Dermatology*, **10**, 337–348.

AlDahlawi, S., Eslami, A., Häkkinen, L., et al. (2006) The αvβ6 integrin plays a role in compromised epidermal wound healing. *Wound Repair and Regeneration*, **14**, 289–297.

Amendt, C., Mann, A., Schirmacher, P., et al. (2002) Resistance of keratinocytes to TGFβ-mediated growth restriction and apoptosis induction accelerates re-epithelialization in skin wounds. *Journal of Cell Science*, **115**, 2189–2198.

Annes, J.P., Rifkin, D.B., Munger, J.S. (2002) The integrin αvβ6 binds and activates latent TGFβ3. *FEBS Letters*, **511**, 65–68.

Antoniades, H.N., Galanopoulos, T., Neville-Golden, J., et al. (1993) Expression of growth factor and receptor mRNAs in skin epithelial cells following acute cutaneous injury. *American Journal of Pathology*, **142**, 1099–1110.

Asai, M., Hattori, C., Szabo, B., et al. (2003) Putative function of ADAM9, ADAM10, and ADAM17 as APP α-secretase. *Biochemical and Biophysical Research Communications*, **301**, 231–235.

Ashcroft, G.S., Yang, X., Glick, A.B., et al. (1999) Mice lacking Smad3 show accelerated wound healing and an impaired local inflammatory response. *Nature Cell Biology*, **1**, 260–266.

Badiavas, E.V., Abedi, M., Butmarc, J., et al. (2003) Participation of bone marrow derived cells in cutaneous wound healing. *Journal of Cellular Physiology*, **196**, 245–250.

Baker, L.L., Chambers, R., DeMuth, S.K., et al. (1997) Effects of electrical stimulation on wound healing in patients with diabetic ulcers. *Diabetes Care*, **20**, 405–412.

Bamberger, C., Schärer, A., Antsiferova, M., et al. (2005) Activin controls skin morphogenesis and wound repair predominantly via stromal cells and in a concentration-dependent manner via keratinocytes. *American Journal of Pathology*, **167**, 733–747.

Banerjee, J., Chan, Y.C., Sen, C.K. (2010) MicroRNAs in skin and wound healing. *Physiological Genomics*, **43**(10), 543–546.

Barker, A.T., Jaffe, L.F., Vanable, J.W. Jr (1982) The glabrous epidermis of cavies contains a powerful battery. *American Journal of Physiology*, **242**, R358–366.

Barreca, A., De Luca, M., Del Monte, P., et al. (1992) In vitro paracrine regulation of human keratinocyte growth by fibroblast-derived insulin-like growth factors. *Journal of Cellular Physiology*, **151**, 262–268.

Basbaum, C.B., Werb, Z. (1996) Focalized proteolysis: spatial and temporal regulation of extracellular matrix degradation at the cell surface. *Current Opinion in Cell Biology*, **8**, 731–738.

Bata-Csorgo, Z., Cooper, K.D., Ting, K.M., et al. (1998) Fibronectin and α5 integrin regulate keratinocyte cell cycling. A mechanism for increased fibronectin potentiation of T cell lymphokine-driven keratinocyte hyperproliferation in psoriasis. *Journal of Clinical Investigation*, **101**, 1509–1518.

Baudoux, B., Castanares-Zapatero, D., Leclercq-Smekens, M., et al. (2000) The tetraspanin CD9 associates with the integrin α6β4 in cultured human epidermal keratinocytes and is involved in cell motility. *European Journal of Cell Biology*, **79**, 41–51.

Beare, A.H., O'Kane S., Krane, S.M., et al. (2003) Severely impaired wound healing in the collagenase-resistant mouse. *Journal of Investigative Dermatology*, **120**, 153–163.

Beaudry, V.G., Ihrie, R.A., Jacobs, S.B., et al. (2010) Loss of the desmosomal component perp impairs wound healing in vivo. *Dermatology Research and Practice*, **2010**, 759731.

Beer, H.D., Bittner, M., Niklaus, G., et al. (2005) The fibroblast growth factor binding protein is a novel interaction partner of FGF-7, FGF-10 and FGF-22 and regulates FGF activity: implications for epithelial repair. *Oncogene*, **24**, 5269–7527.

Berditchevski, F. (2001) Complexes of tetraspanins with integrins: more than meets the eye. *Journal of Cell Science*, **114**, 4143–4151.

Berditchevski, F., Tolias, K.F., Wong, K., et al. (1997) A novel link between integrins, transmembrane-4 superfamily proteins (CD63 and CD81), and phosphatidylinositol 4-kinase. *Journal of Biological Chemistry*, **27**, 2595–2598.

Bevan, D., Gherardi, E., Fan, T.P., et al. (2004) Diverse and potent activities of HGF/SF in skin wound repair. *Journal of Pathology*, **203**, 831–838.

Beyer, T.A., Werner, S., Dickson, C., et al. (2003) Fibroblast growth factor 22 and its potential role during skin development and repair. *Experimental Cell Research*, **287**, 228–236.

Blakytny, R., Jude, E.B., Martin Gibson, J., et al. (2000) Lack of insulin-like growth factor 1 (IGF1) in the basal keratinocyte layer of diabetic skin and diabetic foot ulcers. *Journal of Pathology*, **190**, 589–594.

Blanpain, C., Fuchs, E. (2009) Epidermal homeostasis: a balancing act of stem cells in the skin. *Nature Reviews Molecular Cell Biology*, **10**, 207–217.

Borradori, L., Sonnenberg, A. (1999) Structure and function of hemidesmosomes: more than simple adhesion complexes. *Journal of Investigative Dermatology*, **112**, 411–418.

Borue, X., Lee, S., Grove, J., et al. (2004) Bone marrow-derived cells contribute to epithelial engraftment during wound healing. *American Journal of Pathology*, **165**, 1767–1772.

Boxman, I.L., Ruwhof, C., Boerman, O.C., et al. (1996) Role of fibroblasts in the regulation of proinflammatory interleukin IL-1, IL-6 and IL-8 levels induced by keratinocyte-derived IL-1. *Archives of Dermatological Research*, **288**, 391–398.

Bradshaw, A.D, Reed, M.J., Sage, E.H. (2002) SPARC-null mice exhibit accelerated cutaneous wound closure. *Journal of Histochemistry and Cytochemistry*, **50**, 1–10.

Brauchle, M., Angermeyer, K., Hubner, G., et al. (1994) Large induction of keratinocyte growth factor expression by serum growth factors and pro-inflammatory cytokines in cultured fibroblasts. *Oncogene*, **9**, 3199–3204.

Breuss, J.M., Gallo, J., DeLisser, H.M., et al. (1995) Expression of the β6 integrin subunit in development, neoplasia and tissue repair suggests a role in epithelial remodeling. *Journal of Cell Science*, **108**, 2241–2251.

Brown, L.F., Yeo, K.T., Berse, B., et al. (1992) Expression of vascular permeability factor (vascular endothelial growth factor) by epidermal keratinocytes during wound healing. *Journal of Experimental Medicine*, **176**, 1375–1379.

Brown, L.F., Dubin, D., Lavigne, L., et al. (1993) Macrophages and fibroblasts express embryonic fibronectins during cutaneous wound healing. *American Journal of Pathology*, **142**, 793–801.

Brown, R.L., Ormsby, I., Doetschman, T.C., et al. (1995) Wound healing in the transforming growth factor β1-deficient mouse. *Wound Repair and Regeneration*, **3**, 25–36.

Brown, S.B., Dransfield, I. (2008) Electric fields and inflammation: may the force be with you. *Scientific World Journal*, **8**, 1280–1294.

Bugge, T.H., Kombrinck, K.W., Flick, M.J., et al. (1996) Loss of fibrinogen rescues mice from the pleiotropic effects of plasminogen deficiency. *Cell*, **87**, 709–719.

Bullard, K.M., Lund, L., Mudgett, J.S., et al. (1999) Impaired wound contraction in stromelysin-1 deficient mice. *Annals of Surgery*, **230**, 260–265.

Cambier, S., Mu, D.Z., O'Connell, D., et al. (2000) A role for the integrin αvβ8 in the negative regulation of epithelial cell growth. *Cancer Research*, **60**, 7084–7093.

Carmeliet, P., Schoonjans, L., Kieckens, L., et al. (1994) Physiological consequences of loss of plasminogen activator gene function in mice. *Nature*, **368**, 419–424.

Carter, W.G., Ryan, M.C., Gahr, P.J. (1991) Epiligrin, a new cell adhesion ligand for integrin α3β1 in epithelial basement membranes. *Cell*, **65**, 599–610.

Castilho, R.M., Squarize, C.H., Leelahavanichkul, K., et al. (2010) Rac1 is required for epithelial stem cell function during dermal and oral mucosal wound healing but not for tissue homeostasis in mice. *PLoS One*, **5**, e10503.

Cavani, A., Zambruno, G., Marconi, A., et al. (1993) Distinctive integrin expression in the newly forming epidermis during wound healing in humans. *Journal of Investigative Dermatology*, **101**, 600–604.

Chan, T., Ghahary, A., Demare, J., et al. (2002) Development, characterization, and wound healing of the keratin 14 promoted transforming growth factor-β1 transgenic mouse. *Wound Repair and Regeneration*, **10**, 177–187.

Chen, J.D., Kim, J.P., Zhang, K., et al. (1993) Epidermal growth factor promotes human keratinocyte locomotion on collagen by increasing the α2 integrin subunit. *Experimental Cell Research*, **209**, 216–223.

Chen, J., Diacovo, T.G., Grenache, D.G., et al. (2002) The α2 integrin subunit-deficient mouse: a multifaceted phenotype including defects of branching morphogenesis and hemostasis. *American Journal of Pathology*, **161**, 337–344.

Chernyavsky, A.I., Arredondo, J., Vetter, D.E., et al. (2007) Central role of α9 acetylcholine reseptor in coordinating keratinocyte adhesion and motility at the initiation of epithelialization. *Experimental Cell Research*, **313**, 3542–3555.

Choma, D.P., Pumiglia, K., DiPersio, C.M. (2004) Integrin α3β1 directs the stabilization of a polarized lamellipodium in epithelial cells through activation of Rac1. *Journal of Cell Science*, **117**, 3947–3959.

Chung, C.Y., Erickson, H.P. (1994) Cell surface annexin II is a high affinity receptor for the alternatively spliced segment of tenascin-C. *Journal of Cell Biology*, **126**, 539–548.

Chung, C.Y., Murphy-Ullrich, J.E., Erickson, H.P. (1996) Mitogenesis, cell migration, and loss of focal adhesions induced by tenascin-C interacting with its cell surface receptor, annexin II. *Molecular Biology of the Cell*, **7**, 883–892.

Clayton, E., Doupé, D.P., Klein, A.M., et al. (2007) A single type of progenitor cell maintains normal epidermis. *Nature*, **446**, 185–189.

Cowin, A.J., Adams, D., Geary, S.M., et al. (2006) Wound healing is defective in mice lacking tetraspanin CD151. *Journal of Investigative Dermatology*, **126**, 680–689.

D'Alessio, S., Gerasi, L. and Blasi, F. (2008) uPAR-deficient mouse keratinocytes fail to produce EGFR-dependent laminin-5, affecting migration in vivo and in vitro. *Journal of Cell Science*, **121**, 3922–3932.

Dalvi, N., Thomas, G.J., Marshall, J.F., et al. (2004) Modulation of the urokinase-type plasminogen activator receptor by the β6 integrin subunit. *Biochemical and Biophysical Research Commununications*, **317**, 92–99.

Danilenko, D.M., Ring, B.D., Lu, J.Z., et al. (1995) Neu differentiation factor upregulates epidermal migration and integrin expression in excisional wounds. *Journal of Clinical Investigation*, **95**, 842–851.

Davis, G.E. (1992) Affinity of integrins for damaged extracellular matrix: αvβ3 binds to denatured collagen type I through RGD sites. *Biochemical and Biophysical Research Commununications*, **182**, 1025–1031.

Davis, G.E., Bayless, K.J., Davis, M.J., et al. (2000) Regulation of tissue injury responses by the exposure of matricryptic sites within extracellular matrix molecules. *American Journal of Pathology*, **156**, 1489–1498.

Décline, F., Rousselle, P. (2001) Keratinocyte migration requires α2β1 integrin-mediated interaction with the laminin 5 γ2 chain. *Journal of Cell Science*, **114**, 811–823.

Décline, F., Okamoto, O., Mallein-Gerin, F., et al. (2003) Keratinocyte motility induced by TGF-β1 is accompanied by dramatic changes in cellular interactions with laminin-5. *Cell Motility and the Cytoskeleton*, **54**, 64–80.

Defilippi, P., Olivo, C., Venturino, M., et al. (1999) Actin cytoskeleton organization in response to integrin-mediated adhesion. *Microscopy Research and Technique*, **47**, 67–78.

deHart, G.W., Healy, K.E. and Jones, J.C. (2003) The role of α3β1 integrin in determining the supramolecular organization of laminin-5 in the extracellular matrix of keratinocytes. *Experimental Cell Research*, **283**, 67–79.

DeMali, K.A., Wennerberg, K., Burridge, K. (2003) Integrin signalling to the actin cytoskeleton. *Current Opinion in Cell Biology*, **15**, 572–282.

Di Colandrea, T., Wang, L., Wille, J., et al. (1998) Epidermal expression of collagenase delays wound-healing in transgenic mice. *Journal of Investigative Dermatology*, **111**, 1029–1033.

DiMilla, P.A., Barbee, K., Lauffenburger, D.A. (1991) Mathematical model for the effects of adhesion and mechanics on cell migration speed. *Biophysical Journal*, **60**, 15–37.

DiPersio, C.M. (2007) Double duty for Rac1 in epidermal wound healing. *Science's STKE: Signal Transduction Knowledge Environment*, **2007**, pe33.

DiPersio, C.M., Hodivala-Dilke, K.M., Jaenisch, R., et al. (1997) α3β1 integrin is required for normal development of the epidermal basement membrane. *Journal of Cell Biology*, **137**, 729–742.

Dlugosz, A.A., Cheng, C., Denning, M.F., et al. (1994) Keratinocyte growth factor receptor ligands induce transforming growth factor alpha expression and activate the epidermal growth factor receptor signaling pathway in cultured epidermal keratinocytes. *Cell Growth and Differentation*, **5**, 1283–1292.

Drew, A.F., Liu, H., Davidson, J.M., et al. (2001) Wound-healing defects in mice lacking fibrinogen. *Blood*, **97**, 3691–3698.

D'Souza-Schorey, C., Boettner, B., Van Aelst, L. (1998) Rac regulates integrin-mediated spreading and increased adhesion of T lymphocytes. *Molecular and Cellular Biology*, **18**, 3936–3946.

Echtermeyer, F., Streit, M., Wilcox-Adelman, S., et al. (2001) Delayed wound repair and impaired angiogenesis in mice lacking syndecan-4. *Journal of Clinical Investigation*, **107**, R9-R14.

Efron, P.A., Moldawer, L.L. (2004) Cytokines and wound healing: the role of cytokine and anticytokine therapy in the repair response. *Journal of Burn Care and Rehabilitation*, **25**, 149–160.

Egging, D., van Vlijmen-Willems, I., van Tongeren, T., et al. (2007) Wound healing in tenascin-X deficient mice suggests that tenascin-X is involved in matrix maturation rather than matrix deposition. *Connective Tissue Research*, **48**, 93–98.

El Ghalbzouri, A., Ponec, M. (2004) Diffusible factors released by fibroblasts support epidermal morphogenesis and deposition of basement membrane components. *Wound Repair and Regeneration*, **12**, 359–367.

Ellis, P.D., Hadfield, K.M., Pascall, J.C., et al. (2001) Heparin-binding epidermal-growth-factor-like growth factor gene expression is induced by scrape-wounding epithelial cell monolayers: involvement of mitogen-activated protein kinase cascades. *Biochemical Journal*, **354**, 99–106.

Eming, S.A., Lee, J., Snow, R.G., et al. (1995) Genetically modified human epidermis overexpressing PDGF-A directs the development of a cellular and vascular connective tissue stroma for the use of genetically modified keratinocytes to modulate dermal regeneration. *Journal of Investigative Dermatology*, **105**, 756–763.

Escámez, M.J., Garcia, M., Larcher, F., et al. (2004) An in vivo model of wound healing in genetically modified skin-humanized mice. *Journal of Investigative Dermatology*, **123**, 1182–1191.

Eslami, A., Gallant-Behm, C.L., Hart, D.A., et al. (2009) Expression of integrin αvβ6 and TGF-β in scarless vs scar-forming wound healing. *Journal of Histochemistry and Cytochemistry*, **57**, 543–557.

Falanga, V., Schrayer, D., Cha, J., et al. (2004) Full-thickness wounding of the mouse tail as a model for delayed wound healing: accelerated wound closure in Smad3 knock-out mice. *Wound Repair and Regeneneration*, **12**, 320–326.

Fan, Q., Lee Yee, C., Ohyama, M., et al. (2006) Bone-marrow-derived keratinocytes are not detected in normal skin and only rarely detected in wounded skin in two different murine models. *Experimental Hematology*, **34**, 672–679.

Farooqui, R., Fenteany, G. (2004) Multiple rows of cells behind an epithelial wound edge extend cryptic lamellipodia to collectively drive cell-sheet movement. *Journal of Cell Science*, **118**, 51–63.

Fenteany, G., Janmey, P.A., Stossel, T.P. (2000) Signaling pathways and cell mechanics involved in wound closure by epithelial cell sheets. *Current Biology*, **10**, 831–838.

ffrench-Constant, C., Colognato, H. (2004) Integrins: versatile integrators of extracellular signals. *Trends in Cell Biology*, **14**, 678–686.

ffrench-Constant, C., van de Water, L., Dvorak, H.F., et al. (1989) Re-appearance of an embryonic pattern of fibronectin splicing during wound healing in the adult rat. *Journal of Cell Biology*, **109**, 903–914.

Firth, J.D., Putnins, E.E. (2004) Keratinocyte growth factor 1 inhibits wound edge epithelial cell apoptosis in vitro. *Journal of Investigative Dermatology*, **122**, 222–231.

Forsberg, E., Hirsch, E., Frohlich, L., et al. (1996) Skin wounds and severed nerves heal normally in mice lacking tenascin-C. *Proceedings of the National Academy of Sciences USA*, **93**, 6594–6599.

Frank, D.E., Carter, W.E. (2004) Laminin 5 deposition regulates keratinocyte polarization and persistent migration. *Journal of Cell Science*, **117**, 1351–1363.

Fuchs, E. (2009) Finding one's niche in the skin. *Cell Stem Cell*, **4**, 499–502.

Galiano, R.D., Michaels, J., Dobryansky, M., et al. (2004) Quantitative and reproducible murine model of excisional wound healing. *Wound Repair and Regeneration*, **12**, 485–492.

Gallo, R., Kim, C., Kokenyesi, R., et al. (1996) Syndecans-1 and -4 are induced during wound repair of neonatal but not fetal skin. *Journal of Investigative Dermatology*, **107**, 676–683.

Gallucci, R.M., Simeonova, P.P., Matheson, J.M., et al. (2000) Impaired cutaneous wound healing in interleukin-6-deficient and immunosuppressed mice. *FASEB Journal*, **14**, 2525–2531.

Gardner, S.E., Frantz, R.A., Schmidt, F.L. (1999) Effect of electrical stimulation on chronic wound healing: a meta-analysis. *Wound Repair and Regeneration*, **7**, 495–503.

Garlick, J.A., Taichman, L.B. (1994) Fate of human keratinocytes during reepithelialization in an organotypic culture model. *Laboratory Investigation*, **70**, 916–924.

Geary, S.M., Cowin, A.J., Copeland, B., et al. (2008) The role of the tetraspanin CD151 in primary keratinocyte and fibroblast functions: implications for wound healing. *Experimental Cell Research*, **314**, 2165–2175.

Geer, D.J., Swartz, D.D., Andreadis, S.T. (2004) In vivo model of wound healing based on transplanted tissue-engineered skin. *Tissue Engineering*, **10**, 1006–1017.

George, E.L., Georges-Labouesse, E.N., Patel-King, R.S., et al. (1993) Defects in mesoderm, neural tube and vascular development in mouse embryos lacking fibronectin. *Development*, **119**, 1079–1091.

Ghosh, S., Brown, R., Jones, J.C., et al. (2000) Urinary-type plasminogen activator (uPA) expression and uPA receptor localization are regulated by α3β1 integrin in oral keratinocytes. *Journal of Biological Chemistry*, **275**, 23869–23876.

Giancotti, F.G., Ruoslahti, E. (1999) Integrin signalling. *Science*, **285**, 1028–1032.

Gill, S.E., Parks, W.C. (2008) Metalloproteinases and their inhibitors: regulators of wound healing. *International Journal of Biochemistry and Cell Biology*, **40**, 1334–1347.

Gipson, I.K., Spurr-Michaud, S., Tisdale, A., et al. (1993) Redistribution of the hemidesmosome components α6β4 integrin and bullous pemphigoid antigens during epithelial wound healing. *Experimental Cell Research*, **207**, 86–98.

Goh, Y.Y., Pal, M., Chong, H.C., et al. (2010a) Angiopoietin-like 4 interacts with matrix proteins to modulate wound healing. *Journal of Biological Chemistry*, **285**(43), 32999–3009.

Goh, Y.Y., Pal, M., Chong, H.C., et al. (2010b) Angiopoietin-like 4 interacts with integrins β1 and β5 to modulate keratinocyte migration. *American Journal of Pathology*, **177**(6), 2791–803.

Goldfinger, L.E., Stack, M.S. and Jones, J.C. (1998) Processing of laminin-5 and its functional consequences: role of plasmin and tissue-type plasminogen activator. *Journal of Cell Biology*, **141**, 255–265.

Goldfinger, L.E., Hopkinson, S.B., deHart, G.W., et al. (1999) The α3 laminin subunit, α6β4 and α3β1 integrin coordinately regulate wound healing in cultured epithelial cells and in the skin. *Journal of Cell Science*, **112**, 2615–2629.

Goretsky, M.J., Harriger, M.D., Supp, A.P., et al. (1996) Expression of interleukin-1α, interleukin-6, and basic fibroblast growth factor by cultured skin substitutes before and after grafting to full-thickness wounds in athymic mice. *Journal of Trauma*, **40**, 894–900.

Greenwood, J.A., Murphy-Ullrich, J.E. (1998) Signaling of de-adhesion in cellular regulation and motility. *Microscopy Research and Technique*, **43**, 420–432.

Grenache, D.G., Zhang, Z., Wells, L.E., et al. (2007) Wound healing in the α2β1 integrin-deficient mouse: altered keratinocyte biology and dysregulated matrix metalloproteinase expression. *Journal of Investigative Dermatology*, **127**, 455–466.

Grinnell, F., Ho, C.H., Wysocki, A. (1992) Degradation of fibronectin and vitronectin in chronic wound fluid: analysis by cell blotting, immunoblotting, and cell adhesion assays. *Journal of Investigative Dermatology*, **98**, 410–416.

Grose, R., Hutter, C., Bloch, W., et al. (2002) A crucial role of β1 integrins for keratinocyte migration in vitro and during cutaneous wound repair. *Development*, **129**, 2303–2315.

Grossman, R.M., Krueger, J., Yourish, D., et al. (1989) Interleukin 6 is expressed in high levels in psoriatic skin and stimulates proliferation of cultured human keratinocytes. *Proceedings of the National Academy of Sciences USA*, **86**, 6367–6371.

Grzesiak, J.J., Pierschbacher, M.D. (1995a) Shifts in concentrations of magnesium and calcium in early porcine and rat wound fluids activate the cell migratory response. *Journal of Clinical Investigation*, **95**, 227–233.

Grzesiak, J.J., Pierschbacher, M.D. (1995b) Changes in the concentrations of extracellular Mg^{2+} and Ca^{2+} down-regulate E-cadherin and up-regulate α2β1 integrin function, activating keratinocyte migration on type I collagen. *Journal of Investigative Dermatology*, **104**, 768–774.

Guo, L., Degenstein, L., Fuchs, E. (1996) Keratinocyte growth factor is required for hair development but not for wound healing. *Genes and Development*, **10**, 165–175.

Haapasalmi, K., Zhang, K., Tonnesen, M., et al. (1996) Keratinocytes in human wounds express αvβ6 integrin. *Journal of Investigative Dermatology*, **106**, 42–48.

Haase, I., Evans, R., Pofahl, R., et al. (2003) Regulation of keratinocyte shape, migration and wound reepithelialization by IGF-1- and EGF-dependent signalling pathways. *Journal of Cell Science*, **116**, 3227–3238.

Häkkinen, L., Hildebrand, H.C., Berndt, A., et al. (2000a) Immunolocalization of tenascin-C, α9 integrin subunit, and αvβ6 integrin during wound healing in human oral mucosa. *Journal of Histochemistry and Cytochemistry*, **48**, 985–998.

Häkkinen, L., Uitto, V.J., Larjava, H. (2000b) Cell biology of gingival wound healing. *Periodontology*, **24**, 127–152.

Häkkinen, L., Koivisto, L., Gardner, H., et al. (2004) Increased expression of β6 integrin in skin leads to spontaneous development of chronic wounds. *American Journal of Pathology*, **164**, 229–242.

Harsha, A., Stojadinovic, O., Brem, H., et al. (2008) ADAM12: a potential target for the treatment of chronic wounds. *Journal of Molecular Medicine*, **86**, 961–969.

Hartwig, B., Borm, B., Schneider, H., et al. (2007) Laminin-5-deficient human keratinocytes: defective adhesion results in a saltatory and inefficient mode of migration. *Experimental Cell Research*, **313**, 1575–1587.

Hashimoto, K. (2000) Regulation of keratinocyte function by growth factors. *Journal of Dermatological Science*, **24** (Suppl 1), S46–50.

Haugh, J.M. (2002) Localization of receptor-mediated signal transduction pathways: the inside story. *Molecular Interventions*, **2**, 292–307.

Hauzenberger, D., Olivier, P., Gundersen, D., et al. (1999) Tenascin-C inhibits β1 integrin-dependent T lymphocyte adhesion to fibronectin through the binding of its fnIII 1–5 repeats to fibronectin. *European Journal of Immunology*, **29**, 1435–1447.

Hemler, M.E. (1998) Integrin associated proteins. *Current Opinion in Cell Biology*, **10**, 578–585.

Hennings, H., Michael, D., Cheng, C., et al. (1980) Calcium regulation of growth and differentiation of mouse epidermal cells in culture. *Cell*, **19**, 245–254.

Higashiyama, S., Nanba, D. (2005) ADAM-mediated ectodomain shedding of HB-EGF in receptor cross-talk. *Biochimica et Biophysica Acta*, **1751**, 110–117.

Hodak, E., Gottlieb, A.B., Anzilotti, M., et al. (1996) The insulin-like growth factor 1 receptor is expressed by epithelial cellswith proliferative potential in human epidermis and skin appendages: correlation with epidermal hyperplasia. *Journal of Investigative Dermatology*, **106**, 564–570.

Hodivala-Dilke, K.M., DiPersio, C.M., Kreidberg, J.A., et al. (1998) Novel roles for α3β1 integrin as a regulator of cytoskeletal assembly and as a trans-dominant inhibitor of integrin receptor function in mouse keratinocytes. *Journal of Cell Biology*, **142**, 1357–1369.

Hoffman, J., Twiesselmann, C., Kummer, M.P., et al. (2000) A possible role for the Alzheimer amyloid precursor protein in the regulation of epidermal basal cell proliferation. *European Journal of Cell Biology*, **79**, 905–914.

Hosoya, A., Lee, J.M., Cho, S.W., et al. (2008) Morphological evidence of basal keratinocyte migration during the re-epithelialization process. *Histochemistry and Cell Biology*, **130**, 1165–1175.

Huang, X.Z., Wu, J.F., Cass, D., et al. (1996) Inactivation of the integrin β6 subunit gene reveals a role of epithelial integrins in regulating inflammation in the lung and skin. *Journal of Cell Biology*, **133**, 921–928.

Huang, X., Wu, J., Spong, S., et al. (1998) The integrin αvβ6 is critical for keratinocyte migration on both its known ligand, fibronectin, and on vitronectin. *Journal of Cell Science*, **111**, 2189–2195.

Huang, X., Griffiths, M., Wu, J., et al. (2000) Normal development, wound healing, and adenovirus susceptibility in β5-deficient mice. *Molecular and Cellular Biology*, **20**, 755–759.

Huang, C., Jacobson, K., Schaller, M.D. (2004) MAP kinases and cell migration. *Journal of Cell Science*, **117**, 4619–4628.

Hübner, G., Hu, Q., Smola, H., et al. (1996a) Strong induction of activin expression after injury suggests an important role of activin in wound repair. *Developmental Biology*, **173**, 490–498.

Hübner, G., Brauchle, M., Smola, H., et al. (1996b) Differential regulation of pro-inflammatory cytokines during wound healing in normal and glucocorticoid-treated mice. *Cytokine*, **8**, 548–556.

Hudson, L.G., McCawley, L.J. (1998) Contributions of the epidermal growth factor receptor to keratinocyte motility. *Microscopy Research and Technique*, **43**, 444–455.

Hynes, R.O. (2002) Integrins: bidirectional, allosteric signaling machines. *Cell*, **110**, 673–687.
Illman, S.A., Lohi, J., Keski-Oja, J. (2008) Epilysin (MMP-28) – structure, expression and potential functions. *Experimental Dermatology*, **17**, 897–907.
Impola, U., Toriseva, M., Suomela, S., et al. (2003) Matrix metalloproteinase-19 is expressed by proliferating epithelium but disappears with neoplastic dedifferentiation. *International Journal of Cancer*, **103**, 709–716.
Ingham, K.C., Brew, S.A., Erickson, H.P. (2004) Localization of a cryptic binding site for tenascin on fibronectin. *Journal of Biological Chemistry*, **279**, 28132–28135.
Inoue, M., Kratz, G., Haegerstrand, A., et al. (1995) Collagenase expression is rapidly induced in wound edge keratinocytes after acute injury in human skin, persists during healing and stops at re-epithelialization. *Journal of Investigative Dermatology*, **104**, 479–483.
Inoue, T., Nabeshima, K., Shimao, Y., et al. (1999) Hepatocyte growth factor/scatter factor (HGF/SF) is a regulator of fibronectin splicing in MDCK cells: comparison between the effects of HGF/SF and TGF-β1 on fibronectin splicing at the EDA region. *Biochemical and Biophysical Research Communications*, **260**, 225–231.
Ito, M., Liu, Y., Yang, Z., et al. (2005) Stem cells in the hair follicle bulge contribute to wound repair but not to homeostasis of the epidermis. *Nature Medicine*, **11**, 1351–1354.
Ivaska, J., Heino, J. (2010) Interplay between cell adhesion and growth factor receptors: from the plasma membrane to the endosomes. *Cell and Tissue Research*, **339**, 111–120.
Jang, Y.C., Tsou, R., Gibran, N.S., et al. (2000) Vitronectin deficiency is associated with increased wound fibrinolysis and decreased microvascular angiogenesis in mice. *Surgery*, **127**, 696–704.
Jensen, P.J., Rodeck, U. (1993) Autocrine/paracrine regulation of keratinocyte urokinase plasminogen activator through the TGF-α/EGF receptor. *Journal of Cellular Physiology*, **155**, 333–339.
Jensen, U.B., Lowell, S., Watt, F.M. (1999) The spatial relationship between stem cells and their progeny in the basal layer of human epidermis: a new view based on whole-mount labelling and lineage analysis. *Development*, **126**, 2409–2418.
Jeschke, M.G., Richter, G., Hofstadter, F., et al. (2002) Non-viral liposomal keratinocyte growth factor (KGF) cDNA gene transfer improves dermal and epidermal regeneration through stimulation of epithelial and mesenchymal factors. *Gene Therapy*, **9**, 1065–1074.
Jeschke, M.G., Schubert, T., Klein, D. (2004) Exogenous liposomal IGF-1 cDNA gene transfer leads to endogenous cellular and physiological responses in an acute wound. *American Journal of Physiology – Regulatory, Integrative and Comparative Physiology*, **286**, R958–966.
Johansson, S., Hook, M. (1980) Heparin enhances the rate of binding of fibronectin to collagen. *Biochemical Journal*, **187**, 521–524.
Jones, J.C., Asmuth, J., Baker, S.E., et al. (1994) Hemidesmosomes: extracellular matrix/intermediate filament connectors. *Experimental Cell Research*, **213**, 1–11.
Jones, P.H., Bishop, L.A., Watt, F.M. (1996) Functional significance of CD9 association with β1 integrins in human epidermal keratinocytes. *Cell Adhesion and Communication*, **4**, 297–305.
Jones P.H., Simons B.D., Watt, F.M. (2007) Sic transit gloria: farewell to the epidermal transit amplifying cell? *Cell Stem Cell*, **1**, 371–381.
Juhasz, I., Murphy, G.F., Yan, H.C., et al. (1993) Regulation of extracellular matrix proteins and integrin cell substratum adhesion receptors on epithelium during cutaneous human wound healing in vivo. *American Journal of Pathology*, **143**, 1458–1469.
Kainulainen, T., Häkkinen, L., Hamidi, S., et al. (1998) Laminin-5 expression is independent of the injury and the microenvironment during reepithelialization of wounds. *Journal of Histochemistry and Cytochemistry*, **46**, 353–360.
Kaiser, S., Schirmacher, P., Philipp, A., et al. (1998) Induction of bone morphogenetic protein-6 in skin wounds. Delayed reepitheliazation and scar formation in BMP-6 overexpressing transgenic mice. *Journal of Investigative Dermatology*, **111**, 1145–1152.
Kane, C.J., Hebda, P.A., Mansbridge, J.N., et al. (1991) Direct evidence for spatial and temporal regulation of transforming growth factor beta 1 expression during cutaneous wound healing. *Journal of Cellular Physiology*, **148**, 157–173.
Kaya, G., Rodriguez, I., Jorcano, J.L., et al. (1997) Selective suppression of CD44 in keratinocytes of mice bearing an antisense CD44 transgene driven by a tissue-specific promoter disrupts hyaluronate metabolism in the skin and impairs keratinocyte proliferation. *Genes and Development*, **11**, 996–1007.
Khwaja, A., Rodriguez-Viciana, P., Wennstrom, S., et al. (1997) Matrix adhesion and Ras transformation both activate a phosphoinositide 3-OH kinase and protein kinase B/Akt cellular survival pathway. *EMBO Journal*, **16**, 2783–2793.

Kim, I., Mogford, J.E., Chao, J.D., et al. (2001) Wound epithelialization deficit in the transforming growth factor-alpha knockout mouse. *Wound Repair and Regeneration*, **9**, 386–390.

Kim, J.P., Zhang, K., Kramer, R.H., et al. (1992) Integrin receptors and RGD sequences in human keratinocyte migration: unique anti-migratory function of α3β1 epiligrin receptor. *Journal of Investigative Dermatology*, **98**, 764–770.

Kirchhofer, D., Grzesiak, J., Pierschbacher, M.D. (1991) Calcium as a potential physiological regulator of integrin-mediated cell adhesion. *Journal of Biological Chemistry*, **266**, 4471–4417.

Kirfel, G., Herzog, V. (2004) Migration of epidermal keratinocytes: mechanisms, regulation, and biological significance. *Protoplasma*, **223**, 67–78.

Kirfel, G., Borm, B., Rigort, A., et al. (2002) The secretory β-amyloid precursor protein is a motogen for human epidermal keratinocytes. *European Journal of Cell Biology*, **81**, 664–676.

Koch, R.M., Roche, N.S., Parks, W.T., et al. (2000) Incisional wound healing in transforming growth factor-β1 null mice. *Wound Repair and Regeneration*, **8**, 179–191.

Koivisto, L., Larjava, K., Häkkinen, L., et al. (1999) Different integrins mediate cell spreading, haptotaxis and lateral migration of HaCaT keratinocytes on fibronectin. *Cell Adhesion and Communication*, **7**, 245–257.

Koivisto, L., Häkkinen, L., Matsumoto, K., et al. (2004) Glycogen synthase kinase-3 regulates cytoskeleton and translocation of Rac1 in long cellular extensions of human keratinocytes. *Experimental Cell Research*, **293**, 68–80.

Koivisto, L., Jiang, G., Häkkinen, L., et al. (2006) Keratinocyte migration is dependent on epidermal growth factor receptor signaling and glycogen synthase kinase-3α. *Experimental Cell Research*, **312**, 2791–2805.

Koskela, A., Engström, K., Hakelius, M, et al. (2010) Regulation of fibroblast gene expression by keratinocytes in organotypic skin culture provides possible mechanisms for the antifibrotic effect of reepithelialization. *Wound Repair and Regeneration*, **18**(5), 452–459.

Krampert, M., Bloch, W., Sasaki, T., et al. (2004) Activities of the matrix metalloproteinase stromelysin-2 (MMP-10) in matrix degradation and keratinocyte organization in wounded skin. *Molecular Biology of the Cell*, **15**, 5242–5254.

Kretz, M., Euwens, C., Hombach, S., et al. (2003) Altered connexin expression and wound healing in the epidermis of connexin-deficient mice. *Journal of Cell Science*, **116**, 3443–3452.

Krissansen, G.W. (2001) Integrins: signalling and disease. *Nature Encyclopedia of Life Sciences*, www.els.net, 1–10.

Kugler, M.C., Wei, Y., Chapman, H.A. (2003) Urokinase receptor and integrin interactions. *Current Pharmaceutical Design*, **9**, 1565–1574.

Kummer, C., Wehner, S., Quast, T., et al. (2002) Expression and potential function of β-amyloid precursor proteins during cutaneous wound repair. *Experimental Cell Research*, **280**, 222–232.

Kuwada, S.K., Li, X. (2000) Integrin α5β1 mediates fibronectin-dependent epithelial cell proliferation through epidermal growth factor receptor activation. *Molecular Biology of the Cell*, **11**, 2485–2496.

Kyriakides, T.R., Tam, J.W., Bornstein, P. (1999) Accelerated wound healing in mice with a disruption of the thrombospondin 2 gene. *Journal of Investigative Dermatology*, **113**, 782–787.

Kyriakides, T.R., Wulsin, D., Skokos, E.A., et al. (2009) Mice that lack matrix metalloproteinase-9 display delayed wound healing associated with delayed reepithelization and disordered collagen fibrillogenesis. *Matrix Biology*, **28**, 65–73.

Laplante, A.F., Germain, L., Auger, F.A., et al. (2001) Mechanisms of wound reepithelialization: hints from a tissue-engineered recinstructed skin to long-standing questions. *FASEB Journal*, **15**, 2377–2389.

Larjava, H., Salo, T., Haapasalmi, K., et al. (1993) Expression of integrins and basement membrane components by wound keratinocytes. *Journal of Clinical Investigation*, **92**, 1425–1435.

Larjava, H., Haapasalmi, K., Salo, T., et al. (1996) Keratinocyte integrins in wound healing and chronic inflammation of the human periodontium. *Oral Diseases*, **2**, 77–86.

Larjava, H., Koivisto, L., Häkkinen, L. (2002) Keratinocyte interactions with fibronectin during wound healing. In: *Cell Invasion* (eds. J. Heino, V.-M. Kähäri), pp. 42–64. Landes Biosciences, Eurecah.com, Georgetown, Texas.

Latijnhouwers, M.A., Bergers, M., Veenhuis, R.T., et al. (1998) Tenascin-C degradation in chronic wounds is dependent on serine proteinase activity. *Archives of Dermatological Research*, **290**, 490–496.

Legate, K.R., Fässler, R. (2009) Mechanisms that regulate adaptor binding to beta-integrin cytoplasmic tails. *Journal of Cell Science*, **122**, 187–198.

Legate, K.R., Wickström, S.A., Fässler, R. (2009) Genetic and cell biological analysis of integrin outside-in signaling. *Genes and Development*, **23**, 397–418.

Levine, J.H., Moses, H.L., Gold, L.I., et al. (1993) Spatial and temporal patterns of immunoreactive transforming growth factor β1, β2, and β3 during excisional wound repair. *American Journal of Pathology*, **143**, 368–380.

Levy, V., Lindon, C., Zheng, Y., et al. (2007) Epidermal stem cells arise from the hair follicle after wounding. *FASEB Journal*, **21**, 1358–1366.

Li, W., Henry, G., Fan J., et al. (2004) Signals that initiate, augment, and provide directionality for human keratinocyte motility. *Journal of Investigative Dermatology*, **123**, 622–633.

Liao, Y.F., Gotwals, P.J., Koteliansky, V.E., et al. (2002) The EIIIA segment of fibronectin is a ligand for integrins α9β1 and α4β1 providing a novel mechanism for regulating cell adhesion by alternative splicing. *Journal of Biological Chemistry*, **277**, 14467–14474.

Liaw, L., Birk, D.E., Ballas, C.B., et al. (1998) Altered wound healing in mice lacking a functional osteopontin gene (spp1). *Journal of Clinical Investigation*, **101**, 1468–1478.

Lightner, V.A., Erickson, H.P. (1990) Binding of hexabrachion (tenascin) to the extracellular matrix and substratum and its effect on cell adhesion *Journal of Cell Science*, **95**, 263–277.

Lin, Z.Q., Kondo, T., Ishida, Y., et al. (2003) Essential involvement of IL-6 in the skin wound-healing process as evidenced by delayed wound healing in IL-6-deficient mice. *Journal of Leukocyte Biology*, **73**, 713–721.

Lotz, M.M., Rabinovitz, I., Mercurio, A.M. (2000) Intestinal restitution: progression of actin cytoskeleton rearrangements and integrin function in a model of epithelial wound healing. *American Journal of Pathology*, **156**, 985–996.

Lund, L.R., Rømer, J., Bugge, T.H., et al. (1999) Functional overlap between two classes of matrix-degrading proteases in wound healing *EMBO Journal*, **18**, 4645–4656.

Mackie, E.J., Tucker, R.P. (1999) The tenascin-C knockout revisited. *Journal of Cell Science*, **112**, 3847–3853.

Madlener, M., Mauch, C., Conca, W., et al. (1996) Regulation of the expression of stromelysin-2 by growth factors in keratinocytes: implications for normal and impaired wound healing. *Biochemical Journal*, **320**, 659–664.

Maeda, S., Dean, D.D., Gay, I., et al. (2001) Activation of latent transforming growth factor β1 by stromelysin 1 in extracts of growth plate chondrocyte-derived matrix vesicles. *Journal of Bone and Mineral Research*, **16**, 1281–1290.

Mainiero, F., Pepe, A., Yeon, M., et al. (1996) The intracellular functions of α6β4 integrin are regulated by EGF. *Journal of Cell Biology*, **134**, 241–253.

Mak, K., Manji, A., Gallant-Behm, C., et al. (2009) Scarless healing of oral mucosa is characterized by faster resolution of inflammation and control of myofibroblast action compared to skin wounds in the red Duroc pig model. *Journal of Dermatological Science*, **56**, 168–180.

Mann, A., Breuhahn, K., Schirmacher, P., et al. (2001) Keratinocyte-derived granulocyte-macrophage colony stimulating factor accelerates wound healing: Stimulation of keratinocyte proliferation, granulation tissue formation, and vascularization. *Journal of Investigative Dermatology*, **117**, 1382–1390.

Manohar, A., Shome, S.G., Lamar, J., et al. (2004) α3β1 integrin promotes keratinocyte cell survival through activation of a MEK/ERK signalling pathway. *Journal of Cell Science*, **117**, 4043–4054.

Marchese, C., Chedid, M., Dirsch, O.R., et al. (1995) Modulation of keratinocyte growth factor and its receptor in reepithelializing human skin. *Journal of Experimental Medicine*, **182**, 1369–1376.

Maretzky, T., Reiss, K., Ludwig, A., et al. (2005) ADAM10 mediates E-cadherin shedding and regulates epithelial cell-cell adhesion, migration, and beta-catenin translocation. *Proceedings of the National Academy of Sciences USA*, **102**, 9182–9187.

Margadant, C., Sonnenberg, A. (2010) Integrin-TGF-β crosstalk in fibrosis, cancer and wound healing. *EMBO Reports*, **11**, 97–105.

Margadant, C., Frijns, E., Wilhelmsen, K., et al. (2008) Regulation of hemidesmosome disassembly by growth factor receptors. *Current Opinion in Cell Biology*, **20**, 589–596.

Margadant, C., Raymond, K., Kreft, M., et al. (2009) Integrin α3β1 inhibits directional migration and wound re-epithelialization in the skin. *Journal of Cell Science*, **122**, 278–288.

Margadant, C., Charafeddine, R.A., Sonnenberg, A. (2010) Unique and redundant functions of integrins in the epidermis. *FASEB Journal*, **24**(11), 4133–4152.

Marikovsky, M., Breuing, K., Liu, P.Y., et al. (1993) Appearance of heparin-binding EGF-like growth factor in wound fluid as a response to injury. *Proceedings of the National Academy of Sciences USA*, **90**, 3889–3893.

Mariotti, A., Kedeshian, P.A., Dans, M., et al. (2001) EGF-R signalling through Fyn kinase disrupts the function of integrin α6β4 at hemidesmosomes: role in epithelial cell migration and carcinoma invasion. *Journal of Cell Biology*, **155**, 447–457.

Marti, G., Ferguson, M., Wang, J., et al. (2004) Electroporative transfection with KGF-1 DNA improves wound healing in a diabetic mouse model. *Gene Therapy*, **11**, 1780–1785.

Martin, P. (1997) Wound healing – aiming for perfect skin regeneration. *Science*, **276**, 75–81.

Matsumoto, K., Hashimoto, K., Yoshikawa, K., et al. (1991) Marked stimulation of growth and motility of human keratinocytes by hepatocyte growth factor. *Experimental Cell Research*, **196**, 114–120.

Mauch, C., Zamek, J., Abety, A.N., et al. (2010) Accelerated wound repair in ADAM-9 knockout animals. *Journal of Investigative Dermatology*, **130**, 2120–2130.

McCarthy, D.W., Downing, M.T., Brigstock, D.R., et al. (1996) Production of heparin-binding epidermal growth factor-like growth factor (HB-EGF) at sites of thermal injury in pediatric patients. *Journal of Investigative Dermatology*, **106**, 49–56.

McCawley, L.J., O'Brien, P., Hudson, L.G. (1998) Epidermal growth factor (EGF)- and scatter factor/hepatocyte growth factor (SF/HGF)-mediated keratinocyte migration is coincident with induction of matrix metalloproteinase (MMP)-9. *Journal of Cellular Physiology*, **176**, 255–265.

Meng, X., Klement, J.F., Leperi, D.A., et al. (2003) Targeted inactivation of murine laminin γ2-chain gene recapitulates human junctional epidermolysis bullosa. *Journal of Investigative Dermatology*, **121**, 720–731.

Miller, D.L., Ortega, S., Bashayan, O., et al. (2000) Compensation by fibroblast growth factor 1 (FGF1) does not account for the mild phenotypic defects observed in FGF2 null mice. *Molecular and Cellular Biology*, **20**, 2260–2268.

Mirastschijski, U., Haaksma, C.J., Tomasek, J.J., et al. (2004) Matrix metalloproteinase inhibitor GM 6001 attenuates keratinocyte migration, contraction and myofibroblast formation in skin wounds. *Experimental Cell Research*, **299**, 465–475.

Mitchell, K., Szekeres, C., Milano, V., et al. (2009) α3β1 integrin in epidermis promotes wound angiogenesis and keratinocyte-to-endothelial-cell crosstalk through the induction of MRP3. *Journal of Cell Science*, **122**, 1778–1787.

Miyamoto, S., Teramoto, H., Gutkind, J.S., et al. (1996) Integrins can collaborate with growth factors for phosphorylation of receptor tyrosine kinases and MAP kinase activation: roles of integrin aggregation and occupancy of receptors. *Journal of Cell Biology*, **135**, 1633–1642.

Mohan, R., Chintala, S.K., Jung, J.C., et al. (2002) Matrix metalloproteinase gelatinase B (MMP-9) coordinates and effects epithelial regeneration. *Journal of Biological Chemistry*, **277**, 2065–2072.

Morasso, M.I., Tomic-Canic, M. (2005) Epidermal stem cells: the cradle of epidermal determination, differentiation and wound healing. *Biology of the Cell*, **97**, 173–183.

Morgan, M.R., Humphries, M.J., Bass, M.D. (2007) Synergistic control of cell adhesion by integrins and syndecans. *Nature Reviews Molecular Cell Biology*, **8**, 957–969.

Mori, R., Kondo, T., Ohshima, T., et al. (2002) Accelerated wound healing in tumor necrosis factor receptor p55-deficient mice with reduced leukocyte infiltration. *FASEB Journal*, **16**, 963–974.

Moro, L., Venturino, M., Bozzo, C., et al. (1998) Integrins induce activation of EGF receptor: role in MAP kinase induction and adhesion-dependent cell survival. *EMBO Journal*, **17**, 6622–6632.

Moser, M., Legate, K.R., Zent, R., et al. (2009) The tail of integrins, talin, and kindlins. *Science*, **324**, 895–899.

Moses, M.A., Marikovsky, M., Harper, J.W., et al. (1996) Temporal study of the activity of matrix metalloproteinases and their endogenous inhibitors during wound healing. *Journal of Cellular Biochemistry*, **60**, 379–386.

Mould, A.P., Akiyama, S.K., Humphries, M.J. (1995) Regulation of integrin α5β1-fibronectin interactions by divalent cations. Evidence for distinct classes of binding sites for Mn^{2+}, Mg^{2+}, and Ca^{2+}. *Journal of Biological Chemistry*, **270**, 26270–26277.

Munger, J.S., Harpel, J.G., Giancotti, F.C., et al. (1998) Interactions between growth factors and integrins: latent forms of transforming growth factor-β are ligands for the integrin αvβ1. *Molecular Biology of the Cell*, **9**, 2627–2638.

Munger, J.S., Huang, X., Kawakatsu, H., et al. (1999) The integrin αvβ6 binds and activates latent TGF-β1: a mechanism for regulating pulmonary inflammation and fibrosis. *Cell*, **96**, 319–328.

Munz, B., Gerke, V., Gillitzer, R., et al. (1997) Differential expression of the calpactin I subunits annexin II and p11 in cultured keratinocytes and during wound repair. *Journal of Investigative Dermatology*, **108**, 307–312.

Munz, B., Smola, H., Engelhardt, F., et al. (1999) Overexpression of activin A in the skin of transgenic mice reveals new activities of activin in epidermal morphogenesis, dermal fibrosis and wound repair. *EMBO Journal*, **18**, 5205–5215.

Muro, A.F., Chauhan, A.K., Gajovic, S., et al. (2003) Regulated splicing of the fibronectin EDA exon is essential for proper skin wound healing and normal lifespan. *Journal of Cell Biology*, **162**, 149–160.

Nakanishi, K., Uenoyama, M., Tomita, N., et al. (2002) Gene transfer of human hepatocyte growth factor into rat skin wounds mediated by liposomes coated with the sendai virus (hemagglutinating virus of Japan). *American Journal of Pathology*, **161**, 1761–1772.

Nanney, L.B., King, L.E. (1996) Epidermal growth factor and transforming growth factor-α. In: *The Molecular and Cellular Biology of Wound Repair* (ed. R.A.F. Clark), 2nd edn, pp. 171–194. Plenum Press, New York.

Nickoloff, B.J., Mitra, R.S., Riser, B.L., et al. (1988) A modulation of keratinocyte motility. Correlation with production of extracellular matrix molecules in response to growth promoting and anti-proliferative factors. *American Journal of Pathology*, **132**, 543–551.

Nikolopoulos, S.N., Blaikie, P., Yoshioka, T., et al. (2005) Targeted deletion of the integrin β4 signaling domain suppresses laminin-5-dependent nuclear entry of mitogen-activated protein kinases and NF-κB, causing defects in epidermal growth and migration. *Molecular and Cellular Biology*, **25**, 6090–6102.

Nishiuchi, R., Sanzen, N., Nada, S., et al. (2005) Potentiation of the ligand-binding activity of integrin α3β1 via association with tetraspanin CD151. *Proceedings of the National Academy of Sciences USA*, **102**, 1939–1944.

Niu, J., Gu, X., Turton, J., et al. (1998) Integrin-mediated signalling of gelatinase B secretion in colon cancer cells. *Biochemical and Biophysical Research Communications*, **249**, 287–291.

Noli, C., Miolo, A. (2001) The mast cell in wound healing. *Veterinary Dermatology*, **12**, 303–313.

Nowak, J.A., Polak, L., Pasolli, H.A., et al. (2008) Hair follicle stem cells are specified and function in early skin morphogenesis. *Cell Stem Cell*, **3**, 33–43.

Nwomeh, B.C., Liang, H.X., Cohen, I.K., et al. (1999) MMP-8 is the predominant collagenase in healing wounds and nonhealing ulcers. *Journal of Surgical Research*, **81**, 189–195.

Odland, G., Ross, R. (1968) Human wound repair. I. Epidermal regeneration. *Journal of Cell Biology*, **39**, 135–168.

Oh, J.E., Park, K.H., Noh, H.K., et al. (2002) Decreased expression of α3 and β1 integrin subunits is responsible for differentiation-associated changes in cells behavior in terminally differentiated human oral keratinocytes. *Cell Communication and Adhesion*, **9**, 173–187.

Okamoto, O., Bachy, S., Odenthal, U., et al. (2003) Normal human keratinocytes bind to the α3LG4/5 domain of unprocessed laminin-5 through the receptor syndecan-1. *Journal of Biological Chemistry*, **278**, 44168–44177.

Oksala, O., Salo, T., Tammi, R., et al. (1995) Expression of proteoglycans and hyalyronan during wound healing. *Journal of Histochemistry and Cytochemistry*, **43**, 125–135.

Ortega, S., Ittmann, M., Tsang, S.H., et al. (1998) Neuronal defects and delayed wound healing in mice lacking fibroblast growth factor 2. *Proceedings of the National Academy of Sciences USA*, **95**, 5672–5677.

O'Toole, E.A., Marinkovich, M.P., Hoeffler, W.K., et al. (1997) Laminin-5 inhibits human keratinocyte migration. *Experimental Cell Research*, **233**, 330–339.

Owens, P., Engelking, E., Han, G., et al. (2010) Epidermal Smad4 deletion results in aberrant wound healing. *American Journal of Pathology*, **176**, 122–133.

Palecek, S.P., Loftus, J.C., Ginsberg, M.H., et al. (1997) Integrin-ligand binding properties govern cell migration speed through cell-substratum adhesiveness. *Nature*, **385**, 537–540.

Paller, A.S., Arnsmeier, S.L., Alvarez-Franco, M., et al. (1993) Ganglioside GM3 inhibits the proliferation of cultured keratinocytes. *Journal of Investigative Dermatology*, **100**, 841–845.

Paller, A.S., Arnsmeier, S.L., Chen, J.D., et al. (1995) Ganglioside GT1b inhibits keratinocyte adhesion and migration on a fibronectin matrix. *Journal of Investigative Dermatology*, **105**, 237–242.

Palmer, E.L., Ruegg, C., Ferrando, R., et al. (1993) Sequence and tissue distribution of the integrin α9 subunit, a novel partner of β1 that is widely distributed in epithelia and muscle. *Journal of Cell Biology*, **123**, 1289–1297.

Pankov, R., Yamada, K.M. (2002) Fibronectin at a glance. *Journal of Cell Science*, **115**, 3861–3863.

Paquet-Fifield, S., Schlüter, H., Li, A., et al. (2009) A role for pericytes as microenvironmental regulators of human skin tissue regeneration. *Journal of Clinical Investigation*, **119**, 2795–2806.

Parks, W.C. (1999) Matrix metalloproteinases in repair. *Wound Repair and Regeneration*, **7**, 423–432.

Parks, W.C. (2007) What is the $\alpha2\beta1$ integrin doing in the epidermis? *Journal of Investigative Dermatology*, **127**, 264–266.

Parks, W.C., Wilson, C.L., López-Boado, Y.S. (2004) Matrix metalloproteinases as modulators of inflammation and innate immunity. *Nature Reviews Immunology*, **4**, 617–629.

Patel, G.K., Wilson, C.H., Harding, K.G., et al. (2006) Numerous keratinocyte subtypes involved in wound re-epithelialization. *Journal of Investigative Dermatology*, **126**, 497–502.

Peñas, P.F., García-Díez, A., Sánchez-Madrid, F., et al. (2000) Tetraspanins are localized at motility-related structures and involved in normal human keratinocyte wound healing migration. *Journal of Investigative Dermatology*, **114**, 1126–1135.

Philipp, K., Riedel, F., Sauerbier, M., et al. (2004) Targeting TGF-β in human keratinocytes and its potential role in wound healing. *International Journal of Molecular Medicine*, **14**, 589–593.

Pilcher, B.K., Dumin, J.A., Sudbeck, B.D., et al. (1997) The activity of collagenase-1 is required for keratinocyte migration on a type I collagen matrix. *Journal of Cell Biology*, **137**, 1445–1457.

Pilcher, B.K., Wang, M., Qin, X.J., et al. (1999) Role of matrix metalloproteinases and their inhibition in cutaneous wound healing and allergic contact hypersensitivity. *Annals of the New York Academy of Sciences*, **878**, 12–24.

Porter, J.C., Hogg, N. (1998) Integrins take partners: cross-talk between integrins and other membrane receptors. *Trends in Cell Biology*, **8**, 390–396.

Potten, C.S. (1981) Cell replacement in epidermis (keratopoiesis) via discrete units of proliferation. *International Review of Cytology*, **69**, 271–318.

Price, L.S., Leng, J., Schwartz, M.A., et al. (1998) Activation of Rac and Cdc42 by integrins mediates cell spreading. *Molecular Biology of the Cell*, **9**, 1863–1871.

Pullar, C.E., Baier, B.S., Kariya, Y., et al. (2006) $\beta4$ integrin and epidermal growth factor coordinately regulate electric field-mediated directional migration via Rac1. *Molecular Biology of the Cell*, **17**, 4925–4935.

Putnins, E.E., Firth, J.D., Lohachitranont, A., et al. (1999) Keratinocyte growth factor (KGF) promotes keratinocyte cell attachment and migration on collagen and fibronectin. *Cell Adhesion and Communication*, **7**, 211–221.

Raghavan, S., Bauer, C., Mundschau, G., et al. (2000) Conditional ablation of $\beta1$ integrin in skin. Severe defects in epidermal proliferation, basement membrane formation, and hair follicle invagination. *Journal of Cell Biology*, **150**, 1149–1160.

Rappolee, D.A., Mark, D., Banda, M.J., et al. (1988) Wound macrophages express TGF-α and other growth factors in vivo: Analysis of RNA phenotyping. *Science*, **241**, 708–712.

Reed, M.J., Puolakkainen, P., Lane, T.F., et al. (1993) Differential expression of SPARC and thrombospondin 1 in wound repair: immunolocalization and in situ hybridization. *Journal of Histochemistry and Cytochemistry*, **41**, 1467–1477.

Reiss, M.J., Han, Y.P., Garcia, E., et al. (2010) Matrix metalloproteinase-9 delays wound healing in a murine wound model. *Surgery*, **147**, 295–302.

Repertinger, S.K., Campagnaro, E., Fuhrman, J., et al. (2004) EGFR enhances early healing after cutaneous incisional wounding. *Journal of Investigative Dermatology*, **123**, 982–989.

Reynolds, L.E., Conti, F.J., Lucas, M., et al. (2005) Accelerated re-epithelialization in $\beta3$-integrin-deficient mice is associated with enhanced TGF-$\beta1$ signaling. *Nature Medicine*, **11**, 167–174.

Reynolds, L.E., Conti, F.J., Silva, R., et al. (2008) $\alpha3\beta1$ integrin-controlled Smad7 regulates reepithelialization during wound healing in mice. *Journal of Clinical Investigation*, **118**, 965–974.

Richards, T.S., Dunn, C.A., Carter, W.G., et al. (2004) Protein kinase C spatially and temporally regulates gap junctional communication during human wound repair via phosphorylation of connexin43 on serine368. *Journal of Cell Biology*, **167**, 555–562.

Rodeck, U., Jost, M., Kari, C., et al. (1997) EGF-R dependent regulation of keratinocyte survival. *Journal of Cell Science*, **110**, 113–121.

Rømer, J., Bugge, T.H., Pyke, C., et al. (1996) Impaired wound healing in mice with disrupted plasminogen gene. *Nature Medicine*, **2**, 287–292.

Ruoslahti, E., Pierschbacher, M., Engvall, E., et al. (1982) Molecular and biological interactions of fibronectin. *Journal of Investigative Dermatology*, **79**, 65s–68s.

Russell, A.J., Fincher, E.F., Millman, L., et al. (2003) $\alpha6\beta4$ integrin regulates keratinocyte chemotaxis through differential GTPase activation and antagonism of $\alpha3\beta1$ integrin. *Journal of Cell Science*, **116**, 3543–3556.

Ryan, M.C., Lee, K., Miyashita, Y., et al. (1999) Targeted disruption of the LAMA3 gene in mice reveals abnormalities in survival and late stage differentiation of epithelial cells. *Journal of Cell Biology*, **145**, 1309–1323.

Saarialho-Kere, U.K., Chang, E.S., Welgus, H.G., et al. (1992) Distinct localization of collagenase and tissue inhibitor of metalloproteinases expression in wound healing associated with ulcerative pyogenic granuloma. *Journal of Clinical Investigation*, **90**, 1952–1957.

Saarialho-Kere, U., Kerkelä, E., Jahkola, T., et al. (2002) Epilysin (MMP-28) expression is associated with cell proliferation during epithelial repair. *Journal of Investigative Dermatology*, **119**, 14–21.

Sakai, T., Johnson, K.J., Murozono, M., et al. (2001) Plasma fibronectin supports neuronal survival and reduces brain injury following transient focal cerebral ischemia but is not essential for skin-wound healing and hemostasis. *Nature Medicine*, **7**, 324–330.

Salo, T., Mäkelä, M., Kylmäniemi, M., et al. (1994) Expression of matrix metalloproteinase-2 and -9 during early human wound healing. *Laboratory Investigation*, **70**, 176–182.

Salonurmi, T., Parikka, M., Kontusaari, S., et al. (2004) Overexpression of TIMP-1 under MMP-9 promoter interferes with wound healing in transgenic mice. *Cell and Tissue Research*, **315**, 27–37.

Sanaie, A.R., Firth, J.D., Uitto, V.J., et al. (2002) Keratinocyte growth factor (KGF)-1 and -2 protein and gene expression in human gingival fibroblasts. *Journal of Periodontal Research*, **37**, 66–74.

Sano, S., Chan, K.S., DiGiovanni, J. (2008) Impact of Stat3 activation upon skin biology: a dichotomy of its role between homeostasis and diseases. *Journal of Dermatological Science*, **50**, 1–14.

Santoro, M.M., Gaudino, G., Marchisio, P.C. (2003) The MSP receptor regulates $\alpha6\beta4$ and $\alpha3\beta1$ integrins via 14–3-3 proteins in keratinocyte migration. *Developmental Cell*, **5**, 257–271.

Satoh, Y., Saitoh, D., Takeuchi, A., et al. (2009) ERK2 dependent signaling contributes to wound healing after a partial-thickness burn. *Biochemical and Biophysical Research Communications*, **381**, 118–122.

Sauder, D.N., Kilian, P.L., McLane, J.A., et al. (1990) Interleukin-1 enhances epidermal wound healing. *Lymphokine Research*, **9**, 465–473.

Schaffer, C.J., Nanney, L.B. (1996) Cell biology of wound healing. *International Review of Cytology*, **169**, 151–181.

Schelfhout, V.R.J., Coene, E.D., Delaey, B., et al. (2002) The role of heregulin-α as a motility factor and amphiregulin as a growth factor in wound healing. *Journal of Pathology*, **198**, 523–533.

Schmitz, A., Tikkanen, R., Kirfel, G., et al. (2002) The biological role of the Alzheimer amyloid precursor protein in epithelial cells. *Histochemistry and Cell Biology*, **117**, 171–180.

Schneider, H., Mühle, C., Pacho, F. (2007) Biological function of laminin-5 and pathogenic impact of its deficiency. *European Journal of Cell Biology*, **86**, 701–717.

Scholz, F., Schulte, A., Adamski, F., et al. (2007) Constitutive expression and regulated release of the transmembrane chemokine CXCL16 in human and murine skin. *Journal of Investigative Dermatology*, **127**, 1444–1455.

Schultz, G.S., Wysocki, A. (2009) Interactions between extracellular matrix and growth factors in wound healing. *Wound Repair and Regeneration*, **17**, 153–162.

Seishima, M., Nojiri, M., Esaki, C., et al. (1999) Activin A induces terminal differentiation of cultured human keratinocytes. *Journal of Investigative Dermatology*, **112**, 432–436.

Shaw, T., Martin, P. (2009) Epigenetic reprogramming during wound healing: loss of polcomp-mediated silencing may enable upregulation of repair genes. *EMBO Reports*, **10**, 881–886.

Shirakata, Y., Komurasaki, T., Toyoda, H., et al. (2000) Epiregulin, a novel member of the epidermal growth factor family, is an autocrine growth factor in normal human keratinocytes. *Journal of Biological Chemistry*, **275**, 5748–5753.

Shirakata, Y., Kimura, R., Nanba, D., et al. (2005) Heparin-binding EGF-like growth factor accelerates keratinocyte migration and skin wound healing. *Journal of Cell Science*, **118**, 2363–2370.

Shirasawa, S., Sugiyama, S., Baba, I., et al. (2004) Dermatitis due to epiregulin deficiency and a critical role of epiregulin in immune-related responses of keratinocyte and macrophage. *Proceedings of the National Academy of Sciences USA*, **101**, 13921–13926.

Singh, P., Reimer, C.L., Peters, J.H., et al. (2004) The spatial and temporal expression patterns of integrin $\alpha9\beta1$ and one of its ligands, the EIIIA segment of fibronectin, in cutaneous wound healing. *Journal of Investigative Dermatology*, **123**, 1176–1181.

Singh, P., Chen, C., Pal-Ghosh, S., et al. (2009) Loss of integrin $\alpha9\beta1$ results in defects in proliferation, causing poor re-epithelialization during cutaneous wound healing. *Journal of Investigative Dermatology*, **129**, 217–228.

Sisco, M., Chao, J.D., Kim, I., et al. (2007) Delayed wound healing in Mac-1-deficient mice is associated with normal monocyte recruitment. *Wound Repair and Regeneration*, **15**, 566–571.

Song, B., Zhao, M., Forrester, J.V., et al. (2002) Electrical cues regulate the orientation and frequency of cell division and the rate of wound healing in vivo. *Proceedings of the National Academy of Sciences USA*, **99**, 13577–13582.

Song, B., Zhao, M., Forrester, J., et al. (2004) Nerve regeneration and wound healing are stimulated and directed by an endogenous electrical field in vivo. *Journal of Cell Science*, **117**, 4681–4690.

Steffensen, B., Häkkinen, L., Larjava, H. (2001) Proteolytic events of wound-healing – coordinated interactions among matrix metalloproteinases (MMPs), integrins, and extracellular matrix molecules. *Critical Reviews in Oral Biology and Medicine*, **12**, 373–398.

Steiling, H., Werner, S. (2003) Fibroblast growth factors: key players in epithelial morphogenesis, repair and cytoprotection. *Current Opinion in Biotechnology*, **14**, 533–537.

Stenn, K.S., Malhotra, R. (1992) Epithelialization. In: *Wound Healing. Biochemical and Clinical Aspects* (eds. I.K. Cohe, R.F. Diegelmann, W.J. Lindblad), pp. 115–127. WB Saunders, Philadelphia.

Stepp, M.A. (1999) α9 and β8 integrin expression correlates with the merger of the developing mouse eyelids. *Developmental Dynamics*, **214**, 216–228.

Stepp, M.A., Gibson, H.E., Gala, P.H., et al. (2002) Defects in keratinocyte activation during wound healing in the syndecan-1-deficient mouse. *Journal of Cell Science*, **115**, 4517–4531.

Sterk, L.M., Geuijen, C.A., Oomen, L.C., et al. (2000) The tetraspan molecule CD151, a novel constituent of hemidesmosomes, associates with the integrin α6β4 and may regulate the spatial organization of hemidesmosomes. *Journal of Cell Biology*, **149**, 969–982.

Stoscheck, C.M., Nanney, L.B. and King, L.E. Jr (1992) Quantitative determination of EGF-R during epidermal wound healing. *Journal of Investigative Dermatology*, **99**, 645–649.

Streit, M., Velasco, P., Riccardi, L., et al. (2000) Thrombospondin-1 suppresses wound healing and granulation tissue formation in the skin of transgenic mice. *EMBO Journal*, **19**, 3272–3282.

Streuli, C.H., Akhtar, N. (2009) Signal co-operation between integrins and other receptor systems. *Biochemical Journal*, **418**, 491–506.

Stricklin, G.P., Li, L., Jancic, V., et al. (1993) Localization of mRNAs representing collagenase and TIMP in sections of healing human burn wounds. *American Journal of Pathology*, **143**, 1657–1666.

Stupack, D.G. (2005) Integrins as a distinct subtype of dependence receptors. *Cell Death and Differentiation*, **12**, 1021–1030.

Sullivan, M.M., Puolakkainen, P.A., Barker, T.H., et al. (2008) Altered tissue repair in hevin-null mice: inhibition of fibroblast migration by a matricellular SPARC homolog. *Wound Repair and Regeneration*, **16**, 310–319.

Sung, C.C., O'Toole, E.A., Lannutti, B.J., et al. (1998) Integrin α5β1 expression is required for inhibition of keratinocyte migration by ganglioside GT1b. *Experimental Cell Research*, **239**, 311–319.

Swindle, C.S., Tran, K.T., Johnson, T.D., et al. (2001) Epidermal growth factor (EGF)-like repeats of human tenascin-C as ligands for EGF receptor. *Journal of Cell Biology*, **154**, 459–468.

Tagashira, S., Harada, H., Katsumata, T., et al. (1997) Cloning of mouse FGF10 and up-regulation of its gene expression during wound healing. *Gene*, **197**, 399–404.

Tokumaru, S., Higashiyama, S., Endo, T., et al. (2000) Ectodomain shedding of epidermal growth factor ligands is required for keratinocyte migration in cutaneous wound healing. *Journal of Cell Biology*, **151**, 209–220.

Toledo, M.S., Suzuki, E., Handa, K., et al. (2005) Effect of ganglioside and tetraspanins in microdomains on interaction of integrinswith fibroblast growth factor receptor. *Journal of Biological Chemistry*, **280**, 16227–16234.

Tran, K.T., Griffith, L. and Wells, A. (2004) Extracellular matrix signaling through growth factor receptors during wound healing. *Wound Repair and Regeneration*, **12**, 262–268.

Tredget, E.B., Demare, J., Chandran, G., et al. (2005) Transforming growth factor-β and its effect on reepithelialization of partial-thickness ear wounds in transgenic mice. *Wound Repair and Regeneration*, **13**, 61–67.

Trengove, N.J., Stacey, M.C., MacAuley, S., et al. (1999) Analysis of the acute and chronic wound environments: the role of proteases and their inhibitors. *Wound Repair and Regeneration*, **7**, 442–452.

Trusolino, L., Bertotti, A., Comoglio, P.M. (2001) A signalling adaptor function for α6β4 integrin in the control of HGF-dependent invasive growth. *Cell*, **107**, 643–654.

Tscharntke, M., Pofahl, R., Chrostek-Grashoff, A., et al. (2007) Impaired epidermal wound healing in vivo upon inhibition or deletion of Rac1. *Journal of Cell Science*, **120**, 1480–1490.

Tsuboi, R., Sato, C., Kurita, Y., et al. (1993) Keratinocyte growth factor (FGF-7) stimulates migration and plasminogen activator activity of normal human keratinocytes. *Journal of Investigative Dermatology*, **101**, 49–53.

Uitto, J., Mauviel, A., McGrath, J. (1996) The dermal-epidermal basement membrane zone in cutaneous wound healing. In: *The Molecular and Cellular Biology of Wound Repair* (ed. R.A.F. Clark), 2nd edn, pp. 513–560. Plenum Press, New York.

Usui, M.L., Underwood, R.A., Mansbridge, J.N., et al. (2005) Morphological evidence for the role of suprabasal keratinocytes in wound reepithelialization. *Wound Repair and Regeneration*, **13**, 468–479.

Usui, M.L., Mansbridge, J.N., Carter, W.G., et al. (2008) Keratinocyte migration, proliferation, and differentiation in chronic ulcers from patients with diabetes and normal wounds. *Journal of Histochemistry and Cytochemistry*, **56**, 687–696.

Vaalamo, M., Weckroth, M., Puolakkainen, P., et al. (1996) Patterns of matrix metalloproteinase and TIMP-1 expression in chronic and normally healing human cutaneous wounds. *British Journal of Dermatology*, **135**, 52–59.

Varani, J., Zeigler, M., Dame, M.K., et al. (2001) Heparin-binding epidermal-growth-factor-like growth factor activation of keratinocyte ErbB receptors Mediates epidermal hyperplasia, a prominent side-effect of retinoid therapy. *Journal of Investigative Dermatology*, **117**, 1335–1341.

Vermeij, W.P., Backendorf, C. (2010) Skin cornification proteins provide global link between ROS detoxification and cell migration during wound healing. *PLoS One*, **5**, e11957.

Vogel, B.E., Tarone, G., Giancotti, F.G., et al. (1990) A novel fibronectin receptor with an unexpected subunit composition (αvβ1). *Journal of Biological Chemistry*, **265**, 5934–5937.

Waelti, E.R., Inaebnit, S.P., Rast, H.P., et al. (1992) Co-culture of human keratinocytes on post-mitotic human dermal fibroblast feeder cells: production of large amounts of interleukin 6. *Journal of Investigative Dermatology*, **98**, 805–808.

Wang, M.H., Dlugosz, A.A., Sun, Y., et al. (1996) Macrophage-stimulating protein induces proliferation and migration of murine keratinocytes. *Experimental Cell Research*, **226**, 39–46.

Wang, X., Sun, P., Al-Qamari, A., et al. (2001) Carbohydrate-carbohydrate binding of ganglioside to integrin α5 modulates α5β1 function. *Journal of Biological Chemistry*, **276**, 84326–8444.

Wang, X.J., Han, G., Owens, P., et al. (2006) Role of TGF beta-mediated inflammation in cutaneous wound healing. *Journal of Investigative Dermatology Symposium Proceedings*, **11**, 112–117.

Wang, X.Q., Sun, P., Paller, A.S. (2003) Ganglioside GM3 blocks the activation of epidermal growth factor receptor induced by integrin at specific tyrosine sites. *Journal of Biological Chemistry*, **278**, 48770–48778.

Wankell, M., Munz, B., Hübner, G., et al. (2001) Impaired wound healing in transgenic mice overexpressing the activin antagonist follistatin in the epidermis. *EMBO Journal*, **20**, 5361–5372.

Wary, K.K., Mainiero, F., Isakoff, S.J., et al. (1996) The adaptor protein Shc couples to a class of integrins to the control of cell cycle progression. *Cell*, **87**, 733–743.

Wary, K.K., Mariotti, A., Zurzolo, C., et al. (1998) A requirement for caveolin-1 and associated kinase Fyn in integrin signaling and anchorage-dependent cell growth. *Cell*, **94**, 625–634.

Watt, F.M. (2002) Role of integrins in regulating epidermal adhesion, growth and differentiation. *EMBO Journal*, **21**, 3919–3926.

Weckroth, M., Vaheri, A., Virolainen, S., et al. (2004) Epithelial tissue-type plasminogen activator expression, unlike that of urokinase, its receptor, and plasminogen activator inhibitor-1, is increased in chronic venous ulcers. *British Journal of Dermatology*, **151**, 1189–1196.

Wenczak, B.A., Lynch, J.B., Nanney, L.B. (1992) Epidermal growth factor receptor distribution in burn wounds. *Journal of Clinical Investigation*, **90**, 2392–2401.

Werner, S. (1998) Keratinocyte growth factor: a unique player in epithelial repair processes. *Cytokine and Growth Factor Reviews*, **9**, 153–165.

Werner, S., Peters, K.G., Longaker, M.T., et al. (1992) Large induction of keratinocyte growth factor expression in the dermis during wound healing. *Proceedings of the National Academy of Sciences USA*, **89**, 6896–6900.

Werner, S., Smola, H., Liao, X., et al. (1994) The function of KGF in morphogenesis of epithelium and re-epithelialization of wounds. *Science*, **266**, 819–822.

Werner, S., Krieg, T., Smola, H. (2007) Keratinocyte-fibroblast interactions in wound healing. *Journal of Investigative Dermatology*, **127**, 998–1008.

White, J.M. (2003) ADAMs: modulators of cell-cell and cell-matrix interactions. *Current Opinion in Cell Biology*, **15**, 598–606.

Wikner, N.E., Persichitte, K.A., Baskin, J.B., et al. (1988) Transforming growth factor-β stimulates the expression of fibronectin by human keratinocytes. *Journal of Investigative Dermatology*, **91**, 207–212.

Wipff, P.J., Hinz, B. (2008) Integrins and the activation of latent transforming growth factor beta1 - an intimate relationship. *European Journal of Cell Biology*, **87**, 601–615.

Wong, J.W., Gallant-Behm, C., Wiebe, C., et al. (2009) Wound healing in oral mucosa results in reduced scar formation as compared with skin: evidence from the red Duroc pig model and humans. *Wound Repair and Regeneration*, **17**, 717–729.

Woodley, D.T. (1996) Reepithelialization. In: *The Molecular and Cellular Biology of Wound Repair* (ed. R.A.F. Clark), 2nd edn, pp. 339–354. Plenum Press, New York.

Woodley, D.T., Chen, J.D., Kim, J.P., et al. (1993) Reepithelialization: human keratinocyte locomotion. *Dermatologic Clinics*, **11**, 641–646.

Wysocki, A.B., Grinnell, F. (1990) Fibronectin profiles in normal and chronic wound fluid. *Laboratory Investigation*, **63**, 825–831.

Xie, Y., Gao, K., Häkkinen, L., et al. (2009) Mice lacking β6 integrin in skin show accelerated wound repair in dexamethasone impaired wound healing model. *Wound Repair and Regeneration*, **17**, 326–339.

Yahata, Y., Shirakata, Y., Tokomaru, S., et al. (2006) A novel function of angiotensin II in skin wound healing. Introduction of fibroblast and keratinocyte migration by angiotensin II via heparin-binding epidermal growth factor (EGF)-like growth factor-mediated EGF receptor transactivation. *Journal of Biological Chemistry*, **281**, 13209–13216.

Yang, J.T., Rayburn, H., Hynes, R.O. (1993) Embryonic mesodermal defects in α5 integrin-deficient mice. *Development*, **119**, 1093–1105.

Yang, L., Qiu, C.X., Ludlow, A., et al. (1999) Active transforming growth factor-β in wound repair: determination using a new assay. *American Journal of Pathology*, **154**, 105–11.

Yang, L., Chan, T., Demare, J., et al. (2001) Healing of burn wounds in transgenic mice overexpressing transforming growth factor-β1 in the epidermis. *American Journal of Pathology*, **159**, 2147–2157.

Yates, C.C., Whaley, D., Hooda, S., et al. (2009) Delayed reepithelialization and basement membrane regeneration after wounding in mice lacking CXCR3. *Wound Repair and Regeneration*, **17**, 34–41.

Yokosaki, Y., Palmer, E.L., Prieto, A.L., et al. (1994) The integrin α9β1mediates cell attachment to a non-RGD site in the third fibronectin type III repeat of tenascin. *Journal of Biological Chemistry*, **269**, 26691–26696.

Yoshida, S., Yamaguchi, Y., Itami, S., et al. (2003) Neutralization of hepatocyte growth factor leads to retarded cutaneous wound healing associated with decreased neovascularization and granulation tissue formation. *Journal of Investigative Dermatology*, **120**, 335–343.

Yoshida, S., Matsumoto, K., Tomioka, D., et al. (2004) Recombinant hepatocyte growth factor accelerates cutaneous wound healing in a diabetic mouse model. *Growth Factors*, **22**, 111–119.

Yu, Q., Stamenkovic, I. (2000) Cell surface-localized matrix metalloproteinase-9 proteolytically activates TGF-β and promotes tumor invasion and angiogenesis. *Genes and Development*, **14**, 163–176.

Zambruno, G., Marchisio, P.C., Marconi, A., et al. (1995) Transforming growth factor-β1 modulates β1 and β5 integrin receptors and induces de novo expression of the αvβ6 heterodimer in normal human keratinocytes: implications for wound healing. *Journal of Cell Biology*, **129**, 853–865.

Zhang, K., Kramer, R.H. (1996) Laminin 5 deposition promotes keratinocyte motility. *Experimental Cell Research*, **227**, 309–322.

Zhang, X., Ibrahimi, O.A., Olsen, S.K., et al. (2006) Receptor specificity of the fibroblast growth factor family. The complete mammalian FGF family. *Journal of Biological Chemistry*, **281**, 15694–15700.

Zhang, X.A., Bontrager, A.L., Hemler, M.E. (2001) Transmembrane-4 superfamily proteins associate with activated protein kinase C (PKC) and link PKC to specific β1 integrins. *Journal of Biological Chemistry*, **276**, 25005–25013.

Zhang, Z., Morla, A.O., Vuori, K., et al. (1993) The αvβ1 integrin functions as a fibronectin receptor but does not support fibronectin matrix assembly and cell migration on fibronectin. *Journal of Cell Biology*, **122**, 235–242.

Zhang, Z., Vuori, K., Reed, J.C., et al. (1995) The α5β1 integrin supports survival of cells on fibronectin and up-regulates Bcl-2 expression. *Proceedings of the National Academy of Sciences USA*, **92**, 6161–6165.

Zhao, M. (2009) Electrical fields in wound healing-An overriding signal that directs cell migration. *Seminars in Cell and Developmental Biology* **20**, 674–682.

Zhao, M., Pu, J., Forrester, J.V., et al. (2002) Membrane lipids, EGF receptors, and intracellular signals colocalize and are polarized in epithelial cells moving directionally in a physiological electric field. *FASEB Journal*, **16**, 857–859.

Zhao, M., Song, B., Pu, J., et al. (2003) Direct visualization of a stratified epithelium reveals that wounds heal by unified sliding of cell sheets. *FASEB Journal*, **17**, 397–406.

Zhao, M., Song, B., Pu, J., et al. (2006) Electrical signals control wound healing through phosphatidylinositol-3-OH kinase-gamma and PTEN. *Nature*, **442**, 457–4560.

Zigrino, P., Steiger, J., Fox, J.W., et al. (2007) Role of ADAM-9 disintegrin-cysteine-rich domains in human keratinocyte migration. *Journal of Biological Chemistry*, **282**, 30785–30793.

Zouq, N.K., Keeble, J.A., Lindsay, J., et al. (2009) FAK engages multiple pathways to maintain survival of fibroblasts and epithelia: differential roles for paxillin and p130Cas. *Journal of Cell Science*, **122**, 357–367.

Zweers, M.C., Davidson, J.M., Pozzi, A., et al. (2007) Integrin α2β1 is required for regulation of murine wound angiogenesis but is dispensable for reepithelialization. *Journal of Investigative Dermatology*, **127**, 467–478.

6 Granulation Tissue Formation and Remodeling

Lari Häkkinen, Hannu Larjava and Leeni Koivisto
Faculty of Dentistry, University of British Columbia, Vancouver, Canada

INTRODUCTION

The aim of this chapter is to summarize the key biological processes involved in soft connective tissue wound healing particularly in the context of oral mucosa. In a broader sense, healing of the connective tissue is not a separate, self-driven process, but occurs in a reciprocal interaction with other tissue components and cells, including the epithelium, vasculature and inflammatory cells, and these interactions will also be discussed when relevant.

From a clinical point of view, connective tissue wound healing is a critical process that restores the blood supply, integrity, mechanical strength and function of the injured tissue. While injury to the epithelium alone results in complete tissue regeneration, connective tissue healing especially in skin is usually not optimal, and can lead to scarring. Scar formation depends on the extent and location of the injury, and may involve small esthetically unpleasant scars, or in more severe cases, pathological hyperthrophic or keloid scars that can cause considerable morbidity to the affected individuals (Bayat et al. 2003). Nonhealing or chronic wounds that often associate with prolonged infection or predisposing systemic conditions, including diabetes, display compromised re-epithelialization, connective tissue healing and angiogenesis, and also result in significant morbidity and financial burden to the individuals and society (Harding et al. 2002; Elliott and Hamilton 2011). Remarkably, wound-healing problems in oral mucosa appear to be less dramatic and frequent than those in skin, and possible reasons for this difference are also discussed.

The reader should keep in mind that much of the available information about connective tissue wound healing is based on studies of skin cells or skin wound healing. However, although both skin and oral mucosa are composed of a stratified squamous epithelium (called epidermis in skin) and connective tissue (called dermis in skin), they have certain important structural and functional differences. For instance, while certain areas of oral mucosa contain small salivary glands, different anatomical locations of skin can harbor adnexa (hair follicles, sebaceous glands and sweat glands) and abundant subcutaneous fat (adipose) tissue which are either missing or less abundant in the oral mucosa. Both skin adnexa and adipose tissue hold stem or progenitor cells that may contribute to epidermal and dermal wound healing (Stephens and Genever 2007; Zouboulis et al. 2008; Sellheyer and Krahl 2010). Moreover, the density of vascular capillaries and blood flow appears significantly higher in the oral mucosa compared with skin (Canady et al. 1993). The composition

Oral Wound Healing: Cell Biology and Clinical Management, First Edition. Edited by Hannu Larjava.

of the extracellular matrix (ECM) in the skin and oral mucosal connective tissue is also distinct, and fibroblasts derived from these two tissues have significant functional and phenotypical differences (Schor et al. 1996; Enoch et al. 2010). Human skin thickness, structure and composition is variable depending on body location, and oral mucosa also differs in these aspects at different areas, including non-keratinized lining mucosa containing a loose connective tissue, and keratinized masticatory mucosa composed of a dense connective tissue attached to the underlying bone. Certain anatomical areas of oral cavity also contain specialized cells and tissues, including gustatory mucosa of the tongue and periodontal tissues. Therefore, wound healing in these different locations may have special characteristics that depend on the anatomy and specific cells and tissue components that are involved. Oral mucosa is also bathed by saliva that has a unique molecular composition, microflora and moisture which may promote the wound healing process (Kaufman and Lamster 2000; Stephens and Genever 2007; Reish et al. 2009; Loo et al. 2010), whereas in skin, wound healing occurs in a dry and microbiologically distinct environment, and the wound surface becomes covered with a protective scab (crust). Finally, many of the skin wound healing studies have been performed using loose skin animal models, including mice and other rodents. In rodents, skin is anatomically partially different from human skin, and wound closure is primarily mediated by contraction. This is fundamentally different from tight skinned animals, including humans and pigs, where wound contraction plays a minor role (Gottrup et al. 2000; Chillcott 2008). It is conceivable that in the masticatory oral mucosa where the connective tissue is firmly attached to the underlying bone, wound contraction may play an even lesser role in the wound healing process.

OVERVIEW OF CONNECTIVE TISSUE RESPONSE TO WOUNDING

Soft connective tissue of oral mucosa or skin is formed and maintained by fibroblasts which are the major producers of the collagen-rich ECM. Function of fibroblasts is supported by vasculature formed by endothelial cells and associated cells (pericytes and smooth muscle cells) which supply nutrients and oxygen to the cells. In normal uninjured connective tissue, fibroblasts encounter few signals from their microenvironment (i.e. niche) and, therefore, reside in a relatively dormant, quiescent state, being metabolically active but unable to proliferate. In this state, fibroblasts are firmly attached to their pericellular ECM and slowly synthesize, degrade and organize the ECM to maintain the tissue structure (De Donatis et al. 2010; Lemons et al. 2010). However, cells remain responsive to various signals in their microenvironment. For instance, at least in skin and periodontal ligament, fibroblasts form an interconnected network through cell–cell adhesions which allows them to exchange information directly via gap junctions (Solomon et al. 1988). These connections may allow the cells to respond collectively to changing functional demands. Quiescent fibroblasts are also responsive to paracrine signaling molecules released from other cells present in the connective tissue or in the epithelium (Roosterman et al. 2006; Chong et al. 2009), and they possess receptors for circulating hormones which may affect their function during tissue homeostasis (Schmuth et al. 2007). In addition, there is a continuous, bidirectional interaction between cells and their surrounding ECM, termed dynamic reciprocity, where biochemical and mechanical signals from ECM molecules regulate cell functions through specific receptor–ligand interactions, and this in turn influences the composition and quantity of the ECM produced by the cells (Schultz et al. 2011). For instance, fibroblasts can sense changes

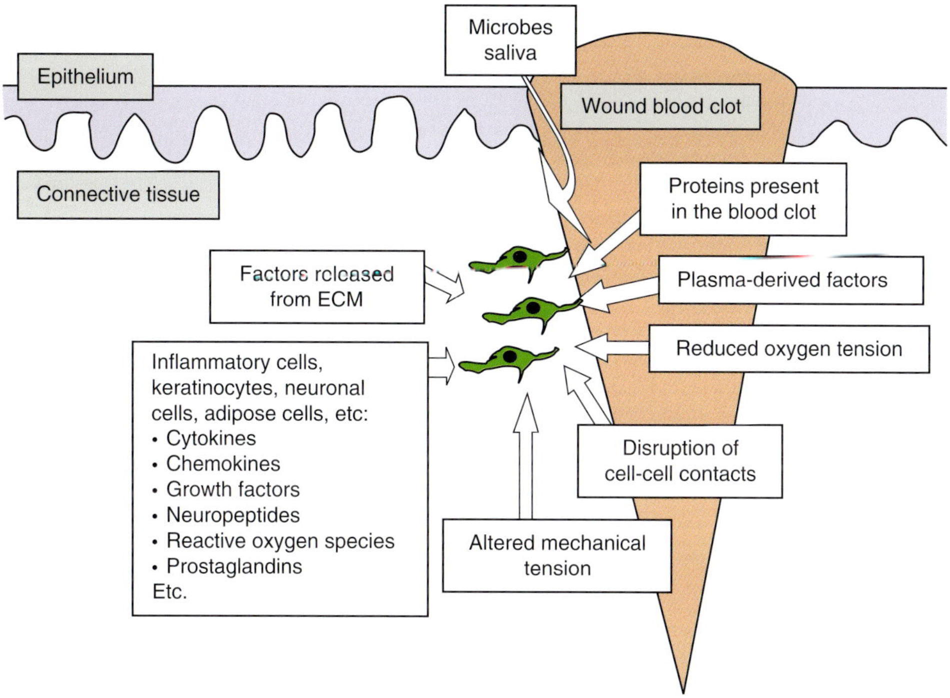

Fig. 6.1 Factors that upon wounding participate in activation of fibroblasts or their progenitor cells to produce granulation tissue.

in the magnitude or direction of mechanical tension in the tissue through specific cell-ECM adhesions mediated by members of the integrin family. This mechanosensory mechanism allows fibroblasts to modulate the ECM to meet changing functional demands (Schwartz 2010). A classical example is the cellular and tissue changes that occur in the periodontal ligament as a response to changing masticatory forces or during orthodontic tooth movement (Meikle 2006; Pavasant and Yongchaitrakul 2011).

Wounding to the tissue induces dramatic changes in the cell's signaling environment, resulting in activation of the cells from the quiescent state (De Donatis et al. 2010; Fig. 6.1). First, upon injury, fibroblasts close to the wound come in contact with microbes that now have access into the tissue and may directly or indirectly by releasing soluble factors interact with fibroblasts and regulate their functions (Hill and Ebersole 1996; Lai et al. 2009; Burke et al. 2010). In oral cavity, molecules present in saliva may also have access to the tissue and fibroblasts (Loo et al. 2010). Second, fibroblasts become exposed to blood-borne cells and factors coming to the area from damaged blood vessels (Clark 1996; Gurtner et al. 2008). Third, fibroblasts experience change in oxygen tension as normal blood supply is disturbed (Tandara and Mustoe 2004). Fourth, cell–cell contacts between fibroblasts are disrupted, breaking the direct cell-to-cell signaling network (Chanson et al. 2005). Fifth, wounding exposes and releases ECM molecules or their components that fibroblasts do not normally encounter (Clark 1996; Gurtner et al. 2008). Sixth, wounding disrupts the mechanical integrity of the tissue and fibroblasts sense the resulting change in the mechanical tension from the ECM (Bush et al. 2008; Schwartz 2010). Seventh, other

Table 6.1 Role of fibroblasts at different stages of wound healing.

Granulation tissue formation
Proliferation
Migration
ECM deposition
Regulation of inflammation, re-epithelialization and angiogenesis
Wound contraction
Differentiation into myofibroblasts
Wound contraction and reorganization of ECM
Remodeling
Downregulate ECM deposition
ECM degradation
Collagen cross-linking
ECM reorganization and maturation
Downregulate cell proliferation
Undergo apoptosis
Assume senescence
Assume quiescent state

cells in the wound area, including inflammatory, epithelial, vascular, adipose and neuronal cells, are activated to secrete or release paracrine factors that modulate fibroblast functions (Barrientos et al. 2008). Eighth, fibroblasts become exposed to new ECM proteins as the fibrin and fibronectin-rich blood clot replaces the regular collagen-rich ECM (Clark 1996; Gurtner et al. 2008).

To quickly start the repair of the connective tissue injury by formation of a granulation tissue, the above-mentioned multiple signals occurring upon wounding need to appropriately activate various fibroblast functions (Table 6.1). This is a very complex process, and regulation of the specificity of the cellular responses to these multiple signals is still poorly understood, but likely depends on the quantity (concentration) and duration of the activating signals, the interplay between multiple simultaneous signals, and cellular context, i.e. cell type and differentiation stage (De Donatis et al. 2010). The activating signals need to initiate fibroblast cell proliferation, prompt the cells to modulate their adhesions to the ECM and provide directional cues to allow cell migration into the injury site filled with the blood clot (also termed provisional wound matrix). Once the cells have migrated into the provisional wound matrix, they need to proliferate again and rapidly produce new granulation tissue ECM to start the repair process. The rapidly formed, primitive, hypercellular granulation tissue serves as a framework for subsequent connective tissue healing. Granulation tissue fibroblasts also participate in regulation of other processes important for wound healing, including inflammation, re-epithelialization and angiogenesis. The granulation tissue rich in cells and poorly organized primitive ECM is finally turned into a mature connective tissue by a slow process called tissue remodeling that ultimately restores the connective tissue structure and function. This process also involves differentiation of fibroblasts into contractile myofibroblasts (Clark 1996). As cell functions need to change fundamentally during granulation tissue formation and remodeling stages, the signaling environment that dictates these functions has to be spatiotemporally well controlled. For the tissue remodeling to occur appropriately, the number of ECM-producing fibroblasts needs to be reduced, and the remaining fibroblasts have to downregulate their active production of new ECM. Instead, they need to be induced to remodel and reorganize the ECM necessary for complete regeneration of the lost tissue to its original form and function. Completion of re-epithelialization that protects the connective tissue from effects of external factors (microbes), angiogenesis that restores oxygen tension and nutrient supply, downregulation of the inflammatory reaction, quantitative and qualitative changes in the growth factors, cytokines and other mediators in the wound area, changes in the composition of ECM, and altered mechanical signals mediated from the ECM all contribute to the changes occurring in fibroblast functions at these stages of wound healing.

The following paragraphs discuss the identity and role of fibroblasts in wound healing, and summarize in more detail the key biological processes involved in various stages of connective tissue wound healing. More detailed description of other aspects of the wound-healing stages can be found elsewhere in this book.

WOUND HEALING STAGES

Wound healing is traditionally divided into stages that describe the key biological processes that dominate the given stage, i.e. hemostasis and blood clot formation, inflammation, re-epithelialization, granulation tissue formation and remodeling of the connective tissue (Clark 1996; Gurtner et al. 2008; Fig. 6.2). The indicated order of the stages follows the order of initiation of each stage relative to the time of injury, but there is considerable overlap between the stages. The duration of each stage depends on the size of the wound. For instance, incisional wounds with good primary closure heal fast by primary intention involving very little granulation tissue formation. This is in contrast to large excisional wounds where ideal primary closure cannot be achieved, and which heal by secondary intention and abundant granulation tissue formation. In this type of wound, epithelium needs to migrate for a considerably longer distance to cover the wound surface, resulting in a longer re-epithelialization stage compared with that of incisional wounds with good primary closure. Accordingly, as healing by secondary intention involves abundant granulation tissue formation, connective tissue healing also takes longer to be completed (Clark 1996). Within a given wound, different parts of the wound can be at a different wound healing stage at the same time. This reflects gradual collective migration of epithelial and connective tissue cells (fibroblasts and endothelial cells) into the wound provisional matrix from the wound edges. Therefore, wound healing in the area closer to the wound edge is progressed to a slightly more advanced stage than in the mid part. Furthermore, connective tissue healing appears to progress faster underneath the wound epithelium than in the deeper parts. This is likely due to an active interplay between epithelial cells and fibroblasts during wound healing (Werner et al. 2007; Koskela et al. 2010; Fig. 6.3). Compared to wound healing in the oral mucosa or skin, timing of wound healing stages can be somewhat different at the tooth–gingiva interface where the cells involved in wound healing originate from the single soft tissue side of the wound.

ORIGIN AND IDENTITY OF WOUND FIBROBLASTS

Fibroblasts are ubiquitous cells found in virtually all tissues, and are broadly defined as adherent cells that have a capacity to synthesize and remodel the collagen-rich ECM (Darby and Hewitson 2007; Sorrell and Caplan 2009). Their importance in wound healing has been

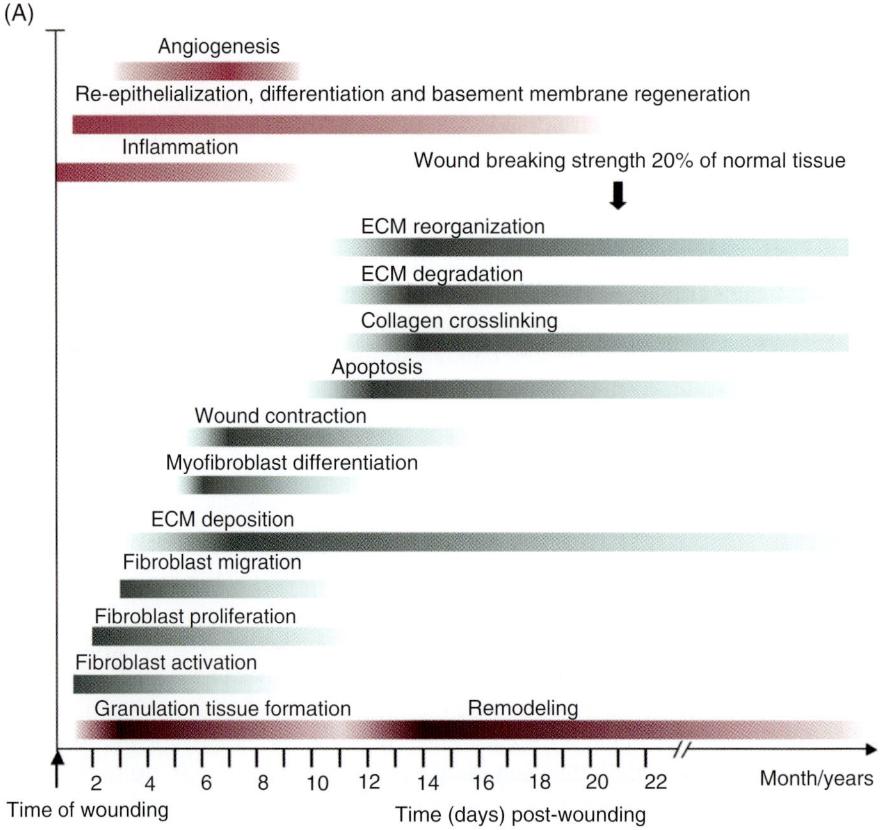

Fig. 6.2 Schematic presentation of timing of the wound healing stages (A), and histological characteristics of full-thickness excisional skin wounds at various stages of wound healing in pig (B). (A) See text for details. (B) In normal, unwounded connective tissue, collagen is organized in the typical basketweave pattern (A–C). Three days post-wounding (D–F), a fibrin clot occupies the wound space, and a scab has formed on the wound surface (D and E). Structurally, the blood clot is devoid of apparent newly deposited fibrillar ECM (F). Most abundant cellular infiltrate localizes to the wound surface and at the base of the wound (D). Seven days after wounding (G–I), epithelium has migrated to cover the entire wound surface (G), and a highly cellular granulation tissue has been formed (G and H). The granulation tissue contains thin, poorly organized, newly deposited fibrillar ECM (I). At day 14 after wounding (J–L), the newly formed connective tissue in the wound area has started to contract, especially in the mid part of the tissue, bringing the wound edges closer together (J). Wound fibroblasts are organized parallel to each other and perpendicular to the wound edges, indicating active, cell-driven wound contraction (K). Fibrillar ECM in the wound area is now composed of thicker, abundant collagen fibers that are organized perpendicular to the wound edges (L). At day 21 after wounding (M–O), wound contraction has progressed further (M). Cell density in the maturing wound connective tissue is reduced compared to day 14 after wounding, but the tissue is still hypercellular as compared to unwounded tissue. At this point, orientation of the wound fibroblasts has partially started to shift from parallel to a more random organization (N). Organization of part of the fibrillar ECM has become more basketweave-like, and the collagen fibers have gained more thickness as compared to earlier time points (O). At day 49 post-wounding (P–R), the wound area is still clearly visible histologically. The connective tissue in the wound area is still hypercellular, and many of the cells remain in parallel orientation, which follows the organization of the collagen in the ECM, indicating presence of a scar (Q). Many of the collagen fibers in the wound area are still thinner than in the unwounded tissue, and they lack the basketweave pattern typical of normal connective tissue (R). NW: non-wounded tissue; D3, D7, D14, D21, D49: tissue samples collected at indicated days post-wounding; A, B, D, E, G, H, J, K, M, N, P, Q: light microscope images of histological sections stained with Movat's pentachrome stain. Green color indicates mature and purple immature collagen; C, F, I, L, O, R: hematoxylin and eosin stained sections viewed under UV-light using the rhodamine channel in a fluorescence microscope. E: epithelium; CT: connective tissue; AT: adipose tissue; M: muscle; FC: fibrin clot; Sc: scab; GT: granulation tissue; WCT: wound connective tissue undergoing remodeling. Magnification bar = 100 μm.

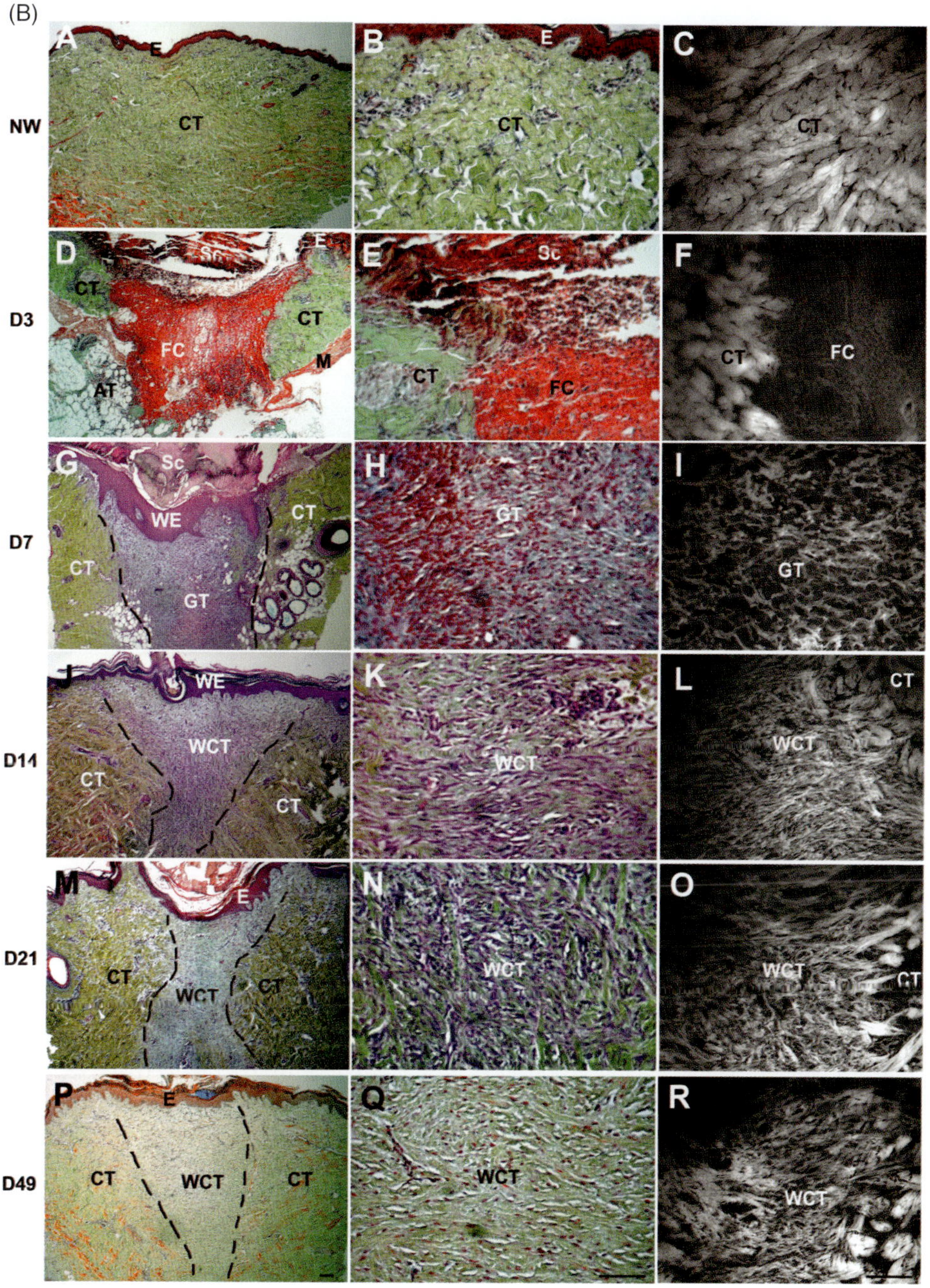

Fig. 6.2 (*Continued*).

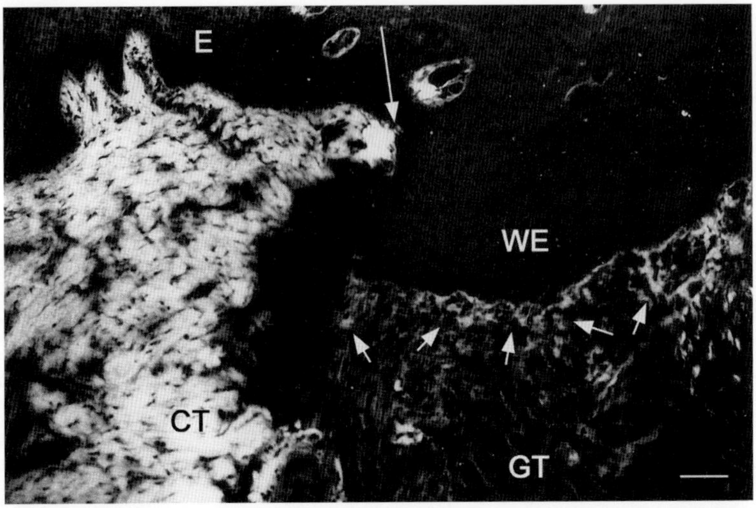

Fig. 6.3 Advanced deposition of extracellular matrix in the granulation tissue beneath the wound epithelium. Image shows a representative hematoxylin and eosin stained section from a human gingival wound biopsy collected 7 days after wounding, and viewed under UV-light using the rhodamine channel in a fluorescence microscope. CT: connective tissue; GT: granulation tissue; E: epithelium; WE: wound epithelium; long arrow: wound edge; short arrows: accumulation of collagen-rich extracellular matrix beneath the wound epithelium. Magnification bar = 100 μm.

well recognized as they invade the wound provisional matrix, modulate inflammation, re-epithelialization and angiogenesis, and serve as the major producers and organizers of connective tissue ECM critical for tissue repair (Nolte et al. 2008). Fibroblasts also play a key role in pathologies associated with wound healing, including chronic, non-healing wounds, keloid or hypertrophic scars and organ fibrosis (Guyot et al. 2006; Toriseva and Kähäri 2009). It is becoming evident that the general term 'fibroblast' widely used in the literature no longer accurately describes all the ECM producing and remodeling cells taking part in the wound healing process. Rather, connective tissue repair involves different fibroblast subsets or fibroblast-like cells originating from various sources.

Past and recent findings have provided evidence that the ECM producing and remodeling cells that populate the wound provisional matrix can originate from both the tissue adjacent to the wound and blood circulation (Stephens and Genever 2007; Nolte et al. 2008; Fig. 6.4). Traditionally, wound fibroblasts have been described as originating from the resident fibroblasts located in the connective tissue close to the injury site which after wounding migrate into the wound provisional matrix (Fathke et al. 2004; Nolte et al. 2008). Interestingly, fibroblasts residing within different areas of skin or oral mucosa are phenotypically heterogeneous and a certain subset may, therefore, have different capacity to be activated, migrate to the wound area and participate in wound healing (Irwin et al. 1994; Sorrell and Caplan 2004, 2009; Werner et al. 2007; Nolte et al. 2008). It is not clear what causes this phenotypical heterogeneity among fibroblasts, but one of the reasons may relate to different origins of the cells during embryonic development (Sorrell and Caplan 2004, 2009). Another reason may relate to differentiation of these cells within the tissue. For instance, cultured human skin and gingival fibroblasts undergo cellular changes indicative of a terminally differentiating cellular lineage (Bayreuther et al. 1991; Häkkinen and Larjava 1992; Nolte

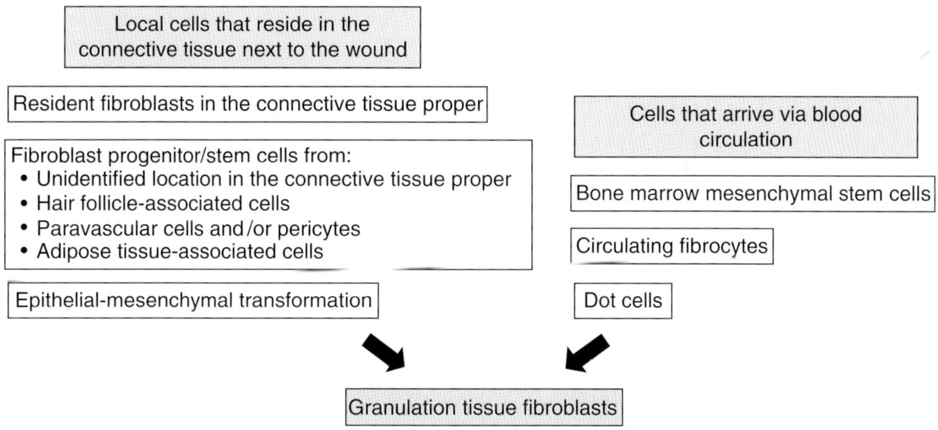

Fig. 6.4 Possible origins of wound granulation tissue fibroblasts.

et al. 2008). However, it is unclear whether these resulting fibroblast subsets are present *in vivo*, and what is their functional significance for wound healing. It is also now well established that skin and different areas of oral mucosal connective tissue contain multipotent mesenchymal progenitor or stem cells, which may account, at least in part, for the phenotypical heterogeneity of fibroblasts in these tissues (Stephens and Genever 2007; Lau et al. 2009; Davies et al. 2010; Fournier et al. 2010; Marynka-Kalmani et al. 2010; Zhang et al. 2010). Mesenchymal progenitor cells can be isolated and cultured from skin or oral mucosal tissue biopsies with essentially similar protocols that have been traditionally used to isolate and culture the classical fibroblasts from these tissues (Lau et al. 2009; Davies et al. 2010; Fournier et al. 2010; Marynka-Kalmani et al. 2010; Zhang et al. 2010). This raises an intriguing possibility that the cells cultured from connective tissue and currently broadly termed 'fibroblasts' are in themselves mesenchymal stem or progenitor cells which under appropriate conditions can undergo differentiation into different mesenchymal cell lineages. Alternatively, fibroblasts residing in the connective tissue may contain a subpopulation of mesenchymal stem cells that share certain properties with fibroblasts (da Silva Meirelles et al. 2008; Nolte et al. 2008; Diaz-Flores et al. 2009). Within the connective tissue *in vivo*, at least two distinct populations of multipotent mesenchymal progenitor cells have been found, residing in skin hair follicles and in perivascular locations, possibly representing pericytes (Jahoda and Reynolds 2001; Diaz-Flores et al. 2009; Lau et al. 2009). Whether these progenitor cells are the same as or different from the above-mentioned connective tissue-derived multipotent progenitor cells established in cell cultures is unclear. Moreover, the importance of these local connective tissue-associated progenitor cells for the wound healing process and outcome remains to be shown. However, these cells are able to find their way to the wound site when administered into the circulation or applied locally, suggesting that they play a role in wound healing (Chunmeng et al. 2004; Nolte et al. 2008). In addition to the multipotent progenitor cells present in the collagen-rich connective tissue proper, adipose tissue associated with the connective tissue may serve as a source for mesenchymal progenitor cells that take part in the wound healing process (Jeong 2010). Furthermore, differentiation of fibroblasts from epithelial cells (epithelial–mesenchymal transformation) has been described (Yan et al. 2010), but its significance for wound healing outcome is unclear.

Fibroblast-like cells involved in wound healing may also derive from blood circulation. For instance, based on animal studies, a variable, but substantial, proportion of wound fibroblasts may originate from bone marrow-derived mesenchymal stem cells (Fathke et al. 2004; Sasaki et al. 2008; Lau et al. 2009; Wu et al. 2010). In addition, a population termed fibrocytes which arise from circulating mononuclear cells can account for up to 10% of fibroblasts in wounds. Interestingly, these cells have characteristics of both hematopoetic and mesenchymal cells. For instance, they express receptors for chemokines that help them to home into wounds, where they undergo phenotypical maturation to function as antigen presenting cells and secrete inflammatory cytokines. In addition, fibrocytes produce several ECM proteins, including collagens, and express receptors, including Endo180 (also called uPARAP or CD280), which are involved in ECM remodeling and produce factors that regulate angiogenesis (Quan et al. 2004; Herzog and Bucala 2010; Bianchetti et al. 2011). Recently, an intriguing small subpopulation of tiny (0.5–1.5 μm in diameter) organisms initially termed Dot cells was isolated from peripheral blood in humans, mice and rats. They express stem cell and germ plasm markers, multiply in cell culture and home into wounds where they regenerate both epidermal and dermal cells, and appear to reduce scar formation in a mouse model (Kong et al. 2008, 2010). The true identity and significance of the germ plasm-like Dot cells for wound healing remain to be determined.

Taken together, fibroblasts and their progenitors form a dynamic and heterogeneous group of cells. It is possible that different subtypes of fibroblasts or their progenitor cells which have distinct origins and phenotypes may perform different functions during wound healing, and their relative proportions may ultimately determine the wound healing outcome. This is supported by findings that myofibroblasts or fibrocytes persist in high numbers in fibrosis and in different types of pathological scars (Yang et al. 2005; Darby and Hewitson 2007), and fibroblasts isolated, for example, from drug-induced or hereditary gingival fibromatosis lesions or from diabetic, non-healing skin ulcers are phenotypically different from cells isolated from corresponding normal tissues (Loot et al. 2002; Trackman and Kantarci 2004; Häkkinen and Csiszar 2007). In addition, fibroblasts present in hypertrophic scar resemble phenotypically fibroblast subpopulations residing in the deep dermal connective tissue (Wang et al. 2008). Finally, experimental delivery of mesenchymal stem cells into wounds improves the wound healing outcome in chronic wounds and reduces scar formation, suggesting that introduction of appropriate cell subpopulations into wounds can be used to prevent or treat wound healing problems (Sorrell and Caplan 2010). Research on fibroblast differentiation and progenitor and subtype characterization has been hampered by lack of specific cell markers. Fibroblasts are poorly antigenic and many of the markers that have been developed are not specific for these cells (Darby and Hewitson 2007; Haniffa et al. 2009). Due to these limitations, in the following paragraphs fibroblasts are defined by using the traditional distinctions of an ECM producing and remodeling cell. Advances in developing fibroblast and fibroblast subtype-specific antibodies and cell markers would allow better understanding of the mechanisms of normal and aberrant wound healing.

GRANULATION TISSUE FORMATION

New connective tissue begins to form approximately 2–4 days after wounding, and it is called granulation tissue due to its granular appearance when examined visually. It consists mainly of components of the blood clot, fibroblasts and their progenitor cells that have homed into the area, new loose and primitive connective tissue ECM produced by wound fibroblasts, new and forming blood vessels and inflammatory cells. The composition of the primitive ECM in the granulation tissue has certain similarities with connective tissue during fetal development, and functionally it serves as a scaffold that contains cells and molecules that are necessary for subsequent tissue maturation into normal connective tissue (Clark 1996; Gurtner et al. 2008; Larson et al. 2010). Approximately 7–10 days after injury, the granulation tissue stage gradually shifts into the reorganization and remodeling phase of connective tissue wound healing.

Activation of connective tissue cells

In order to form granulation tissue, fibroblasts and/or their progenitor cells need to proliferate, change their gene expression, release their adhesions to the pericellular ECM, be directionally attracted and migrate into the blood clot that occupies the wound space. The cells that enter the wound during the initial inflammatory stage, namely platelets and leukocytes (neutrophils, lymphocytes, mast cells, macrophages), and epithelial and neuronal cells residing at or close to the wound area play a key role in orchestrating this process. The inflammatory stage starts immediately after wounding and lasts usually until about 7–10 days after injury. Cell populations shift during this stage so that neutrophils may account for the majority of the leukocytes during the early acute inflammation, but starting around day 3 concomitant with advancing re-epithelialization, macrophages, lymphocyte subsets and mast cells start to accumulate in greater numbers in the wound area (Eming et al. 2007; Shiota et al. 2010). Wound keratinocytes also take part in this process by secreting inflammatory mediators, including chemokines (small, structurally related chemotactic cytokines), such as monocyte chemotactic protein-1 (MCP-1 or CCL2) and interferon inducible protein-10 (IP-10 or CXCL10), and cytokines (secreted factors primarily expressed by immune cells that regulate gene expression of target cells), such as interleukin-1 (IL-1) and tumor necrosis factor-α (TNF-α), which attract inflammatory cells into the wound (Gibran et al. 1997; Werner and Grose 2003; Barrientos et al. 2008; Roupé et al. 2010; Table 6.2). The inflammatory cells arriving at the wound site release several soluble growth factors (secreted factors that regulate cell growth and gene expression), cytokines and chemokines which are key factors in regulating fibroblast proliferation, chemotaxis, migration and gene expression necessary for granulation tissue formation (Table 6.2). In addition, signaling molecules, including prostaglandins, released by damaged cells, activate and recruit connective tissue cells, including mesenchymal progenitor cells, into the wound (Werner and Grose 2003; Li et al. 2010). During wound healing there is an active cross-talk between inflammatory cells and fibroblasts, and activated fibroblasts can secrete chemokines, cytokines and prostaglandins, which in turn modulate the inflammatory response (Buckley et al. 2001; Werner and Grose 2003; Flavell et al. 2008).

In addition to inducing secretion of inflammatory cytokines, injury causes a release of reactive oxygen species (ROS) such as oxygen ions, peroxides and unstable intermediates in lipid peroxidation. The primary source of ROS is inflammatory cells, but also epithelial and connective tissue cells can produce them (Schäfer and Werner 2008). In high concentrations, ROS can prevent cell proliferation and cause further tissue damage, but at lower concentrations they can serve as powerful signaling molecules participating in regulation of cell survival and gene expression, and they appear to induce a pro-fibrogenic response in various cells involved in wound healing (Novo and Parola 2008). The action of ROS is balanced by several anti-oxidants expressed by the wound cells, including superoxide

Table 6.2 Key growth factors, cytokines and chemokines that regulate fibroblast functions during wound healing.[1]

Molecules		Sources[2]	Major effects on fibroblasts[2]
Growth factors	CCN2 (connective tissue growth factor or CTGF)	Fibroblasts	Promotes proliferation, migration and ECM synthesis
	EGF (epidermal growth factor)	Platelets, macrophages, fibroblasts, plasma, saliva	Promotes migration, proliferation and collagenase expression and modulates ECM deposition (either suppresses or increases depending on ECM signaling)
	FGF-2 (basic fibroblast growth factor or bFGF)	Macrophages, mast cells, keratinocytes, endothelial cells, fibroblasts	Promotes migration, proliferation, ECM and collagenase synthesis
	IGF-1 (insulin-like growth factor-1)	Plasma, platelets, keratinocytes, endothelial cells, fibroblasts	Promotes proliferation and ECM deposition
	NGF (nerve growth factor)	Mast cells, eosinophils, keratinocytes, fibroblasts	Promotes migration, myofibroblast differentiation and collagen contraction
	PDGF (platelet-derived growth factor)	Platelets, macrophages, keratinocytes, endothelial cells, fibroblasts	Promotes migration, proliferation, ECM and collagenase synthesis
	TGF-α (transforming growth factor-α)	Platelets, macrophages, keratinocytes, eosinophils	Promotes proliferation
	TGF-β1, -β2 and -β3 (transforming growth factor-β)	Platelets, macrophages, lymphocytes, mast cells, keratinocytes, fibroblasts	Proliferation (either promotes or suppresses depending on concentration), promotes migration, myofibroblast differentiation and ECM synthesis, reduces collagenase activity
Cytokines	IL-1 (interleukin-1)	Neutrophils, monocytes and macrophages, keratinocytes, endothelial cells, fibroblasts, mast cells, T and B lymphocytes	Promotes proliferation
	IL-4	Mast cells	Promotes proliferation
	IL-6	Macrophages, neutrophils, lymphocytes, keratinocytes, mast cells, fibroblasts	Promotes proliferation
	TNF-α (tumor necrosis factor-α)	Neutrophils, macrophages, keratinocytes, fibroblasts	Proliferation (either promotes or suppresses depending on concentration), promotes expression of proteolytic enzymes, suppresses myofibroblast differentiation and collagen expression
Chemokines	CCL2 (monocyte chemotactic protein-1 or MCP-1)	Keratinocytes, macrophages	Promotes TGF-β, collagen, collagenase and TIMP-1 expression
	CXCL8 (IL-8)	Neutrophils, macrophages, keratinocytes, lymphocytes	Promotes gap-junctional communication and granulation tissue maturation, inhibits collagen contraction
	CXCL10 (interferon inducible protein 10 or IP-10)	Keratinocytes, macrophages	Inhibits migration
	CXCL11 (IP-9)	Keratinocytes, macrophages	Inhibits migration, promotes ECM remodeling

[1]Colige et al. 1988, 1992; Kiritsy et al. 1993; Buck et al. 1996; Engelhardt et al. 1998; Gillitzer and Goebeler 2001; Micera et al. 2001; Werner and Grose 2003; Moyer et al. 2002; Broughton et al. 2006; Goldberg et al. 2007; Yates et al. 2007; Barrientos et al. 2008; Grimstad et al. 2011.
[2]Based on cell culture and/or *in vivo* findings.

Table 6.3 Key neuropeptides released upon wounding that regulate fibroblast functions.[1]

Molecule	**Major effects on fibroblasts[2]**
α-Melanocyte stimulating hormone (α-MSH)	Promotes IL-8 and collagenase expression, suppresses TGF-β-induced collagen expression
Angiotensin II (ANG II)	Promotes collagen remodeling, collagen contraction and integrin expression
Calcitonin gene-related peptide (CGRP)	Promotes proliferation
Corticotropin releasing hormone (CRH)	Promotes proliferation
Neurokinin A (NKA)	Promotes proliferation
Neurotensin (NT)	Promotes proliferation
Secretoneurin (SN)	Promotes migration
Substance P (SP)	Promotes proliferation and migration

[1]Ziche et al. 1990; Kähler et al. 1996; Kiss et al. 1999; Steinhoff et al. 2003; Bohm and Luger 2004; Scarpa et al. 2005; Roosterman et al. 2006; Slominski et al. 2006; Sorrell and Caplan 2009; da Silva et al. 2010.
[2]Based on cell culture and/or *in vivo* findings.

dismutase, catalase and various peroxidases. Expression of these inhibitory ROS-scavenging molecules is tightly spatiotemporally regulated during wound healing (Steiling et al. 1999).

Damage to the tissue also disrupts normal blood flow, resulting in ischemia. Tissue cells are sensitive to changes in oxygen levels, and decreased (hypoxic) or increased (hyperoxic) oxygen tension compared to the normal (normoxic) state causes fundamental changes in key signaling pathways that regulate cell proliferation (Sen and Roy 2010). Acute, short-term hypoxia has beneficial effects to the early wound healing events. In particular, it promotes angiogenesis and activates connective tissue cells, including mesenchymal and adipose tissue-derived stem cells and fibroblasts, and induces their proliferation and ECM and growth factor production (Falanga et al. 2002; Boraldi et al. 2007; Grayson et al. 2007; Lee et al. 2009). However, chronic, long-lasting ischemia is detrimental and can lead to development of non-healing chronic wounds. For instance, chronic hypoxia can suppress re-epithelialization as well as myofibroblast differentiation and function. Chronic ischemia also causes increased collagen accumulation and fibrosis, but because of reduced collagen stability and increased protease expression, the wound connective tissue becomes mechanically weak and susceptible to ulceration (Dalton et al. 2007; Modarressi et al. 2010). Thus, short-term hypoxic condition is one of the mechanisms that promote cell proliferation and early granulation tissue formation, but the oxygen tension needs to be restored to normoxic level rather quickly by angiogenesis to allow subsequent wound healing events to progress appropriately.

In addition to inflammatory cells, other cells present in the tissue participate in the activation of fibroblasts for wound healing. During early granulation tissue formation, sensory and sympathetic peripheral nerves close to the wound edges release neuropeptides which control vascular responses and inflammation and influence proliferation of many cells, including fibroblasts, involved in the repair process (Roosterman et al. 2006; da Silva et al. 2010; Table 6.3). Also other cells involved in wound healing can secrete neuropeptides, including keratinocytes, fibroblasts and endothelial cells (Steinhoff et al. 2003), but these cannot completely compensate for neuronal cell-derived mediators as denervation of rat skin delays re-epithelialization and wound contraction (Fukai et al. 2005). In addition, wound keratinocytes secrete paracrine factors which activate fibroblasts (Table 6.2). Activated fibroblasts can in turn produce factors that promote re-epithelialization, including keratinocyte growth factor (KGF or FGF7), epidermal growth factor (EGF), hepatocyte growth factor/scatter factor (HGF) and transforming growth factor-β (TGF-β), providing a feedback system where re-epithelialization controls connective tissue healing and vice versa. In chronic, non-healing wounds and scar formation, this feedback system is disturbed (Beer et al. 2000; Werner and Grose 2003; Conway et al. 2006; Ghahary and Ghaffari 2007; Werner et al. 2007; Koskela et al. 2010).

Cell proliferation

There are at least two major groups of connective tissue cells that actively proliferate during wound healing. This is based on a classical study using detection of radioactively labeled thymidine in proliferating cells in experimental incisional skin wounds in pigs (Oliver 1979). One group of proliferating cells can be noted 2 days after injury immediately next to the wound margin, and consists of cells residing in the connective tissue proper, around blood vessels and in the connective tissue associated with adnexa. Although the exact identity of these cells remains unknown, they likely represent fibroblasts and endothelial cells. Moreover, based on the tissue location, some of them may correspond to the more recently described hair follicle-associated and paravascular mesenchymal stem cell populations (Jahoda and Reynolds 2001; Diaz-Flores et al. 2009; Lau et al. 2009). Another group of proliferating cells resides within granulation tissue already at day 1 (Oliver 1979). The identity of these cells is also unclear, but they are likely derived from circulation. Both the cells at the wound margin and in the granulation tissue sustain active proliferation for up to about 7 days after wounding, followed by a sharp decline in the number of proliferating cells at day 9 (Oliver 1979). Thus, the cells at the wound margin are activated within 2 days after injury to proliferate and feed new cells into the granulation tissue. Once in the granulation tissue, connective tissue cells continue to proliferate to quickly populate the granulation tissue and provide new cells to deposit ECM and re-establish vasculature.

Proliferation of fibroblasts and/or their progenitor cells is initiated and regulated by a combined action of growth factors, cytokines and other factors released during the early inflammatory stage (Table 6.2). The inflammatory process, and, hence, the cytokine and growth factor environment can be further modulated by changes in the composition of the extracellular matrix in the wound. For instance, within hours after wounding, expression of enzymes for hyaluronan (a large secreted glycosaminoglycan) synthesis is increased in fibroblasts and keratinocytes at the wound edge (Mack et al. 2011; Table 6.4). As a result, there is a significant increase in hyaluronan accumulation in the ECM at wound margins at day 3 after wounding (Mack et al. 2011). At this early stage, hyaluronan plays a role in regulating the inflammatory response, but the exact mechanism remains unclear as reduced expression of hyaluronan can result in either increased or decreased inflammation (Mack et al. 2011; Wight and Potter-Perigo 2011). These apparently contradictory effects of hyaluronan on inflammation may depend on the heterogeneity of hyaluronan structure. Hyaluronan can be produced by three different enzymes, namely hyaluronan synthase-1 (Has1), Has2 or Has3, in a cell-specific manner, and the average polymer length, and possibly function, of the product from each of the enzymes during wound healing may be spatiotemporally different (Mack et al. 2011).

In addition to affecting inflammation, ECM composition impacts fibroblast proliferation in response to growth factors and cytokines. This process involves a complex interplay between intracellular signaling cascades initiated by binding of growth factors or cytokines to their specific receptors and interaction of ECM molecules with their receptors, such as

Table 6.4 Approximate time of first appearance, peak expression and long-term accumulation of key ECM molecules or molecules involved in collagen cross-linking during wound healing.[1]

Molecule	Appears first time[2]	Peak expression[2]	Long-term accumulation[2]
Collagens			
Total collagen	SW[3]: day 3	SW: day 7–14	SW: increases fast until 21 days followed by a slower accumulation phase up to 90 days. Remains elevated for years in pathological scars
Type I collagen	SW: day 3–5	SW: day 7–14	SW: increases fast until 21 days followed by a slower accumulation phase up to 90 days. Remains elevated for years in pathological scars
Type III collagen	SW: day 3	SW: day 5–7	SW: accumulation increases until day 22
Type V collagen	SW: day 3	SW: day 21	SW: after day 21 gradually declines for at least up to 90 days. Remains elevated in pathological scars
Glycosaminoglycans and proteoglycans			
Hyaluronan	SW: within hours at the wound edge, at day 3 within the wound	SW: day 5	SW: starts to decrease in abundance between day 5 and 10, after that remains unaltered
Decorin	OMW[4]: day 3	OMW: day 7–14	OMW: remains elevated for at least 60 days
Biglycan	OMW: day 3	OMW: day 14–28	OMW: returns to the level of unwounded tissue by day 60
Fibromodulin	OMW: day 3	OMW: increased accumulation from day 3 up to at least day 60	OMW: remains elevated for at least 60 days
Adhesive glycoproteins			
Cellular EDA fibronectin	SW/OMW: day 3	SW/OMW: day 7–14	SW: remains elevated at least for 49 days OMW: returns to the level of unwounded tissue by day 35
Cellular EDB fibronectin	OMW: not present at day 3	OMW: day 7	OMW: gradually reduced after day 7, but remains elevated at least for 28 days
Matricellular proteins			
SPARC	SW: day 3	SW: day 7	SW: remains strongly upregulated at least for 14 days. Highly expressed in established scars
Thrombospondin-1	SW: 12 hours	SW: day 1–2	SW: undetectable by day 5
Thrombospondin-2	SW: day 3	SW: day 7–10	SW: starts to decrease after day 14
Tenascin-C	OMW and SW: day 3 (connective tissue next to the wound)	OMW and SW: day 7 in the wound granulation tissue	SW: returns to the level of unwounded tissue by day 35; OMW: remains elevated at least for 49 days
Tenascin-X	SW: day 7	SW: day 14	N/A[5]

(*Continued*)

Table 6.4 (*Continued*).

Molecule	Appears first time[2]	Peak expression[2]	Long-term accumulation[2]
Periostin	SW: day 3 in the connective tissue next to the wound, not detected in the granulation tissue	SW: day 7 in the granulation tissue	SW: returns to the level of unwounded tissue by day 28. Remains elevated in pathological scars
CCN1 (Cyr61)	SW: day 1	SW: day 7	SW: returns to the level of unwounded tissue by day 14
CCN2 (CTGF)	SW: day 3	SW: day 7	SW: returns to the level of unwounded tissue by day 14
CCN3 (Nov)	SW: remains below unwounded tissue until day 28.		
Collagen cross-linking and related enzymes			
Lysyl hydroxylase-2 (LH-2)	N/A	SW: day 7	SW: remains elevated at least for 28 days. LH-2-mediated collagen cross-links remain elevated at least for 8 weeks
Lysyl oxidase (LOX)	N/A	SW: peak expression at day 3, peak activity at day 10	SW: expression remains elevated at least for 21 days. Activity remains high for years in pathological scars
Transglutaminase	SW: day 1	SW: day 4	SW: returns to level of unwounded tissue by day 9. Remains upregulated in fibrosis
Cross-linked collagen	N/A	SW: day 21	SW: remains elevated for years in pathological scars

[1]Bentley 1967; Clore et al. 1979; Hering et al. 1983; Reed et al. 1993; Clarck 1996; Fushida-Takemura et al. 1996; Haroon et al. 1999; Kyriakides et al. 1999; Bradshaw and Sage 2001; Agah et al. 2004; Verderio et al. 2004; Egging et al. 2007; Ulrich et al. 2007; Honardoust et al. 2008; Jackson-Boeters et al. 2009; Kyriakides and MacLauchlan 2009; Wong et al. 2009; Zhou et al. 2010; Mack et al. 2011; Rittié et al. 2011.
[2]Time after wounding.
[3]SW: information based on studies on skin wound healing.
[4]OMW: information based on studies on oral mucosal wound healing.
[5]N/A: data not available or contradictory.

integrins and CD44 (Ivaska and Heino 2010; Meran et al. 2011). For example, hyaluronan regulates TGF-β1-mediated induction of skin fibroblast proliferation by a mechanism that requires EGF receptor (EGFR) and CD44 (receptor for hyaluronan) coupling. Curiously though, this mechanism depends on the cellular context as TGF-β1 reduces cell proliferation in oral mucosal fibroblasts and this effect does not depend on CD44 (Meran et al. 2011). In addition, integrin-mediated cell adhesion to ECM is required and promotes the pro-mitotic effect of growth factors, including platelet-derived growth factor (PDGF), a potent fibroblast mitogen during wound healing (Schneller et al. 1997).

Disruption of gap junctional communication due to tissue injury or by factors released during wound healing may also contribute to fibroblast activation and proliferation and promote granulation tissue formation. As mentioned above, at least in skin and periodontal ligament, fibroblasts form a network in which the cells are directly connected to each other with connexin-mediated gap junctions. This allows transfer of signaling molecules directly between the cells (Shore et al. 1981; Solomon et al. 1988; Su et al. 1997). The exact role of gap junctions in tissue maintenance in fibroblasts is not completely clear, but they may help to maintain the cells in the quiescent state by a mechanism where they transfer inhibitory microRNAs between the cells (Lim et al. 2011). Injury to connective tissue breaks this gap-junctional transfer of the inhibitory molecules between the cells. Interestingly, PDGF also blocks gap-junctional communication, and this is a prerequisite for its mitogenic effect (Moorby and Gherardi 1999). Accordingly, blocking of gap junction function using connexin-mimetic peptides accelerates fibroblast proliferation and granulation tissue formation (Mori et al. 2006; Ghatnekar et al. 2009).

Cell migration

Connective tissue cell migration into the wound provisional matrix starts around day 3 after wounding. Migration of fibroblasts and endothelial cells occurs at the same time, allowing the forming blood vessels to supply appropriate nutrients and oxygen for the advancing fibroblasts (Clark 1996; Gurtner et al. 2008). Reciprocally, angiogenesis is partly regulated by fibroblasts that secrete pro-angiogenic factors, including vascular endothelial growth factor (VEGF), basic fibroblast growth factor (bFGF or FGF-2) and TGF-β, and produce ECM proteins, including fibronectin, collagen and tenascin-C, which are conducive for endothelial cell migration and angiogenesis (Li et al. 2003; Werner and Grose 2003; Flavell et al. 2008). As compared to migration of inflammatory cells, fibroblast migration is slow, about 0.5–1 μm/minute (Schneider and Haugh 2006). In order to populate the wound provisional matrix, fibroblasts need to release their adhesions to the existing pericellular matrix, express appropriate receptors that are conducive for cell migration on the ECM proteins present in the connective tissue and in the wound provisional matrix, and be directionally attracted to the wound. These processes are supported by expression of proteases that process the ECM and by production of novel ECM molecules that promote fibroblast migration (Clark 1996; Gurtner et al. 2008; Brábek et al. 2010).

In normal connective tissue, fibroblasts are attached to a fibrillar ECM mesh that contains an abundance of structural proteins such as cross-linked type I collagen and elastin produced by fibroblasts themselves. In addition, fibroblast pericellular matrix harbors multidomain adhesive proteins, including cellular fibronectin, glycosaminoglycans (hyaluronan) and proteoglycans (e.g. small leucine-rich proteoglycans, versican, heparan sulfate proteoglycans) which mediate or modulate cell adhesion to the collagen-rich ECM (Chen and Abatangelo 1999; Heino and Käpylä 2009; Brábek et al. 2010). In contrast, the major ECM component in the blood clot is fibrin. It forms thin, loosely organized fibers that are cross-linked by transglutaminase and harbor plasma-derived adhesive glycoproteins fibronectin and vitronectin, and a matricellular protein thrombospondin-1 released from degranulating platelets entrapped in the clot (Clark 1996; Verderio et al. 2004; Stocum 2006). The clot may also contain some type I, III and IV collagens presumably derived from infiltrating monocytes (Lindblad 1998). The ECM proteins present in the fibroblast microenvironment serve as a conduit for cell migration into the wound. Therefore, in order to migrate, fibroblasts need to modify their interaction with the existing ECM and be able to recognize and interact with the novel proteins present in the wound provisional matrix. Fibroblasts use mainly receptors of the integrin family for this purpose.

Integrins form a family of integral cell membrane proteins. Each integrin is composed of an α and a β subunit which form a heterodimer that has an extracellular, transmembrane and cytoplasmic domain and links ECM to the cytoskeleton. There are 18 different α and 8 different β subunits that can combine in a cell-specific manner to produce in total 24 different integrin $\alpha\beta$ heterodimers. To interact with the very different ECM components in the connective tissue and wound provisional matrix the cells adjust their integrin expression and function accordingly (Friedl and Bröcker 2000; Heino and Käpylä 2009). In general, cell culture studies have shown that it is the interplay between adhesive and anti-adhesive interactions between fibroblast surface receptors and ECM molecules that determine whether the cells will remain stationary or migrate. For example, cells that are too strongly or too weakly attached to the ECM cannot migrate, while cells with intermediate adhesion strength are migratory (Heino and Käpylä 2009). Accordingly, in order to migrate, the cells have to release their existing, relatively strong and stable integrin-mediated adhesions to the ECM. This may be accomplished by modifying integrin expression and function, by modulating the composition of the ECM ligands for integrins or by controlled focalized proteolytic remodeling of the ECM (Heino and Käpylä 2009; Toriseva and Kähäri 2009).

To modulate integrin function, cells use so-called inside-out and outside-in signaling mechanisms to change integrin conformation to coordinately release and activate their grip on the ECM molecules. This process is regulated by soluble growth factors present in the wound, composition of the integrin ECM ligands and mechanosensory or other intracellular signaling events (Heino and Käpylä 2009). It appears that the cytoplasmic integrin-associated adaptor molecule, kindlin-2, is critical for integrin activation in fibroblasts, and it directs cell migration by coordinating the maturation of distinct cell–ECM adhesions (so-called focal adhesions) and organization of the cytoskeleton (He et al. 2011). In order to invade the wound, cells also need to adjust their integrin expression to interact with novel proteins present in the provisional matrix. Consequently, expression of integrins of the αv and $\beta 1$ families is increased in the granulation tissue fibroblasts. Certain cytokines expressed at this stage of wound healing, including TGF-$\beta 1$ and PDGF, potently regulate the expression of several key integrins, including $\alpha 2\beta 1$ (major collagen receptor), $\alpha 5\beta 1$ (fibronectin and CCN3/Nov receptor), $\alpha v\beta 3$ (fibrinogen and CCN1/Cyr61 receptor) and $\alpha v\beta 5$ (vitronectin and CCN1/Cyr61 receptor) in fibroblasts (Ignotz and Massagué 1987; Roberts et al. 1988; Heino et al. 1989; Ignotz et al. 1989; Kirchberg et al. 1995; Gailit et al. 1996, 1997; Memmo McKeown-Longo 1998; Grzeszkiewicz et al. 2001; Noszczyk et al. 2002; Lin et al. 2005; van Beurden et al. 2006; Martinez-Ferrer et al. 2010). In addition to integrins, cell surface hyaluronan receptors (e.g. CD44 and RHAMM), proteoglycans (e.g. syndecan-4) and integrin-associated molecules (e.g. CD151) collaborate with integrins to mediate and regulate fibroblast migration into wounds (Lovvorn et al. 1998; Clark et al. 2004; Lin et al. 2005; Tolg et al. 2006; Geary et al. 2008). Disruption of cell-to-cell gap junctional connexin-mediated communication also promotes fibroblast migration into the granulation tissue (Mori et al. 2006; Wright et al. 2009). However, this effect may relate to the pro-migratory signaling functions of the connexin molecules rather than to the gap junctional functions *per se* (Behrens et al. 2010).

To facilitate cell migration, fibroblasts use focalized proteolysis to help release their adhesion to the pericellular ECM and to remodel the ECM (Toriseva and Kähäri 2009; Brábek et al. 2010). The mode of fibroblast migration is different from leukocytes, which appear to use a more dynamic ameboid migration which does not require extensive ECM remodeling (Friedl and Bröcker 2000). In contrast, fibroblasts use focalized proteolytic ECM remodeling to develop dynamic cell adhesions needed for cell migration. In addition, focalized proteolysis cleaves impeding collagen and other fibrillar ECM components present in the connective tissue and in the blood clot. As this process is limited to the pericellular matrix close to the cell–ECM contact sites it allows the cells to maintain the overall integrity of the matrix as a conduit for cell migration (Hotary et al. 2002; Sabeh et al. 2009a, 2009b).

This cell migration-related focalized proteolysis is different from the action of secreted collagenases of the matrix metalloproteinase (MMP) family, including MMP-1, MMP-2, MMP-8 and MMP-13, that are considered to be responsible for bulk collagen degradation associated with ECM remodeling at the later stages of wound healing (Sabeh et al. 2009a, 2009b). The cell surface-associated, membrane-type MMPs (MT-MMPs) play a key role in the focalized ECM remodeling during fibroblast migration. For instance, MT1-MMP (MMP-14) is required for cell migration in a matrix that is rich in cross-linked collagen, such as normal connective tissue. When cells reach the fibrin and fibronectin-rich wound provisional matrix, they may also utilize MT2-MMP and MT3-MMP, as well as serine proteases, such as the plasminogen activator–plasminogen system, to aid migration (Greiling and Clark 1997; Hotary et al. 2002). The function of various MMPs is regulated by the action of other proteases that participate in MMP activation, including serine proteases, and balanced with the presence of tissue inhibitors of MMPs (TIMPs) (Ravanti and Kähäri 2000; Toriseva and Kähäri 2009). In addition to their well-recognized proteolytic capacity, MMPs may regulate cell migration by non-catalytic means. For instance, pro-forms of MMP-2 and MMP-9 can enhance chemotactic cell migration *in vitro*. In addition, MMPs can interact with integrins and regulate apoptosis and cell survival (Kessenbrock et al. 2010). However, the significance of these non-catalytic functions of MMPs for wound healing *in vivo* remains to be elucidated.

Fibroblast migration from surrounding tissues into the wound is guided by soluble chemotactic mediators released from inflammatory cells and ECM. PDGF-induced chemotaxis provides a well-described example of some of the key signaling pathways involved in this process (De Donatis et al. 2010). At the start of the granulation tissue formation, the blood clot releases chemotactic signals, including PDGF from platelets and macrophages (Schneider and Haugh 2006). The resulting chemotactic gradient induces asymmetric localization of PDGF receptors and signaling molecules, including 3′-phosphorylated phosphoinositide lipids, at the fibroblast plasma membrane facing the highest PDGF concentration. This allows concentrated activation of downstream signaling pathways at the leading (front) edge of the cell as well as appropriate reorganization of the actin cytoskeleton required for the directed cell migration into the wound (Schneider and Haugh 2006). Cell–ECM interactions mediated by integrins modulate the growth factor signaling necessary for chemotaxis and migration (Ivaska and Heino 2010). For instance, the PDGF-induced chemotactic signaling and migration of mesenchymal stem cells is enhanced by $\alpha5\beta1$ integrin-mediated cell adhesion to fibronectin (Hauck et al. 2000; Veevers-Lowe et al. 2011). In addition, integrin-mediated mechanosensory signaling which senses stiffness gradients in the ECM can participate in guiding cell migration towards the wound (Grinnell and Petroll 2010).

Proteases play a role in granulation tissue formation also by modulating the abundance and quality of signaling molecules present in the wounds. For example, proteases produced by inflammatory, epithelial and connective tissue cells process cytokines and chemokines and can either activate or inactivate their function (Gill and Parks 2008; Wolf et al. 2008). In addition, proteases, including MMP-2, MMP-9 and plasmin, can release and activate latent growth factors, such as TGF-β, which are stored in the pericellular matrix and when activated by the release promote fibroblast migration and other functions (Toriseva and Kähäri 2009). MMPs also process ECM, basement membrane and provisional wound matrix components to expose cryptic functional sequences (matricryptins), such as EGF-like repeats present in laminin-5 or functional sequences of elastin and type IV and XVIII collagens (Tran et al. 2005; Ricard-Blum and Ballut 2011). Matricryptins can regulate various key functions in wound healing, including cell proliferation, migration and angiogenesis (Tran et al. 2005;

Ricard-Blum and Ballut 2011). Apart from proteolytic processing, cryptic sites in ECM proteins can also be exposed when cells that are attached to the ECM by integrins actively pull and deform the matrix proteins during cell migration or matrix organization and remodeling (Ricard-Blum and Ballut 2011). A classical example is a process where integrin-mediated conformational changes expose cryptic sites in the fibronectin molecule required for deposition of a stabilized fibrillar fibronectin matrix (Singh et al. 2010). Certain ECM proteins also possess signaling components (matrikines), such as EGF-like repeats present in the matricellular protein tenascin-C or distinct EGF-receptor binding region of the small leucine-rich proteoglycan decorin, which do not require proteolytic processing to interact with growth factor or cytokine receptors (Tran et al. 2005; Schultz and Wysocki 2009; Eckes et al. 2010; Pagano and Reboud-Ravaux 2011).

To facilitate migration, cells also secrete new ECM proteins (Table 6.4). Although the ECM is composed of several adhesion proteins, it appears that fibronectin is required for fibroblast migration in the connective tissue and in the provisional wound matrix (Greiling and Clark 1997). For instance, wound edge fibroblasts, granulation tissue fibroblasts and macrophages secrete cellular extra domain A (EDA)-fibronectin. This fibronectin isoform contains a distinct EIIIA domain that supports integrin-mediated cell adhesion and migration better than plasma fibronectin which lacks this domain (Manabe et al. 1997; Singh et al. 2004; Singh et al. 2010). In addition, other newly expressed ECM proteins promote migration. As discussed above, hyaluronan starts to accumulate in the connective tissue next to the wound and inside the granulation tissue at the same time that fibroblasts are actively migrating into the wound. To support migration, cells interact with hyaluronan using CD44 and RHAMM receptors (Tolg et al. 2006). In addition, hyaluronan can induce expression of MMPs in fibroblasts required for cell migration (David-Raoudi et al. 2008). Around day 3 after injury, connective tissue cells close to the wound edge also strongly deposit tenascin-C in the ECM, which may support their migration (Trebaul et al. 2007; Table 6.4). As pointed out above, tenascin-C is a matrikine that contains EGF-like sequences which bind to EGF-receptor (Swindle et al. 2001). EGF-receptor signaling is an important stimulator of fibroblast migration (Nishimura and Terranova 1996; Ellis et al. 1997). In addition, tenascin-C is an anti-adhesive protein that modulates cell adhesion to the ECM, presumably allowing development of dynamic cell adhesions necessary for migration (Halfter et al. 1990; Trebaul et al. 2007). Interestingly, tenascin-C contains a cryptic site that can be released by MMP-2 cleavage, and this fragment can induce activation of β1 integrins, possibly further promoting cell migration (Saito et al. 2007).

Taken together, appropriate stimulatory and chemotactic factors, the selection, abundance and activation state of cell surface ECM receptors that the cells express, composition of the adhesive and anti-adhesive molecules in the pericellular matrix, as well as the presence of appropriate proteases all play a key role in cell migration into the wound provisional matrix.

Matrix deposition and wound contraction

Collagen deposition

Once fibroblasts have migrated into the granulation tissue, their primary role is to rapidly produce new connective tissue ECM to re-establish tissue strength and function. It appears that fibroblast migration into the wound provisional matrix continues along an increasing but relatively low concentration gradient of a given chemoattractant, e.g. EGF, TGF-β and PDGF. When the ligand concentration in the wound provisional matrix reaches a higher threshold level and/or becomes homogenous around the cell, migration stops, and the same signaling molecules, i.e. EGF, TGF-β and PDGF, induce cells to start other functions, including proliferation, ECM deposition and remodeling (De Donatis et al. 2010). This results in a highly hypercellular granulation tissue where fibroblasts are synthetically very active producing increased amounts of ECM (Clark 1996; Gurtner et al. 2008). In addition to the above-mentioned PDGF, EGF and TGF-β1, matrix deposition is driven by the actions of insulin-like growth factor-1 (IGF-1), FGF-2 (bFGF) and connective tissue growth factor (CTGF or CCN2) present in the granulation tissue (Colige et al. 1988; Pierce et al. 1999; Werner and Grose 2003; Berrientos et al. 2008; Table 6.2). Based on a model of granulation tissue formation in rat skin, accumulation of total collagen increases fast up to 21 days after injury, followed by a period of slower deposition that can last for at least 90 days (Hering et al. 1983; Table 6.4). The major fibrillar collagen produced early in the granulation tissue formation is type III. However, within days type I collagen accumulation speeds up, reaching a peak at day 7–14 when it accounts for at least 75% of total collagen in the granulation tissue (Clore et al. 1979; Hering et al. 1983). The proportion of type III collagen remains relatively constant from day 7 to 90, averaging about 22% of total collagen. In addition, other fibrillar collagens are deposited, but they account only for a minor proportion of total collagen in the wounds. For instance, deposition of type V collagen increases up to day 21 post-wounding, when it accounts for about 3% of total collagen, followed by a gradual decline at least up to 90 days (Hering et al. 1983; Table 6.4). Interestingly, in fetal lamb skin wounds that heal without scarring, deposition of collagen is initially faster, and the proportions of type III and type V collagen relative to type I are elevated compared to scar-forming adult skin wounds (Lovvorn et al. 1999).

Deposition of non-structural ECM components

As mentioned above, granulation tissue fibroblasts produce initially a primitive, unorganized and structurally weak ECM that resembles connective tissue during fetal development, suggesting that this ECM serves as a template that guides subsequent tissue maturation (Buchanan et al. 2009; Rozario and DeSimone 2010). For instance, fibroblasts synthesize abundantly cellular EDA and EDB fibronectins (Larjava et al. 2002; Wong et al. 2009; Table 6.4). The latter fibronectin isoform contains the extra domain B (EDB) which is missing from other fibronectin isoforms. Although its function remains elusive, EDB fibronectin may regulate fibroblast growth and granulation tissue angiogenesis (Ronca et al. 2009). As discussed above, EDA fibronectin is an important molecule that mediates cell adhesion to the ECM and supports fibroblast migration. In the granulation tissue, EDA fibronectin is actively assembled by the fibroblasts into a three-dimensional fibrillar network at the cell surface. As fibronectin harbors binding sites for various ECM proteins, including collagen, it also controls deposition and organization of the collagen-rich pericellular ECM. Furthermore, through integrin-mediated signaling, EDA fibronectin regulates fibroblast gene expression and differentiation into myofibroblasts (Serini et al. 1998; Leiss et al. 2008; Singh et al. 2010). Hyaluronan, a large polymeric glycosaminoglycan that is present abundantly in fetal skin, is also secreted into the early granulation tissue ECM (Buchanan et al. 2009). As mentioned above, it regulates inflammation, promotes cell migration into the wound and collaborates with growth factors to modulate cell proliferation (Chen and Abatangelo 1999; Meran et al. 2011). In addition, it helps diffusion of nutrients and other molecules to the cells when vascularization has not yet been restored. Its amount in the wound granulation tissue peaks around day 5 after wounding, followed by a gradual decline

(Bentley 1967; Table 6.4). Interestingly, in fetal skin wounds that display scarless healing, hyaluronan levels remain elevated long after wounding (Longaker et al. 1991; Larson et al. 2010). The exact role of hyaluronan in scar formation remains to be shown, but it may suppress scar formation due to the property of certain hyaluronan fragments to stimulate expression of type III collagen and TGF-β3 (David-Raoudi et al. 2008). The presumed antifibrotic effect of type III collagen is based on findings that targeted deletion of type III collagen in mice results in increased accumulation of ECM during the remodeling stage, and that cryptic peptides derived from type III collagen promote recruitment of progenitor cells into wounds (Agrawal et al. 2011; Volk et al. 2011). Administration of TGF-β3 into wounds has also been shown to reduce scar formation (Occleston et al. 2008). Curiously, however, certain hyaluronan fragments have also pro-fibrogenic effects and promote expression of type I collagen and pro-fibrotic TGF-β1 (David-Raoudi et al. 2008; Buchanan et al. 2009).

At the later stages of granulation tissue formation and coinciding with the most active collagen deposition and remodeling, connective tissue cells also produce abundantly various matricellular proteins (Table 6.4). They are non-structural ECM components that associate with the structural proteins at the pericellular matrix and include SPARC (also called osteonectin or BM-40), hevin, thrombospondin-1 and -2, tenascin-C and -X, periostin and the Cyr-CTGF-Nov-family (CCN-family) proteins (Chiodoni et al. 2010). Like hyaluronan and certain fibronectin isoforms, many of these proteins are also strongly expressed during fetal development, but re-emerge in adult tissues during tissue remodeling and repair. In addition to modulating cell–ECM interactions, they bind and regulate the activity of cytokines and growth factors and may also interact with growth factor receptors expressed by wound cells (Hamilton 2008; Chiodoni et al. 2010). For instance, two closely related matricellular proteins, SPARC and hevin, regulate ECM deposition and organization during wound healing. Spatiotemporal expression of hevin during wound healing is not known, but increased SPARC abundance can be noted 3 days after injury at the wound edge, and it shows peak accumulation in the granulation tissue at day 7 (Reed et al. 1993; Table 6.4). Both SPARC and hevin are anti-adhesive molecules suppressing cell migration, and SPARC also inhibits cell cycle progression. In fact, deletion of these molecules promotes wound healing, and their increased expression is associated with reduced angiogenesis and scar formation (Bradshaw and Sage 2001; Bradshaw et al. 2002; Barker et al. 2005; Sullivan et al. 2008).

Thrombospondin-1 is fast released into the blood clot from the α-granules of platelets in the early wound healing stage, while thrombospondin-2 is produced more slowly by fibroblasts during granulation tissue formation, with peak accumulation at day 7–10 after wounding (Kyriakides et al. 1999; Agah et al. 2004; Kyriakides and MacLauchlan 2009; Table 6.4). Thrombospondins can interact with cells in various ways, as several receptors for these molecules have been described, including integrins, proteoglycans and lipoprotein receptors. Thrombospondin-1 is an important activator of the immunomodulatory and fibrogenic growth factor TGF-β1. It also controls angiogenesis and appears to regulate fibroblast migration, important for granulation tissue formation. In contrast, thrombospondin-2 regulates fibroblast–ECM interactions, influencing ECM remodeling. It also inhibits angiogenesis, and mice deficient in the expression of thrombospondin-2 exhibit increased vascularization of wounds (Kyriakides and MacLauchlan 2009).

As discussed above, around day 3 after wounding, tenascin-C is produced abundantly at the connective tissue close to the wound edge, where it may help fibroblast recruitment to the wound. However, by day 7 when fibroblasts have populated the granulation tissue, tenascin-C expression is strongly downregulated in the tissues surrounding the wound.

Instead, it is now strongly expressed in the granulation tissue (Table 6.4). This coincides with gradually increased mechanical stiffness within the granulation tissue caused by myofibroblasts actively depositing collagen and reorganizing it by contraction (Häkkinen et al. 2000b; Wong et al. 2009). Tenascin-C gene has a promotor region that is responsive to mechnosensory signaling, which provides a possible explanation for its increased expression during wound contraction (Chiquet-Ehrismann and Chiquet 2003). Although the function of tenascin-C in granulation tissue remains elusive, it contains several binding sites for fibronectin, and regulates fibronectin assembly into a three-dimensional fibrillar matrix (To and Midwood 2011). Moreover, certain peptide fragments derived from tenascin-C degradation appear to inhibit fibroblast migration (Trebaul et al. 2007). Therefore, degradation of tenascin-C during the remodeling phase of wound healing may prevent further recruitment of fibroblasts into the wound site. Curiously, abundant expression of tenascin-C has been associated with both keloid scars and scarless wound healing in fetal skin, human oral mucosa and spinal cord injury (Whitby et al. 1991; Sible et al. 1995; Dalkowski et al. 1999; Wong et al. 2009; Chen et al. 2010). Thus, the role of tenascin-C in fibrosis and scar formation remains to be shown. Spatiotemporal expression of the closely related tenascin-X during wound healing is somewhat unclear. However, in general its abundance appears to be greatly reduced as compared to unwounded connective tissue during wound healing. It first appears in the wound granulation tissue at day 7 post-wounding, with clearly increased accumulation at day 14 (Egging et al. 2007; Table 6.4). Targeted deletion of tenascin-X results in significantly reduced breaking strength of wounds without any apparent effect on collagen abundance or wound closure rate. Therefore, tenascin-X may be a regulator of biomechanical properties of the tissue (Egging et al. 2007). Interestingly, in a model of radiation-induced fibrosis in skin, the level of tenascin-C was significantly elevated, while expression of tenascin-X remained unaltered compared to normal tissue, suggesting that these two closely related molecules may have opposing properties to regulate tissue fibrosis (Geffrotin et al. 1998).

Periostin was initially discovered in the periosteum during fracture healing, but more recently it has been found in other connective tissues, including skin and periodontal ligament (Hamilton 2008; Elliott and Hamilton 2011). In acute wounds, periostin is strongly expressed at the dermo-epidermal junction at the wound margin at day 3 after wounding. It also quickly starts to appear in the granulation tissue, with peak accumulation at day 7 and returning to the level of normal tissue at day 28 (Jackson-Boeters et al. 2009; Zhou et al. 2010; Table 6.4). Periostin can bind to other ECM molecules, including tenascin-C and collagen, and it regulates cell adhesion, proliferation and migration. It also has significant pro-fibrotic functions as it promotes collagen deposition, fibrillogenesis and cross-linking, and it may play a role in MMP-mediated activation of TGF-β, myofibroblast differentiation and wound contraction. Accordingly, periostin is highly expressed in the connective tissue stroma in pathological scars (Hamilton 2008; Zhou et al. 2010; Elliott and Hamilton 2011).

The CCN family of matricellular proteins contains three major members, namely CCN1 (also called Cyr61), CCN2 (CTGF) and CCN3 (Nov), which can be upregulated as a response to growth factors, such as TGF-β1, or to cellular stress and hypoxia during granulation tissue formation (Leask and Abraham 2006; Kular et al. 2011). During dermal wound healing, CCN1 and CCN2 expression peak at day 7 after wounding, returning to the normal low level found in unwounded tissue by day 14. In contrast, CCN3 remains downregulated in the dermal wounds until 28 days post-wounding (Rittié et al. 2011; Table 6.4). CCN proteins mediate cell interactions to other ECM molecules, although there are no specific high affinity receptors for these proteins. Instead, cells interact with these molecules via many different types of receptors which include certain integrins and cell surface heparan sulfate proteoglycans (Leask and Abraham 2006). In general, CCN proteins regulate several key aspects of wound healing, including cell adhesion and migration, matrix deposition, angiogenesis and differentiation, but they are also involved in pathological scar formation and fibrosis (Leask and Abraham 2006; Kular et al. 2011).

In addition to their role in directly regulating functions of wound fibroblasts and ECM organization, many of the ECM molecules secreted into the granulation tissue also sequester and modulate the activity of growth factors and cytokines, such as TGF-β, PDGF, VEGF, TNF-α, HGF, FGF, IGF and interleukins. The above ECM molecules include small leucine-rich proteoglycans decorin, biglycan and fibromodulin, heparan sulfate proteoglycans, fibronectin, SPARC, thrombospondin, hyaluronan, vitronectin and collagens (Macri et al. 2007). Therefore, it is conceivable that, depending on their spatiotemporal expression and specific biological functions, these ECM molecules may contribute to pathological scar formation or promote scarless healing. Further studies are needed to unravel their exact role in wound healing.

Myofibroblast differentiation

Wound contraction is the process that brings wound edges closer together, thereby reducing the surface area that needs to be covered with new epithelium. In human skin, contraction can account for about 50% of wound closure, but in rodents it is more extensive and makes up to 90% of the wound closure (Stocum 2006). Wound contraction also brings collagen fibrils together and organizes them perpendicular to the wound edges, increasing the mechanical strength of the tissue (Clark 1996; Gurtner et al. 2008; Schultz et al. 2011). The contraction is an active process mediated by differentiation of wound cells into myofibroblasts. These cells have characteristics of contractile smooth muscle cells and express α-smooth muscle actin (Tomasek et al. 2002; Hinz 2010). It is not completely clear what the principal progenitor cells for myofibroblasts in the granulation tissue are, although differentiation of myofibroblasts from local fibroblasts has been well documented. In addition, myofibroblasts may originate from other cells, including mesenchymal stem cells, endothelial cells, pericytes, fibrocytes and epithelial cells (Hinz and Gabbiani 2010; Quaggin and Kapus 2011; Schrimpf and Duffield 2011). Myofibroblast differentiation starts when granulation tissue is well established around day 7 after wounding, and it is a gradual process whereby fibroblasts or their progenitor cells assume a proto-myofibroblast phenotype which is then turned into a fully differentiated myofibroblast (Clark 1996; Tomasek et al. 2002). Myofibroblast differentiation is coordinately regulated by distinct cell–ECM interactions, growth factors and mechanosensory signals present in the granulation tissue. Interaction of cells with cellular EDA fibronectin, but not plasma fibronectin, via α5β1 and αvβ3 integrins and at least in lung fibroblasts by α4β7 integrin, and stimulation by TGF-β1 are necessary for myofibroblast differentiation (Serini et al. 1998; Lygoe et al. 2007; Eyden 2008; Kohan et al. 2010). In addition, integrin-mediated mechanosensory signaling caused by strain from the wound ECM promotes this process (Hattori et al. 2009; Hinz 2010). Other factors present in wounds, including hyaluronan, osteopontin, periostin, vitronectin, endothelin, angiotensin, PDGF and CCN2 (CTGF), as well as functional connexin-43 gap junctions have also been associated with myofibroblast differentiation (Asazuma-Nakamura et al. 2009; Simpson et al. 2009; Webber et al. 2009; Leask 2010; Elliott and Hamilton 2011). In addition, MMPs regulate the differentiation process as MMP inhibitors block myofibroblast differentiation *in vivo* (Mirastschijski et al. 2004, 2010), but the exact mechanism is unclear.

In contrast to the above-mentioned pro-differentiation factors, certain inflammatory mediators, including TNF-α, can inhibit myofibroblast differentiation (Goldberg et al. 2007). Thus, extended inflammation may postpone myofibroblast differentiation, delaying the wound healing process.

Multiple mechanisms regulate wound contraction. In the granulation tissue, myofibroblasts are attached to a polymerized fibronectin network that serves as a bridge between cells and newly synthesized collagen fibrils. In order to attach to this fibronectin-rich matrix, fibroblasts use integrins of the β1 and αv families (Clark 1996). In addition, fibroblasts can use their collagen receptors, including α1β1, α2β1 and α11β1 integrins and discoidin domain receptor-2 (DDR2), to interact directly with collagen (Vogel et al. 2006; Schultz et al. 2011). While DDR2-mediated interaction with collagen regulates myofibroblast differentiation, collagen deposition and cross-linking, as well as tensile strength of the wound (Olaso et al. 2011), integrins play a more direct role in mediating wound contraction. Wound contraction is achieved when myofibroblasts attach to the collagen fibrils with their integrins and pull the fibrils in alignment perpendicularly to wound edges using their actin-rich cytoskeleton (Clark 1996; Tomasek et al. 2002). In addition, fibroblasts can rearrange and contract collagen-rich ECM when they pull collagen during cell migration (Grinnell and Petroll 2010). Based mostly on studies utilizing an *in vitro* model of collagen gel contraction by fibroblasts, contraction can be induced by several wound growth factors, including TGF-β1, PDGF and endothelin, and inhibited by inflammatory mediators, such as IL-1α, TNF-α and interferon-γ (Clark et al. 1989; Guidry and Hook 1991; Tingström et al. 1991; Irwin et al. 1998; Zhu et al. 2001). Wound contraction is also aided by cadherin-mediated cell–cell adhesions between myofibroblasts, possibly allowing the cells to function as a coordinated unit (Follonier et al. 2008). At this stage of wound healing, gap junctional cell–cell communication that was disrupted upon wounding, and that was mostly absent from migrating fibroblasts, is also re-established between myofibroblasts. As mentioned above, gap junctions may promote myofibroblast differentiation, but there are contradicting findings whether gap junctions could be involved in mediating wound contraction (Gabbiani et al. 1978; Ehrlich et al. 2000; Follonier et al. 2008; Mori et al. 2006). Wound contraction may also require action of MMPs as this process is suppressed in MMP-13 knockout mice (Hattori et al. 2009). In addition, as MMP inhibitors block myofibroblast differentiation, they also reduce wound contraction (Mirastschijski et al. 2004, 2010). The exact mechanism of how MMPs may regulate wound contraction remains to be shown.

Transforming growth factor-β

As mentioned above, deposition of ECM molecules in the granulation tissue is regulated by growth factors, including TGF-β isoforms and PDGF, which are abundantly present in wounds (Werner and Grose 2003; Clark 1996). In general, PDGF appears to promote secretion of hyaluronan and certain proteoglycans, while TGF-βs induce production of fibronectin, collagens and proteoglycans (Hyytiäinen et al. 2004). TGF-β1, -β2 and -β3 isoforms are multifunctional cytokines that are spatiotemporally strongly upregulated during wound healing (Berrientos et al. 2008). Particularly TGF-β1 is released initially into wounds by platelets. It is also expressed by lymphocytes, macrophages, keratinocytes, mast cells and fibroblasts at the later stages of wound healing (Berrientos et al. 2008). The above-mentioned three different TGF-β isoforms have overlapping functions, regulating fibroblast proliferation, migration, ECM deposition, myofibroblast differentiation, wound contraction and downregulation of MMP expression (Clark 1996; Berrientos et al. 2008). In addition, TGF-βs are potent modulators of the immunological responses during wound healing (Berrientos et al. 2008). While increased or prolonged activity of TGF-β1 has been strongly associated with extended myofibroblast differentiation, increased matrix accumulation and scar formation, TGF-β3 appears to prevent myofibroblast differentiation and scarring, but the exact mechanism remains to be shown (Ferguson and O'Kane 2004; Waddington et al. 2010).

TGF-βs are usually secreted in a latent form comprised of TGF-β, latency-associated peptide (LAP) and latent TGF-β binding protein (LTBP). Latent TGF-β binds to the ECM where it remains stored until cells process it for activation (Hyytiäinen et al. 2004). Activation of TGF-β is key to its biological function, and in principle can occur via a proteolytic release of TGF-β from the latent complex, by conformational changes produced by interaction of integrins with the latent TGF-β or by a combination of these mechanisms (Jenkins 2008; Wipff and Hinz 2008; Margadant and Sonnenberg 2010). In any case, the role of integrins appears crucial in this process *in vivo* (Margadant and Sonnenberg 2010). LAP of TGF-β1 and TGF-β3 contains the Arg-Gly-Asp (RGD) sequence which can be recognized by integrins, including α5β1, αvβ3, αvβ5, αvβ6 and αvβ8. TGF-β activation by β1 integrins and most of the αv integrins is accomplished by cytoskeletal tractional forces that are transmitted via integrins to the latent TGF-β complex. These forces cause conformational changes that allow TGF-β to interact with its receptor. In contrast, αvβ8 integrin activates TGF-β by recruiting MT1-MMP and inducing a proteolytical release of active TGF-β (Margadant and Sonnenberg 2010). It remains unclear, however, whether this interaction is relevant for wound healing, as there are no reports describing expression of αvβ8 integrin in the granulation tissue. Integrin αvβ3 can also bind MMP-2 and MMP-9, both capable of proteolytic TGF-β activation, but the physiological relevance of this mechanism remains also unclear (Margadant and Sonnenberg 2010). In general, the non-proteolytic TGF-β activation is a controlled, focalized process and exposes TGF-β to the same or immediately nearby cells, while the proteolytic process releases TGF-β which can reach cells further away.

The cellular processes that mediate TGF-β activation specifically during wound healing are not completely understood, but several mechanisms may be involved. For instance, during granulation tissue formation, wound keratinocytes residing on the surface of forming granulation tissue express strongly αvβ6 integrin, an important keratinocyte-specific activator of ECM-associated latent TGF-β1 and TGF-β3 (Annes et al. 2002, 2004). ECM deposition and maturation progress faster in the granulation tissue immediately beneath the wound epithelium than in the other parts of the granulation tissue (Fig. 6.3). Therefore, keratinocyte αvβ6-mediated activation of TGF-β may provide paracrine TGF-β for the subepithelial fibroblasts. This TGF-β could directly, or indirectly by inducing further autocrine TGF-β secretion in fibroblasts, promote fibroblast proliferation, migration and ECM deposition at this location (Eslami et al. 2009). Integrins may also be involved in TGF-β activation by granulation tissue fibroblasts. For instance, deletion of β1 integrins specifically in fibroblasts suppresses wound closure, granulation tissue formation, ECM deposition and myofibroblast differentiation through a mechanism that is linked to abnormal TGF-β activation (Liu et al. 2010). In addition to β1 integrins, αvβ3 and αvβ5 which can also activate latent TGF-β are expressed by wound fibroblasts (Wipff and Hinz 2008). As discussed above, TGF-β upregulates expression of β1 and αv integrins (Margadant and Sonnenberg 2010). Thus, there is a reciprocal relationship between TGF-β and integrin expression and function in wound healing that is likely to be important for ECM deposition and remodeling.

The activation of TGF-β is balanced by mechanisms that modulate this process. ECM molecules (decorin, biglycan, fibromodulin, thrombospondins, fibronectin, transglutaminase and fibrillin) can bind latent or active TGF-β to either support or inhibit its activation

(Macri et al. 2007; Schaefer and Iozzo 2008). For instance, the small leucine-rich proteoglycan decorin reduces organ fibrosis through its ability to bind and inactivate pro-fibrotic TGF-β1, and possibly CCN2/CTGF (Schaefer and Iozzo 2008; Vial et al. 2011). Targeted deletion of fibromodulin results in increased TGF-β3 activity in skin wounds (Zheng et al. 2011).

Taken together, the abundance of cells secreting TGF-β, the repertoire of integrins that can activate TGF-β expressed by wound cells and the relative abundance of proteases and certain ECM molecules that modulate TGF-β activation may contribute to regulation of TGF-β activity and, hence, wound healing outcome.

CONNECTIVE TISSUE REMODELING

Wound remodeling stage turns the abundant and poorly organized granulation tissue ECM into a mature connective tissue. At the peak of granulation tissue formation the tissue is highly hypercellular with fibroblasts, macrophages, myofibroblasts and neovasculature, and wound contraction is underway. At this stage, ECM secretion by fibroblasts exceeds degradation, resulting in accumulation of ECM (Clark 1996; Gurtner et al. 2008). Remodeling starts when wound contraction has assembled the collagen fibrils into thicker bundles and aligned them perpendicularly to the wound edges. The timing of the start of this stage depends on the size of the wound and whether the wound healing occurs by primary or secondary intention. When very little granulation tissue is formed, wound contraction can occur already around day 3–5 post-wounding, but in larger wounds healing by secondary intention, it may take 7–14 days, or more, to commence. After wound contraction, ECM production and degradation is gradually balanced, and many of the molecules present in granulation tissue are replaced with more mature connective tissue. For instance, type III collagen abundantly present in the early granulation tissue is degraded and replaced with type I collagen (Clark 1996; Gurtner et al. 2008). During the remodeling stage, collagen cross-linking also gradually increases, improving the stability of the tissue. There is also a gradual maturation of the tissue so that the aligned collagen fiber bundles are reorganized to the typical and more resilient basketweave organization found in normal connective tissue. In an ideal case, this process of remodeling and maturation fully restores the integrity, structure and function of the tissue. However, this is a slow process, and based on animal studies the breaking strength of the wound may be only about 20% of the final strength after 21 days. After that, remodeling continues slowly and can last for months or in some cases for years (Clark 1996; Gurtner et al. 2008).

As mentioned above, if remodeling does not lead to complete structural regeneration of the tissue, scar formation may occur. In the mildest form, scars may contain some excess of collagen-rich ECM where collagen is organized in thick parallel bundles instead of the mechanically more versatile and stronger basketweave that is present in normal tissue. Therefore, scars can gain at best only about 70–80% of the breaking strength of normal skin. However, in more severe cases, ECM deposition and degradation is not balanced, leading to progressive ECM accumulation and formation of pathological scars, namely keloids or hyperthrophic scars in the skin (Hardy 1989; Clark 1996; Slemp and Kirschner 2006; Stocum 2006; Gurtner et al. 2008; Wolfram et al. 2009; Wight and Potter-Perigo 2011). Therefore, biological processes that regulate ECM abundance and organization are critical for appropriate wound healing outcome. At least four different mechanisms likely contribute to these processes. First, the number of cells secreting ECM is reduced. Second, cells degrade and remodel ECM components to reduce their abundance. Third, ECM is reorganized and its stability is increased by appropriate collagen cross-linking. Fourth, secretion of ECM by the cells is downregulated.

Downregulation of cell proliferation and cellularity

Cellularity of the tissue is reduced during the remodeling stage as there is a strong decrease in the abundance of pro-mitogenic growth factors, cytokines and chemokines present in the tissue as compared to the granulation tissue formation stage. This is due to a reduction in the number of inflammatory cell subsets that produce many of these factors (Clark 1996; Werner and Grose 2003; Eming et al. 2007; Gurtner et al. 2008). One of the main reasons for suppression of inflammatory cell numbers is the overall reduction in the levels of pro-inflammatory signals in the wound. Moreover, expression of mediators that actively suppress or resolve inflammation, including lipoxins, resolvins, meresins and cytokines such as IL-10, is induced during wound healing (Sato et al. 1999; Peranteau et al. 2008; Serhan 2011). As mentioned previously, proteases produced by fibroblasts and other wound healing cells also cleave chemokines, changing their function to suppress inflammation (Gillitzer and Goebeler 2001; Tran et al. 2005; Gill and Parks 2008; Manicone and McGuire 2008).

Cell proliferation is also reduced because of emergence of signals that suppress proliferation or induce apoptosis. During wound remodeling, the composition of the ECM changes both quantitatively and qualitatively, and this impacts on fibroblast proliferation (Clark 1996; Gurtner et al. 2008; Schultz et al. 2011). For example, there is an increased accumulation of small leucine-rich proteoglycans in the ECM, which in addition to regulating appropriate collagen fibrillogenesis, organization and remodeling, serve as negative regulators of pro-mitogenic TGF-β signaling and can regulate certain intracellular signaling pathways that suppress cell proliferation (Häkkinen et al. 2000c; Bhide et al. 2005; Honardoust et al. 2008; Iozzo and Schaefer 2010). In addition, mechanosensory signaling from ECM regulates fibroblast growth and survival. During the remodeling stage, gradually increased collagen accumulation and wound contraction results in organization of the collagen-rich ECM along the stress lines perpendicular to the wound edges. During this process, increased integrin-mediated mechanosensory signaling keeps cells in an active state where they proliferate and deposit more ECM. This process continues until the compliance of the ECM reaches a balance with the surrounding tissues. The resulting reduction in mechanosensory signaling then reduces cell proliferation and ECM deposition (Carlson and Thompson 2004; Grinnell and Petroll 2010; Provenzano and Keely 2011; Schultz et al. 2011). Some wound cells, including myofibroblasts and cells forming blood vessels, are also driven into apoptosis, contributing to the reduced cellularity and vascularity of the tissue (Desmoulière et al. 1997). The mechanisms that induce apoptosis in the wound remodeling stage are not very well understood, but altered cell–ECM interactions and reduced mechanosensory signaling may play a part in this process (Carlson and Thompson 2004; Provenzano and Keely 2011). Thus, once granulation tissue has been formed, multiple signals from inflammatory and other cells and ECM need to be coordinated to reduce cell proliferation and, hence, the number of ECM producing cells.

ECM degradation

Remodeling of ECM involves deposition of new ECM molecules, albeit at a slower rate than during granulation tissue formation, and degradation of the excess collagen-rich ECM (Singer and Clark 1999). ECM degradation allows normalization of the tissue composition both qualitatively and quantitatively, and it may also facilitate reorganization of the ECM. Proteolytic degradation mediated particularly by MMPs has been considered as the main mechanism to reduce ECM abundance and help appropriate reorganization of the ECM (Gill and Parks 2008; Toriseva and Kähäri 2009). As discussed above, MMPs can reside as cell membrane anchored molecules (MT-MMPs) that mediate focalized proteolysis or they can be secreted into the ECM, where they are responsible for the bulk ECM degradation further away from cells. In addition, secreted MMPs can bind to cell surface molecules, including integrins and proteoglycans, which can target MMP function to the pericellular location (Murphy and Nagase 2011). As mentioned above, function of MMPs is generally regulated by the activation of the latent molecules by proteases, including plasmin, by inhibitory or modulatory molecules, including TIMPs, and by factors that regulate their expression (Toriseva and Kähäri 2009). Expression of MMPs during wound healing is tightly spatiotemporally regulated, and many MMPs, including collagenases MMP-1, -8 and -13, gelatinases MMP-2 and -9, stromelysins MMP-3 and -10, as well as cell membrane-associated MT1-MMP, are expressed most abundantly during the early inflammatory, re-epithelialization and granulation tissue formation stages. Furthermore, MMP-2, MMP-9 and MT1-MMP are also expressed in the remodeling stage (Ulrich et al. 2007; Gill and Parks 2008; Toriseva and Kähäri 2009). In addition to being regulated by the growth factors and cytokines present in the wound (Table 6.2), cell–ECM interactions modulate MMP expression (Gill and Parks 2008; Toriseva and Kähäri 2009). For instance, when fibroblasts experience mechanical strain from the ECM they actively produce ECM proteins, but little matrix degrading proteases, including MMPs. When strain from the ECM relaxes, as occurs during the remodeling stage of wound healing, the gene expression changes to favor expression of proteolytic enzymes over ECM proteins. This may allow the cells to remodel the forming connective tissue and degrade excess proteins, thus helping to normalize the tissue composition and organization (Clark 1996; Gill and Parks 2008; Gurtner et al. 2008; Toriseva and Kähäri 2009; Grinnell and Petroll 2010; Schultz et al. 2011). It appears that it is the balance between MMPs and their inhibitors (TIMPs) that may in part determine whether wound healing results in abnormal accumulation of ECM, i.e. scar, or not (Gill and Parks 2008; Toriseva and Kähäri 2009). For instance, fetal skin wound healing that does not produce scars has increased levels of MMPs relative to TIMPs compared to scar-forming adult skin (Dang et al. 2003).

Interestingly, though, recent findings have suggested that proteolytic bulk degradation of ECM by MMPs is not necessarily essential for remodeling during wound healing. For instance, in mice engineered to express collagenase-resistant collagen, wound re-epithelialization, myofibroblast differentiation and wound contraction are impaired, but the wounds eventually heal without apparent differences in scar formation compared to similar wounds in control animals (Beare et al. 2003). This supports the idea that MMPs may be more important for the initial inflammation, re-epithelialization and granulation tissue formation stages of wound healing than for ECM remodeling. This is further supported by findings from wound healing studies using broad-spectrum MMP inhibitors or MMP-3, MMP-9 and MMP-13 knockout animals. In these studies, the early wound healing events, including inflammation, re-epithelialization, myofibroblast differentiation and wound contraction were affected, but no major changes were reported in the remodeling stage and scar formation (Bullard et al. 1999; Mirastschijski et al. 2004; Hattori et al. 2009; Kyriakides et al. 2009). These studies were performed in mouse skin, however, where scar formation is rare and wound healing occurs by mechanisms that are partially different from those in human skin (Gottrup et al. 2000; Chillcott 2008). In addition, it is possible that functional redundancy between proteases compensates for lack of certain MMPs. Interestingly, however, recent findings have provided further proof that MMPs are more important in regulation of inflammation by cleaving chemokines and other inflammatory mediators and their receptors rather than degrading ECM during wound remodeling (Gill and Parks 2008). MMP-mediated cleavage either reduces or increases the activity of inflammatory mediators during early wound healing (Gill and Parks 2008; Toriseva and Kähäri 2009). Indirectly, this may be important for wound healing outcome as early inflammation determines the progression of the remodeling stage. For instance, fetal skin or oral mucosal wounds that heal without scarring show reduced inflammatory response compared to adult skin wounds that form scars (Sciubba et al. 1978; Szpaderska et al. 2003; Mak et al. 2009; Namazi et al. 2011).

As proteolytic bulk degradation of ECM alone may not mediate wound remodeling, there may be other mechanisms that participate in this process. Various studies have provided evidence that wound cells, mainly macrophages and fibroblasts, are able to phagocytose and endocytose ECM molecules for intracellular degradation by lysosomal enzymes, including cystein proteinase cathepsin-K (McGaw 1986; East and Isacke 2002; Rünger et al. 2007; Quintanilla-Dieck et al. 2009). For instance, collagen phagocytosis and endocytosis can be mediated by several cell surface receptors, including $\alpha 2\beta 1$ integrins and Endo180/uPARAP, respectively, which are expressed by wound cells (Lee et al. 1996; Honardoust et al. 2006). Interestingly, collagen internalization by these receptors is promoted by initial focalized proteolytic processing by MT1-MMP, although other collagenases may also be involved (Lee et al. 2006, 2007; Madsen et al. 2007; Messaritou et al. 2009; Shi et al. 2010; Murphy and Nagase 2011). Collagen internalization by fibroblasts is further modulated by other ECM molecules. For instance, the small leucine-rich proteoglycan decorin that avidly binds to collagen and is abundantly expressed during the remodeling stage of wound healing suppresses collagen phagocytosis by fibroblasts (Bhide et al. 2005; Honardoust et al. 2008). Thus, it is the collaboration of focalized proteolysis by MMPs, and maybe other proteases, with phagocytosis and endocytosis mechanisms and the molecular composition of the ECM that are important for appropriate remodeling. However, more studies are needed to address the role of these processes in wound remodeling *in vivo*.

ECM reorganization and increased stability by collagen cross-linking

Tissue breaking strength depends mostly on appropriate collagen fibrillogenesis, intermolecular collagen cross-linking and orientation of collagen fiber bundles (Clark 1996; Gurtner et al. 2008). Therefore, mechanisms that regulate these processes are critical for rapid restoration of connective tissue strength and function after wounding. Initially, type I collagen is secreted into the granulation tissue as poorly organized, thin fibrils that have limited number of intermolecular cross-links, rendering it easily soluble (Lovvorn et al. 1999). Fibrillogenesis of type I collagen is an active process driven by wound fibroblasts and requires the presence of fibronectin, type III and V collagen and expression of fibronectin and collagen-binding integrins by fibroblasts (Liu et al. 1997; Kadler et al. 2008). In addition, many proteins present in the granulation tissue can modulate lateral assembly, size and organization of the collagen fibrils into thicker fiber bundles. These include small leucine-rich proteoglycans decorin, biglycan and fibromodulin as well as matricellular proteins SPARC, thrombospondin-2 and tenascin-X which are expressed in the wounds at the time of wound contraction and/or during tissue remodeling (Reed et al. 1993; Agah et al. 2004; Egging et al. 2007; Rentz et al. 2007; Kadler et al. 2008; Honardoust et al. 2008;

Kyriakides and MacLauchlan 2009; Kalamajski and Oldberg 2010; Table 6.4). In addition to appropriate collagen fibrillogenesis, remodeling involves spatial reorientation of the existing and forming collagen fibrils. Based on cell culture studies using cancer cells, this process depends on tractional forces created by the cells to the collagen via the cytoskeleton–integrin–ECM link and focalized proteolysis mediated by MT1-MMP (Kirmse et al. 2011), but it is unclear whether the same mechanism is functional in wound fibroblasts.

To further stabilize ECM during remodeling, cells present in the granulation tissue, including fibroblasts, endothelial cells and macrophages, produce enzymes that promote intermolecular cross-linking of type I collagen. To this end, they secrete enzymes such as lysyl hydroxylases (LH-1, LH-2, LH-3), lysyl oxidase (LOX) and transglutaminase-2 which mediate the intermolecular cross-linking and gradually turn collagen insoluble and more resistant to degradation (Mercer et al. 2003; Verderio et al. 2004; Lopez et al. 2010). Expression of these enzymes is spatiotemporally regulated during wound healing (Table 6.4). In animal skin wound models, LOX and LH-2 mRNAs were significantly elevated at day 3 and 7 post-wounding, respectively, and remained elevated for at least 3 weeks (Fushida-Takemura et al. 1996). However, in a similar model, LOX activity peaked at day 10 (Szauter et al. 2005). These findings complement findings from a rat skin granulation tissue model showing a gradual increase in stabilization of collagen fibrils with a peak at 3 weeks (Hering et al. 1983). In pig skin wounds, LH-2-dependent collagen cross-links were elevated still 8 weeks after wounding (Ulrich et al. 2007). Secreted transglutaminase appears first in granulation tissue at day 1 and reaches peak activity around day 4 post-wounding (Haroon et al. 1999; Verderio et al. 2004; Table 6.4). In the provisional wound matrix, transglutaminase is initially attached to fibronectin where it helps to form a polymeric fibronectin matrix that supports subsequent collagen fibrillogenesis and cell adhesion to fibronectin. Its secretion is strongly induced by factors present in wounds, including TGF-β and hypoxia (Verderio et al. 2004). Transglutaminase-mediated collagen cross-linking also enhances cell adhesion to collagen and makes it more resistant to proteolytic degradation (Chau et al. 2005). Thus, intermolecular cross-linking of collagen by LOX, LHs and transglutaminase appears to start early during granulation tissue formation and progresses fast for at least 3 weeks post-wounding in skin.

Although collagen cross-linking is important for the initial wound stability, excess cross-linking may contribute to scar formation. Accordingly, cell culture studies suggest that increased or prolonged transglutaminase activity may render collagen less susceptible to proteolytic remodeling, resulting in collagen accumulation (Verderio et al. 2004). In further support of this idea, fetal lamb skin wounds that heal without scar formation contain a reduced amount of cross-linked collagen as compared to scar-forming adult skin wounds (Lovvorn et al. 1999). Moreover, levels of the collagen cross-linking enzymes are elevated and can remain at a high level for several months or years in established scars (Verderio et al. 2004; Szauter et al. 2005; van den Bogaerdt et al. 2009). Interestingly, transglutaminase can also store TGF-β in the ECM and participate in its activation, promoting excess collagen deposition by fibroblasts, thus potentially further contributing to pathological scar formation (Verderio et al. 2004).

Downregulation of ECM production

During the remodeling stage, ECM deposition is suppressed by coordinated changes in soluble signaling molecules and cell–ECM interactions. For instance, during the remodeling stage, there is a reduction in pro-fibrotic TGF-β1 and TGF-β2 as the cell populations, including macrophages and fibroblasts, which produce this growth factor, are reduced. In addition, it is likely that secretion of TGF-β by the remaining connective tissue cells is downregulated due to a decrease in the level of cytokines that stimulate TGF-β expression (Levine et al. 1993; Gold et al. 1997; Yang et al. 1999; Beanes et al. 2003; Eslami et al. 2009). Moreover, as mentioned above, reduced tension experienced by the cells from the ECM induces integrin-mediated signaling that suppresses ECM deposition and promotes expression of MMPs, potentially contributing to shifting the balance from ECM deposition to ECM remodeling (Grinnell and Petroll 2010). In addition, signals mediated from the ECM can potently change the response of fibroblasts to growth factors. For instance, EGF can either induce or suppress collagen expression, depending on the organization and quality of the ECM (Colige et al. 1988). Cell–ECM interactions also modulate matrix deposition and remodeling by yet another mechanism. Recent findings have suggested that myofibroblasts that play an active part in ECM deposition are driven into senescence during the remodeling phase (Jun and Lau 2010a, 2010b). In the senescent state, proliferation of the cells ceases, their ECM production is downregulated and they start producing ECM degrading enzymes. Myofibroblast senescence is promoted by the matricellular protein CCN1 (Cyr61) which induces intracellular ROS generation through cell surface heparan sulfate proteoglycans and α6β1 integrin-mediated signaling, but also other factors are likely to be involved (Jun and Lau 2010a, 2010b).

RE-EMERGENCE OF QUIESCENT FIBROBLAST PHENOTYPE

Normal connective tissue does not contain many myofibroblasts, while they appear to persist abundantly in different types of pathological scars and in tissue fibrosis (Germain et al. 1994; Darby and Hewitson 2007; Hinz and Gabbiani 2010). Therefore, for optimal tissue regeneration, myofibroblasts may need to be ultimately replaced by fibroblasts with low metabolic activity that will be able to re-establish and maintain the tissue structure. Curiously, though, oral mucosal wounds in the palate that display reduced histological and clinical scar formation compared to skin wounds harbor elevated numbers of myofibroblasts (Mak et al. 2009). Therefore, the regulation of myofibroblast function rather than their presence *per se* may be more critical for the wound-healing outcome. As described above, induction of senescence and apoptosis of myofibroblasts may be two mechanisms that help to modulate myofibroblast function and abundance, respectively, during the remodeling stage of wound healing (Hinz and Gabbiani 2010). However, very little is known about the biological mechanisms that ultimately lead to re-establishment of the quiescent fibroblast cell phenotype of normal connective tissue responsible for tissue maintenance and homeostasis. It is possible that the local pericellular microenvironment (i.e. niche) established during the remodeling stage determines the phenotype and function of the resident cells. Alternatively, the local tissue microenvironment may provide signals that help to recruit new fibroblast subsets or their progenitor cells to replace the myofibroblasts during the remodeling stage. Interestingly, apoptotic cells can promote mesenchymal progenitor cell proliferation (Li et al. 2010). Thus, apoptotic myofibroblasts may recruit new fibroblast progenitor cells into the tissue which, under the influence of an appropriately established pericellular niche, acquire the quiescent phenotype required for complete tissue regeneration and maintenance. Finding out more details about the factors that regulate these processes may be key to prevent pathological scarring where fibroblast populations actively producing ECM, including myofibroblasts, seem to persist.

SPECIFIC FEATURES OF ORAL MUCOSAL WOUND HEALING

For a long time there has been a general notion among clinicians that wounds in oral mucosa heal fast and do not often involve wound healing complications or scar formation. These clinical ideas have been recently supported with systematic studies using rodent and pig wound healing models showing that, indeed, oral mucosal wound healing progresses faster and results in significantly reduced clinical and histological scar formation compared to similar skin wounds (Sciubba et al. 1978; Szpaderska et al. 2003, 2005; Mak et al. 2009; Wong et al. 2009). The reason for this differential wound healing outcome in oral mucosa and skin is not completely clear.

However, it has been suggested that during evolution selection pressures favored fast skin wound closure, which protected tissues from microbial infection but lead to suboptimal connective tissue healing and scar formation (Ferguson and O'Kane 2004). As discussed above, in scars, the organization and structure of the excessively produced connective tissue ECM is not optimal, and the tissue tensile strength is reduced compared to normal tissue. However, although being esthetically problematic and structurally somewhat weaker, small scars allow the tissue, and hence the individual, to function usually rather normally (Bayat et al. 2003; Corr et al. 2009). Based on this idea, one could further speculate that during evolution, there may have been even greater selection pressures for faster and better wound regeneration in the oral mucosa compared to skin as delayed wound healing or scarring in the oral cavity might have been more detrimental to the survival of an individual by compromising appropriate nutrient intake.

Nevertheless, previous and more recent studies have provided some clues about the cellular mechanisms which may explain favorable wound healing in the oral mucosa. It is possible that the pericellular ECM niche where the cells reside before wounding and which is critical for regulation of cell functions during the initial stages of wound healing is different in oral mucosa and skin, favoring fast and complete wound regeneration (Macri et al. 2007; Daley et al. 2008). Surprisingly, little is known about differences in the pericellular ECM in oral mucosa and skin *in vivo*, although it appears that there are quantitative and qualitative differences between certain molecules, including sulfated glycosaminoglycans, heparan, chondroitin, dermatan and keratan sulfate, hyaluronan, type III collagen and tenascin-C (Pedlar 1984; Bronson et al. 1988; Wong et al. 2009). In contrast, several studies have shown that fibroblasts isolated from oral mucosa and skin have several inherent phenotypical differences, including a different capability for collagen remodeling, distinct secretion patterns for certain ECM molecules, different growth, migration and cell adhesion properties, as well as differential expression of ECM receptors and response to growth factors. Consequently, the phenotype of oral mucosal fibroblasts exhibits similarities to fetal-type fibroblasts which contributes to scar-free healing in fetal skin (Bronson et al. 1988; Kähäri et al. 1991; Schor et al. 1996; Stephens et al. 1996; al-Khateeb et al. 1997; Ravanti et al. 1999; Häkkinen et al. 2000b; Stephens et al. 2001a, 2001b; Ferguson and O'Kane 2004; van Beurden et al. 2005: Shannon et al. 2006; McKeown et al. 2007; Nolte et al. 2008; Enoch et al. 2009, 2010; Meran et al. 2011; Table 6.5). These inherent differences may derive from a distinct embryonic developmental program between skin and oral mucosal fibroblasts, as the former are derived from mesodermal mesenchymal cells and the latter from cells associated with the neural crest (Breau et al. 2008). Of note, palatal mucosa harbors abundantly neural-crest-related stem cells which may promote fast wound healing and tissue regeneration (Widera et al. 2009).

Table 6.5 Differences between adult skin and oral mucosal fibroblasts, ECM and wound healing response.[1]

Adult skin	Adult oral mucosa
Fibroblasts *in vitro*	
Slower fibroblast migration	Faster fibroblast migration
Slower collagen gel contraction	Faster collagen gel contraction
Lower expression of HGF/SF and KGF	Higher expression of HGF/SF and KGF
Lower expression of MMP-2 and MMP-3	Higher expression of MMP-2 and MMP-3
TGF-β promotes proliferation	TGF-β suppresses proliferation
Shorter proliferative lifespan	Longer proliferative lifespan
Quantitative and qualitative differences in production of hyaluronan and sulfated glycosaminoglycans	
Connective tissue ECM	
Less tenascin-C	Abundantly tenascin-C
Less hyaluronan	More hyaluronan
Quantitative and qualitative differences in sulfated glycosaminoglycans	
Acute wound healing	
Dry, contaminated environment	Moist (saliva), contaminated environment
Strong and prolonged inflammation	More rapid, short and weaker inflammation
Slower re-epithelialization	Faster re-epithelialization
Strong angiogenesis response	Moderate angiogenesis response
High expression of VEGF	Lower expression of VEGF
TGF-β1/TGF-β3 isoform ratio higher	TGF-β1/TGF-β3 isoform ratio lower
Results in scar formation	Results in minimal scar formation
Fundamental differences in the expression of MMPs, peptidases, cytokines and chemokines	

[1]Sciubba et al. 1978; Bronson et al. 1988; Kähäri et al. 1991; Bodner et al. 1992; Schor et al. 1996; Stephens et al. 1996, 2001a, 2001b; Yang et al. 1996; al-Khateeb et al. 1997; Ravanti et al. 1999; Häkkinen et al. 2000b; Szpaderska et al. 2003, 2005; Ferguson and O'Kane 2004; van Beurden et al. 2005: Shannon et al. 2006; McKeown et al. 2007; Nolte et al. 2008; Schrementi et al. 2008; Enoch et al. 2009, 2010; Eslami et al. 2009; Chen et al. 2010; Meran et al. 2011.

Other mechanisms that may promote scarless healing include the presence of saliva and differential inflammatory response in the oral mucosa. Saliva contains factors, including cytokines and growth factors such as EGF, TGF-β and IGF, that are known to promote wound healing (Häkkinen et al. 2000b; Loo et al. 2010). Furthermore, lack of saliva results in delayed oral wound closure, further suggesting that it is beneficial for wound healing (Bodner et al. 1992; Yang et al. 1996). However, the effect of saliva on scar formation is less clear.

Rapid and mild inflammatory response at the early stages of wound healing in the oral mucosa may also be beneficial for the wound healing outcome. Oral mucosal wounds in pigs and rodents that heal faster than skin wounds also show a reduced inflammatory response, including a reduced recruitment of neutrophils, mast cells, macrophages and T-cells (Sciubba et al. 1978; Szpaderska et al. 2003; Mak et al. 2009; Chen et al. 2010). Similar to non-scarring fetal skin wounds, wounds in the oral mucosa demonstrate reduced levels of certain cytokines in the first days following injury, including the pro-fibrotic TGF-β1 and the pro-inflammatory interleukins and TNF-α (Szpaderska et al. 2003; Chen et al. 2010). Furthermore, the level of antifibrotic TGF-β3 relative to pro-fibrotic TGF-β1 appears to be elevated in oral mucosal wounds as compared to skin wounds (Schrementi et al. 2008; Eslami et al. 2009).

Recently, global gene expression profiles were compared in experimental skin and oral mucosal (tongue) wounds using a murine model (Chen et al. 2010). The findings further confirmed fundamental site-specific genetic differences in the wound healing responses between these two tissues, and showed that the general gene expression response to wounding in oral mucosa was more rapid, shorter and less pronounced than in skin. Interestingly, the basal expression of many of the genes involved in wound healing was higher in the non-wounded oral mucosal tissue compared to skin, suggesting that cells in the oral mucosa are primed for a fast wound healing response (Chen et al. 2010). This may, at least partially, depend on cellular and anatomical differences between skin and oral mucosa. For instance, as mentioned above, the number of vascular capillaries and blood flow are higher in oral mucosa than in skin, possibly allowing a faster wound healing response (Canady et al. 1993). In addition, normal buccal oral mucosal epithelium contains 34 times more T-cells than skin epithelium, possibly contributing to the fast inflammatory response in the oral mucosa (van Loon et al. 1989). Many of the studies comparing skin and oral mucosal wound healing are, however, from loose skinned animals in which skin wound healing occurs by different mechanisms compared to tight skinned animals such as humans and pigs. Nevertheless, comparing the molecular and cellular differences between oral mucosal and skin healing may help to identify novel mechanisms that may be used to improve aberrant wound healing in skin.

CONCLUSIONS

Wound healing is a complex process that involves interactions of multiple inflammatory and tissue resident cells, soluble and structural molecules and mechanical forces generated at the cell–ECM interface. The timing, combination, magnitude or abundance and duration of these interactions ultimately determine the wound-healing outcome. Remarkable advances have been made in the past decade in understanding some of these processes. In addition, different models to assess mechanisms that lead to the ideal wound healing result (wound regeneration) in contrast to situations where wound healing outcome is compromised (non-healing chronic wounds or excessive wound healing involving scar formation) have provided important information that may be used to develop novel strategies to promote regeneration and alleviate wound healing problems. In spite of this progress, more detailed understanding of the cellular and molecular interactions is needed to translate this knowledge to efficiently and predictably promote tissue regeneration.

ACKNOWLEDGMENTS

This work was supported by the Canadian Institutes for Health Research.

REFERENCES

Agah, A., Kyriakides, T.R., Letrondo, N., et al. (2004) Thrombospondin 2 levels are increased in aged mice: consequences for cutaneous wound healing and angiogenesis. *Matrix Biology,* **22** (7), 539–547.

Agrawal, V., Tottey, S., Johnson, S.A., et al. (2011) Recruitment of progenitor cells by an ECM cryptic peptide in a mouse model of digit amputation. *Tissue Engineering Part A*, May 12. [Epub ahead of print] al-Khateeb, T., Stephens, P., Shepherd, J.P., et al. (1997) An investigation of preferential fibroblast wound repopulation using a novel in vitro wound model. *Journal of Periodontology,* **68** (11), 1063–1069.

Annes, J.P., Rifkin, D.B., Munger, J.S., et al. (2002) The integrin alphaVbeta6 binds and activates latent TGFbeta3. *FEBS Letters,* **511** (1–3), 65–68.

Annes, J.P., Chen, Y., Munger, J.S., et al. (2004) Integrin alphaVbeta6-mediated activation of latent TGF-beta requires the latent TGF-beta binding protein-1. *Journal of Cell Biology,* **165** (5), 723–734.

Asazuma-Nakamura, Y., Dai, P., Harada, Y., et al. (2009) Cx43 contributes to TGF-beta signaling to regulate differentiation of cardiac fibroblasts into myofibroblasts. *Experimental Cell Research,* **315** (7), 1190–1199.

Barker, T.H., Framson, P., Puolakkainen, P. et al. (2005) Matricellular homologs in the foreign body response: hevin suppresses inflammation, but hevin and SPARC together diminish angiogenesis. *American Journal of Pathology,* **166** (3), 923–933.

Barrientos, S., Stojadinovic, O., Golinko, M.S., et al. (2008) Growth factors and cytokines in wound healing. *Wound Repair and Regeneration,* **16** (5), 585–601.

Bayat, A., McGrouther, D.A., Ferguson, M.W. (2003) Skin scarring. *BMJ* **326** (7380), 88–92.

Bayreuther, K., Francz, P.I., Gogol, J., et al. (1991) Differentiation of primary and secondary fibroblasts in cell culture systems. *Mutation Research,* **256** (2–6), 233–242.

Beanes, S.R., Dang, C., Soo, C., et al. (2003) Skin repair and scar formation: the central role of TGF-beta. *Expert Reviews in Molecular Medicine,* **5** (8), 1–22.

Beare, A.H., O'Kane, S., Krane, S.M., et al. (2003) Severely impaired wound healing in the collagenase-resistant mouse. *Journal of Investigative Dermatology,* **120** (1), 153–163.

Beer, H.D., Gassmann, M.G., Munz, B., et al. (2000) Expression and function of keratinocyte growth factor and activin in skin morphogenesis and cutaneous wound repair. *Journal of Investigative Dermatology Symposium Proceedings,* **5** (1), 34–39.

Behrens, J., Kameritsch, P., Wallner, S., et al. (2010) The carboxyl tail of Cx43 augments p38 mediated cell migration in a gap junction-independent manner. *European Journal of Cell Biology,* **89** (11), 828–838.

Bentley, J.P. (1967) Rate of chondroitin sulfate formation in wound healing. *Annals of Surgery,* **165** (2), 186–191.

Bhide, V.M., Laschinger, C.A., Arora, P.D., et al. (2005) Collagen phagocytosis by fibroblasts is regulated by decorin. *Journal of Biological Chemistry,* **280** (24), 23103–23113.

Bianchetti, L., Barczyk, M., Cardoso, J., et al. (2011) Extracellular matrix remodelling properties of human fibrocytes. *Journal of Cellular and Molecular Medicine,* May 20. [Epub ahead of print]

Bodner, L., Dayan, D., Oberman, M., et al. (1992) Healing of experimental wounds in sialadenectomized rat. *Journal of Clinical Periodontology,* **19** (5), 345–347.

Bohm, M., Luger, T.A. (2004) Melanocortins in fibroblast biology – current update and future perspective for dermatology. *Experimental Dermatology,* **13** (Suppl. 4), 16–21.

Boraldi, F., Annovi, G., Carraro, F., et al. (2007) Hypoxia influences the cellular cross-talk of human dermal fibroblasts. A proteomic approach. *Biochimica et Biophysica Acta,* **1774** (11), 1402–1413.

Brábek, J., Mierke, C.T., Rösel, D., et al. (2010) The role of the tissue microenvironment in the regulation of cancer cell motility and invasion. *Cell Communication and Signaling,* **8**, 22.

Bradshaw, A.D., Sage, E.H. (2001) SPARC, a matricellular protein that functions in cellular differentiation and tissue response to injury. *Journal of Clinical Investigation,* **107** (9), 1049–1054.

Bradshaw, A.D., Reed, M.J., Sage, E.H. (2002) SPARC-null mice exhibit accelerated cutaneous wound closure. *Journal of Histochemistry and Cytochemistry,* **50** (1), 1–10.

Breau, M.A., Pietri, T., Stemmler, M.P., et al. (2008) A nonneural epithelial domain of embryonic cranial neural folds gives rise to ectomesenchyme. *Proceeding of National Academy of Sciences USA,* **105** (22), 7750–7755.

Bronson, R.E., Argenta, J.G., Siebert, E.P., et al. (1988) Distinctive fibroblastic subpopulations in skin and oral mucosa demonstrated by differences in glycosaminoglycan content. *In Vitro Cellular and Developmental Biology,* **24** (11), 1121–1126.

Broughton, G. 2nd, Janis, J.E., Attinger, C.E. (2006) The basic science of wound healing. *Plastic and Reconstructive Surgery,* **117** (7 Suppl.), 12S–34S.

Buchanan, E.P., Longaker, M.T., Lorenz, H.P. (2009) Fetal skin wound healing. *Advances in Clinical Chemistry,* **48**, 137–161.

Buck, M., Houglum, K., Chojkier, M. (1996) Tumor necrosis factor-alpha inhibits collagen alpha1(I) gene expression and wound healing in a murine model of cachexia. *American Journal of Pathology,* **149** (1) 195–204.

Buckley, C.D., Pilling, D., Lord, J.M., et al. (2001) Fibroblasts regulate the switch from acute resolving to chronic persistent inflammation. *Trends in Immunology,* **22** (4), 199–204.

Bullard, K.M., Lund, L., Mudgett, J.S., et al. (1999) Impaired wound contraction in stromelysin-1-deficient mice. *Annals of Surgery,* **230** (2), 260–265.

Burke, J.P., Cunningham, M.F., Watson, R.W., et al. (2010) Bacterial lipopolysaccharide promotes profibrotic activation of intestinal fibroblasts. *British Journal of Surgery,* **97** (7), 1126–1134.

Bush, J.A., Ferguson, M.W., Mason, T., et al. (2008) Skin tension or skin compression? Small circular wounds are likely to shrink, not gape. *Journal of Plastic, Reconstructive and Aesthetic Surgery,* **61** (5), 529–534.

Canady, J.W., Johnson, G.K., Squier, C.A. (1993) Measurement of blood flow in the skin and oral mucosa of the rhesus monkey (*Macaca mulatta*) using laser Doppler flowmetry. *Comparative Biochemistry and Physiology. Comparative Physiology,* **106** (1), 61–63.

Carlson, M.A., Thompson, J.S. (2004) Wound splinting modulates granulation tissue proliferation. *Matrix Biology,* **23** (4), 243–250.

Chanson, M., Derouette, J.P., Roth, I., et al. (2005) Gap junctional communication in tissue inflammation and repair. *Biochimica et Biophysica Acta,* **1711** (2), 197–207.

Chau, D.Y., Collighan, R.J., Verderio, E.A., et al. (2005) The cellular response to transglutaminase-cross-linked collagen. *Biomaterials,* **26** (33); 6518 6529.

Chen, J., Joon Lee, H., Jakovcevski, I., et al. (2010) The extracellular matrix glycoprotein tenascin-C is beneficial for spinal cord regeneration. *Molecular Therapy,* **18** (10), 1769–1777.

Chen, L., Arbieva, Z.H., Guo, S., et al. (2010) Positional differences in the wound transcriptome of skin and oral mucosa. *BMC Genomics,* **11**, 471.

Chen, W.Y., Abatangelo, G. (1999) Functions of hyaluronan in wound repair. *Wound Repair and Regeneration,* **7** (2), 79–89.

Chillcott, R.P. (2008) Cutaneous anatomy and function. In: *Principles and Practice of Skin Toxicology* (eds. Chilcott, R.P., Price, S.), pp. 2–16. John Wiley, Mississauga, Ontario, Canada.

Chiodoni, C., Colombo, M.P., Sangaletti, S. (2010) Matricellular proteins: from homeostasis to inflammation, cancer, and metastasis. *Cancer Metastasis Reviews,* **29** (2), 295–307.

Chiquet-Ehrismann, R., Chiquet, M. (2003) Tenascins: regulation and putative functions during pathological stress. *Journal of Pathology,* **200** (4), 488–499.

Chong, H.C., Tan, M.J., Philippe, V., et al. (2009) Regulation of epithelial-mesenchymal IL-1 signaling by PPARbeta/delta is essential for skin homeostasis and wound healing. *Journal of Cell Biology,* **184** (6), 817–831.

Chunmeng, S., Tianmin, C., Yongping, S., et al. (2004) Effects of dermal multipotent cell transplantation on skin wound healing. *Journal of Surgical Research,* **121** (1), 13–19.

Clark, R.A.F. (1996) *The Molecular and Cellular Biology of Wound Repair*, 2nd edn. Plenum Press, New York, London.

Clark, R.A., Folkvord, J.M., Hart, C.E., et al. (1989) Platelet isoforms of platelet-derived growth factor stimulate fibroblasts to contract collagen matrices. *Journal of Clinical Investigation,* **84** (3), 1036–1040.

Clark, R.A., Lin, F., Greiling, D., et al. (2004) Fibroblast invasive migration into fibronectin/fibrin gels requires a previously uncharacterized dermatan sulfate-CD44 proteoglycan. *Journal of Investigative Dermatology,* **122** (2), 266–277.

Clore, J.N., Cohen, I.K., Diegelmann, R.F. (1979) Quantitation of collagen types I and III during wound healing in rat skin. *Proceedings of the Society for Experimental Biology and Medicine. Society for Experimental Biology and Medicine New York,* **161** (3), 337–340.

Colige, A., Nusgens, B., Lapiere, C.M. (1988) Effect of EGF on human skin fibroblasts is modulated by the extracellular matrix. *Archives of Dermatological Research,* **280** (Suppl.), S42–46.

Colige, A.C., Lambert, C.A., Nusgens, B.V., et al. (1992) Effect of cell-cell and cell-matrix interactions on the response of fibroblasts to epidermal growth factor in vitro. Expression of collagen type I, collagenase, stromelysin and tissue inhibitor of metalloproteinases. *Biochemical Journal,* **285** (Pt 1), 215–221.

Conway, K., Price, P., Harding, K.G., et al. (2006) The molecular and clinical impact of hepatocyte growth factor, its receptor, activators, and inhibitors in wound healing. *Wound Repair and Regeneration,* **14** (1), 2–10.

Corr, D.T., Gallant-Behm, C.L., Shrive, N.G., et al. (2009) Biomechanical behavior of scar tissue and uninjured skin in a porcine model. *Wound Repair and Regeneration,* **17** (2), 250–259.

da Silva, L., Carvalho, E., Cruz, M.T. (2010) Role of neuropeptides in skin inflammation and its involvement in diabetic wound healing. *Expert Opinion in Biological Therapy,* **10** (10), 1427–1439.

da Silva Meirelles, L., Caplan, A.I., Nardi, N.B. (2008) In search of the in vivo identity of mesenchymal stem cells. *Stem Cells,* **26** (9), 2287–2299.

Daley, W.P., Peters, S.B., Larsen, M. (2008) Extracellular matrix dynamics in development and regenerative medicine. *Journal of Cell Science,* **121** (Pt 3), 255–264.

Dalkowski, A., Schuppan, D., Orfanos, C.E., et al. (1999) Increased expression of tenascin C by keloids in vivo and in vitro. *British Journal of Dermatology,* **141** (1), 50–56.

Dalton, S.J., Whiting, C.V., Bailey, J.R., et al. (2007) Mechanisms of chronic skin ulceration linking lactate, transforming growth factor-beta, vascular endothelial growth factor, collagen remodeling, collagen stability, and defective angiogenesis. *Journal of Investigative Dermatology,* **127** (4), 958–968.

Dang, C.M., Beanes, S.R., Lee, H., et al. (2003) Scarless fetal wounds are associated with an increased matrix metalloproteinase-to-tissue-derived inhibitor of metalloproteinase ratio. *Plastic and Reconstructive Surgery,* **111** (7), 2273–2285.

Darby, I.A., Hewitson, T.D. (2007) Fibroblast differentiation in wound healing and fibrosis. *International Review of Cytology,* **257**, 143–179.

David-Raoudi, M., Tranchepain, F., Deschrevel, B., et al. (2008) Differential effects of hyaluronan and its fragments on fibroblasts: relation to wound healing. *Wound Repair and Regeneration,* **16** (2), 274–287.

Davies, L.C., Locke, M., Webb, R.D., et al. (2010) A multipotent neural crest-derived progenitor cell population is resident within the oral mucosa lamina propria. *Stem Cells and Development,* **19** (6), 819–830.

De Donatis, A., Ranaldi, F., Cirri, P. (2010) Reciprocal control of cell proliferation and migration. *Cell Communication and Signaling,* **8**, 20.

Desmoulière, A., Badid, C., Bochaton-Piallat, M.L., et al. (1997) Apoptosis during wound healing, fibrocontractive diseases and vascular wall injury. *International Journal of Biochemistry and Cell Biology,* **29** (1), 19–30.

Diaz-Flores, L. Jr., Gutierrez, R., Madrid, J.F., et al. (2009) Adult stem cells and repair through granulation tissue. *Frontiers in Bioscience,* **14**, 1433–1470.

East, L., Isacke, C.M. (2002) The mannose receptor family. *Biochimica et Biophysica Acta,* **1572** (2–3), 364–386.

Eckes, B., Nischt, R., Krieg, T. (2010) Cell-matrix interactions in dermal repair and scarring. *Fibrogenesis and Tissue Repair,* **3**, 4.

Egging, D., van Vlijmen-Willems, I., van Tongeren, T., et al. (2007) Wound healing in tenascin-X deficient mice suggests that tenascin-X is involved in matrix maturation rather than matrix deposition. *Connective Tissue Research,* **48** (2), 93–98.

Ehrlich, H.P., Gabbiani, G., Meda, P. (2000) Cell coupling modulates the contraction of fibroblast-populated collagen lattices. *Journal of Cellular Physiology,* **184** (1), 86–92.

Elliott, C.G., Hamilton, D.W. (2011) Deconstructing fibrosis research: do pro-fibrotic signals point the way for chronic dermal wound regeneration? *Journal of Cell Communication and Signaling,* Apr 19. [Epub ahead of print]

Ellis, I., Banyard, J., Schor, S.L. (1997) Differential response of fetal and adult fibroblasts to cytokines: cell migration and hyaluronan synthesis. *Development,* **124** (8), 1593–1600.

Eming, S.A., Krieg, T., Davidson, J.M. (2007) Inflammation in wound repair: molecular and cellular mechanisms. *Journal of Investigative Dermatology,* **127** (3), 514–525.

Engelhardt, E., Toksoy, A., Goebeler, M., et al. (1998) Chemokines IL–8, GROα, MCP–1, IP–10, and Mig are sequentially and differentially expressed during phase-specific infiltration of leukocyte subsets in human wound healing. *American Journal of Pathology,* **153**, 1849–1860.

Enoch, S., Wall, I., Peake, M., et al. (2009) Increased oral fibroblast lifespan is telomerase-independent. *Journal of Dental Research,* **88** (10), 916–921.

Enoch, S., Peake, M.A., Wall, I., et al. (2010) 'Young' oral fibroblasts are geno/phenotypically distinct. *Journal of Dental Research,* **89** (12), 1407–1413.

Eslami, A., Gallant-Behm, C.L., Hart, D.A., et al. (2009) Expression of integrin alphavbeta6 and TGF-beta in scarless vs scar-forming wound healing. *Journal of Histochemistry and Cytochemistry,* **57** (6), 543–557.

Eyden, B. (2008) The myofibroblast: phenotypic characterization as a prerequisite to understanding its functions in translational medicine. *Journal of Cellular and Molecular Medicine,* **12** (1), 22–37.

Falanga, V., Zhou, L., Yufit, T. (2002) Low oxygen tension stimulates collagen synthesis and COL1A1 transcription through the action of TGF-beta1. *Journal of Cellular Physiolology,* **191** (1), 42–50.

Fathke, C., Wilson, L., Hutter, J., et al. (2004) Contribution of bone marrow-derived cells to skin: collagen deposition and wound repair. *Stem Cells,* **22** (5), 812–822.

Ferguson, M.W., O'Kane, S. (2004) Scar-free healing: from embryonic mechanisms to adult therapeutic intervention. *Philosophical Transactions of the Royal Society of London. Series B, Biological Sciences,* **359** (1445), 839–850.

Flavell, S.J., Hou, T.Z., Lax, S. (2008) Fibroblasts as novel therapeutic targets in chronic inflammation. *British Journal of Pharmacology,* **153** (Suppl. 1), S241–246.

Follonier, L., Schaub, S., Meister, J.J., et al. (2008) Myofibroblast communication is controlled by intercellular mechanical coupling. *Journal of Cell Science,* **121** (Pt 20), 3305–3316.

Fournier, B.P., Ferre, F.C., Couty, L., et al. (2010) Multipotent progenitor cells in gingival connective tissue. *Tissue Engineering Part A,* **16** (9), 2891–2899.

Friedl, P., Bröcker, E.B. (2000) The biology of cell locomotion within three-dimensional extracellular matrix. *Cellular and Molecular Life Sciences,* **57** (1), 41–64.

Fukai, T., Takeda, A., Uchinuma, E. (2005) Wound healing in denervated rat skin. *Wound Repair and Regeneration,* **13** (2), 175–180.

Fushida-Takemura, H., Fukuda, M., Maekawa, N., et al. (1996) Detection of lysyl oxidase gene expression in rat skin during wound healing. *Archives of Dermatological Research,* **288** (1), 7–10.

Gabbiani, G., Chaponnier, C., Hüttner, I. (1978) Cytoplasmic filaments and gap junctions in epithelial cells and myofibroblasts during wound healing. *Journal of Cell Biology,* **76** (3), 561–568.

Gailit, J., Xu, J., Bueller, H., et al. (1996) Platelet-derived growth factor and inflammatory cytokines have differential effects on the expression of integrins alpha 1 beta 1 and alpha 5 beta 1 by human dermal fibroblasts in vitro. *Journal of Cellular Physiology,* **169** (2), 281–289.

Gailit, J., Clarke, C., Newman, D., et al. (1997) Human fibroblasts bind directly to fibrinogen at RGD sites through integrin alpha(v)beta3. *Experimental Cell Research,* **232** (1), 118–126.

Geary, S.M., Cowin, A.J., Copeland, B., et al. (2008) The role of the tetraspanin CD151 in primary keratinocyte and fibroblast functions: implications for wound healing. *Experimental Cell Research,* **314** (11–12), 2165–2175.

Geffrotin, C., Tricaud, Y., Crechet, F., et al. (1998) Unlike tenascin-X, tenascin-C is highly up-regulated in pig cutaneous and underlying muscle tissue developing fibrosis after necrosis induced by very high-dose gamma radiation. *Radiation Research,* **14** (5), 472–481.

Germain, L., Jean, A., Auger, F.A., et al. (1994) Human wound healing fibroblasts have greater contractile properties than dermal fibroblasts. *Journal of Surgical Research,* **57** (2), 268–273.

Ghahary, A., Ghaffari, A. (2007) Role of keratinocyte-fibroblast cross-talk in development of hypertrophic scar. *Wound Repair and Regeneration,* **15** (Suppl. 1), S46–53.

Ghatnekar, G.S., O'Quinn, M.P., Jourdan, L.J., et al. (2009) Connexin43 carboxyl-terminal peptides reduce scar progenitor and promote regenerative healing following skin wounding. *Regenerative Medicine,* **4** (2), 205–223.

Gibran, N.S., Ferguson, M., Heimbach, D.M., et al. (1997) Monocyte chemoattractant protein-1 mRNA expression in the human burn wound. *Journal of Surgical Research,* **70** (1), 1–6.

Gill, S.E., Parks, W.C. (2008) Metalloproteinases and their inhibitors: regulators of wound healing. *International Journal of Biochemistry and Cell Biology,* **40** (6–7), 1334–1347.

Gillitzer, R., Goebeler, M. (2001) Chemokines in cutaneous wound healing. *Journal of Leukocyte Biology,* **69** (4), 513–521.

Gold, L.I., Sung, J.J., Siebert, J.W., et al. (1997) Type I (RI) and type II (RII) receptors for transforming growth factor-beta isoforms are expressed subsequent to transforming growth factor-beta ligands during excisional wound repair. *American Journal of Pathology,* **150** (1), 209–222.

Goldberg, M.T., Han, Y.P., Yan, C., et al. (2007) TNF-alpha suppresses alpha-smooth muscle actin expression in human dermal fibroblasts: an implication for abnormal wound healing. *Journal of Investigative Dermatology,* **127** (11), 2645–2655.

Gottrup, F., Agren, M.S., Karlsmark, T. (2000) Models for use in wound healing research: a survey focusing on in vitro and in vivo adult soft tissue. *Wound Repair and Regeneration,* **8** (2), 83–96.

Grayson, W.L., Zhao, F., Bunnell, B., et al. (2007) Hypoxia enhances proliferation and tissue formation of human mesenchymal stem cells. *Biochemical and Biophysical Research Communications,* **358** (3), 948–953.

Greiling, D., Clark, R.A. (1997) Fibronectin provides a conduit for fibroblast transmigration from collagenous stroma into fibrin clot provisional matrix. *Journal of Cell Science,* **110** (Pt 7), 861–870.

Grimstad, O., Sandanger, O., Ryan, L., et al. (2011) Cellular sources and inducers of cytokines present in acute wound fluid. *Wound Repair and Regeneration,* **19** (3), 337–347.

Grinnell, F., Petroll, WM. (2010) Cell motility and mechanics in three-dimensional collagen matrices. *Annual Review of Cell and Developmental Biology,* **26**, 3353–3361.

Grzeszkiewicz, T.M., Kirschling, D.J., Chen, N., et al. (2001) CYR61 stimulates human skin fibroblast migration through Integrin alphavbeta 5 and enhances mitogenesis through integrin alpha vbeta 3, independent of its carboxyl-terminal domain. *Journal of Biological Chemistry,* **276** (24), 21943–21950.

Guidry, C., Hook, M. (1991) Endothelins produced by endothelial cells promote collagen gel contraction by fibroblasts. *Journal of Cell Biology,* **115** (3), 873–880.

Gurtner, G.C., Werner, S., Barrandon, Y., et al. (2008) Wound repair and regeneration. *Nature,* **453** (7193), 314–321.

Guyot, C., Lepreux, S., Combe, C., et al. (2006) Hepatic fibrosis and cirrhosis: the (myo)fibroblastic cell subpopulations involved. *International Journal of Biochemistry and Cell Biology,* **38** (2), 135–151.

Häkkinen, L., Csiszar, A. (2007) Hereditary gingival fibromatosis: characteristics and novel putative pathogenic mechanisms. *Journal of Dental Research,* **86** (1), 25–34.

Häkkinen, L., Larjava, H. (1992) Characterization of fibroblast clones from periodontal granulation tissue in vitro. *Journal of Dental Research,* **71** (12), 1901–1907.

Häkkinen, L., Hildebrand, H.C., Berndt, A., et al. (2000a) Immunolocalization of tenascin-C, alpha9 integrin subunit, and alphavbeta6 integrin during wound healing in human oral mucosa. *Journal of Histochemistry and Cytochemistry,* **48** (7), 985–998.

Häkkinen, L., Uitto, V.J., Larjava, H. (2000b) Cell biology of gingival wound healing. *Periodontology,* **24**, 127–152.

Häkkinen, L., Strassburger, S., Kähäri, V.M., et al. (2000c) A role for decorin in the structural organization of periodontal ligament. *Laboratory Investigation,* **80** (12), 1869–1880.

Halfter, W., Liverani, D., Vigny, M., et al. (1990) Deposition of extracellular matrix along the pathways of migrating fibroblasts. *Cell Tissue Research,* **262** (3), 467–481.

Hamilton, D.W. (2008) Functional role of periostin in development and wound repair: implications for connective tissue disease. *Journal of Cell Communication and Signaling,* **2** (1–2), 9–17.

Haniffa, M.A., Collin, M.P., Buckley, C.D., et al. (2009) Mesenchymal stem cells: the fibroblasts' new clothes? *Haematologica,* **94** (2), 258–263.

Harding, K.G., Morris, H.L., Patel, G.K. (2002) Science, medicine and the future: healing chronic wounds. *BMJ,* **324** (7330), 160–163.

Hardy, M.A. (1989) The biology of scar formation. *Physical Therapy,* **69** (12), 1014–1024.

Haroon, Z.A., Hettasch, J.M., Lai, T.S., et al. (1999) Tissue transglutaminase is expressed, active, and directly involved in rat dermal wound healing and angiogenesis. *FASEB Journal*, **13** (13), 1787–1795.

Hattori, N., Mochizuki, S., Kishi, K., et al. (2009) MMP-13 plays a role in keratinocyte migration, angiogenesis, and contraction in mouse skin wound healing. *American Journal of Pathology,* **175** (2), 533–546.

Hauck, C.R., Hsia, D.A., Schlaepfer, D.D. (2000) Focal adhesion kinase facilitates platelet-derived growth factor-BB-stimulated ERK2 activation required for chemotaxis migration of vascular smooth muscle cells. *Journal of Biological Chemistry,* **275** (52), 41092–41099.

He, Y., Esser, P., Schacht, V., et al. (2011) Role of kindlin-2 in fibroblast functions: implications for wound healing. *Journal of Investigative Dermatology,* **131** (1), 245–256.

Heino, J., Käpylä, J. (2009) Cellular receptors of extracellular matrix molecules. *Current Pharmaceutical Design,* **15** (12), 1309–1317.

Heino, J., Ignotz, R.A., Hemler, M.E., et al. (1989) Regulation of cell adhesion receptors by transforming growth factor-beta. Concomitant regulation of integrins that share a common beta 1 subunit. *Journal of Biological Chemistry,* **264** (1), 380–388.

Hering, T.M., Marchant, R.E., Anderson, J.M. (1983) Type V collagen during granulation tissue development. *Experimental and Molecular Pathology,* **39** (2), 219–229.

Herzog, E.L., Bucala, R. (2010) Fibrocytes in health and disease. *Experimental Hematology,* **38** (7), 548–556.

Hill, S.J., Ebersole, J.L. (1996) The effect of lipopolysaccharide on growth factor-induced mitogenesis in human gingival fibroblasts. *Journal of Periodontology,* **67** (12), 1274–1280.

Hinz, B. (2010) The myofibroblast: paradigm for a mechanically active cell. *Journal of Biomechanics,* **43** (1), 146–155.

Hinz, B., Gabbiani, G. (2010) Fibrosis: recent advances in myofibroblast biology and new therapeutic perspectives. *F1000 Biology Reports,* **2**, 78.

Honardoust, H.A., Jiang, G., Koivisto, L., et al. (2006) Expression of Endo180 is spatially and temporally regulated during wound healing. *Histopathology,* **49** (6), 634–648.

Honardoust, D., Eslami, A., Larjava, H., et al. (2008) Localization of small leucine-rich proteoglycans and transforming growth factor-beta in human oral mucosal wound healing. *Wound Repair and Regeneration,* **16** (6), 814–823.

Hotary, K.B., Yana, I., Sabeh, F., et al. (2002) Matrix metalloproteinases (MMPs) regulate fibrin-invasive activity via MT1-MMP-dependent and -independent processes. *Journal of Experimental Medicine,* **195** (3), 295–308.

Hyytiäinen, M., Penttinen, C., Keski-Oja, J. (2004) Latent TGF-beta binding proteins: extracellular matrix association and roles in TGF-beta activation. *Critical Reviews in Clinical Laboratory Sciences,* **4** (3), 233–264.

Ignotz, R.A., Massagué, J. (1987) Cell adhesion protein receptors as targets for transforming growth factor-beta action. *Cell,* **51** (2), 189–197.

Ignotz, R.A., Heino, J., Massagué, J. (1989) Regulation of cell adhesion receptors by transforming growth factor-beta. Regulation of vitronectin receptor and LFA-1. *Journal of Biological Chemistry,* **264** (1), 389–392.

Iozzo, R.V., Schaefer, L. (2010) Proteoglycans in health and disease: novel regulatory signaling mechanisms evoked by the small leucine-rich proteoglycans. *FEBS Journal,* **277** (19), 3864–3875.

Irwin, C.R., Picardo,. M, Ellis, I., et al. (1994) Inter- and intra-site heterogeneity in the expression of fetal-like phenotypic characteristics by gingival fibroblasts: potential significance for wound healing. *Journal of Cell Science,* **107** (Pt 5), 1333–1346.

Irwin, C.R., Myrillas, T., Smyth, M., et al. (1998) Regulation of fibroblast-induced collagen gel contraction by interleukin-1beta. *Journal of Oral Pathology and Medicine,* **27** (6), 255–259.

Ivaska, J., Heino, J. (2010) Interplay between cell adhesion and growth factor receptors: from the plasma membrane to the endosomes. *Cell and Tissue Research,* **33** (1), 111–120.

Jackson-Boeters, L., Wen, W., Hamilton, D.W. (2009) Periostin localizes to cells in normal skin, but is associated with the extracellular matrix during wound repair. *Journal of Cell Communication and Signaling,* **3** (2), 125–133.

Jahoda, C.A., Reynolds, A.J. (2001) Hair follicle dermal sheath cells: unsung participants in wound healing. *Lancet,* **358** (9291), 1445–1448.

Jenkins, G. (2008) The role of proteases in transforming growth factor-beta activation. *International Journal of Biochemistry and Cell Biology,* **40** (6–7), 1068–1078.

Jeong, J.H. (2010) Adipose stem cells and skin repair. *Current Stem Cell Research and Therapy,* **5** (2), 137–140.

Jun, J.I., Lau, L.F. (2010a) The matricellular protein CCN1 induces fibroblast senescence and restricts fibrosis in cutaneous wound healing. *Nature Cell Biology,* **12** (7), 676–685.

Jun, J.I., Lau, L.F. (2010b) Cellular senescence controls fibrosis in wound healing. *Aging,* **2** (9), 627–631.

Kadler, K.E., Hill, A., Canty-Laird, E.G. (2008) Collagen fibrillogenesis: fibronectin, integrins, and minor collagens as organizers and nucleators. *Current Opinion in Cell Biology,* **20** (5), 495–501.

Kähäri, V.M., Larjava, H., Uitto, J. (1991) Differential regulation of extracellular matrix proteoglycan (PG) gene expression. Transforming growth factor-beta 1 up-regulates biglycan (PGI), and versican (large fibroblast PG) but down-regulates decorin (PGII) mRNA levels in human fibroblasts in culture. *Journal of Biological Chemistry,* **266** (16), 10608–10615.

Kähler, C.M., Bellmann, R., Reinisch, N., et al. (1996) Stimulation of human skin fibroblast migration by the neuropeptide secretoneurin. *European Journal of Pharmacology,* **304** (1–3), 135–139.

Kalamajski, S., Oldberg, A. (2010) The role of small leucine–rich proteoglycans in collagen fibrillogenesis. *Matrix Biology,* **29** (4), 248–253.

Kaufman, E., Lamster, I.B. (2000) Analysis of saliva for periodontal diagnosis – a review. *Journal of Clinical Periodontology,* **27** (7), 453–465.

Kessenbrock, K., Plaks, V., Werb, Z. (2010) Matrix metalloproteinases: regulators of the tumor microenvironment. *Cell,* **141** (1), 52–67.

Kirchberg, K., Lange, T.S., Klein, E.C., et al. (1995) Induction of beta 1 integrin synthesis by recombinant platelet-derived growth factor (PDGF-AB) correlates with an enhanced migratory response of human dermal fibroblasts to various extracellular matrix proteins. *Experimental Cell Research,* **220** (1), 29–35.

Kiritsy, C.P., Lynch, A.B., Lynch, S.E. (1993) Role of growth factors in cutaneous wound healing: a review. *Critical Reviews in Oral Biology and Medicine,* **4** (5), 729–760.

Kirmse, R., Otto, H., Ludwig, T. (2011) Interdependency of cell adhesion, force generation and extracellular proteolysis in matrix remodeling. *Journal of Cell Science,* **124** (11), 1857–1866.

Kiss, M., Kemény, L., Gyulai, R., et al. (1999) Effects of the neuropeptides substance P, calcitonin gene–related peptide and alpha-melanocyte-stimulating hormone on the IL-8/IL-8 receptor system in a cultured human keratinocyte cell line and dermal fibroblasts. *Inflammation,* **23** (6), 557–567.

Kohan, M., Muro, A.F., White, E.S., et al. (2010) EDA-containing cellular fibronectin induces fibroblast differentiation through binding to alpha4beta7 integrin receptor and MAPK/Erk 1/2-dependent signaling. *FASEB Journal,* **24** (11), 4503–4512.

Kong, W., Li, S., Longaker, M.T., et al. (2008) Blood-derived small Dot cells reduce scar in wound healing. *Experimental Cell Research,* **314** (7), 1529–1539.

Kong, W., Li, S., Lorenz, H.P. (2010) Germ plasm-like Dot cells maintain their wound regenerative function after in vitro expansion. *Clinical Experimental Pharmacology and Physiology,* **37** (4), e136–144.

Koskela, E., Engstrom, K., Hakelius, M., et al. (2010) Regulation of fibroblast gene expression by keratinocytes in organotypic skin culture provides possible mechanisms for the antifibrotic effect of reepithelialization. *Wound Repair and Regeneration,* **18** (5), 452–459.

Kular, L., Pakradouni, J., Kitabgi, P., et al. (2011) The CCN family: a new class of inflammation modulators? *Biochimie,* **93** (3), 377–388.

Kyriakides, T.R., Maclauchlan, S. (2009) The role of thrombospondins in wound healing, ischemia, and the foreign body reaction. *Journal of Cell Communication and Signaling,* **3** (3–4), 215–225.

Kyriakides, T.R., Tam, J.W., Bornstein, P. (1999) Accelerated wound healing in mice with a disruption of the thrombospondin 2 gene. *Journal of Investigative Dermatology,* **113** (5), 782–787.

Kyriakides, T.R., Wulsin, D., Skokos, E.A., et al. (2009) Mice that lack matrix metalloproteinase-9 display delayed wound healing associated with delayed reepithelization and disordered collagen fibrillogenesis. *Matrix Biology,* **28** (2), 65–73.

Lai, Y., Di Nardo, A., Nakatsuji, T., et al. (2009) Commensal bacteria regulate Toll-like receptor 3-dependent inflammation after skin injury. *Nature Medicine,* **15** (12), 1377–1382.

Larjava, H., Koivisto, L., Häkkinen, L. (2002) Keratinocyte interactions with fibronectin during wound healing. In: *Cell Invasion* (eds Heino, J., Kähäri, V-M.), pp. 42–64. Landes Biosciences, Eurekah.com, Georgetown, Texas, USA.

Larson, B.J., Longaker, M.T., Lorenz, H.P. (2010) Scarless fetal wound healing: a basic science review. *Plastic and Reconstructive Surgery,* **126** (4), 1172–1180.

Lau, K., Paus, R., Tiede, S., et al. (2009) Exploring the role of stem cells in cutaneous wound healing. *Experimental Dermatology,* **18** (11), 921–933.

Leask, A. (2010) Potential therapeutic targets for cardiac fibrosis: TGFbeta, angiotensin, endothelin, CCN2, and PDGF, partners in fibroblast activation. *Circulation Research,* **106** (11), 1675–1680.

Leask, A., Abraham, D.J. (2006) All in the CCN family: essential matricellular signaling modulators emerge from the bunker. *Journal of Cell Science,* **119** (Pt 23), 4803–4810.

Lee, E.Y., Xia, Y., Kim, W.S., et al. (2009) Hypoxia-enhanced wound-healing function of adipose-derived stem cells: increase in stem cell proliferation and up-regulation of VEGF and bFGF. *Wound Repair and Regeneration,* **17** (4), 540–754.

Lee, H., Overall, C.M., McCulloch, C.A., et al. (2006) A critical role for the membrane-type 1 matrix metalloproteinase in collagen phagocytosis. *Molecular Biology of the Cell,* **17** (11), 4812–4826.

Lee, H., Sodek, K.L., Hwang, Q., et al. (2007) Phagocytosis of collagen by fibroblasts and invasive cancer cells is mediated by MT1-MMP. *Biochemical Society Transactions,* **35** (Pt 4), 704–706.

Lee, W., Sodek, J., McCulloch, C.A. (1996) Role of integrins in regulation of collagen phagocytosis by human fibroblasts. *Journal of Cellular Physiology,* **168** (3), 695–704.

Leiss, M., Beckmann, K., Girós, A., et al. (2008) The role of integrin binding sites in fibronectin matrix assembly in vivo. *Current Opinion in Cell Biology,* **20** (5), 502–507.

Lemons, J.M., Feng, X.J., Bennett. B.D., et al. (2010) Quiescent fibroblasts exhibit high metabolic activity. *PLOS Biology,* **8** (10), e1000514.

Levine, J.H., Moses, H.L., Gold, L.I., et al. (1993) Spatial and temporal patterns of immunoreactive transforming growth factor beta 1, beta 2, and beta 3 during excisional wound repair. *American Journal of Pathology,* **143** (2), 368–380.

Li, F., Huang, Q., Chen, J., et al. (2010) Apoptotic cells activate the "phoenix rising" pathway to promote wound healing and tissue regeneration. *Science Signaling,* **3** (110), ra13.

Li, J., Zhang, Y.P., Kirsner, R.S. (2003) Angiogenesis in wound repair: angiogenic growth factors and the extracellular matrix. *Microscopy Research and Technique,* **60** (1), 107–114.

Lim, P.K., Bliss, S.A., Patel, S.A., et al. (2011) Gap junction-mediated import of microRNA from bone marrow stromal cells can elicit cell cycle quiescence in breast cancer cells. *Cancer Research,* **71** (5), 1550–1560.

Lin, C.G., Chen, C.C., Leu, S.J., et al. (2005) Integrin-dependent functions of the angiogenic inducer NOV (CCN3): implication in wound healing. *Journal of Biological Chemistry,* **280** (9), 8229–8237.

Lin, F., Ren, X.D., Doris,. G, et al. (2005) Three-dimensional migration of human adult dermal fibroblasts from collagen lattices into fibrin/fibronectin gels requires syndecan-4 proteoglycan. *Journal of Investigative Dermatology,* **124** (5), 906–913.

Lindblad, W.J. (1998) Perspective article: collagen expression by novel cell populations in the dermal wound environment. *Wound Repair and Regeneration,* **6** (3), 186–193.

Liu, S., Xu, S.W., Blumbach, K., et al. (2010) Expression of integrin beta1 by fibroblasts is required for tissue repair in vivo. *Journal of Cell Science,* **123** (Pt 21), 3674–3682.

Liu, X., Wu, H., Byrne, M., et al. (1997) Type III collagen is crucial for collagen I fibrillogenesis and for normal cardiovascular development. *Proceedings of the National Academy of Sciences USA,* **94** (5), 1852–1856.

Longaker, M.T., Chiu, E.S., Adzick, N.S., et al. (1991) Studies in fetal wound healing. V. A prolonged presence of hyaluronic acid characterizes fetal wound fluid. *Annals of Surgery,* **213** (4), 292–296.

Loo, J.A., Yan, W., Ramachandran, P., et al. (2010) Comparative human salivary and plasma proteomes. *Journal of Dental Research,* **89** (10), 1016–1023.

Loot, M.A., Kenter, S.B., Au, F.L., et al. (2002) Fibroblasts derived from chronic diabetic ulcers differ in their response to stimulation with EGF, IGF-I, bFGF and PDGF-AB compared to controls. *European Journal of Cell Biology,* **81** (3), 153–160.

López, B., González, A., Hermida, N., et al. (2010) Role of lysyl oxidase in myocardial fibrosis: from basic science to clinical aspects. *American Journal of Physiology, Heart and Circulatory Physiology*, **299** (1), H1–9.

Lovvorn, H.N. 3rd, Cass, D.L., Sylvester, K.G., et al. (1998) Hyaluronan receptor expression increases in fetal excisional skin wounds and correlates with fibroplasia. *Journal of Pediatric Surgery,* **33** (7), 1062–1069

Lovvorn, H.N. 3rd, Cheung, D.T., Nimni, M.E., et al. (1999) Relative distribution and crosslinking of collagen distinguish fetal from adult sheep wound repair. *Journal of Pediatric Surgery,* **34** (1), 218–223.

Lygoe, K.A., Wall, I., Stephens, P., et al. (2007) Role of vitronectin and fibronectin receptors in oral mucosal and dermal myofibroblast differentiation. *Biology of the Cell,* **99** (11), 601–614.

Mack, J.A., Feldman, R.J., Itano, N., et al. (2011) Enhanced inflammation and accelerated wound closure following tetraphorbol ester application or full-thickness wounding in mice lacking hyaluronan synthases Has1 and Has3. *Journal of Investigative Dermatology*, 18 August, doi: 10.1038/jid.2011.248. [Epub ahead of print]

Macri, L., Silverstein, D., Clark, R.A. (2007) Growth factor binding to the pericellular matrix and its importance in tissue engineering. *Advanced Drug Delivery Reviews,* **59** (13), 1366–1381.

Madsen, D.H., Engelholm, L.H., Ingvarsen, S., et al. (2007) Extracellular collagenases and the endocytic receptor, urokinase plasminogen activator receptor-associated protein/Endo180, cooperate in fibroblast-mediated collagen degradation. *Journal of Biological Chemistry,* **82** (37), 27037–27045.

Mak, K., Manji, A., Gallant-Behm, C., et al. (2009) Scarless healing of oral mucosa is characterized by faster resolution of inflammation and control of myofibroblast action compared to skin wounds in the red Duroc pig model. *Journal of Dermatological Science,* **5** (3), 168–180.

Manabe, R., Ohe, N., Maeda, T., et al. (1997) Modulation of cell-adhesive activity of fibronectin by the alternatively spliced EDA segment. *Journal of Cell Biology,* **139** (1), 295–307.

Manicone, A.M., McGuire, J.K. (2008) Matrix metalloproteinases as modulators of inflammation. *Seminars in Cell and Developmental Biology,* **19** (1), 34–41.

Margadant, C., Sonnenberg, A. (2010) Integrin-TGF-beta crosstalk in fibrosis, cancer and wound healing. *EMBO Reports,* **11** (2), 97–105.

Martinez-Ferrer, M., Afshar-Sherif, A.R., Uwamariya, C., et al. (2010) Dermal transforming growth factor-beta responsiveness mediates wound contraction and epithelial closure. *American Journal of Pathology,* **176** (1), 98–107.

Marynka-Kalmani, K., Treves, S., Yafee, M., et al. (2010) The lamina propria of adult human oral mucosa harbors a novel stem cell population. *Stem Cells,* **28** (5), 984–995.

McGaw, W.T. (1986) The effect of tension on collagen remodelling by fibroblasts: a stereological ultrastructural study. *Connective Tissue Research,* **14** (3), 229–235.

McKeown, S.T., Barnes, J.J., Hyland, P.L., et al. (2007) Matrix metalloproteinase-3 differences in oral and skin fibroblasts. *Journal of Dental Research,* **86** (5), 457–462.

Meikle, M.C. (2006) The tissue, cellular, and molecular regulation of orthodontic tooth movement: 100 years after Carl Sandstedt. *European Journal of Orthodontics,* **28** (3), 221–240.

Memmo, L.M., McKeown-Longo, P. (1998) The alphavbeta5 integrin functions as an endocytic receptor for vitronectin. *Journal of Cell Science,* **111** (Pt 4), 425–433.

Meran, S., Luo, D.D., Simpson, R., et al. (2011) Hyaluronan facilitates transforming growth factor-β1 dependent proliferation via CD44 and epidermal growth factor-receptor interaction *Journal of Biological Chemistry,* **286** (20), 17618–17630.

Mercer, D.K., Nicol, P.F., Kimbembe, C., et al. (2003) Identification, expression, and tissue distribution of the three rat lysyl hydroxylase isoforms. *Biochemical and Biophysical Research Communications,* **307** (4), 803–809.

Messaritou, G., East, L., Roghi, C., et al. (2009) Membrane type-1 matrix metalloproteinase activity is regulated by the endocytic collagen receptor Endo180. *Journal of Cell Science,* **122** (Pt 22), 4042–4048.

Micera, A., Vigneti, E., Pickholtz, D., et al. (2001) Nerve growth factor displays stimulatory effects on human skin and lung fibroblasts, demonstrating a direct role for this factor in tissue repair. *Proceedings of the National Academy of Sciences USA,* **98** (11), 6162–6167.

Mirastschijski, U., Haaksma, C.J., Tomasek, J.J., et al. (2004) Matrix metalloproteinase inhibitor GM 6001 attenuates keratinocyte migration, contraction and myofibroblast formation in skin wounds. *Experimental Cell Research,* **299** (2), 465–475.

Mirastschijski, U., Schnabel, R., Claes, J., et al. (2010) Matrix metalloproteinase inhibition delays wound healing and blocks the latent transforming growth factor-beta1-promoted myofibroblast formation and function. *Wound Repair and Regeneration,* **18** (2), 223–234.

Moorby, C.D., Gherardi, E. (1999) Expression of a Cx43 deletion mutant in 3T3 A31 fibroblasts prevents PDGF-induced inhibition of cell communication and suppresses cell growth. *Experimental Cell Research,* **249** (2), 367–376.

Mori, R., Power, K.T., Wang, C.M., et al. (2006) Acute downregulation of connexin43 at wound sites leads to a reduced inflammatory response, enhanced keratinocyte proliferation and wound fibroblast migration. *Journal of Cell Science,* **119** (Pt 24), 5193–5203.

Moyer, K.E., Saggers, G.C., Allison, G.M., et al. (2002) Effects of interleukin-8 on granulation tissue maturation. *Journal of Cellular Physiology,* **193** (2), 173–179.

Murphy, G., Nagase, H. (2011) Localizing matrix metalloproteinase activities in the pericellular environment. *FEBS Journal,* **278** (1), 2–15.

Namazi, M.R., Fallahzadeh, M.K., Schwartz, R.A. (2011) Strategies for prevention of scars: what can we learn from fetal skin? *International Journal of Dermatology,* **50** (1), 85–93.

Nishimura, F., Terranova, V.P. (1996) Comparative study of the chemotactic responses of periodontal ligament cells and gingival fibroblasts to polypeptide growth factors. *Journal of Dental Research,* **75** (4), 986–992.

Nolte, S.V., Xu, W., Rennekampff, H.O., et al. (2008) Diversity of fibroblasts – a review on implications for skin tissue engineering. *Cells, Tissues, Organs,* **187** (3), 165–176.

Noszczyk, B.H., Klein, E., Holtkoetter, O., et al. (2002) Integrin expression in the dermis during scar formation in humans. *Experimental Dermatology,* **11** (4), 311–318.

Novo, E., Parola, M. (2008) Redox mechanisms in hepatic chronic wound healing and fibrogenesis. *Fibrogenesis and Tissue Repair,* **1** (1), 5.

Occleston, N.L., O'Kane, S., Goldspink, N., et al. (2008) New therapeutics for the prevention and reduction of scarring. *Drug Discovery Today,* **13** (21–22), 973–981.

Olaso, E., Lin, H.C., Wang, L.H., et al. (2011) Impaired dermal wound healing in discoidin domain receptor 2-deficient mice associated with defective extracellular matrix remodeling. *Fibrogenesis and Tissue Repair,* **4** (1), 5.

Oliver, R.F. (1979) An autoradiographic study of 3H-thymidine incorporation and distribution in the dermis of healing skin incisions in the pig. *British Journal of Experimental Pathology,* **60** (1), 65–71.

Pagano, M., Reboud-Ravaux, M. (2011) Cryptic activities of fibronectin fragments, particularly cryptic proteases. *Frontiers in Bioscience,* **16**, 698–706.

Pavasant, P., Yongchaitrakul, T. (2011) Role of mechanical stress on the function of periodontal ligament cells. *Periodontology,* **56** (1), 154–165.

Pedlar, J. (1984) Biochemistry of glycosaminoglycans in the skin and oral mucosa of the rat. *Archives of Oral Biology,* **29** (8), 591–597.

Peranteau, W.H., Zhang, L., Muvarak, N., et al. (2008) IL-10 overexpression decreases inflammatory mediators and promotes regenerative healing in an adult model of scar formation. *Journal of Investigative Dermatology,* **128** (7), 1852–1860.

Pierce, G.F., Vande Berg, J., Rudolph, R., et al. (1999) Platelet-derived growth factor-BB and transforming growth factor beta 1 selectively modulate glycosaminoglycans, collagen, and myofibroblasts in excisional wounds. *American Journal of Pathology,* **138** (3), 629–646.

Provenzano, P.P., Keely, P.J. (2011) Mechanical signaling through the cytoskeleton regulates cell proliferation by coordinated focal adhesion and Rho GTPase signaling. *Journal of Cell Science,* **124** (Pt 8), 1195–1205.

Quaggin, S.E., Kapus, A. (2011) Scar wars: mapping the fate of epithelial-mesenchymal-myofibroblast transition. *Kidney International,* Mar 23. [Epub ahead of print]

Quan, T.E., Cowper, S., Wu, S.P., et al. (2004) Circulating fibrocytes: collagen-secreting cells of the peripheral blood. *International Journal of Biochemistry and Cell Biology,* **36** (4), 598–606.

Quintanilla-Dieck, M.J., Codriansky, K., Keady, M., et al. (2009) Expression and regulation of cathepsin K in skin fibroblasts. *Experimental Dermatology,* **18** (7), 596–602.

Ravanti, L., Kähäri, V.M. (2000) Matrix metalloproteinases in wound repair (review). *International Journal of Molecular Medicine,* **6** (4), 391–407.

Ravanti, L., Häkkinen, L., Larjava, H., et al. (1999) Transforming growth factor-beta induces collagenase-3 expression by human gingival fibroblasts via p38 mitogen-activated protein kinase. *Journal of Biological Chemistry,* **274** (52), 37292–37300.

Reed, M.J., Puolakkainen, P., Lane, T.F., et al. (1993) Differential expression of SPARC and thrombospondin 1 in wound repair: immunolocalization and in situ hybridization. *Journal of Histochemistry and Cytochemistry,* **41** (10), 1467–1477.

Reish, R.G., Zuhaili, B., Bergmann, J., et al. (2009) Modulation of scarring in a liquid environment in the Yorkshire pig. *Wound Repair and Regeneration,* **17** (6), 806–816.

Rentz, T.J., Poobalarahi, F., Bornstein, P., et al. (2007) SPARC regulates processing of procollagen I and collagen fibrillogenesis in dermal fibroblasts. *Journal of Biological Chemistry*, **282** (30), 22062–22071.

Ricard-Blum, S., Ballut, L. (2011) Matricryptins derived from collagens and proteoglycans. *Frontiers in Bioscience,* **16**, 674–697.

Rittié, L., Perbal, B., Castellot, J.J. Jr, et al. (2011) Spatial–temporal modulation of CCN proteins during wound healing in human skin in vivo. *Journal of Cell Communication and Signaling,* **5** (1), 69–80.

Roberts, C.J., Birkenmeier, T.M., McQuillan, J.J., et al. (1988) Transforming growth factor beta stimulates the expression of fibronectin and of both subunits of the human fibronectin receptor by cultured human lung fibroblasts. *Journal of Biological Chemistry,* **263** (10), 4586–4592.

Ronca, R., Sozzani, S., Presta, M., et al. (2009) Delivering cytokines at tumor site: The immunocytokine-conjugated anti-EDB-fibronectin antibody case. *Immunobiology,* **214** (9–10), 800–810

Roosterman, D., Goerge, T., Schneider, S.W., et al. (2006) Neuronal control of skin function: the skin as a neuroimmunoendocrine organ. *Physiological Reviews,* **86** (4), 1309–1379.

Roupé, K.M., Nybo, M., Sjöbring, U., et al. (2010) Injury is a major inducer of epidermal innate immune responses during wound healing. *Journal of Investigative Dermatology,* **130** (4), 1167–1177.

Rozario, T., DeSimone, DW. (2010) The extracellular matrix in development and morphogenesis: a dynamic view. *Developmental Biology,* **341** (1), 126–140.

Rünger, T.M., Quintanilla-Dieck, M.J., Bhawan, J. (2007) Role of cathepsin K in the turnover of the dermal extracellular matrix during scar formation. *Journal of Investigative Dermatology,* **127** (2), 293–297.

Sabeh, F., Li, X.Y., Saunders, T.L., et al. (2009a) Secreted versus membrane-anchored collagenases: relative roles in fibroblast-dependent collagenolysis and invasion. *Journal of Biological Chemistry,* **284** (34), 23001–23011.

Sabeh, F., Shimizu-Hirota, R., Weiss, S.J. (2009b) Protease-dependent versus -independent cancer cell invasion programs: three-dimensional amoeboid movement revisited. *Journal of Cell Biology,* **185** (1), 11–19.

Saito, Y., Imazeki, H., Miura, S., et al. (2007) A peptide derived from tenascin-C induces beta1 integrin activation through syndecan-4. *Journal of Biological Chemistry,* **282** (48), 34929–34937.

Sasaki, M., Abe, R., Fujita, Y., et al. (2008) Mesenchymal stem cells are recruited into wounded skin and contribute to wound repair by transdifferentiation into multiple skin cell type. *Journal of Immunology,* **180** (4), 2581–2587.

Sato, Y., Ohshima, T., Kondo, T. (1999) Regulatory role of endogenous interleukin-10 in cutaneous inflammatory response of murine wound healing. *Biochemical and Biophysical Research Communications,* **265** (1), 194–199.

Scarpa, R.C., Carraway, R.E., Cochrane, D.E. (2005) Insulin-like growth factor (IGF) induced proliferation of human lung fibroblasts is enhanced by neurotensin. *Peptides,* **26** (11), 2201–2210.

Schaefer, L., Iozzo, R.V. (2008) Biological functions of the small leucine-rich proteoglycans: from genetics to signal transduction. *Journal of Biological Chemistry,* **283** (31), 21305–21309.

Schäfer, M., Werner, S. (2008) Oxidative stress in normal and impaired wound repair. *Pharmacological Research,* **58** (2), 165–171.

Schmuth, M., Watson, R.E., Deplewski, D., et al. (2007) Nuclear hormone receptors in human skin. *Hormone and Metabolic Research,* **39** (2), 96–105.

Schneider, I.C., Haugh, J.M. (2006) Mechanisms of gradient sensing and chemotaxis: conserved pathways, diverse regulation. *Cell Cycle,* **5** (11), 1130–1134.

Schneller, M., Vuori, K., Ruoslahti, E. (1997) Alphavbeta3 integrin associates with activated insulin and PDGFbeta receptors and potentiates the biological activity of PDGF. *EMBO Journal*, **16** (18), 5600–5607.

Schor, S.L., Ellis, I., Irwin C.R., et al. (1996) Subpopulations of fetal-like gingival fibroblasts: characterisation and potential significance for wound healing and the progression of periodontal disease. *Oral Diseases,* **2** (2), 155–166.

Schrementi, M.E., Ferreira, A.M., Zender, C., et al. (2008) Site-specific production of TGF-beta in oral mucosal and cutaneous wounds. *Wound Repair and Regeneration,* **16** (1), 80–86.

Schrimpf, C., Duffield, J.S. (2011) Mechanisms of fibrosis: the role of the pericyte. *Current Opinion in Nephrology and Hypertension,* **20** (3), 297–305.

Schultz, G.S., Wysocki, A. (2009) Interactions between extracellular matrix and growth factors in wound healing. *Wound Repair and Regeneration,* **17** (2), 153–162.

Schultz, G.S., Davidson, J.M., Kirsner, R.S., et al. (2011) Dynamic reciprocity in the wound microenvironment. *Wound Repair and Regeneration,* **19** (2), 134–148.

Schwartz, M.A. (2010) Integrins and extracellular matrix in mechanotransduction. *Cold Spring Harbor Perspectives in Biology,* **2** (12), a005066.

Sciubba, J.J., Waterhouse, J.P., Meyer, J. (1978) A fine structural comparison of the healing of incisional wounds of mucosa and skin. *Journal of Oral Pathology,* **7** (4), 214–227.

Sellheyer, K., Krahl, D. (2010) Skin mesenchymal stem cells: prospects for clinical dermatology. *Journal of the American Academy of Dermatology,* **63** (5), 859–865.

Sen, C.K., Roy, S. (2010) Oxygenation state as a driver of myofibroblast differentiation and wound contraction: hypoxia impairs wound closure. *Journal of Investigative Dermatology,* **130** (12), 2701–2703.

Serhan, C.N. (2011) The resolution of inflammation: the devil in the flask and in the details. *FASEB Journal,* **25**, 1441–1448.

Serini, G., Bochaton-Piallat, M.L., Ropraz, P., et al. (1998) The fibronectin domain ED-A is crucial for myofibroblastic phenotype induction by transforming growth factor-beta1. *Journal of Cell Biology,* **142** (3), 873–881.

Shannon, D.B., McKeown, S.T., Lundy, F.T., et al. (2006) Phenotypic differences between oral and skin fibroblasts in wound contraction and growth factor expression. *Wound Repair and Regeneration,* **14** (2), 172–178.

Shi, F., Harman, J., Fujiwara, K., et al. (2010) Collagen I matrix turnover is regulated by fibronectin polymerization. *American Journal of Physiology Cell Physiology,* **298** (5), C1265–1275.

Shiota, N., Nishikori, Y., Kakizoe, E., et al. (2010) Pathophysiological role of skin mast cells in wound healing after scald injury: study with mast cell-deficient W/W(V) mice. *International Archives of Allergy and Immunology,* **151** (1), 80–88.

Shore, R.C., Berkovitz, B.K., Moxham, B.J. (1981) Intercellular contacts between fibroblasts in the periodontal connective tissues of the rat. *Journal of Anatomy,* **133** (Pt 1), 67–76.

Sible, J.C., Rettig, W.J., Eriksson, E., et al. (1995) Gene expression of tenascin is altered in normal scars and keloids. *Wound Repair and Regeneration,* **3** (1), 37–48.

Simpson, R.M., Meran, S., Thomas, D., et al. (2009) Age-related changes in pericellular hyaluronan organization leads to impaired dermal fibroblast to myofibroblast differentiation. *American Journal of Pathology,* **175** (5), 1915–1928.

Singer, A.J., Clark, R.A. (1999) Cutaneous wound healing. *New England Journal of Medicine,* **341** (10), 738–746.

Singh, P., Reimer, C.L., Peters, J.H, et al. (2004) The spatial and temporal expression patterns of integrin alpha9beta1 and one of its ligands, the EIIIA segment of fibronectin, in cutaneous wound healing. *Journal of Investigative Dermatology,* **123** (6), 1176–1181.

Singh, P., Carraher, C., Schwarzbauer, J.E. (2010) Assembly of fibronectin extracellular matrix. *Annual Reviews in Cell and Developmental Biology,* **26**, 397–419.

Slemp, A.E., Kirschner, R.E. (2006) Keloids and scars: a review of keloids and scars, their pathogenesis, risk factors, and management. *Current Opinion in Pediatrics,* **18** (4), 396–402.

Slominski, A., Zbytek, B., Pisarchik, A., et al. (2006) CRH functions as a growth factor/cytokine in the skin. *Journal of Cellular Physiology,* **206** (3), 780–791.

Solomon, D., Saurat, J.H., Media, P. (1988) Cell-to-cell communication within intact human skin. *Journal of Clinical Investigation,* **82** (1), 248–254.

Sorrell, J.M., Caplan, A.I. (2004) Fibroblast heterogeneity: more than skin deep. *Journal of Cell Science,* **117** (Pt 5), 667–675.

Sorrell, J.M., Caplan, A.I. (2009) Fibroblasts-a diverse population at the center of it all. *International Review of Cell and Molecular Biology,* **276**, 161–214.

Sorrell, J.M., Caplan, A.I. (2010) Topical delivery of mesenchymal stem cells and their function in wounds. *Stem Cell Research and Therapy,* **1** (4), 30.

Steiling, H., Munz, B., Werner, S., et al. (1999) Different types of ROS-scavenging enzymes are expressed during cutaneous wound repair. *Experimental Cell Research,* **247** (2), 484–494.

Steinhoff, M., Ständer, S., Seeliger, S., et al. (2003) Modern aspects of cutaneous neurogenic inflammation. *Archives of Dermatology,* **139** (11), 1479–1488.

Stephens, P., Genever, P. (2007) Non-epithelial oral mucosal progenitor cell populations. *Oral Diseases* **13** (1), 1–10.

Stephens, P., Davies, K.J., al-Khateeb, T., et al. (1996) A comparison of the ability of intra-oral and extra-oral fibroblasts to stimulate extracellular matrix reorganization in a model of wound contraction. *Journal of Dental Research,* **75** (6), 1358–1364.

Stephens, P., Davies, K.J., Occleston, N., et al. (2001a) Skin and oral fibroblasts exhibit phenotypic differences in extracellular matrix reorganization and matrix metalloproteinase activity. *British Journal of Dermatology,* **144** (2), 229–237.

Stephens, P., Hiscox, S., Cook, H., et al. (2001b) Phenotypic variation in the production of bioactive hepatocyte growth factor/scatter factor by oral mucosal and skin fibroblasts. *Wound Repair and Regeneration,* **9** (1), 34–43.

Stocum, D.L. (2006) *Regenerative Biology and Medicine*. Academic Press, Burlington, Maryland, USA.

Su, M., Borke, J.L., Donahue, H.J., et al. (1997) Expression of connexin 43 in rat mandibular bone and periodontal ligament (PDL) cells during experimental tooth movement. *Journal of Dental Research,* **76** (7), 1357–1366.

Sullivan, M.M., Puolakkainen, P.A., Barker, T.H., et al. (2008) Altered tissue repair in hevin-null mice: inhibition of fibroblast migration by a matricellular SPARC homolog. *Wound Repair and Regeneration,* **16** (2), 310–319.

Swindle, C.S., Tran, K.T., Johnson, T.D., et al. (2001) Epidermal growth factor (EGF)-like repeats of human tenascin-C as ligands for EGF receptor. *Journal of Cell Biology,* **154** (2), 459–468.

Szauter, K.M., Cao, T., Boyd, C.D., et al. (2005) Lysyl oxidase in development, aging and pathologies of the skin. *Pathologie-Biologie,* **53** (7), 448–456.

Szpaderska, A.M., Zuckerman, J.D., DiPietro, L.A. (2003) Differential injury responses in oral mucosal and cutaneous wounds. *Journal of Dental Research,* **82** (8), 621–626.

Szpaderska, A.M., Walsh, C.G., Steinberg, M.J., et al. (2005) Distinct patterns of angiogenesis in oral and skin wounds. *Journal of Dental Research,* **84** (4), 309–314.

Tandara, A.A., Mustoe, T.A. (2004) Oxygen in wound healing – more than a nutrient. *World Journal of Surgery,* **28** (3), 294–300.

Tingström, A., Heldin, C.H., Rubin, K. (1992) Regulation of fibroblast-mediated collagen gel contraction by platelet-derived growth factor, interleukin-1 alpha and transforming growth factor-beta 1. *Journal of Cell Science,* **102** (Pt 2), 315–322.

To, W.S., Midwood, K.S. (2011) Identification of novel and distinct binding sites within tenascin-C for soluble and fibrillar fibronectin. *Journal of Biological Chemistry,* **286** (17), 14881–14891.

Tolg, C., Hamilton, S.R., Nakrieko, K.A., et al. (2006) Rhamm-/- fibroblasts are defective in CD44-mediated ERK1,2 motogenic signaling, leading to defective skin wound repair. *Journal of Cell Biology,* **175** (6), 1017–1028.

Tomasek, J.J., Gabbiani, G., Hinz, B., et al. (2002) Myofibroblasts and mechano-regulation of connective tissue remodelling. *Nature Reviews Molecular Cell Biology,* **3** (5), 349–363.

Toriseva, M., Kähäri, V.M. (2009) Proteinases in cutaneous wound healing. *Cellular and Molecular Life Sciences,* **66** (2), 203–224.

Trackman, P.C., Kantarci, A. (2004) Connective tissue metabolism and gingival overgrowth. *Critical Reviews in Oral Biology and Medicine,* **15** (3), 165–175.

Tran, K.T., Lamb, P., Deng, J.S. (2005) Matrikines and matricryptins: Implications for cutaneous cancers and skin repair. *Journal of Dermatological Science,* **40** (1), 11–20.

Trebaul, A., Chan, E.K., Midwood, K.S. (2007) Regulation of fibroblast migration by tenascin-C. *Biochemical Society Transactions,* **35** (Pt 4), 695–697.

Ulrich, M.M., Verkerk, M., Reijnen, L., et al. (2007) Expression profile of proteins involved in scar formation in the healing process of full-thickness excisional wounds in the porcine model. *Wound Repair and Regeneration,* **15** (4), 482–490.

van Beurden, H.E., Von den Hoff, J.W., Torensma, R., et al. (2005) Myofibroblasts in palatal wound healing: prospects for the reduction of wound contraction after cleft palate repair. *Journal of Dental Research,* **84** (10), 871–880.

van Beurden, H.E., Snoek, P.A., Hoff, J.W., et al. (2006) In vitro migration and adhesion of fibroblasts from different phases of palatal wound healing. *Wound Repair and Regeneration,* **14** (1), 66–71.

van den Bogaerdt, A.J., van der Veen, V.C., van Zuijlen, P.P., et al. (2009) Collagen cross-linking by adipose-derived mesenchymal stromal cells and scar-derived mesenchymal cells: are mesenchymal stromal cells involved in scar formation? *Wound Repair and Regeneration,* **17** (4), 548–558.

van Loon, L.A., Krieg, S.R., Davidson, C.L., et al. (1989) Quantification and distribution of lymphocyte subsets and Langerhans cells in normal human oral mucosa and skin. *Journal of Oral Pathology and Medicine,* **18** (4), 197–201.

Veevers-Lowe, J., Ball, S.G., Shuttleworth, A., et al. (2011) Mesenchymal stem cell migration is regulated by fibronectin through α5β1-integrin-mediated activation of PDGFR-{beta} and potentiation of growth factor signals. *Journal of Cell Science,* **124** (Pt 8), 1288–1300.

Verderio, E.A., Johnson, T., Griffin, M. (2004) Tissue transglutaminase in normal and abnormal wound healing: review article. *Amino Acids,* **26** (4), 387–404.

Vial, C., Gutierrez, J., Santander, C., et al. (2011) Decorin interacts with CTGF/CCN2 through LRR12 inhibiting its biological activity. *Journal of Biological Chemistry,* Mar 23. [Epub ahead of print]

Vogel, W.F., Abdulhussein, R., Ford, C.E. (2006) Sensing extracellular matrix: an update on discoidin domain receptor function. *Cellular Signaling,* **18** (8), 1108–1116.

Volk, S.W., Wang, Y., Mauldin, E.A., et al. (2011) Diminished type III collagen promotes myofibroblast differentiation and increases scar deposition in cutaneous wound healing. *Cells, Tissues, Organs,* Jan 19. [Epub ahead of print]

Waddington, S.N., Crossley, R., Sheard, V., et al. (2010) Gene delivery of a mutant TGFβ3 reduces markers of scar tissue formation after cutaneous wounding. *Molecular Therapy,* **18** (12), 2104–2111.

Wang, J., Dodd, C., Shankowsky, H.A., et al. (2008) Deep dermal fibroblasts contribute to hypertrophic scarring. *Laboratory Investigation,* **88** (12), 1278–1290.

Webber, J., Meran, S., Steadman, R., et al. (2009) Hyaluronan orchestrates transforming growth factor-beta1-dependent maintenance of myofibroblast phenotype. *Journal of Biological Chemistry,* **284** (14), 9083–9092.

Werner, S., Grose, R. (2003) Regulation of wound healing by growth factors and cytokines. *Physiological Reviews,* **83** (3), 835–780.

Werner, S., Krieg, T., Smola, H. (2007) Keratinocyte-fibroblast interactions in wound healing. *Journal of Investigative Dermatology,* **127** (5), 998–1008.

Whitby, D.J., Longaker, M.T., Harrison, M.R., et al. (1991) Rapid epithelialisation of fetal wounds is associated with the early deposition of tenascin. *Journal of Cell Science,* **99** (Pt 3), 583–586.

Widera, D., Zander, C., Heidbreder, M., et al. (2009) Adult palatum as a novel source of neural crest-related stem cells. *Stem Cells,* **27** (8), 1899–1910.

Wight, T.N., Potter-Perigo, S. (2011) The extracellular matrix: an active or passive player in fibrosis. *American Journal of Physiology Gastrointestinal and Liver Physiology,* Apr 21. [Epub ahead of print]

Wipff, P.J., Hinz, B. (2008) Integrins and the activation of latent transforming growth factor beta1 – an intimate relationship. *European Journal of Cell Biology,* **87** (8–9), 601–615.

Wolf, M., Albrecht, S., Märki, C. (2008) Proteolytic processing of chemokines: implications in physiological and pathological conditions. *International Journal of Biochemistry and Cell Biology,* **40** (6–7), 1185–1198.

Wolfram, D., Tzankov, A., Pülzl, P., et al. (2009) Hypertrophic scars and keloids – a review of their pathophysiology, risk factors, and therapeutic management. *Dermatological Surgery,* **35** (2), 171–181.

Wong, J.W., Gallant-Behm, C., Wiebe, C., et al. (2009) Wound healing in oral mucosa results in reduced scar formation as compared with skin: evidence from the red Duroc pig model and humans. *Wound Repair and Regeneration,* **17** (5), 717–729.

Wright, C.S., van Steensel, M.A., Hodgins, M.B., et al. (2009) Connexin mimetic peptides improve cell migration rates of human epidermal keratinocytes and dermal fibroblasts in vitro. *Wound Repair and Regeneration,* **17** (2), 240–249

Wu, Y., Zhao, R.C., Tredget, E.E. (2010) Concise review: bone marrow-derived stem/progenitor cells in cutaneous repair and regeneration. *Stem Cells,* **28** (5), 905–915.

Yan, C., Grimm, W.A., Garner, W.L., et al. (2010) Epithelial to mesenchymal transition in human skin wound healing is induced by tumor necrosis factor-alpha through bone morphogenic protein-2. *American Journal of Pathology,* **176** (5), 2247–2258.

Yang, J., Tyler, L.W., Donoff, R.B., et al. (1996) Salivary EGF regulates eosinophil-derived TGF-alpha expression in hamster oral wounds. *American Journal of Physiology,* **270** (1 Pt 1), G191–202.

Yang, L., Qiu, C.X., Ludlow, A., et al. (1999) Active transforming growth factor-beta in wound repair: determination using a new assay. *American Journal of Pathology,* **154** (1), 105–111.

Yang, L., Scott, P.G., Dodd, C., et al. (2005) Identification of fibrocytes in postburn hypertrophic scar. *Wound Repair and Regeneration,* **13** (4), 398–404.

Yates, C.C., Whaley, D., Kulasekeran, P., et al. (2007) Delayed and deficient dermal maturation in mice lacking the CXCR3 ELR-negative CXC chemokine receptor. *American Journal of Pathology,* **171** (2), 484–495.

Zhang, Q.Z., Su, W.R., Shi, S.H., et al. (2010) Human gingiva-derived mesenchymal stem cells elicit polarization of m2 macrophages and enhance cutaneous wound healing. *Stem Cells,* **28** (10), 1856–1868.

Zheng, Z., Nguyen, C., Zhang, X., et al. (2011) Delayed wound closure in fibromodulin-deficient mice is associated with increased TGF-β3 signaling. *Journal of Investigative Dermatology,* **131** (3), 769–778.

Zhou, H.M., Wang, J., Elliott, C., et al. (2010) Spatiotemporal expression of periostin during skin development and incisional wound healing: lessons for human fibrotic scar formation. *Journal of Cell Communication and Signaling,* **4** (2), 99–107.

Zhu, Y.K., Liu, X.D., Sköld, M.C., et al. (2001) Cytokine inhibition of fibroblast-induced gel contraction is mediated by PGE(2) and NO acting through separate parallel pathways. *American Journal of Respiratory Cell and Molecular Biology,* **25** (2), 245–253.

Ziche, M., Morbidelli, L., Pacini, M., et al. (1990) NK1-receptors mediate the proliferative response of human fibroblasts to tachykinins. *British Journal of Pharmacology,* **100** (1), 11–14.

Zouboulis, C.C., Adjaye, J., Akamatsu, H., et al. (2008) Human skin stem cells and the ageing process. *Experimental Gerentology,* **43** (11), 986–997.

7 Angiogenesis and Wound Healing: Basic Discoveries, Clinical Implications and Therapeutic Opportunities

Peter J. Polverini

University of Michigan, School of Dentistry, 1011 N. University, Ann Arbor, MI, USA

INTRODUCTION

The ability to restore injured tissues to an optimal state of function and health requires the participation of a highly orchestrated series of cellular and molecular events. Because of the increased metabolic demand that accompanies wound healing, a variety of nutrients, inflammatory cells, cytokines, chemokines and matrix molecules must be rapidly transported to and efficiently deployed throughout the wound site. There is perhaps no better or more efficient means of delivery than through the countless tributaries of new blood vessels that define the angiogenic response. This chapter describes studies that revealed some of the earliest mechanistic insights into angiogenesis. The cellular and molecular processes that coordinate angiogenesis will be described in some detail along with a description of some of the more recently identified regulatory molecules and signaling networks that have been implicated in the angiogenic response.

It is well established that an aberrant angiogenic response contributes to the pathogenesis of a number of diseases and can dramatically influence the course of wound healing. The consequences of a dysregulated angiogenic response and its role in the pathogenesis of an aberrant wound healing in diabetes mellitus will be discussed. Lastly, the chapter highlights the potential for new cellular, protein and tissue engineering strategies in the treatment of angiogenesis-dependent disorders.

HOW BLOOD VESSELS DEVELOP

Angiogenesis is among the most fundamental of physiological processes (Polverini 1995; Carmeliet 2000, 2003) and is central to how tissues respond to injury (Singer and Clark 1999; Diegelmann and Evans 2004; Goldman 2004; Bauer et al. 2005; Martin and Leibovich 2005; Gurtner et al. 2008). Endothelial cells, the cells that comprise the innermost lining of all blood vessels, are relatively quiescent cells. The average turnover time for vascular endothelium is generally measured in years (Engerman et al. 1967; Denekamp 1984; Tannock and Hayashi 1972). However, when endothelial cells are exposed to physiological

Oral Wound Healing: Cell Biology and Clinical Management, First Edition. Edited by Hannu Larjava.

or pathologic stimuli they rapidly enter the cell cycle, where their growth rate approaches that of some bone marrow cell populations and may exceed the replicative capacity of some tumor cells (Folkman 1985a, 1985b). Despite the dramatic growth response associated with physiologic angiogenesis, this process is transient and strictly limited in time and space (Folkman 1985a, 1985b; Polverini 1995; Carmeliet 2003). This is particularly true for cutaneous wounds where, once the heighten metabolic demands of the healing tissue have been met, the rich network of blood vessels that comprises granulation tissue rapidly regresses, returning the vascular bed to pre-injury levels (Singer and Clark 1999; Eming et al. 2007; Gurtner et al. 2008). To put this process into a proper context it is first important to understand how new blood vessels form in adult tissues.

New capillary blood vessels develop in three ways: by sprouting from pre-existing capillary vessels; by forming new blood vessels de novo through the incorporation of bone marrow derived endothelial precursor cells (EPCs) (Carmeliet 2000, 2003; Phelps and Garcia 2009); and, as has been recently shown, by incorporating circulating monocytes that have transdifferentiated into endothelial cells (Kim et al. 2009).

In sprouting angiogenesis, the advancing tip of migrating endothelial cells initiates sprouting by first degrading the basement membrane that surrounds the activated endothelial cell and laying down a provisional extracellular matrix. Distal to the advancing edge of migrating endothelial cells, a wave of proliferating endothelial cells extends the incipient new vessels where they eventually connect with adjacent vessels (Polverini 1995; Carmeliet 2000). The nascent blood vessels develop lumens and go on to form transluminal pillars with neighboring vessels though a process known as intussusception (Djonov et al. 2003; Makanya et al. 2009). As the network of new blood vessels mature they are stabilized by the apposition of pericytes and smooth muscle cells (Carmeliet 2003; Djonov et al. 2003; Makanya et al. 2009). This process is driven by a complex network of growth factors, chemokines and proteolytic enzymes that work to coordinate and refine the branching process and stabilize the new microvascular network (Eming et al. 2007; Bicknell and Harris 2004; Adams and Alitalo 2007). All of this is tempered by cell, matrix and blood derived inhibitors that work to ensure a stable supply of new blood vessels and when called upon can virtually bring the angiogenic response to a standstill by halting endothelial proliferation and migration and inducing endothelial cell apoptosis (Ribatti 2009; Nyberg et al. 2005).

Vasculogenesis is a process in which new blood vessels develop from EPCs that originate in the bone marrow and find their way into the circulation (Rafii and Lyden 2003; Asahara and Kawamoto 2004). These precursor endothelial cells are recruited to sites of active angiogenesis where they differentiate into mature endothelial cells (Carmeliet 2003). Once thought to be a process restricted to embryonic development, it is now known to play a role, albeit controversial, in adult angiogenic responses (Purhonen et al. 2008). Asahara and colleagues initially identified EPCs by isolating and culturing mononuclear blood cells from human peripheral blood using magnetic beads against CD34, an endothelial cell surface antigen (Asahara and Kawamoto 2004). Adult vasculogenesis continues to be an area of intense controversy. The extent to which EPCs are incorporated into angiogenic vessels and contribute significantly to adult neovascular responses remains to be determined. EPCs secrete a number of proangiogenic mediators and thus may play a key role in promoting angiogenesis by stimulating endothelial proliferation and migration as well as helping to direct the homing of bone marrow and circulating EPCs to sites of angiogenesis (Rafii and Lyden 2003; Asahara and Kawamoto 2004). More germane to this review, Suh et al. (2005) showed that EPCs introduced into wounds can accelerate healing by promoting the influx of angiogenic macrophages. Galiano and colleagues (2004) showed that when vascular endothelial growth factor (VEGF) was applied topically to wounds in diabetic mice, it accelerated wound healing in part by mobilizing EPCs to the wound site.

More recently, using GFP-expressing transgenic mice parabiosed with non-GFP mice, Kim and colleagues (2009) demonstrated that following dermal wounding the majority of GFP-positive cells populating angiogenic vessels also expressed F4/80, a well-known macrophage marker, suggesting that the principal cell types homing to angiogenic sites were circulating monocytes. This work confirmed earlier observations by Urbich et al. (2003) and Rehman et al. (2003) who were among the first to implicate monocytes/macrophages as putative angiogenic endothelial precursor cells.

EARLY MECHANISTIC INSIGHTS INTO THE ANGIOGENIC RESPONSE: FROM SOLID TUMORS TO CHRONIC INFLAMMATION AND WOUND HEALING

Given what we know today about the complexity of the angiogenic response it is remarkable how, despite the lack of experimental sophistication, much of what we know about the mechanisms and mediators that underlie the process of new blood vessel growth was proposed more than 70 years ago (Clark and Clark 1932; Clark 1939; Ide et al. 1939; Algire 1943a, 1943b; Algire et al. 1945).

Angiogenesis is a distinctive feature of wound repair (Singer and Clark 1999; Bauer et al. 2005; Martin and Leibovich 2005; Eming et al. 2007). Early studies employing wound chambers revealed that new blood vessels grew in a precisely organized manner in an environment rich in proteins and cells (Clark 1939; Algire 1943a, 1943b).

Although angiogenesis was known to be a feature of inflammation and wound repair for many years, most of the early studies on wound angiogenesis were largely observational in nature. However, in the late 1960s and early 1970s great strides were made in advancing our understanding of angiogenic response. Perhaps no single individual was more influential than Judah Folkman (Ribatti 2008). Virtually everything we know today about the angiogenic response can be traced to the visionary studies of Folkman and a handful of predecessors and contemporaries. His pioneering studies in tumor angiogenesis began in the late 1960s and are regarded today as some of the most seminal work in this field (Gimbrone et al. 1969, 1972, 1973, 1974a, 1973b; Folkman et al. 1971). Despite early inroads into defining the mechanism and mediators of tumor angiogenesis, comparable data on physiological angiogenesis, in particular chronic inflammation and would healing, were lacking (Polverini et al. 1977).

Much of the early work on endothelial proliferation and angiogenesis in chronic inflammation provided only a glimpse into potential mechanisms (Willms-Kretschmer et al. 1967; Anderson et al. 1975; Courtade et al. 1975; Sidky and Auerbach 1975; Dvorak et al. 1976; Sholley et al. 1977). A variety of agents were implicated in mediating angiogenesis, including vasoactive mediators of inflammation generated at the site of injury or, alternatively, by cytotoxic factors released from inflammatory cells (Sholley et al. 1977). It was also reported that various inflammatory cells that populated the wound site were the source of 'angiogenic factors' (Sidky and Auerbach 1975; Polverini et al. 1977, 1978; Sholley et al. 1977).

For example, Sidky and Auerbach reported that capillary proliferation occurred in local graft-versus-host reaction in the skin of mice, suggesting that this angiogenic response was induced by immunocompetent donor lymphocytes (Sidky and Auerbach 1975). In a study of peroxidase-induced arthritis in the articular joints of rabbits, Graham and Shannon (1972a, 1972b) noted that endothelial mitoses were observed coincidental with active lymphoid cell migration into the inflamed joints. Anderson et al. (1975) showed extensive proliferation of post-capillary venular endothelium in lymph nodes draining allografted skin sites and suggested that this amplification of the vascular surface area may aid in the recirculation of sensitized lymphoid cells. Klintworth and colleagues using the transparent rabbit cornea as a model system showed that corneal neovascularization induced by silver nitrate wounds was invariably accompanied by an infiltrate rich in neutrophils, thus implicating these cells in mediating angiogenesis (Fromer and Klintworth 1975a, 1975b, 1976).

In the early 1970s, Leibovich and Ross were investigating the role that macrophages played during wound repair. At that time the prevailing view was that macrophages were primarily scavenger cells. In a series of seminal publications, they showed that macrophages played an equally if not more important role in wound healing by stimulating mesenchymal cell proliferation (Leibovich and Ross 1975, 1976). These studies along with others revealed that macrophages were capable of elaborating both inhibitory and stimulatory factors, which affect the growth and differentiation of several mesenchymal cell types (Calderon et al. 1974; Calderon and Unanue 1975; Leibovich and Ross 1975, 1976; Unanue 1976).

A direct link between macrophages and angiogenesis was suggested by Clark et al. (1976), who showed that macrophages injected into the transparent rabbit cornea could elicit an angiogenic response, although they were unable to demonstrate unequivocally the direct involvement of macrophages in mediating angiogenesis. The answer as to whether macrophages were the source of an angiogenic mediator was revealed in a study by Polverini et al. (1978). They showed that macrophages or their culture fluids could directly stimulate angiogenesis in the absence of other inflammatory cell populations. This study was the first to establish that macrophages, an indispensible component of chronic inflammation and wound healing, could directly stimulate angiogenesis. It is now well established that macrophages are a central figure in wound angiogenesis (Sunderkötter et al. 1991, 1994; Adamson 2009; Dong et al. 2009).

Macrophages are among the most versatile cells that accumulate at sites of injury. They are professional phagocytes that are efficient at engulfing micro-organisms and cellular debris (van Furth et al. 1972; Pollard 2009). They also secrete a wide array of chemokines, cytokines and immunomodulatory molecules (Pollard 2009). Macrophages have a number of important trophic functions including the initiation and patterning of neovascular networks both in adult tissues and embryos (Lobov et al. 2005; Bergmann et al. 2006; Rao et al. 2007). Once recruited to the wound site monocytes differentiate into macrophages and become activated, thereby acquiring the capacity to influence virtually every facet of the wound response (Lingen 2001; Bauer et al. 2005; Martin and Leibovich 2005; Eming et al. 2007).

Macrophages influence angiogenesis in several ways. They facilitate sprouting angiogenesis, recruit EPCs and influence the branching morphology of new vessels and vessel remodeling (Pollard 2009). As oxygen levels become reduced macrophages are induced to produce the endothelial mitogen and survival factor VEGF as well as a number of more generic cytokines and chemokines that directly stimulate endothelial proliferation and migration (Lingen 2001; Grunewald et al. 2006; Pollard 2009). They also produce metalloproteinases that enable new blood vessels to move through a developing matrix, and macrophages can also recruit other cells including stromal fibroblast, keratinocytes to produce mediators of angiogenesis. Macrophages also help temper wound angiogenesis through the production of angiogenesis inhibitors (DiPietro and Polverini 1993; DiPietro et al. 1996). The continued presence of macrophages well beyond the peak proliferative phase of angiogenesis suggests that macrophages play a key role in establishing the permanent architectural design that comprises the mature microvascular network. Indeed, VEGF, a principal mediator of wound angiogenesis, has been shown to play a role not only in the initial stages of angiogenesis but also in maintaining vessel integrity over time (Ceradini et al. 2004; Grunewald et al. 2006).

There are a number of important environmental queues that function to initiate the angiogenic response during the healing process. These stimuli activate a process known as the 'angiogenic switch'. The angiogenic switch was first shown to be a critical stage in tumor progression. During tumor development the key event that initiates the expression of angiogenic activity by tumor cells was shown to be linked to loss of key tumor suppressor genes (Restinejad et al. 1989). In this case, loss or inactivation of the p53 tumor suppressor was shown to be associated with a failure to produce the endogenous angiogenesis inhibitor thrombospondin 1. The resulting local imbalance in angiogenic stimulators and inhibitors manifested as sustained angiogenesis. Subsequent studies have both confirmed and revealed other important events that contribute to this phenomenon (Hanahan and Folkman 1996). Recent evidence suggests that a comparable physiologic angiogenic switch occurs during wound healing. Leibovich and colleagues have shown that the accumulation of the purine nucleotide adenosine in the wound environment in conjunction with specific Toll-like receptors on the surface of macrophages can switch macrophages from a proinflammatory phenotype to an angiogenic, anti-inflamatory phenotype by downregulating production of inflammatory cytokines and upregulating production of angiogenic mediators (Leibovich et al. 2002; Pinhal-Enfield et al. 2003).

THE ROLE OF OTHER INFLAMMATORY CELLS IN ANGIOGENESIS

It is well understood that synergistic cross-talk between inflammatory cells and activated host cells plays a pivotal role in orchestrating the wound response including angiogenesis (Singer and Clark 1999; Lingen 2001; Eming et al. 2007; Gurtner et al. 2008). While there have been numerous studies of the role of myeloid cells in tumor angiogenesis, comparable data on their role in physiological wound healing are generally lacking. Nevertheless, there is mounting evidence that many myeloid cell populations are a rich source of angiogenic mediators and inhibitors and thus may have a role in wound angiogenesis.

Chronic wounds are invariably populated by large numbers of lymphocytes. These cells produce a number of mediators, such as VEGF, bFGF and HGF, that stimulate angiogenesis. Apart from their role in immune surveillance both CD4 and CVD8 lymphocytes have been associated with angiogenic responses in tumors. However, their role in angiogenic responses that accompany chronic inflammation and wound healing remains largely unexplored (Ahn and Brown 2009).

Mast cells are known to contain a number of potential mediators of angiogenesis stored in secretory granules. Mediators such as VEGF, FGF-2, TNF-α and TGF-β and several chemokines have been shown to stimulate angiogenesis following their accumulation at sites of inflammation. Additionally these cells are rich in serine protease which can activate a cascade of proteolytic enzymes that create important corridors for new vessels to populate. Heparin, the most abundant glycosaminoglycan, plays a key role in sequestering angiogenic mediators at the wound site and concentrating their availability while enhancing the potency of many mitogenic and chemotactic endothelial cells (Lingen 2001; Ribatti et al 2009).

Neutrophils are among the most abundant cells at sites of inflammation and during wound healing. These cells have long been implicated as a potential source of angiogenic mediators (Graham and Shannon 1972a 1972b; Fromer and Klintworth 1975a, 1975b, 1976; Sidky and Auerbach 1975). Neutrophils are an abundant source of proteolytic enzymes. As such they are good candidates for initiating many of the early steps in the angiogenic response (Murdoch et al. 2008; Tazzyman et al. 2009). Activated neutrophils also secrete a number of pro-angiogenic factors. Pro-inflammatory factors such as TNFα induce neutrophil degranulation, releasing VEGF and inflammatory chemokines such as CXCR1 and 8 from intracellular stores, which subsequently induces endothelial cell proliferation and can induce tubule formation *in vitro*. The release of both proinflammatory molecules, soluble angiogenic mediators and proteolytic enzyme such as matrix metalloproteinases can contribute significantly to both initiating as well as sustaining angiogenesis (Murdoch et al. 2008; Tazzyman et al. 2009).

Except for certain types of parasitic infections, local and systemic allergic phenomena, and tumors, eosinophils are infrequent components of uncomplicated inflammation reactions and wound healing (Kumar and Abbas et al. 2009). However, recent reports suggest that eosinophils may have a role in tumor angiogenesis (Munitz and and Levi-Schaffer 2004). Freshly isolated human blood eosinophils or supernatants from cultured eosinophils induce endothelial cell proliferation *in vitro* and angiogenesis. Eosinophils contain VEGF and many other angiogenic mediators in their secretory granules and decoy antibodies directed against one or more of these mediators can block eosinophil mediated angiogenesis (Horiuchi and Weller 1997; Munitz and Levi-Schaffer 2004).

Dendritic cells are crucial regulators of adaptive immune responses and play an important role as antigen presenting cells. They also possess the unique ability to induce both primary and secondary T- and B-cell responses as well as immune tolerance (Banchereau and Steinman 1998). Dendritic cells produce a number of cytokines, several of which have known angiogenic activity and can be recruited to the tumor site by many of these same angiogenic mediators (Curiel et al. 2004; Murdoch et al. 2008). More recently, Gottfried et al. (2007) reported that tumor associated dendritic cells can differentiate into endothelial-like cells and thus contribute to tumor angiogenesis.

MATRIX MOLECULES

The highly orchestrated and coordinated nature of the angiogenic response is dependent to a great extent on how proangiogenic mediators engage the extracellular matrix (ECM) (Li et al. 2003; Schultz and Wysocki 2009). The appropriate scheduling of endothelial proliferation and migration and the incorporation and differentiation of endothelial precursors into nascent vessels requires the participation of a variety of ECM components, including fibronectin, collagen, vitronectin, tenascin and laminin (Ruoslahti and Yamaguchi 1991; Witt and Lander 1994; Feng et al. 1999; Li et al. 2003).

Integrins, a family of heterodimeric transmembrane proteins located on the surface of cells, are the principal means by which cells communicate with the extracellular matrix. Working synergistically with proangiogenic signaling molecules, integrins play a central role in wound angiogenesis (Sepp et al. 1994; Giancotti and Ruoslahti 1999). The αvβ1 integrins are essential in facilitating angiogenic responses. For example, α1β1 has been shown to be essential for VEGF mediated angiogenic signaling (Senger et al. 1997) and antibodies directed against $\alpha v\beta 3$ impair fibroblast growth factor-2 (FGF-2) mediated angiogenesis (Brooks et al. 1994). The $\alpha v\beta 3$ integrin receptor is among the most important in wound angiogenesis (Brooks et al. 1994). $\alpha V\beta 3$ expression can be detected in the provisional and mature matrix surrounding blood vessels and on proliferating endothelial cells during neovascularization of skin wounds (Brooks et al. 1994). The significance of these observations is further substantiated by studies which showed that blocking this integrin receptor blocks angiogenesis (Christofidou-Solomidou et al. 1997).

In summary, there is a critical interdependence of angiogenic mediators and integrin signaling during wound healing. The coordinated regulation of these key components is essential for the timely induction and resolution of wound angiogenesis and many other aspects of wound healing.

VASCULAR ENDOTHELIAL GROWTH FACTOR AND THE MODERN ERA OF ANGIOGENESIS RESEARCH

The recognition that tumor cells secreted a 'mediator of angiogenesis' led to a flurry of research activity directed at identifying this presumptive 'angiogenesis factor'. However, it was the discovery of VEGF that propelled the field forward and established the identity of the first endothelial specific mediator of angiogenesis (Otrock et al. 2007; Nieves et al. 2009). The initial breakthrough came in a report by Dvaork that described a tumor-secreted factor that enhanced vessel leakiness and ascites fluid accumulation (Senger et al. 1983, 1986). Parallel work in other laboratories described an angiogenic mitogen, VEGF, which would turn out to be identical to vascular permeability factor (VPF). Thus VPF became VEGF (Leung et al. 1989). Early studies of endothelial growth factors and angiogenesis mediators that preceded the discovery of VEGF as well as work in subsequent years revealed an increasing number of endothelial growth factors and signaling networks that contributed to one or more phases in the angiogenic response. A number of excellent detailed reviews of angiogenic mediators and signaling networks are available. The following paragraphs will focus on the role VEGF in angiogenesis in general and wound angiogenesis specifically.

The VEGF is a homodimeric glycoprotein that consists of six family members: VEGF-A, B, C, D and E and placental growth factor (PLGF) (Nieves et al. 2007; Otrock et al. 2007). The human VEGF gene produces eight isoforms generated through alternative splicing. The isoforms $VEGF_{121}$, $VEGF_{145}$, $VEGF_{165}$, $VEGF_{189}$ and $VEGF_{206}$ are referred to as VEGF-A, B, C, D, and E respectively (Bicknell and Harris 2004; Nieves et al. 2007; Ahmed and Bicknell 2009). Forms of VEGF bearing the heparin sulfate-binding domain are sequestered on cell surfaces or embedded in the extracellular matrix. VEGF-A, on the other hand, is freely diffusible and tends to be in greatest abundance at sites of injury. The various isoforms suggest that VEGF may have a role not only in initiating angiogenesis in adult tissues but also in maintaining long-term vascular stability and homeostasis (Ng et al. 2001; Lee et al. 2007; Nieves et al. 2007). The central importance of VEGF in early development was revealed in studies which showed that deletion of a single VEGF allele in mice resulted in embryonic lethality (Fong et al. 1995; Ng et al. 2001). VEGF binds to two high affinity tyrosine kinase receptors Flt-1 (VEGFR-1) and KDR (VEGFR-2) on the surface of endothelial cells (Fong et al. 1995; Otrock et al. 2007). Engagement of VEGFR-2 is primarily associated with capillary assembly and differentiation, while signaling through VEGFR-1 is associated with increased vascular permeability, induction of matrix metalloproteinases in smooth muscle cells, neutrophil, monocyte and macrophage activation, chemotaxis and endothelial survival (Berse et al. 1992; Nissen et al. 1995; Clauss et al. 1996; Gaudry et al. 1997; Barrientos et al. 2008; Zhang et al. 2009).

One of the most potent inducers of VEGF during wound healing is hypoxia (Shweiki et al. 1992; Namiki et al. 1995; Detmar et al. 1997). As metabolic demand increases in injured tissues and oxygen tension is lowered VEGF production is stimulated in a variety of cells at the wound site (Bao et al. 2009). Additionally, hypoxia preferentially stimulates expression of the VEGF receptor Flt-1 (VEGFR1) which influences the function of a number of inflammatory cells as mentioned earlier. Perhaps more importantly is the role of VEGF and VEGFR1 in endothelial cell survival (Nör et al. 1999, 2000a, 2000b; Zhang et al. 2009). This is of critical importance during wound neovascularization where growing blood vessels are subjected to intermittent stress and a host of potentially lethal stimuli at the wound site (Katoh et al. 1995; Nör et al. 1999). It has recently been reported that tumor associated endothelial cells expressing the survival protein Bcl-2 transiently acquire the resistance phenotype (Kumar et al. 2004, 2007). As a result, endothelial cells are protected from potentially lethal endogenous and exogenous toxins at the tumor site. This raises the possibility that Bcl-2 may confer this same resistance phenotype on endothelial cells during wound angiogenesis, giving them a much needed, albeit temporary, survival advantage.

Many cell types at the wound site produce VEGF-A including endothelial cells, fibroblasts, smooth muscle cells platelets, neutrophils and macrophages (Detmar et al. 1997; Gaudry et al. 1997; Banks 1998; Barrientos et al. 2008). VEGF functions to promote angiogenesis at several stages during the wound response (Nissen et al. 1998). Following injury, platelets release VEGF that promotes endothelial proliferation and migration (Banks et al. 1998). Macrophages attracted to the wound site produce TNF-α which in turn induces VEGF expression in a host of resident cell populations including keratinocytes and fibroblasts (Frank et al. 1995). As proinflammatory, immunomodulatory and angiogenic mediators accumulate at the wound site and as the hypoxic gradient is established, VEGF expression is further enhanced. The resulting neovascular network restores tissue perfusion and helps drive tissue regeneration. Clearly, there are a number of other mediator systems that participate at various stages of wound neovascularization. Precisely how these various mediators synergize with VEGF to coordinate wound neovascularization remains the subject of considerable interest and speculation.

SIGNALING NETWORKS OF POTENTIAL IMPORTANCE IN WOUND NEOVASCULARIZATION

The next paragraphs describe several mediators and signaling molecules that have recently been linked to angiogenesis. For the most part, these molecules and signaling pathways are involved in developmental processes during embryogenesis, in particular neuronal development. Many of these signaling molecules share properties that either repel or repress certain endothelial cell functions and in some case can have both stimulatory as well as inhibitory functions depending on the type of ligand–receptor pairing. Many of them potentiate the function of angiogenic mediators such as VEGF. Although the evidence is just beginning to emerge, a number of studies suggest that at least some of these molecules may have a role in regulating physiological angiogenic responses such as in wound healing.

The semaphorins are a group of eight membrane-bound glycoproteins that are categorized according to their amino acid sequence. Originally described in invertebrates, these glycoproteins provide both repulsive and attractive cues for certain types of neurons. Among the semaphorins identified, Semaphorin 3 has been most widely linked with angiogenesis, where it has been reported to have repellant-like activity for endothelial cells, while Semaphorin 6 can block VEGF and FGF-mediated endothelial migration (Bicknell and Harris 2004; Klagsbrun and Eichmann 2005; Ahmed and Bicknell 2009).

The neuropilins (NP) were originally shown to be receptors of class 3 semaphorins (Kolodkin et al. 1997; Klagsbrun and Eichmann 2005). Mice deficient in the NP1 gene develop severe cardiovascular defects and abnormal vascular patterning (Kawasaki et al. 1999). NP1 also exists in a soluble form where it functions as a co-receptor of VEGF-C by signaling through VEGFR-2. Overexpression of NP1 signaling collaboratively with VEGF accelerates tumor growth presumably by increasing tumor neovascular density. NP2 has also been shown to have an important regulatory role for VEGF (Miao et al. 1999; Neufeld et al. 2005).

The plexins are large transmembrane glycoproteins whose cysteine-rich extracellular domains share regions of homology with scatter factor receptor Met (Gu et al. 2005; Neufeld et al. 2007). Members of the Plexin B subclass bind to either the membrane bound or soluble members of the semaphorin family. Type A plexins normally associate with Neuropilins to form functional receptors while Plexin B1 complexes with scatter factor and this complex potentiates the effects of VEGF (Toyofuku et al. 2004).

The ephrins are membrane bound ligands and their tyrosine kinase Eph receptors participate in neuronal development. The ephrins and their receptors are divided into two classes, A and B, with a penchant for a promiscuous binding. Their role in neovascularization has been demonstrated genetically where truncated forms of EphB2 or 4 lead to defects in vascular morphogenesis and aberrant capillary branching and patterning during embryonic development. Several Ephs and their receptors are present on vascular endothelium including ephrinA1, which participates in TNF-α induced inflammatory neovascularization, and ephrinB1, which promotes capillary assembly. Additionally several of the ephrins have been shown to block VEGF mediated angiogenic responses (Pandey et al. 1995; Adams 2002; Yancopoulos et al. 2004).

Notch signaling, originally discovered as a developmentally regulated gene in Drosophila, has critical roles in regulating cell fate (Bicknell and Harris 2004; Ahmed and Bicknell 2009). Notch's role in neovascularization is best revealed in the Alagille syndrome, which is characterized by a functional loss of a Notch ligand (Kalaria et al. 2002; Shawber et al. 2003; Sullivan and Bicknell 2003). All of the Notch receptors and their jagged and delta ligands are expressed on one or more cell types that comprise the vascular system, although Notch is ordinarily expressed in the arterial system and venous systems with delta also reported to be endothelial specific (Shawber et al. 2003). The Notch receptors and the delta ligands play an important role as transcriptional regulators of angiogenesis where they function to block differentiation and negatively regulate angiogenesis (Zeng et al. 2005). Jagged-1 is expressed at high levels during endothelial regeneration and plays an important role in directional migration of endothelial cells (Bicknell and Harris 2004; Ahmed and Bicknell 2009).

The Netrins are a family of highly conserved secreted proteins that function primarily as attractants. Originally they were shown to play a role in axon guidance but more recently have been implicated in angiogenesis where they function through the uncoordinated-5 (UNC5) receptor families. Netrins 1, 2 and 4 mediate endothelial migration, proliferation and tube formation. They have been shown to initiate vessel formation and accelerate revascularization of ischemic tissues in mice. UNC receptors are present on the vascular system during embryogenesis and primarily localize to the arterial circulation and on 'tip' cells where they are believed to provide guidance during capillary branching. Inactivation of UNC leads to embryonic lethality and defective capillary branching (Wilson et al. 2006; Ahmed and Bicknell 2009).

Roundabouts (Robos) are transmembrane proteins that function as receptors for the 'Slit' protein family of ligands. Originally, the Robos and Slits were thought to be restricted to cells of neural lineage where they mediate repulsive signaling and axon guidance during neural patterning. Four Robos have been identified, with Robo4 implicated in vascular guidance. However, the precise role of Roundabouts and Slits in neovascularization is controversial because some members of this receptor ligand family have been linked to the inhibition of endothelial cell migration and thus to the inhibition of angiogenesis (Klagsbrun and Eichmann 2005; Legg et al. 2008; Ahmed and Bicknell 2009).

Hedgehog is a 19-kDa heparin binding protein that is tethered to the surface of cells through cholesterol. There are three homologs of Hedgehog: Sonic, Desert and Indian. Hedgehog signals through the patch receptor, which activates the Gli family of transcription factors, Gli 1, 2 and 3. In adult tissues Gli and its downstream target smoothen is transcriptionally repressed. Mutations in Patch prevent Hedgehog from repressing Gli and smoothen resulting in unscheduled growth. Hedgehog signaling is crucial during development. Postnatal defects in Hedgehog signaling results in variable morphologic abnormalities and the development of a range of tumors (Jacob and Lum 2007). Hedgehog has been reported to have a role in angiogenesis and vascular patterning where hyperactivity of Sonic Hedgehog in zebrafish embryos is associated with hypervascularization and defective arteriogenesis (Pola et al. 2001; Nagase et al. 2008; Ahmed and Bicknell 2009).

Lastly, Sprouty (Spry) is an intracellular protein originally discovered in Drosophila as a repressor of FGF signaling during tracheal development. Spry consists of four human and four mouse homologs. Because of its role in tracheal branching there was speculation that it may also have a role in determining the branching morphology of capillary beds. Direct evidence for Spry in angiogenesis was revealed when Spry-4 was overexpressed in mouse embryos. The affected embryos showed reduced sprouting and incompletely developed hearts. Spry-4 appears to mediate its effects by reducing bFGF and VEGF MAP kinase phosphorylation and thus suppresses endothelial cell proliferation and migration. Thus Spry may function as a developmentally regulated check on neovascular growth and branching (Lee et al. 2001; Sullivan and Bicknell 2003; Ahmed and Bicknell 2009; Taniguchi et al. 2009).

INHIBITORS OF ANGIOGENESIS: IMPORTANT COUNTERWEIGHTS IN WOUND NEOVASCULARIZATION

Endogenous inhibitors of angiogenesis are comprised primarily of proteins or fragments of proteins that are present in various tissues and in the circulation (Ribatti 2009). These inhibitors can be detected in the blood as well as the extracellular compartments where they serve as vital checks on endothelial repair and the activity of proangiogenic mediators.

Many endogenous inhibitors of angiogenesis are fragments of larger matrix molecules that are stored in the extracellular matrix and released following activation of metalloproteinases (MMPs), cathepsins or elastases (van Hinsbergh et al. 2006) In addition to matrix-derived inhibitors are those inhibitors derived from fragments of coagulation factors, certain growth factors and cytokines and a host of metabolites and hormone fragments. Many of the endogenous inhibitors require proteolytic activation to function (van Hinsbergh et al. 2006). In addition to blocking cell proliferation, most of the endogenous inhibitors induce cell death via the intrinsic and/or extrinsic apoptosis pathways. Nevertheless, despite inroads made these past 20 years in the identification and understanding of the mechanism of action of many of these inhibitors, there is still research that needs to be done to understand how these inhibitors work and how their function is coordinated with proangiogenic mediators.

In 1989 Bouck and colleagues made the seminal observation that inactivation or loss of a tumor suppressor gene, in this case p53, was linked to the 'angiogenic switch' in tumors. This switch to the angiogenic phenotype was attributed to loss of an important matrix molecule, thrombospondin 1 (TSP-1) (Rastinejad et al. 1989; Good et al. 1990). Thus began the search for other naturally occurring inhibitors of angiogenesis. A number of excellent comprehensive reviews on endogenous angiogenesis inhibitors have been published recently (Nyberg et al. 2005; Sato 2006; Zhang and Lawler 2007; Ribatti 2009). In this chapter I will limit my comments to the thrombospondins as a prototype inhibitor of wound angiogenesis (Armstrong and Bornstein 2003; Adams and Lawler 2004).

The TSPs are modular heparin-binding matricellular proteins that influence the proliferation, migration, differentiation and survival of a number of cell types including endothelial cells (Nör et al. 2000; Armstrong and Bornstein 2003; Adams and Lawler 2004). TSP-1 was the first of the thrombospondins discovered to have angiostatic and proapoptotic activity for endothelial cells (Rastinejad et al. 1989; Good et al. 1990; Nör et al. 2000). Later, TSP-2 was found to have similar anti-angiogenic properties. Neither of the other TSPs (TSP-3/COMP) were found to inhibit angiogenesis (Armstrong and Bornstein 2003). A deficiency of TSP-1 and/or TSP-2 has a profound effect on several important aspects of wound healing (Streit et al. 2000; Agah et al. 2002; Nör et al. 2005). TSP-1-deficient mice show impaired wound healing with persistent granulation tissue, decreased collagen content over time and delayed arrival of macrophages compared to wild-type littermates. Nör and colleagues (2005) showed that the number of microvessels in wounds of TSP-1-deficient mice is approximately two-fold greater than in wild-type littermates 10 days after injury. Topical application of TSP-1, or KRFK (a peptide derived from TSP-1 that activates latent TGF-β1), to wounds of TSP-1-deficient mice rescued wild-type patterns of wound repair and partially restored local levels of TGF-β1 expression. Topical application of anti-TGF-β antibody impaired the ability of KRFK to rescue normal patterns of wound neovascularization in TSP-1-deficient mice. This suggest that TSP-1-mediated activation of local TGF-β1 is an important step in this process (Murphy-Ullrich and Poczatek 2000). More recently TSP-1 has been shown to be important in macrophage recruitment and phagocytic function (Kirsch et al. 2009). TSP-2 inhibits endothelial cell migration and tube formation, as well as increasing endothelial cell-specific apoptosis through an 80-kDa fragment in the N-terminal region of the molecule (Noh et al. 2003).

The observation that TSP-1 is a potent endogenous inhibitor of angiogenesis has prompted several groups to explore its therapeutic application. The discovery of specific anti-angiogenic regions within the TSP-1 molecule has enabled the development of recombinant proteins and synthetic peptides with greater stability for use in clinical trials.

Endogenous inhibitors of angiogenesis are important in maintaining the angiogenic balance that influences the rate of new blood vessel formation in both physiological and pathological conditions. The existence of numerous endogenous inhibitors of angiogenesis and their overlapping effects on angiogenic response suggest an important redundancy in the system that may regulate angiogenesis at various stages in the wound healing process.

It is tempting to speculate that both intrinsic inhibitory factors such as sprouty and extrinsic inhibitors such as TSP1 and 2 may work in a coordinate manner to temper and downregulate angiogenesis with great precision in a number of physiological settings such as wound healing.

THE ROLE OF ABERRANT WOUND ANGIOGENESIS IN THE PATHOGENESIS OF DIABETES MELLITUS

Stasis ulcers and persistent wounds that heal slowly or not at all are pathognomonic of diabetes. A diabetic patient subjected to an otherwise minor injury runs the risk of developing a chronic non-healing wound or worse, amputation of digits or an entire limb. These greatly out of proportion consequences to simple injury are all too often the result in a patient suffering from diabetes mellitus. Many of the untoward events that accompany wound healing in diabetic patients can be attributed to an inadequate inflammatory and angiogenic response (Falanga 2005; Brem and Tomic-Canic 2007).

Deficiencies in a number of important aspects of the wound response are evident in diabetic patients. These include a reduction in the production of essential growth factors (Falanga 2005; Galkowska et al. 2006; Goren et al. 2006; Brem and Tomic-Canic 2007), an angiogenic response that is prolonged and arrested at the proliferative-non-differentiation stage (Galiano et al. 2004; Falanga 2005), ineffective debridement of tissues, defective collagen maturation and collagen accumulation (Lobmann et al. 2002; Maruyama et al. 2007), and a failure to completely epithelialize skin or mucosal wounds, thus compromising the barrier function of skin (Stojadinovic et al. 2005). The overall quality and quantity of granulation tissue is markedly reduced (Lobmann et al. 2002) in diabetic wounds resulting in an uncoordinated healing response at the cellular and molecular level (Brem and Tomic-Canic 2007; Stojadinoviv et al. 2007).

Several aspects of the angiogenic response are abnormal in diabetes. First, sprouting angiogenesis tends to be delayed due to aberrant endothelial activation (Falanga 2005; Brem and Tomic-Canic 2007). Endothelial proliferation and migration are compromised resulting in impaired neovascularization. Mobilization of bone marrow derived EPCs is ineffective, thus preventing EPCs from reaching the wound site in significant numbers. There is some evidence suggesting that reduced mobilization of EPCs and the contribution of new EPCs to neovascular responses is minimized, thus contributing to an ineffective neovascular response. During ischemia stromal cell derived factor-1α (SDF-1α) is normally upregulated. Gallagher et al. (2007) reported that iNOS, an important mediator of EPC mobilization and SDF-1α expression, is streptozotocin-induced in diabetic wounds in mice. Diabetic endothelial cells tend to be resistant to the proangiogenic and prosurvival effects of VEGF and EPCs are ineffective in migrating to sites of neovascularization (Galiano et al. 2004; Waltenberger 2009).

The incidence of microvascular disease is greatly enhanced in patients with diabetes, particularly those with type 1 diabetes as compared to non-diabetic patients. In addition to functional abnormalities associated with angiogenic responses, diabetic blood vessels suffer from a variety of structural and functional abnormalities. These abnormalities include a reduction in capillary size, thickening of the basement membrane and hyalinosis of arterioles. The thickening of the basement membrane interferes with physiological fluid exchange and cellular migration, and contributes to a decreased capacity to confront infections (Falanga 2005; Brem and Tomic-Canic 2007). Collectively these structural and functional defects in diabetic endothelial cells are perhaps among the most important factors that contribute to aberrant wound healing in diabetic patients.

CONCLUSIONS

Figure 7.1 depicts the complex integration of cellular and molecular events that are required for a coordinated angiogenic response and thus successful wound healing. Current options for treating complicated wounds or diseased compromised or injured tissues are few and far between. However, future approaches to therapeutic vascularization show great promise. Advances in the development of target deliveries of growth factors and growth inhibitors as well as innovative cell and protein based therapies suggest new opportunities for improving pathologic wound healing. Approaches to re-engineering the angiogenic response are likely to employ multiple modalities that combine emerging cell, protein and metabolic therapies. Additionally, advances in regenerative medicine, stem cell biology and the development of bioactive matrices and 'smart' materials have enormous potential for creating an optimal environment for angiogenesis to occur without the constraints imposed by a disease compromised environment, as in diabetes and intractable inflammatory disorders such as

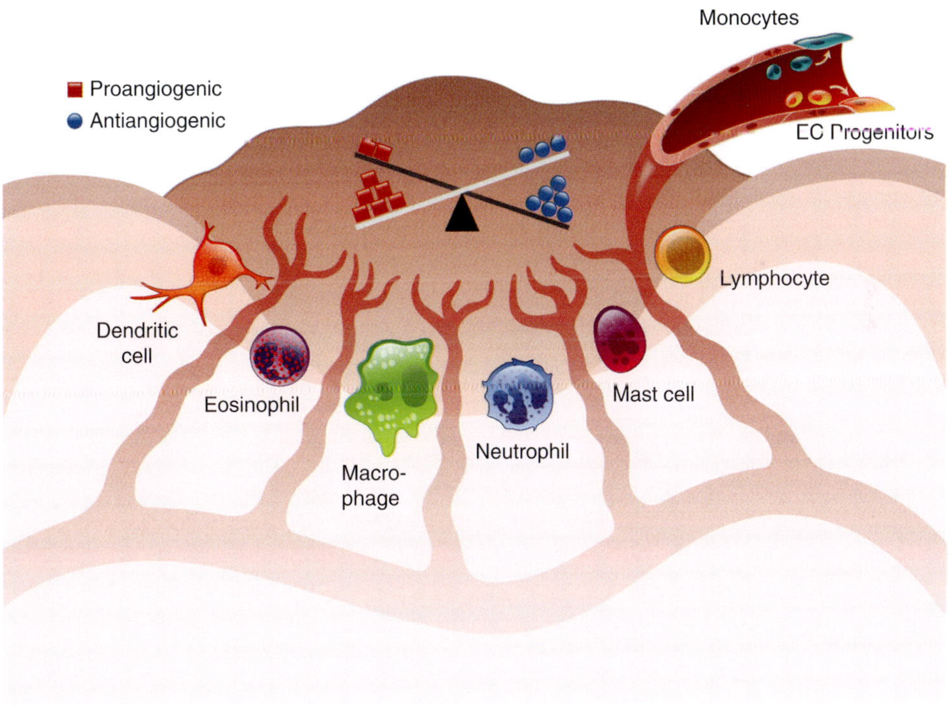

Fig. 7.1 This cartoon depicts the proposed contribution of a variety of inflammatory cell populations in the induction and maintenance of wound neovascularization. The balance between proangiogenic and anti-angiogenic mediators ultimately determines when angiogenesis is both initiated and terminated. The long-term maintenance of the microvasculature and intermittent endothelial repair is also under the control of one or more proangiogenic and anti-angiogenic mediators. How these mediators are coordinated temporally remains to be determined.

rheumatoid arthritis. As work progresses in all of these areas, we can expect a broader spectrum of therapies will be made available to patients.

REFERENCES

Adams, J.C., Lawler, J. (2004) The thrombospondins. *International Journal of Biochemistry and Cell Biology* **36**: 961–968.

Adams, R.H. (2002) Vascular patterning by Eph receptor tyrosine kinases and ephrins. *Seminars in Cell and Developmental Biology* **13**(1): 55–60.

Adams, R.H., Alitalo, K. (2007) Molecular regulation of angiogenesis and lymphangiogenesis. *Nature Reviews Molecular Cell Biology* **8**: 464–478.

Adamson, R. (2009) Role of macrophages in normal wound healing; an overview. *Journal of Wound Care* **18**: 349–351.

Agah, A., Kyriakides, T.R., Lawler, J. Bornstein, P. (2002) The lack of thrombospondin 1 (TSP1) dictates the course of wound healing in double-TSP1/TSP2-null mice. *American Journal of Pathology* **161**: 831–839.

Ahmed, Z., Bicknell, R. (2009) Angiogenic signaling pathways. In: (eds S. Martin, C. Murray) *Angiogenesis Protocols*, 2nd edn. Humana Press, New York.

Ahn, G.-O., Brown, J.M. (2009) Role of endothelial progenitors and other bone marrow derived cells in the development of the tumor vasculature *Angiogenesis* **12**: 159–164.

Algire, G.H. (1943a) An adaptation of the transparent-chamber technique to the mouse. *Journal of the National Cancer Institute* **4**: 1–11.

Algire, G.H. (1943b) Microscopic studies of the early growth of a transplantable melanoma of the mouse, using the transparent-chamber technique. *Journal of the National Cancer Institute* **4**: 13–20.

Algire, G.H., Chalkley, H.W., Legallais, F.Y., Park, H.D. (1945) Vascular reactions of normal and malignant tumors in vivo. I. Vascular reactions of mice to wounds and to normal and neoplastic transplants. *Journal of the National Cancer Institute* **6**: 73–85.

Anderson, N.D., Anderson, A.O., Wyllie, R.G. (1975) Microvascular changes in lymph nodes draining skin allografts. *American Journal of Pathology* **81**: 131–141.

Asahara, T., Kawamoto, A. (2004) Endothelial progenitor cells for postnatal vasculogenesis. *American Journal of Physiology, Cell Physiology* **287**: C572–C579.

Banchereau, J., Steinman, R.M. (1998) Dendritic cells and the control of immunity. *Nature* **392**: 245–252.

Banks, R.E., Forbes, M.A., Kinsey, S.E., et al. (1998) Release of the angiogenic cytokine vascular endothelial growth factor (VEGF) from platelets: significance for VEGF measurements and cancer biology. *British Journal of Cancer* **77**: 956–964.

Baron, M., Aslam, H., Flasza, M., et al. (2002) Multiple levels of Notch signal regulation. *Molecular Membrane Biology* **19**: 27–38.

Barrientos, S., Stojadinovic O., Golinko, M.S., et al. (2008) Growth factors and cytokines in wound healing. *Wound Repair and Regeneration* **16**: 585–601.

Bauer, S.M., Bauer, R.J., Velazquez, O.C. (2005) Angiogenesis, vasculogenesis, and induction of healing in chronic wounds. *Vascular and Endovascular Surgery* **39**: 293–306.

Bergmann, C.E., Hoefer, I.E., Meder, B., et al. (2006) Arteriogenesis depends on circulating monocytes and macrophage accumulation and is severely depressed in op/op mice. *Journal of Leukocyte Biology* **80**: 59–65.

Berse, B., Brown, L.F., Van de Water, L., et al. (1992) Vascular permeability factor (vascular endothelial growth factor) gene is expressed differentially in normal tissues, macrophages, and tumors. *Molecular Biology of the Cell* **3**(2): 211–220.

Bicknell, R., Harris, A.L. (2004) Novel angiogenic signaling pathways and vascular targets. *Annual Review of Pharmacology and Toxicology* **44**: 219–238.

Brem, H., Tomic-Canic, M. (2007) Cellular and molecular basis of wound healing in diabetes. *Journal of Clinical Investigation* **117**: 1219–1222.

Brooks, P.C., Clark, R.A., Cheresh, D.A. (1994) Requirement of vascular integrin alpha v beta 3 for angiogenesis. *Science* **264**: 569–571.

Calderon, J., Unanue, E.R. (1975) Two biological activities regulating cell proliferation found in cultures of peritoneal exudate cells. *Nature* **31**: 359–361.

Calderon, J., Williams, R.T., Unanue, E.R. (1974) An inhibitor of cell proliferation released by cultures of macrophages. *Proceedings of the National Academy of Sciences USA* **71**: 4273–4277.

Callahan, R., Egan, S.E. (2004) Notch signaling in mammary development and oncogenesis. *Neoplasia* **9**: 145–163.

Carmeliet, P. (2000) Mechanisms of angiogenesis and arteriogenesis. *Nature Medicine* **6**: 389–395.

Carmeliet, P. (2003) Angiogenesis in health and disease. *Nature Medicine* **9**: 653–660.

Ceradini, D.J., Kulkarni, A.R., Callaghan, M.J., et al. (2004) Progenitor cell trafficking is regulated by hypoxic gradients through HIF-1 induction of SDF-1. *Nature Medicine* **10**: 858–864.

Cheng, N., Brantley, D.M., Chen, J. (2002) The ephrins and Eph receptors in angiogenesis. *Cytokine Growth Factor Reviews* **13**: 75–85.

Clark, E.R. (1939) Microscopic observations on the growth of blood capillaries in the living mammal. *American Journal of Anatomy* **64**: 251–299.

Clark, E.R. (1981) Studies on the growth of blood vessels from the tail of the frog. *American Journal of Anatomy* **23**: 37–88.

Clark, E.R., Clark, E.L. (1932) Observations on living preformed blood vessels as seen in a transparent chamber inserted into the rabbit ear. *American Journal of Anatomy* **49**: 441–447.

Clark, R.A., Stone, R.D., Leung, D.Y.K., et al. (1976) Role of macrophages in wound healing. *Surgical Forum* **27**: 16–18.

Clark, R.A., Tonnesen, M.G., Gailit, J., et al. (1996) Transient functional expression of alpha v beta 3 on vascular cells during wound repair. *American Journal of Pathology* **148**: 1407–1421.

Courtade, E.T., Tsuda, T., Thomas, C.R., et al. (1975) Capillary density in developing and healing tuberculosis lesions produced by BCG in rabbits. *American Journal of Pathology* **78**: 243–252.

Crawford, S.E., Stellmach, V., Murphy-Ullrich, J.E., et al. (1998) Thrombospondin-1 is a major activator of TGFB-1 in vivo. *Cell* **93**: 1159–1170.

Curiel, T. J., Cheng, P., Mottram, P., et al. (2004) Dendritic cell subsets differentially regulate angiogenesis in human ovarian cancer. *Cancer Research* **64**: 5535–5538.

Dong, Z.M., Alpin, A.C., Nicosia, R.F. (2009) Regulation of angiogenesis by macrophages, dendritic cells and circulating monocytes. *Current Pharmaceutical Design* **15**: 365–379.

Dawson, D.W., Pearce, S.F., Zhong, R., Silverstein, R.L., Frazier, W.A., Bouck, N.P. (1997) CD36 mediates the in vitro inhibitory effects of thrombospondin-1 on endothelial cells. *Journal of Cell Biology* **138**: 707–717.

Denekamp, J. (1984) Vasculature as a target for tumor therapy. *Progress in Applied Microbiology* **4**: 28–38.

Diegelmann, R.F., Evans, M.C. (2004) Wound healing: an overview of acute, fibrotic and delayed healing. *Frontiers in Biosciences* **9**: 283–289.

DiPietro, L.A., Polverini, P.J. (1993) Angiogenic macrophages produce the angiogenic inhibitor thrombospondin 1. *American Journal of Pathology* **143**: 678–684.

DiPietro, L.A., Nissen, N.N., Gamelli, R.L., et al (1996) Thrombospondin 1 synthesis and function in wound repair. *American Journal of Pathology* **148**: 1851–1860.

Djonov, V., Baum, O., Burri, P.H. (2003) Vascular remodeling by intussusceptive angiogenesis. *Cell and Tissue Research* **314**: 107–117.

Dvorak, A.M., Mihm, M.C., Dvorak, H.F. (1976) Morphology of delayed-type-hypersensitivity reactions in man. II. Ultra structural alterations affecting the microvasculature and the tissue mast cells. *Laboratory Investigation* **34**: 179–186.

Eming, S.A., Brachvogel, B., Odorisio, T., et al. (2007) Regulation of angiogenesis: wound healing as a model. *Progress in Histochemistry and Cytochemistry* **42**: 115–170.

Engerman, R.L., Pfaffenbach, D., Davis, M.D. (1967) Cell turnover of capillaries. *Laboratory Investigation* **17**: 738–743.

Falanga, V. (2005) Wound healing and its impact in the diabetic foot. *Lancet* **366**: 1736–1743.

Feng, X., Clark, R.A., Galanakis, D., Tonnesen, M.G. (1999) Fibrin and collagen differentially regulate human dermal microvascular endothelial cell integrins: stabilization of alphav/beta3 mRNA by fibrin 1. *Journal of Investigative Dermatology* **113**: 913–919.

Folkman, J. (1972) Tumor dormancy in vivo by prevention of neovascularization. *Journal of Experimental Medicine* **136**: 261–276.

Folkman, J. (1985a) Tumor angiogenesis. *Advances in Cancer Research* **43**: 175–203.

Folkman, J. (1985b) Toward an understanding of angiogenesis: search and discovery. *Prospectives in Biology and Medicine* **9**: 10–36.

Folkman, J., Merler, E., Abernathy, C., Williams, G. (1971) Isolation of a tumor factor responsible for angiogenesis. *Journal of Experimental Medicine* **133**: 275–288.

Fong, G.H., Rossant, J., Gertsenstein, M., et al. (1995) Role of the Flt-1 receptor tyrosine kinase in regulating the assembly of vascular endothelium. *Nature* **376**: 66–70.

Frank, S., Hubner, G., Breier, G., et al. (1995) Regulation of vascular endothelial growth factor expression in cultured keratinocytes. Implications for normal and impaired wound healing. *Journal of Biological Chemistry* **270**: 12607–12613.

Fromer, C.H., Klintworth, G.K. (1975a) An evaluation of the role of leukocytes in the pathogenesis of experimentally induced corneal neovascularization. *American Journal of Pathology* **79**: 537–554.

Fromer, C.H., Klintworth, G.K. (1975b) An evaluation of the role of leukocytes in the pathogenesis of experimentally induced corneal neovascularization. II. Studies on the effect of leukocyte elimination on corneal neovascularization. *American Journal of Pathology* **81**: 531–544.

Fromer, C.H., Klintworth, G.K. (1976) An evaluation of the role of leukocytes in the pathogenesis of experimentally induced corneal neovascularization. III. Studies related to the vasoproliferative capability of polymorphonuclear leukocytes and lymphocytes. *American Journal of Pathology* **82**: 157–170.

Galiano, R.D., Tepper, O.M., Pelo, C.R., et al. (2004) Topical vascular endothelial growth factor accelerates diabetic wound healing through increased angiogenesis and by mobilizing and recruiting bone marrow-derived cells. *American Journal of Pathology* **164**: 1935–1947.

Galkowska, H., Wojewodzka, U., Olszewski, W.L. (2006) Chemokines, cytokines, and growth factors in keratinocytes and dermal endothelial cells in the margin of chronic diabetic foot ulcers. *Wound Repair and Regeneration* **14**: 558–565.

Gallagher, K.A., Liu, Z.J., Xiao, M., et al. (2007) Diabetic impairments in NO-mediated endothelial progenitor cell mobilization and homing are reversed by hyperoxia and SDF-1α. *Journal of Clinical Investigations* **117**: 1249–1259.

Gaudry, M., Bregerie, O., Andrieu, V., et al. (1997) Intracellular pool of vascular endothelial growth factor in human neutrophils. *Blood* **90**: 4153–4161.

Goldman, R. (2004) Growth factors and chronic wound healing: past, present, and future. *Advances in Skin Wound Care* **17**: 24–35.

Gottfried, E., Kreutz, M., Haffner, S., et al. (2007) Differentiation of human tumour-associated dendritic cells into endothelial-like cells: an alternative pathway of tumor angiogenesis. *Journal of Immunology* **65**: 329–335.

Goren, I., Muller, E., Pfeilschifter, J., et al. (2006) Severely impaired insulin signaling in chronic wounds of diabetic ob/ob mice: a potential role of tumor necrosis factor-alpha. *American Journal of Pathology* **168**: 765–777.

Graham, R.C., Shannon, S. (1972a) Peroxidase arthritis. I. An immunologically mediated inflammatory response with ultrastructural cytochemical localization of antigen and specific antibody. *American Journal of Pathology* **67**: 69–82.

Graham, R.C., Shannon, S. (1972b) Peroxidase arthritis. II. Lymphoid cell-endothelial interactions during developing immunologic inflammatory responses. *American Journal of Pathology* **69**: 7–14.

Greenblatt, M., Shubik, P. (1968) Tumor angiogenesis: transfilter diffusion studies in the hamster by the transparent chamber technique. *Journal of the National Cancer Institute* **41**: 111–124.

Grunewald, M., Avraham, I., Dor, Y., et al. (2006) VEGF-induced adult neovascularization: recruitment, retention, and role of accessory cells. *Cell* **124**: 175–189.

Gu, C., Yoshida, Y., Livet, J., et al. (2005) The semaphorin 3E and plexin-D1 control vascular pattern independently of neuropilins. *Science* **307**: 265–268.

Gurtner, G.C., Werner, S., Barrandon, Y., et al. (2008) Wound repair and regeneration. *Nature* **453**: 314–321.

Hanahan, D., Folkman, J. (1996) Patterns and emerging mechanisms of the angiogenic switch during tumorigenesis. *Cell* **86**: 353–364.

Horiuchi, T., Weller, P.F. (1997) Expression of vascular endothelial growth factor by human eosinophils: upregulation by granulocyte macrophage colony stimulating factor and interleukin-5. *American Journal Respiratory Cellular and Molecular Biology* **17**: 70–77.

Ide, A.G., Baker, N.H., Warren, S.L. (1939) Vascularization of the brown pearce rabbit epithelioma transplant as seen in the transparent ear chamber. *American Journal of Gastroenterology* **42**: 891–899.

Jacob, L., Lum, L. (2007) Deconstructing the hedgehog pathway in development and disease. *Science* **318**: 66–68.

Kalaria, R.N., Low, W.C., Oakley, A.E., et al. (2002) CADASIL and genetics of cerebral ischaemia. *Journal of Neural Transmission Supplement* **63**: 75–90.

Kawasaki, T., Kitsukawa, T., Bekku, Y., et al. (1999) A requirement for neuropilin -1 in embryonic vessel formation. *Development* **126**: 4895–4902.

Kim, S.J., Kim, J.S., Papadopoulos, J. et al. (2009) Circulating monocytes expressing CD**31**: implications for acute and chronic angiogenesis. *American Journal of Pathology* **174**: 1972–1980.

Klagsbrun, M., Eichmann, A. (2005) A role for axon guidance receptors and ligands in blood vessel development and tumor angiogenesis. *Cytokine Growth Factor Reviews* **16**: 535–548.

Kolodkin, A.L., Levengood, D.V., Rowe, E.G., et al. (1997) Neuropilin is a semaphorin III receptor. *Cell* **90**: 753–762.

Kumar, P., Miller, A.I., Polverini, P.J. (2004) p38 MAPK mediates gamma-irradiation-induced endothelial cell apoptosis and VEGF protects endothelial cells through PI3K-Akt-Bcl-2 pathway. *Journal of Biological Chemistry* **279**: 43352–43360.

Kumar, P., Benedict, R., Kumar, B., et al. (2007) Bcl-2 protects endothelial cells against gamma-radiation via a cytochrome c independent signaling pathway. *Cancer Research* **67**: 1193–1202.

Lee, S., Chen, T.T., Barber, C.L., et al. (2007) Autocrine VEGF signaling is required for vascular homeostasis. *Cell* **130**: 691–703.

Lee, S.H., Schloss, D.J., Jarvis, L., et al. (2001) Inhibition of angiogenesis by mouse sprouty protein. *Journal of Biological Chemistry* **276**: 4128–4133.

Legg, J.A., Herbert, J.M., Clissold, P., et al. (2008) Slits and roundabouts in cancer, tumour angiogenesis and endothelial migration. *Angiogenesis* **11**: 13–21.

Leibovich, S.J., Ross, R. (1975) The role of the macrophage in wound repair: a study with hydrocortisone and antimacrophage serum. *American Journal of Pathology* **78**: 71–100.

Leibovich, S.J., Chen, J.F., Pinhal-Enfield, G., et al. (2002) Synergistic up-regulation of vascular endothelial growth factor expression in murine macrophages by adenosine A2A receptor agonists and endotoxin. *American Journal of Pathology* **160**: 2231–2244.

Leung, D.W., Cachianes, G., Kuang, W.J., et al. (1989) Vascular endothelial growth factor is a secreted angiogenic mitogen. *Science* **246**: 1306–1309.

Li, J., Zhang, Y.-P., Kirsner, R.S. (2003) Angiogenesis in wound repair: angiogenic growth factors and the extracellular matrix. *Microscopy Research and Techniques* **60**: 107–114.

Lingen, M.W. (2001) Role of leukocytes and endothelial cells in the development of angiogenesis in inflammation and wound healing. *Archives of Pathology and Laboratory Medicine* **125**: 67–71.

Lobmann, R., Ambrosch, A., Schultz, G., et al. (2002) Expression of matrix metalloproteinases and their inhibitors in the wounds of diabetic and non-diabetic patients. *Diabetologia* **45**: 1011–1016.

Lobov, I.B., Rao, S., Carroll, T.J., et al. (2005) WNT7b mediates macrophage induced programmed cell death in patterning of the vasculature. *Nature* **437**: 417–421.

Maione, F., Molla, F., Claudia Meda, F.C., et al. (2009) Semaphorin 3A is an endogenous angiogenesis inhibitor that blocks tumor growth and normalizes tumor vasculature in transgenic mouse models. *Journal of Clinical Investigation* **11**: 3356–3372.

Makanya, A.N., Hlushchuk, R., Djonov, V.G. (2009) Intussusceptive angiogenesis and its role in vascular morphogenesis, patterning, and remodeling. *Angiogenesis* **12**: 113–123.

Martin, P., Leibovich, S.J. (2005) Inflammatory cells during wound repair: the good, the bad and the ugly. *Trends in cell Biology* **15**: 599–607.

Miao, H.Q., Soker, S., Feiner, L., et al. (1999) Neuropilin-1 expression by tumor cells promotes tumor angiogenesis and progression. *FASEB Journal* **14**: 2532–2539.

Munitz, A., Levi-Schaffer, F. (2004) Eosinophils: 'new' roles for 'old' cells. *Allergy* 59(3): 268–75. Review.

Murdoch, C., Muthana, M., Coffelt, S.B., et al. (2008) The role of myeloid cells in the promotion of tumor angiogenesis. *Nature Reviews Cancer* **8**: 618–631.

Murphy-Ullrich, J.E., Poczatek, M. (2000) Activation of latent TGF-b by thrombospondin-**1**: mechanisms and physiology. *Cytokine Growth Factor Reviews* **11**: 59–69.

Nagase, T., Nagase, M., Machida, M., et al. (2008) Hedgehog signaling in vascular development. *Angiogenesis* **11**: 71–77.

Namiki, A., Brogi, E., Kearney, M., et al. (1995) Hypoxia induces vascular endothelial growth factor in cultured human endothelial cells. *Journal of Biological Chemistry* **270**: 31189–31195.

Neufeld, G., Lange, T., Varshavsky, A. et al. (2007) Semaphorin signaling in vascular and tumor biology. *Advances in Experimental Medicine and Biology* **600**: 118–131.

Pandey, A., Shao, H., Marks, R.M., et al. (1995) The role of B61, the ligand for the *Eck* receptor tyrosine kinase, in TNF-alpha-induced angiogenesis. *Science* **268**: 567–569.

Park, Y.W., Kang, Y.M., Butterfield, J., et al. (2004) Thrombospondin 2 functions as an endogenous regulator of angiogenesis and inflammation in rheumatoid arthritis. *American Journal of Pathology* **165**: 2087–2098.

Phelps, E.A., Garcia, A.J. (2009) Update on therapeutic vascularization strategies. *Regenerative Medicine* **4**: 65–80.

Pinhal-Enfield, G., Ramanathan, M., Hasko, G., et al. (2003) An angiogenic switch in macrophages involving synergy between Toll-like receptors 2, 4, 7 and 9 and adenosine A2A receptors. *American Journal of Pathology* **163**: 711–721.

Pola, R., Ling, L.E., Silver, M., et al. (2001) The morphogen Sonic hedgehog is an indirect angiogenic agent upregulating two families of angiogenic growth factors. *Nature Medicine* **7**: 706–711.

Pollard, J. (2009) Trophic macrophages in development and disease. *Nature Reviews Immunology* **9**: 259–270.

Polverini, P.J. (1995) The pathophysiology of angiogenesis. *Critical Reviews in Oral Biology* **6**: 230–247.

Polverini, P.J., Cotran, R.S., Sholley, M.M. (1977) Endothelial proliferation in the delayed hypersensitivity reaction: an autoradiographic study. *Journal of Immunology* **118**: 529–532.

Purhonen, S., Palm, J., Rossi, D., et al. (2008) Bone marrow-derived circulating endothelial precursors do not contribute to vascular endothelium and are not needed for tumor growth. *Proceeding of the National Academy of Sciences USA* **105**: 6620–6625.

Rafii, S., Lyden, D. (2003) Therapeutic stem and progenitor cell transplantation for organ vascularization and regeneration. *Nature Medicine* **9**: 702–712.

Rao, S., Lobov, I.B., Vallance, J.E., et al. (2007) Obligatory participation of macrophages in an angiopoietin 2-mediated cell death switch. *Development* **134**: 4449–4458.

Rehman, J., Li, J., Orschell, C.M., March, K.L. (2003) Peripheral blood "endothelial progenitor cells" are derived from monocyte/macrophages and secrete angiogenic growth factors. *Circulation* **107**: 1164–1169.

Restinejad, F., Polverini, P.J., Bouck, N. (1989) Regulation of the activity of a new inhibitor of angiogenesis by a cancer suppressor gene. *Cell* **56**: 345–355.

Ribatti, D. (2008) Judah Folkman, a pioneer in the study of angiogenesis. *Angiogenesis* **11**: 3–10.

Ribatti, D. (2009) Endogenous inhibitors of angiogenesis a historical review. *Leukemia Research* **33**: 638–644.

Ribatti, D., Crivellato, E., Molica, S. (2009) Mast cells and angiogenesis in haematological malignancies. *Leukemia Research* **33**: 876–879.

Ruoslahti, E., Yamaguchi, Y. (1991) Proteoglycans as modulators of growth factor activities. *Cell* **64**: 867–869.

Sato, Y. (2006) Update on endogenous inhibitors of angiogenesis. *Endothelium* **13**: 147–155.

Schultz, G.S., Wysocki, A. (2009) Interactions between extracellular matrix and growth factors in wound healing. *Wound Repair and Regeneration* **17**: 153–162.

Senger, D.R., Galli, S.J., Dvorak, A.M., et al. (1983) Tumor cells secrete a vascular permeability factor that promotes accumulation of ascites fluid. *Science* **219**: 983–985.

Senger, D.R., Perruzzi, C.A., Feder, J., et al. (1986) A highly conserved vascular permeability factor secreted by a variety of human and rodent tumor cell lines. *Cancer Research* **46**: 5629–5632.

Senger, D.R., Claffey, K.P., Benes, J.E., et al. (1997) Angiogenesis promoted by vascular endothelial growth factor: regulation through alpha1beta1 and alpha2beta1 integrins. *Proceedings of the National Academy of Sciences USA* **94**: 13612–13617.

Sepp, N.T., Li, L.J., Lee, K.H., et al. (1994) Basic fibroblast growth factor increases expression of the alpha v beta 3 integrin complex on human microvascular endothelial cells. *Journal of Investigative Dermatology* **103**: 295–299.

Shawber, C.J., Das, I., Francisco, E., et al. (2003) Notch signaling in primary endothelial cells. *Annals of the New York Academy of Sciences* **995**: 162–170.

Sholley, M.M., Cavallo, T., Cotran, R.S. (1977) Endothelial proliferation in inflammation, I. autoradiographic studies following thermal injury to the skin of normal rats. *American Journal of Pathology* **89**: 277–296.

Singer, A.J., Clark, R.A. (1999) Cutaneous wound healing. *New England Journal of Medicine* **341**: 738–746.

Stojadinovic, O., Brem, H., Vouthounis, C., et al. (2005) Molecular pathogenesis of chronic wounds: the role of beta-catenin and c-myc in the inhibition of epithelialization and wound healing. *American Journal of Pathology* **167**: 59–69.

Streit, M., Velasco, P., Riccardi, L., et al. (2000) Thrombospondin-1 suppresses wound healing and granulation tissue formation in the skin of transgenic mice. *EMBO Journal* **19**: 3272–3282.

Suh, W., Kim, K.L., Kim, J.M., et al. (2005) Transplantation of endothelial progenitor cells accelerates dermal wound healing with increased recruitment of monocytes/macrophages and neovascularization. *Stem Cells* **23**: 1571–1578.

Sunderkötter, C., Goebeler, M., Schulze-Osthoff, K., et al. (1991) Macrophage-derived angiogenesis factors. *Pharmacology Therapeutics* **51**: 195–216.

Sunderkötter, C., Steinbrink, K., Goebeler, M., et al. (1994) Macrophages and angiogenesis. *Journal of Leukocyte Biology* **55**: 410–422.

Swift, M.R., Weinstein, B.M. (2009) Arterial-venous specification during development. *Circulation Research* **104**: 576–588.

Taniguchi, K., Ishizaki, T., Sugiyama, Y., et al. (2009) Sprouty4 deficiency potentiates Ras-independent angiogenic signals and tumor growth. *Cancer Science* **100**: 1648–1654.

Tannock, I.F., Hayashi, S. (1972) The proliferation of capillary endothelial cells. *Cancer Research* **32**: 77–82.

Toyofuku, T., Zhang, H., Kumanogoh, A., et al. (2004) Dual roles of Sema6D in cardiac morphogenesis through region-specific association of its receptor, Plexin-A1 with offtrack and vascular endothelial growth factor receptor type 2. *Genes and Development* **18**: 435–447.

Unanue, E.R. (1976) Secretory function of mononuclear phagocytes a review. *American Journal of Pathology* **83**: 396–418.

Urbich, C., Heeschen, C., Aicher, A., et al. (2003) Relevance of monocytic features for neovascularization capacity of circulating endothelial progenitor cells. *Circulation* **108**: 2511–2516.

van Furth, R., Cohn, Z.A., Hirsch, J.G., Humphrey, J.H., Spector, W.G., Langevoort, H.L. (1972) The mononuclear phagocyte system: a new classification of macrophages, monocytes, and their precursor cells. *Bulletin of the World Health Organization* **46**(6): 845–852.

van Hinsbergh, V.W., Engelse, M.A., Quax, P.H. (2006) Pericellular proteases in angiogenesis and vasculogenesis. *Arteriosclerosis, Thrombosis and Vascular Biology* **26**(4): 716–728.

Waltenberger, J. (2009) VEGF resistance as a molecular basis to explain the angiogenesis paradox in diabetes mellitus. *Biochemical Society Transactions* **37**: 1167–1170.

Willms-Kretschmer, K., Flax, M.H., Cotran, R.S. (1967) The fine structure of the vascular response in hapten-specific delayed hypersensitivity and contact dermatitis. *Laboratory Investigation* **17**: 334–339.

Wilson, B.D., Li, M., Park, K.W., et al. (2006) Netrins promote developmental and therapeutic angiogenesis. *Science* **313**: 640–644.

Witt, D.P., Lander, A.D. (1994) Differential binding of chemokines to glycosaminoglycan subpopulations. *Current Biology* **4**: 394–400.

Zeng, Q., Li, S., Chepeha, D., et al. (2005) Crosstalk between tumor and endothelial cells promotes tumor angiogenesis by MAPK activation of Notch signaling. *Cancer Cell* **8**: 1–11.

Zhang, X., Lawler, J. (2007) Thrombospondin-based antiangiogenic therapy. *Microvascular Research* **74**: 90–99.

Zhang, Z., Neiva, K.G., Lingen, M.W., et al. (2009) VEGF-dependent tumor angiogenesis requires inverse and reciprocal regulation of VEGFR1 and VEGFR2. *Cell Death and Differentiation* **17**(3): 499–512.

8 Wound Healing of Extraction Sockets

Roberto Farina and Leonardo Trombelli

Research Centre for the Study of Periodontal and Peri-implant Diseases, University of Ferrara, Ferrara, Italy

HEALING OF EXTRACTION SOCKETS

Histological aspects

The extraction of a tooth initiates a series of reparative processes involving both hard tissue (i.e. alveolar bone) and soft tissues (periodontal ligament, gingiva). The biological events occurring during the healing of an extraction socket and their chronological sequence have been studied in different animal models (e.g. Yoshiki and Langeland 1968; Kuboki et al. 1988; Hsieh et al. 1994; Lin et al. 1994; Lekic et al. 2001; Cardaropoli et al. 2003, 2005; Kanyama et al. 2003; Sato and Takeda 2007), and these studes have helped to characterize the tissues involved in the healing process of extraction sockets. According to the existing literature, a gross classification of these tissues can be as following: blood clot (BC), consisting of erythrocytes and leukocytes embedded in a fibrin network; granulation tissue (GT), rich in newly formed vascular structures, inflammatory cells and erythrocytes; provisional matrix (PM), presenting densely packed mesenchymal cells, collagen fibers and vessels but no or only scattered inflammatory cells; woven bone (WB), consisting of fingerlike projections of immature bone embedded in a primary spongiosa; lamellar bone and marrow (LB/BM), i.e. lamellae of mature, mineralized bone harboring secondary osteons surrounded by marrow spaces rich in vessels, adipocytes, mesenchymal cells and inflammatory cells.

The different animal models share a common sequence of post-extraction healing events involving the above-listed tissues, yet with a different timing. In other words, in such animal experiments new tissue formation in the socket follows a well-defined course. Immediately after tooth extraction, the socket fills with blood and BC formation occurs. The BC fills the socket up to the soft tissue margins of the wound. Portions of the severed periodontal ligament, containing large numbers of mesenchymal cells, fibers and blood vessels, are in direct contact with the BC. In the center of the BC, firstly, and in the marginal portions of the BC, secondly, erythrocytes undergo lysis by coagulative necrosis. Starting from the marginal portion of the socket, several areas of the BC are progressively replaced by GT. Later on, the residual principal fibers of the severed periodontal ligament, which are perpendicular to the surface of the hard tissue wall and inserted in the bundle bone, accompany the formation of a PM towards the

Oral Wound Healing: Cell Biology and Clinical Management, First Edition. Edited by Hannu Larjava.

center of the extraction socket. The PM replaces in part the fiber bundles of the periodontal ligament as well as residues of the BC and GT.

The coronal portion of the extraction socket is progressively covered by a plug of well-organized fibrous connective tissue, partially lined with epithelial cells. The active synthesis and deposition of collagen fibers to form the PM anticipates the deposition of mineralized tissue. At this time, several osteoclasts are present in the marrow spaces within the bundle bone lining the socket as well as in the Volkmann canals, sustaining the remodeling process of the socket. The progressive loss of the periodontal ligament and the bundle bone is paralleled by the deposition of an osteoid matrix and its progressive mineralization within the socket. The mineral apposition rate, mineralizing surface and mineral formation rate tend to decrease from the lingual to the buccal regions. In several areas, the resorption of the bundle bone leads to a communication between the bone marrow spaces of the neighboring interdental septa and the newly formed WB in the socket. The trabeculae of WB extend from the old bone of the socket walls towards the center of the wound, and are often associated with the deposition of newly formed blood vessels. The formation of WB progressively restricts the presence of PM to the central portion of the socket. This time interval coincides with the highest content in mineralized tissue of the extraction socket. Osteoclasts are present on the socket walls up to surface of the native LB of the crestal region lateral to the extraction socket, but the osteoclastic resorbing activity involves also the trabeculae of newly formed WB, indicating that the process of modeling/remodeling of the newly formed bone has begun. The bridge sealing the socket progressively matures in a newly formed hard tissue bridge, mainly composed of WB, separating the repaired marginal mucosa from the extraction socket. Further, most of the WB in the socket apical of the bridge is replaced with LB and BM. The marginal hard tissue bridge is then reinforced by layers of lamellar bone deposited on the top of the previously formed woven bone. Concomitantly, collagen fibers from the lining mucosa become inserted in the new 'cortical' bone and, hence, a periosteum-like structure is established. At this stage of healing, the entire region of the extraction socket apical to the socket sealing bridge is characterized by a high content of well-organized BM and trabeculae of LB.

Socket repair after tooth extraction has also been studied in humans (Claflin 1936; Mangos 1941; Christopher 1942; Amler et al. 1960; Amler et al. 1964; Boyne 1966; Amler 1969; Evian et al. 1982; Trombelli et al. 2008). Immediately after tooth extraction, the socket fills with blood and BC formation occurs (Amler 1969). Within the first week after tooth removal, the BC that first filled the socket space is almost entirely remodeled and replaced with granulation tissue. After 1 week of tissue modeling, deposition of mineralized tissue begins (Amler et al. 1960; Amler 1969). After 2–4 weeks, erythrocytes scattered in between mesenchymal cells can still be observed, although typical structured BC formations are not anymore (Fig. 8.1a). At this phase of healing, GT and PM were shown to represent the dominating tissues, constituting on average about 30% and 50% of the total tissue filling the socket (Trombelli et al. 2008; Fig. 8.1b). Within 6–8 weeks of healing, most of the GT is replaced with PM and WB and the marginal portion of the socket harbors islands of immature WB (Amler et al. 1960; Evian et al. 1982; Trombelli et al. 2008; Fig. 8.1c). In specimens obtained between 6 and 8 weeks, PM and WB were shown to occupy about 60% and 35% of the tissue sample respectively (Trombelli et al. 2008). PM and WB also dominate in the late phase of healing (12–24 weeks), while LB/BM is less frequently observed and less represented, if present (Fig. 8.1d). Thus, the bone organization and architecture is often not completed at 24 weeks after tooth extraction (Fig. 8.2).

(a)

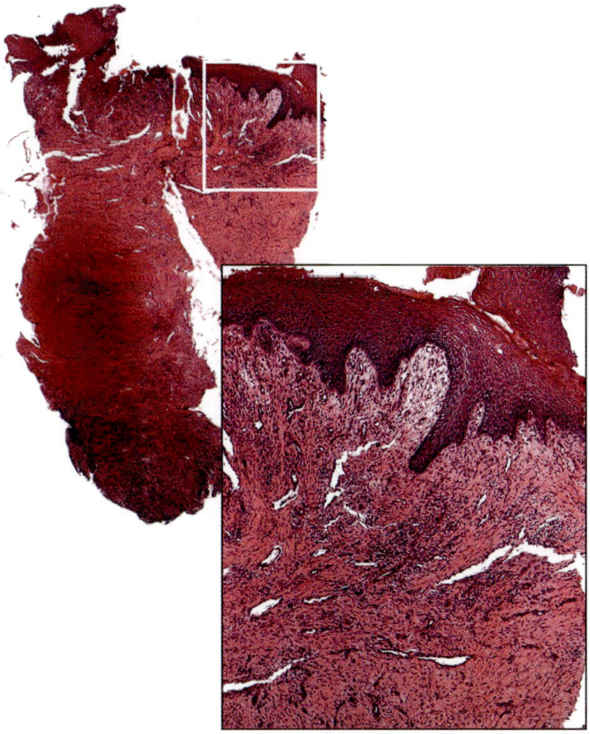

(b)

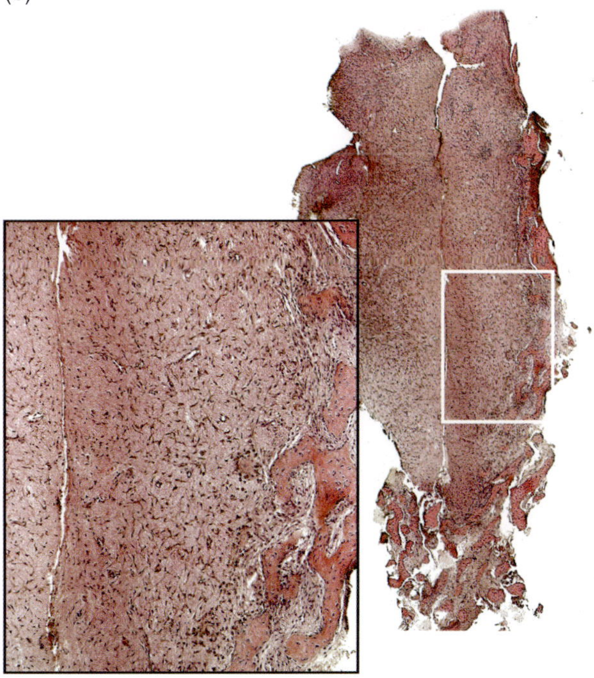

Fig. 8.1 Histological aspects of the spontaneous wound healing process of extraction sockets. (a) A biopsy obtained after 3 weeks of healing. The tissue is rich in vessels, fibroblasts and inflammatory cells and is characterized as granulation tissue. Original magnification × 2.5. (b) A biopsy obtained after 4 weeks of healing. The provisional matrix comprises mesenchymal cells, densely packed fibers and vessels. Only a few inflammatory cells can be observed. Original magnification × 2.5.

(c)

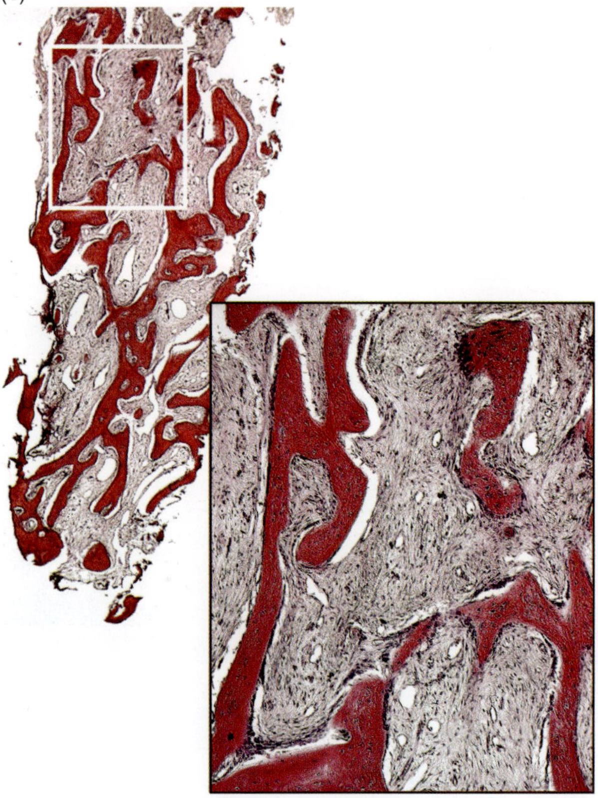

(d)

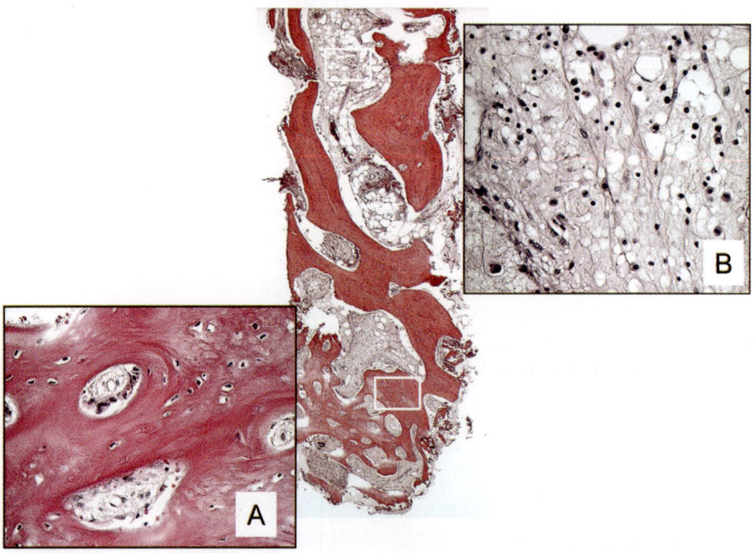

Fig. 8.1 (c) Decalcified section obtained from a biopsy sampled after 6 weeks of healing. Note the presence of trabeculae of immature woven bone that occur in a cell- and fibre-rich provisional matrix. Original magnification × 2.5. (d) Biopsy obtained from an extraction wound representing 12 weeks of healing. The tissue comprises more mature bone: woven bone and lamellar bone that reside in a non-mineralized matrix. Original magnification × 2.5. [Reprinted from Trombelli, L., Farina, R., et al. (2008). Modeling and remodeling of human extraction sockets. *J Clin Periodontol* **35**: 630–639.]

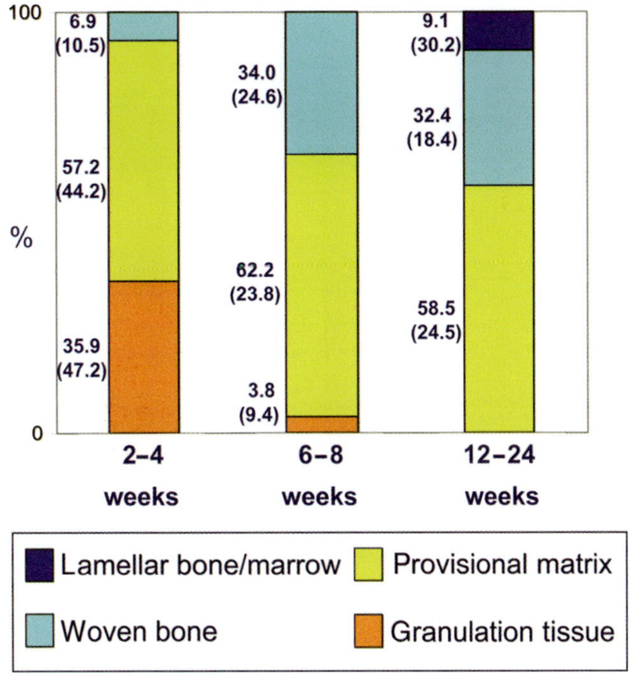

Fig. 8.2 Distribution (mean percentage, standard deviation in parenthesis) of the tissue components (granulation tissue, provisional matrix, woven bone, lamellar bone/bone marrow) at different stages of the healing (i.e. 2–4 weeks, 6–8 weeks and 12–24 weeks) of human extraction sockets. [Reprinted from Trombelli, L., Farina, R., et al. (2008). Modeling and remodeling of human extraction sockets. *J Clin Periodontol* **35**: 630–639.]

Clinical aspects

Previous animal studies have demonstrated that the alveolar socket undergoes substantial dimensional alterations after tooth extraction. In a dog model, Araújo and Lindhe (2005) evaluated the processes of bone modeling and remodeling occurring following tooth extraction as well as the dimensional alterations of the buccal and lingual wall of the socket with associated biological events. Over an 8-week observation interval, a marked osteoclastic activity was observed, resulting in bone resorption at the crestal region of both the buccal and the lingual bone wall. While at 1 week following tooth extraction the thinner buccal bone wall was located coronal to the lingual wall, after 2, 4, and 8 weeks of healing the buccal crest was found consistently apical of its lingual counterpart (Araújo and Lindhe 2005). Consistent with these observations, several human studies have confirmed that the alveolar process undergoes atrophy following the loss of single or multiple teeth in humans (Pietrokovski and Massler 1967; Johnson 1969; Schropp et al. 2003; Pietrokovski et al. 2007; Figs. 8.3a–e). When edentulous sites were evaluated on dried skulls, the crest of the edentulous surface was found to shift lingually when compared to the original position of the teeth before extraction. From the bucco-lingual view, the residual ridge formed a concavity or went straight between the alveolar crests of the adjacent remaining teeth (Pietrokovski 1975).

A recent systematic review has evaluated the extent of the dimensional changes in height and width of the alveolar bone occurring after tooth extraction in humans (Van der Weijden et al. 2009). Twelve studies were included and used for data extraction. Of the selected studies, six were randomized controlled clinical trials, four studies were controlled clinical

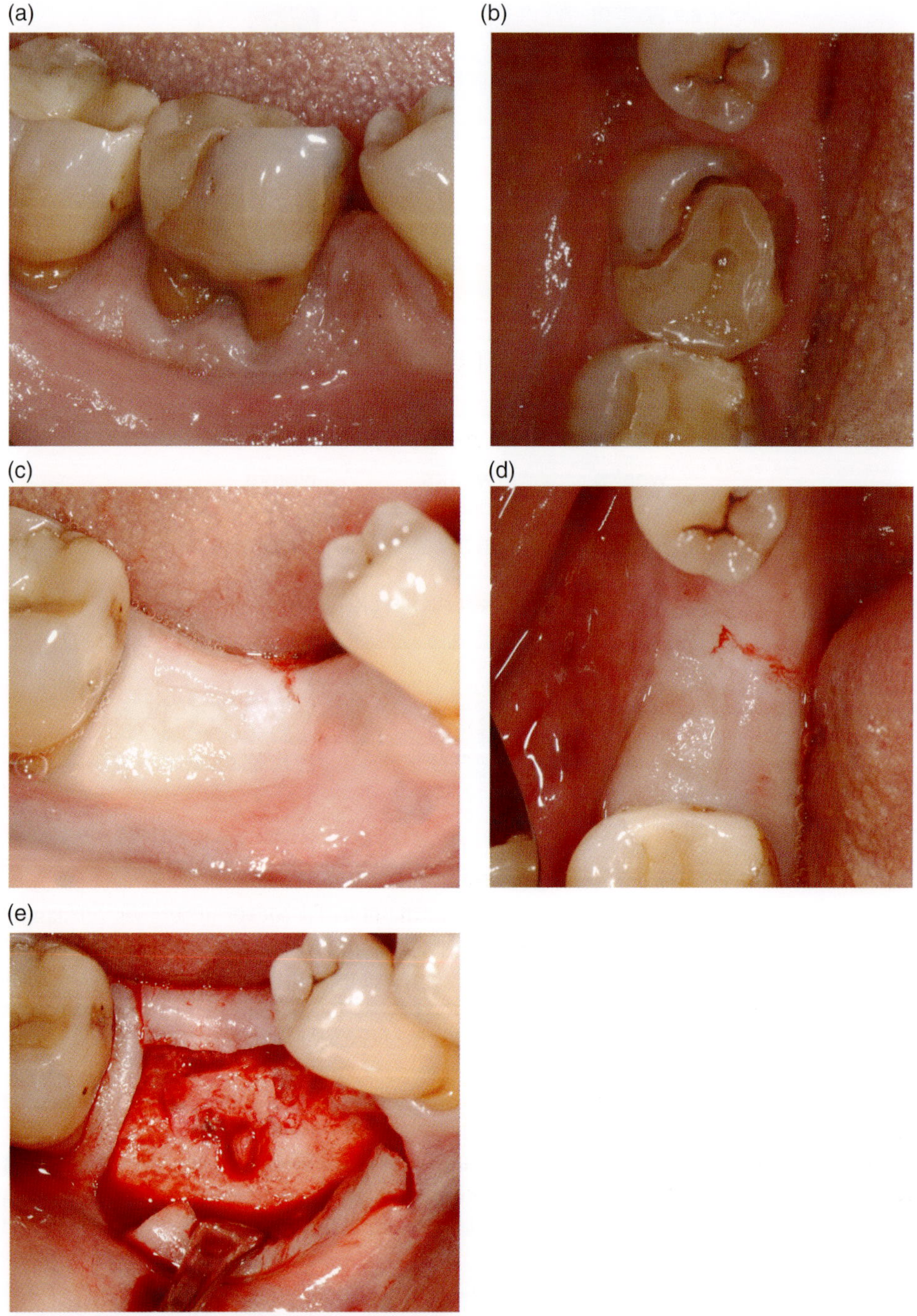

Fig. 8.3 Dimensional alterations of the ridge occurring at 6 months following tooth extraction. (a, b) Lower first molar candidate to extraction in a frontal and occlusal view. (c, d) After 6 months of healing, the site shows a marked volumetric change, mostly due to the loss of the buccal cortical plate. (e) Note the incomplete mineralization of the most coronal part of the extraction socket.

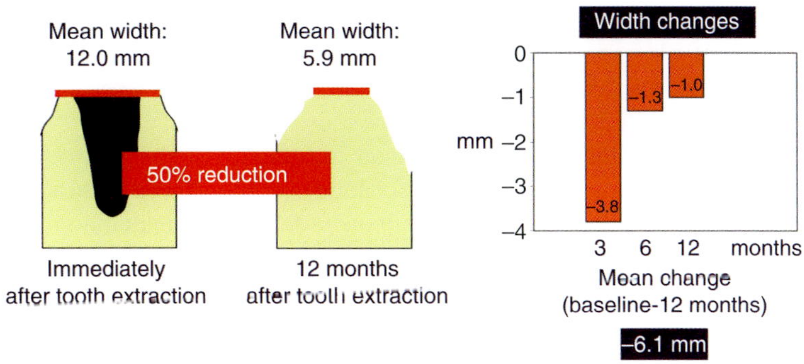

Fig. 8.4 Mean changes of the bucco-lingual ridge width as assessed on cast models over a period of 12 months following tooth extraction. [Based on data from Schropp, L., Wenzel, A., et al. (2003). Bone healing and soft tissue contour changes following single-tooth extraction: a clinical and radiographic 12-month prospective study. *Int J Periodont Restor Dent* **23**: 313–323.]

trials, one study was a case series and one study was a prospective clinical trial. Most of the extracted data concerned control groups/teeth in studies that evaluated the effect of different therapies on the dimensional alterations of extraction sockets. Most studies evaluated the effect of tooth extraction at anterior and premolar sites. Over an evaluation period of 3–12 months after tooth extraction, a weighted mean reduction in height of 1.67 mm was reported for the buccal wall, while the loss at the lingual counterpart was 2.03 mm. At the approximal aspects of the neighboring teeth, a mean loss of 0.64 mm was reported. Socket fill in height as measured relative to the original socket floor was on average 2.57 mm. When dimensional changes in height and width of the alveolar socket were investigated on radiographs, clinical measurements of change in bone height were substantially confirmed at all extraction socket aspects. The weighted mean reduction in width of the alveolar ridges, as clinically and radiographically assessed, was 3.87 mm and 1.21 mm, respectively (Van der Weijden et al. 2009).

Interestingly, a recent study evaluated the contribution of vertical ridge resorption to the difference in bone height (measured as the distance between the alveolar crest and the sinus floor) between edentulous and contralateral dentate posterior maxillary sites. Such contribution was 76% at first premolar sites, 54% at second premolar sites, 80% at first molar sites and 75% at second molar site. The residual difference in bone height between dentate and edentulous sites was explained by the pneumatization of the maxillary sinus floor (Farina et al. 2011).

The dimensional modifications in the profile of the gingival tissues occurring over a period of 12 months after tooth extraction were studied on cast models in the premolar and molar regions of 46 patients (Schropp et al. 2003; Fig. 8.4). Marked alterations were generally observed after tooth removal. Immediately after tooth extraction, the most occluso-buccal point was located on average 1.3 mm more apically than the occluso-oral point. After 12 months of healing, this difference was reduced to 0.2 mm as a result of a tissue gain of 0.3 mm buccally and a tissue loss of 0.8 mm orally. Most of the tissue gain occurred between 3 and 12 months following extraction, whereas almost the entire tissue loss took place during the first 3 months. An average reduction in ridge width of approximately 50% was found, i.e. from 12.0 mm to 5.9 mm, of which two-thirds occurred during the first 3 months of healing. The results of this study indicate that substantial modifications of the soft tissue profile occur during the first months after tooth removal, but the process of remodeling may continue up to 12 months after tooth extraction (Schropp et al. 2003).

FACTORS INFLUENCING THE HEALING OF EXTRACTION SOCKETS

Despite the results from the animal and human histological studies delineating a well-defined tendency of each tissue component to change over time, these studies also revealed great inter-individual variation with respect to tissue formation and maturation. In particular, it was observed that whereas a provisional connective tissue seems to form consistently within the first weeks of healing, the interval during which mineralized bone is laid down is much less predictable (Trombelli et al. 2008). This variability in the wound healing process is also paralleled by a large variation in the dimensional alteration of the healing socket. The reason for this variation is presently not understood but may be linked to different factors which may be, at least in part, related to patient and site characteristics as well as surgical variables.

Smoking

According to the results of a 6-month prospective study (Saldanha et al. 2006), smoking may negatively affect the extent of the dimensional reduction occurring after tooth extraction. Based on Saldanha et al.'s observations, an additional reduction of 0.5 mm in bone height may be expected following tooth extraction in smokers compared to non-smokers. However, the mechanisms by which tobacco smoke interferes with post-extraction wound healing are presently not understood.

Flapless tooth extraction

It is well established that the elevation of a full-thickness flap (muco-periostal flap) may cause loss of attachment and resorption of bone (for a review see Heitz-Mayfield et al. 2002). The reported crestal bone loss after a full-thickness flap elevation is approximately 0.6 mm (Wood et al. 1972). In a dog model of post-extraction healing, an additional volumetric shrinkage of 0.5–0.7 mm was observed 2 months after flap elevation and tooth extraction compared to flapless tooth extraction, mostly due to an increased resorption of the buccal wall of the socket. At 4 months, the observed differences were substantially unaltered (Fickl et al. 2008a). Recently, however, a study by Araújo and Lindhe (2009a) reported that both flap and flapless groups showed similar post-extraction dimensional alterations when compared with the corresponding tooth site, thus suggesting that the difference between flap and flapless procedures may disappear after 6-month healing periods.

Location of the edentulous site

When an intra-subject comparison of the extent of vertical ridge resorption was performed between dentate and contralateral edentulous maxillary posterior sextants on computerized tomography scans, second premolar and second molar edentulous sites showed a more apical position of the alveolar crest compared to dentate sites (Farina et al. 2011). This observation seems to suggest that vertical ridge resorption may occur with a different pattern depending on the location of the extraction site. Consistent with these findings, data obtained from a large cohort of subjects reported that the alveolar crest resorption [calculated as the distance from the alveolar crest to an ideal line passing through the cemento-enamel junction

(CEJ) of the missing teeth] was different among posterior maxillary edentulous sites. A statistically significant effect of edentulous site on alveolar resorption was observed, with second molar sites showing a higher resorption compared to first and second premolar sites (Pramstraller et al. 2011). When the changes in the height of the alveolar crest occurring after tooth extraction were measured on soft tissues, however, height loss was not significantly different in premolar compared to molar post-extraction sites (Schropp et al. 2003).

In the study by Farina et al. (2011), the site location significantly affected the difference in ridge width between dentate and contralateral edentulous sites. Pramstraller et al. (2011) reported a statistically significant effect of edentulous site location on residual ridge width, with molar sites showing a significantly greater width than premolar sites. Post-extraction dimensional variations, as measured on soft tissues, revealed a greater bucco-lingual collapse of the alveolar ridge in molar sites compared to premolar sites (Schropp et al. 2003).

Single versus multiple extractions

In a study conducted on a large sample of dried skulls, a more pronounced concavity was frequently observed in multiple adjacent edentulous sites compared to single tooth edentulous sites (Pietrokovski 1975). Consistently, when the absence of teeth adjacent to the edentulous site was evaluated as a predictor variable for the dimensions of the alveolar ridge, the absence of both teeth mesial and distal to the edentulous site negatively influenced both the extent of vertical alveolar crest resorption and the bucco-lingual ridge width (Pramstraller et al. 2011). These observations are supported by the results of a recent systematic review, reporting a detrimental effect of tooth extraction on alveolar bone height at the approximal aspects of the teeth adjacent to the lacuna, resulting in a bone loss of 0.64 mm (Van der Weijden et al. 2009).

Chlorhexidine mouth rinse following tooth extraction

It was previously reported that patients rinsing with a chlorhexidine digluconate mouth rinse for 30 days after tooth extraction showed a 0.06-mm reduction in bone height after tooth extraction, while patients rinsing with a placebo solution lost almost 1 mm over a 6-month period (Brägger et al. 1994). The mechanisms by which chlorhexidine exerts a protective effect towards dimensional alterations of the post extraction socket are presently unknown.

HEALING OF EXTRACTION SOCKETS FOLLOWING IMMEDIATE IMPLANT PLACEMENT

Immediate implant (II) placement consists of the insertion of an implant into a fresh extraction socket. II placement has been proposed primarily to reduce the number of surgical interventions needed to perform an implant-supported rehabilitation and shorten the treatment time. In addition, it was previously advocated that II placement could potentially reduce the extent of alveolar bone resorption after tooth loss.

The placement of an implant into a fresh extraction socket usually results in the direct bone-to-implant contact in the apical, narrowest part of the alveolus, providing the apical osseous anchorage to ensure a high degree of initial mechanical stability, while resulting in a circumferential gap in the most coronal portion. IIs have been repeatedly shown to have success and survival rates similar to implants placed into a healed socket (Stafford 2009).

In this chapter, only the healing dynamics occurring following II placement as well as the factors influencing the healing pattern following the insertion of the implant will be taken into consideration.

Histological aspects

Animal studies have shown that the bone-to-implant gap which is observed after II placement may heal with apposition of newly formed bone (Fujii et al. 1998; Rimondini et al. 2005). In particular, the deposition of immature mineralized tissue may be observed during the first days after immediate implantation (Fujii et al. 1998), and the circumferential gap between the socket walls is progressively filled with newly formed bone and paralleled by an increase in the bone-to-implant contact (Rimondini et al. 2005). During the healing process, the epithelium remains confined to the area of the alveolar crest and never migrates much deeper with respect to the top of the alveolar bone level (Rimondini et al. 2005). In humans, histologic specimens retrieved from healed extraction sites with IIs showed the formation of a sulcular epithelium, an epithelial attachment as well as the organization of a dense, well-vascularized supracrestal connective tissue (Cornelini 2000).

Clinical aspects

In a dog model, a partial loss of osseo-integration was observed at 3 months from implant placement as a result of tissue modeling, determining a resorption of the buccal bone wall with an apical displacement of more than 2 mm (Araújo et al. 2006a). When the 3-month variations in the height of the buccal and lingual socket walls were compared with sites where IIs had been placed and non-implanted post-extraction sites, no significant difference was observed (Araújo et al. 2005). Thus, II placement seems not to prevent the dimensional alterations of the alveolar crest occurring after tooth extraction.

The dimensional alterations of extraction sites implanted immediately after tooth removal have also been studied in humans (Covani et al. 2003, 2004a; Botticelli et al. 2004). Previous authors have observed that narrow peri-implant defects tend to heal spontaneously with bone fill up to their complete closure (Covani et al. 2003). Differently, wider (exceeding 1.5 mm) horizontal peri-implant defects heal by connective tissue apposition rather than by direct bone-to-implant contact. This connective tissue interface, however, seals even the largest gap with the formation of a barrier which is resistant to probe penetration (Covani et al. 2004a, 2004b). In a recent study by Sanz et al. (2010), the healing of defects surrounding either cylindrical or tapered implants placed immediately after the extraction of a maxilllary incisor, canine or premolar was evaluated at 16 weeks after implant placement. The results of the study showed that peri-implant defects around IIs resolved with a substantial spontaneous defect fill. In particular, the horizontal gap was reduced by 63–80% at the buccal and 58–70% at the palatal aspect, respectively, while the vertical gap was reduced by 65–69% at the buccal and 58–70% at the palatal aspect, respectively (Sanz et al. 2010; Figs. 8.5a–e). The resolution, either partial or complete, of the peri-implant gap, however, is accompanied by a marked bone resorption from the outside of the ridge as well as a loss in ridge height (Covani et al. 2003; Botticelli et al. 2004; Sanz et al. 2010; Figs. 8.5a–e). After 4 months of healing, Botticelli et al. (2004) reported a horizontal reduction of 56% and 30% of the thickness at the buccal and lingual/palatal socket walls, respectively, while Covani et al. (2003) reported that the mean distance between buccal bone and lingual bone decreased from 10.5 ± 1.52 mm at the time of implant placement to 6.8 ± 1.33 mm at second-stage

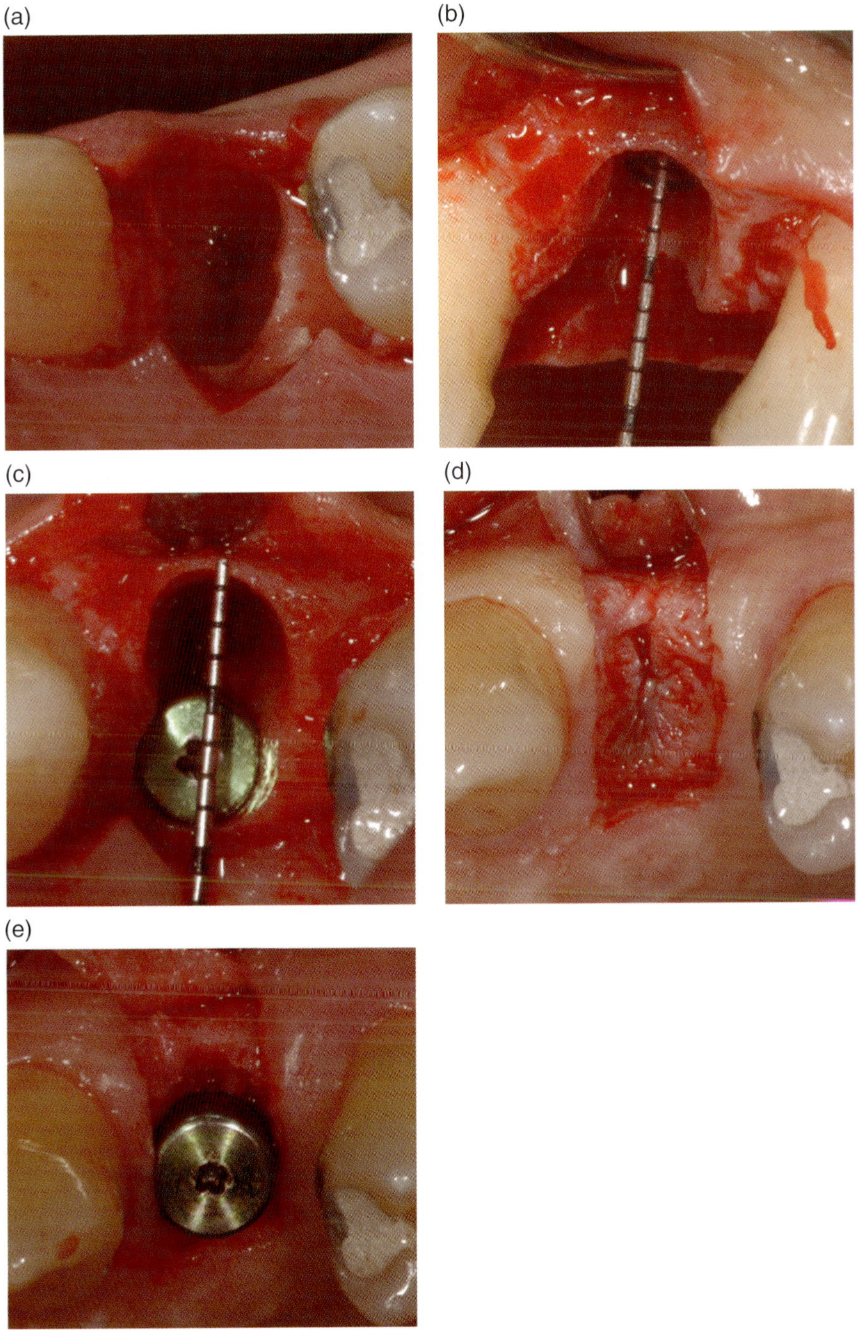

(a) (b) (c) (d) (e)

Fig. 8.5 Spontaneous healing of the bone-to-implant gap around an immediate implant. (a) Extraction socket as observed immediately after the removal of a first maxillary premolar. (b, c) An implant is positioned in the socket immediately after tooth removal. Note that the implant position has been kept more palatal with respect to the center of the socket, and the head of the implant is positioned apical to the bone crest. (d) At the surgical re-entry performed at 3 months following implant placement, the bone-to-implant gap has healed with a substantial spontaneous vertical and horizontal bone fill. (e) A marked resorption of the outer aspect of the buccal cortical plate is also visible.

surgery. In the study by Botticelli et al. (2004), mean vertical reduction of ridge height amounted to 0.3 mm, 0.6 mm, 0.2 mm, and 0.5 mm at the buccal, lingual/palatal, mesial and distal aspects of the socket, respectively.

Healing determinants of extraction sockets after immediate implant placement

A high within-subject variability in the extent of osseo-integration and filling of the bone-to-implant gap with newly formed bone was observed in humans (Wilson et al. 1998), sustaining the role of local, site-specific factors as determinants of the healing of extraction sockets after II placement. Some of these determinants have been identified and their role is depicted in the following sections.

Presence of peri-radicular infection at the time of tooth extraction

In a dog model, Chang et al. (2009) studied the healing of IIs placed in extraction sites with experimentally induced peri-radicular lesions compared to infection-free sites. The results of the study indicated that implants may heal with a high bone-to-implant contact in the absence of complications and implant loss irrespective of the presence of a peri-radicular infection, provided that the extraction socket is carefully debrided before implant installation (Chang et al. 2009). In a human study by Ferrus et al. (2010), at 4-month second-stage surgery IIs placed in periodontitis sites showed a mean vertical defect fill of 60% compared to 83% in non-periodontitis sites. At implant placement, however, the mean vertical depth of the buccal gap was significantly greater at the non-periodontitis than at the periodontitis sites (7.9 mm vs. 5.3 mm). Moreover, periodontitis and non-periodontitis sites showed a similar pattern of healing in terms of horizontal ridge reduction and horizontal gap fill (Ferrus et al. 2010). Overall, these results seem to indicate that the presence of a chronic infection in the extraction socket is not an absolute contraindication for II placement.

Implant location (maxilla/mandible)

A study conducted on mongrel dogs reported the histologic and histomorphometric results concerning bone healing around 13 IIs placed in maxillary and mandibular premolar extraction sockets (Parr et al. 1993). Maxillary implants showed a lower amount of bone apposition around the implants and a greater variability in osseous healing compared to mandibular implants (Parr et al. 1993). At present, however, no specifically designed human studies have evaluated the dental arch as an outcome determinant of IIs.

Implant location (anterior/posterior)

The results of a study conducted on beagle dogs revealed significant differences in the mean extent of bone loss occurring at the buccal crest at 8 weeks after implant placement, being more pronounced at the third premolar site compared to the fourth premolar site. As a potential explanation, the authors advocate that the dimension of the socket might influence the process of wound healing of implants placed into fresh extraction sockets, with more bone loss in the narrower sockets (Vignoletti et al. 2009). Recently, a human study evaluated the differences in the clinical outcomes, as clinically assessed at surgical re-entry at 4 months after implant installation, between IIs placed in anterior (incisor, canine) and posterior (premolar) sites (Ferrus et al. 2010). The results indicated that the mean reduction of the height of the buccal bone crest was, although not statistically significant, twice as large at the anterior than at the posterior sites (−1.4 mm vs. −0.7 mm). In addition, the mean horizontal gap fill was significantly greater at posterior than anterior sites (1.8 mm vs. 1.1 mm). Anterior and posterior sites did not differ significantly in terms of resorption from the outer aspect of the ridge and vertical gap fill (Ferrus et al. 2010). Overall, these results seem to indicate that the implant location (anterior/posterior) is a healing determinant of extraction sockets implanted immediately after tooth removal, with a tendency of anterior sites to show a greater resorption of the buccal wall and a greater horizontal defect fill.

Thickness of the socket bone walls

In a dog model, marked alterations of both the buccal and lingual walls of the socket were observed at 4 and 12 weeks after II installation (Araújo et al. 2006b). However, the thinner, buccal wall underwent a significantly greater apical displacement (> 2 mm) during healing, suggesting an association between the thickness of the socket walls and the extent of bone resorption after II placement (Araújo et al. 2006b). In a human study using a multivariate approach, the size of the residual gap was dependent on the thickness of the bone crest (Tomasi et al. 2010). In particular, a smaller horizontal gap (difference: 0.25 mm), a smaller resorption of the outer surface of the crest (difference 0.45 mm) as well as a smaller reduction of the height of the bony crest (difference 0.59 mm) were observed at the time of re-entry at sites with a thick (> 1 mm) buccal wall compared with sites with a thin (≤ 1 mm) wall. On the palatal aspect, the presence of a thick palatal wall in comparison to a thin wall had a significant impact on the horizontal gap at the time of re-entry, with a reduction of 0.2 mm (Tomasi et al. 2010). Consistently, Ferrus et al. (2010) observed a substantial degree of gap fill at sites where the buccal bone wall was thick (>1 mm) after a 4-month period of healing. Overall, the results from the above-mentioned study indicate that thick (> 1 mm) bone walls favor a greater defect fill when compared to thin (≤ 1 mm) bone walls in sites where IIs have been placed. These findings seem to be of clinical relevance when considering that a thickness ≤ 1 mm of the buccal and/or palatal socket wall is a rather common clinical condition, especially at the anterior and premolar region (Huynh-Ba et al. 2010).

Gingival biotype

In a retrospective study conducted on patients treated with IIs placed with a flapless approach, recession of > 10% of the length of the central incisor crown occurred at 6 out of 25 thin biotype sites compared to 2 out of 19 thick biotype sites (Chen et al. 2009). In a recent prospective study, IIs placed in patients with a thin periodontal biotype showed more mucosal recession than implants placed in cases of thick periodontal tissues (Cordaro et al. 2009).

Flap versus flapless surgery

A study conducted on beagle dogs suggested that II insertion without flap elevation (flapless procedure) may significantly reduce the extent of bone resorption at the buccal aspect when compared to flap surgery and concomitant implant placement (Blanco et al. 2008). In particular, at 3 months after implant placement, IIs placed with a flapless approach showed a mean distance from the peri-implant mucosa margin to the first bone-implant contact at the buccal aspect of 3.02 mm compared to 3.69 mm in the flap group, the difference being statistically significant. No significant differences were found between groups in terms of mucosal recession, percentage of bone-to-implant contact and failure rate (Blanco et al. 2008). In 33 patients with teeth extracted for endodontic or periodontal lesions and replaced with IIs or early implants, a tendency towards lower mean bone loss was observed with the flapless protocol (–0.74 mm) versus flap protocol (–1.02 mm) (Villa and Rangert 2007). At present, however, no randomized clinical trials comparing flapless and flap approaches for the placement of IIs are available.

Submerged versus transmucosal protocol

A randomized controlled clinical trial compared the clinical outcomes of submerged vs. transmucosal tapered IIs. Submerged implants were surgically exposed 8 weeks after the first surgery, then provisionalized at 12 weeks after the first surgery. Soft tissue recession occurred after II placement regardless of submerged or non-submerged implant healing. However, statistically significant differences in the mean value of keratinized tissue height were observed after surgery, with submerged implants showing lower amounts of keratinized tissue when compared with transmucosal implants (mean reduction of KT at year follow-up: transmucosal group: 0.2 mm, submerged group: 1.3 mm) (Cordaro et al. 2009).

Implant micro- and macro-geometry

Previous animal studies failed to find significant differences in the healing pattern after 6 weeks when placing four different implant systems with different micro- and macro-geometry in fresh extraction sockets (de Sanctis et al. 2009). In a dog model, the resorption of the alveolar crest was more marked both at the buccal and lingual aspects of root-form wide implants than at standard cylindrical implants. However, the distance between the alveolar crest and the most coronal bone-to-implant contact, the remaining gap between the implant surface and the inner surface of the alveolar crest, and the defect area represented by the intrabony component characterizing the residual peri-implant defect were significantly smaller around cylindrical implants (Caneva et al. 2010).

When comparing implant systems with different micro- and macro-geometry, no differences in clinical outcomes were observed in a human study (Evans and Chen 2008). In contrast, in a randomized controlled parallel-group multicenter study where cylindrical or tapered implants were used to immediately replace maxillary teeth (Sanz et al. 2010), the mean percentage reduction in the horizontal gap size was greater for cylindrical compared to tapered implants at both buccal (80% vs. 63%) and palatal (70% vs 58%) aspects after 16 weeks of healing.

Different studies have specifically evaluated the effect of the surface characteristics of the implant on post-extraction healing dynamics. In an animal study where IIs were installed in experimental defects, reproducing the peri-implant gap observed in natural fresh extraction sockets, the marginal defects around rough surface implants healed with substantial bone fill and a high degree of osseo-integration. In contrast, healing at turned implants was characterized by incomplete bone fill and the presence of a connective tissue zone between the implant and the newly formed bone. The mean distance between the implant margin and the basis of the residual bone-to-implant gap was lower than 1 mm for implants with a rough surface but higher than 3 mm for implants with a turned surface, the difference being statistically significant (Botticelli et al. 2005). Consistently, grit-blasted implants with retention elements performed better in terms of bone–implant contact and amount of regenerated bone when compared to implants with a machined surface without retention elements in an immediate implantation protocol (Rasmusson et al. 2001). Some animal studies explored the influence of different surface treatments on the outcomes of IIs. A pilot study conducted on mongrel dogs suggested that bone-to-implant gaps around IIs with a hydroxyapatite coating may heal with a higher bone-to-implant contact compared to gaps surrounding titanium plasma-sprayed implants after 8 weeks of healing (Karabuda et al. 1999). The results of two recent studies conducted on beagle dogs showed that an enhanced nano-topography of the implant surface has a limited effect on the II surgical protocol. In particular, sites implanted with fixtures characterized by a nano-surface topography exhibited less buccal bone resorption (about 0.3 mm) than the control sites (about 1 mm) at 8 weeks following placement (Vignoletti et al. 2009). Overall, the results of the above-mentioned studies seem to indicate that a rough implant surface and the presence of macroscopic retention elements on the fixture may enhance the healing and limit the dimensional alterations of extraction sockets implanted immediately after tooth removal.

Implant-to-abutment connection

In a case series of 22 patients, 22 implants of 5.5-mm platform diameter were placed in fresh extraction sockets and the bone-to-implant gap was filled with bovine bone matrix and collagen (Canullo et al. 2009). A provisional crown was adapted and adjusted for non-functional immediate positioning to a 3.8-mm-diameter abutment (platform switching group) or a 5.5-mm-diameter abutment (control group). Two months later, definitive prosthetic rehabilitation was performed. Over a mean follow-up of 25 months, a decrease in gingival recession of 0.18 mm was observed in the platform switching group, while a recession increase of 0.45 mm was observed in control group. In contrast, the mean value of bone filling was similar between the two groups (Canullo et al. 2009). At present, however, no specifically designed study has evaluated the impact of implant-to-abutment connection on the healing of extraction sockets implanted immediately after tooth removal without the use of reconstructive techniques.

Morphology and dimensions of the peri-implant defect

Vertical (corono-apical) dimension of the peri-implant defect

In a study by Covani et al. (2007), all bone-to-implant gaps had healed completely 6 months after II placement. The pattern of bone healing around the neck of the implants showed an absence of peri-implant defects, with the vertical distance between the implant shoulder and bone crest ranging from 0 to 2 mm (Covani et al. 2007). In a study by Tomasi et al. (2010), the size of the 4-month residual vertical gap between the shoulder of the implant and the base of the defect was found to be correlated with its baseline value at implant placement. The deeper the initial vertical gap, the deeper the residual vertical gap.

Horizontal (bone-to-implant) dimension of the peri-implant defect

The dimension of the horizontal gap has been positively correlated with the dimension of the residual horizontal gap at 4 months after II placement, at both buccal and lingual aspect (Tomasi et al. 2010). It is well established that small gaps between implant surface and socket wall have a sufficient potential for spontaneous healing (Schropp and Isidor 2008a, 2008b). In this respect, it was previously demonstrated that sites with a horizontal gap of 2 mm or less may heal by spontaneous, complete bone fill (Chen et al. 2004). Although sites with a large (> 1 mm) horizontal bone-to-implant gap have greater healing potential in terms of percentage horizontal defect fill compared to sites with a shallow (≤ 1 mm) gap (Ferrus et al. 2010), peri-implant horizontal gaps exceeding 1.5 mm spontaneously healed by connective tissue apposition, rather than by direct bone-to-implant contact (Covani et al. 2004a). For gaps exceeding 3 mm, a limited reparative potential was observed, with a residual gap ranging from 0.5 mm to 1.5 mm in a substantial proportion of sites at 4-month surgical re-entry (Botticelli et al. 2004).

The displacement of implant position on the bucco-lingual axis may influence the healing pattern of the peri-implant gap. In this respect, it was previosuly demonstrated that the decrease of the buccal gap by the buccal displacement of the implant position resulted in a 0.22-mm apical displacement of the buccal crest for every millimeter of the implant in buccal direction from the center of the alveolus (Tomasi et al. 2010). In a recent animal study, implants installed in a lingual position with respect to the center of fresh extraction sockets showed a lower exposure above the alveolar crest of the endosseous portion of the implant when compared to implants placed in the center of the socket (Caneva et al. 2010). Overall, the available pertinent studies seem to suggest that the greater the horizontal bone-to-implant gap, the greater the extent of spontaneous horizontal defect resolution. For defects with a horizontal gap ≤ 1 mm, defect fill is often sufficient to ensure a complete resolution of the defect.

Bone dehiscence

A damaged buccal bone wall was found to be a risk indicator for a recession of the facial mucosal margin on IIs (Chen and Buser 2009). In a 12-month controlled clinical trial, 15 subjects received transmucosal IIs in molar sites with a considerable (height and width ≥3 mm) buccal bone dehiscence. Although bone dehiscences were treated with a reconstructive technique in conjunction with implant placement, significantly higher pocket probing depth and relative attachment level were observed in these sites compared to sites without bone dehiscences (Siciliano et al. 2009).

Corono-apical position of the implant head

In a recent animal study, implants installed into fresh extraction sockets 1 mm deeper than the level of the buccal alveolar crest and in a lingual position with respect to the center of the alveolus showed a lower exposure above the alveolar crest of the endosseous (rough) portion of the implant when compared to implants placed at the level of the alveolar crest and in the center of the socket (Caneva et al. 2010). In a recent human study, more apically positioned IIs showed less implant exposure at the buccal aspect when compared to implants with a shoulder positioned more closely to the alveolar crest (Tomasi et al. 2010).

Implant loading: immediate versus delayed protocol

In a human histologic split-mouth report, Guida et al. (2008) evaluated the 6-month healing pattern of an immediately loaded II and compared the results with those observed in a non-loaded II. The results of the study indicated that both implants became osseointegrated and clinically stable. No differences were observed in terms of bone-to-implant contact. Around the loaded implant, a more compact, mature, well-organized peri-implant bone was found with many areas of remodeling and some osteons, whereas the bone tissue surrounding the unloaded implant was constituted of only thin bone trabeculae (Guida et al. 2008). Controlled clinical studies indicate that the bone level changes of dental implants placed in fresh extraction sockets and restored immediately are comparable to those obtained in a delayed loading group (Crespi et al. 2008). A recent systematic review reported the results of 10 clinical trials comparing immediate loading of single implant units in fresh extraction sites versus a healed ridge (Atieh et al. 2009). The meta-analysis of all the included studies revealed a significantly higher bone gain in the immediate placement group, with a mean difference of 1.96 mm with respect to the implants placed in a healed ridge. However, a significantly higher risk of implant failure (risk ratio of 3.62) was observed for implants placed in fresh extraction sockets compared to implants placed in a healed ridge (Atieh et al. 2009). Differently, the results of recent controlled clinical trials indicate that immediately loaded IIs splinted in a full-arch restoration have the same extent of peri-implant bone loss and a similarly high (> 95%) survival rate both at 1 year (Pieri et al. 2009) and 5 years (Jaffin et al. 2007) after placement/loading. Even though favorable and predictable results were reported for the immediate implantation and provisionalization of implants both from biologic and clinical points of view, these results should be carefully considered. A recent systematic review stated that maintaining the midfacial gingival margin may be more problematic with an immediate placement and loading protocol, since post-extraction bone remodeling and therefore marginal gingival changes will occur irrespective of the timing of the placement of an implant (De Rouck et al. 2008). In addition, the long-term impact of this remodeling is currently unclear and needs to be elucidated in future research. At present, therefore, II placement and provisionalization should be restricted to specific cases and should be approached with caution in the anterior zone (De Rouck et al. 2008).

DOES THE USE OF RECONSTRUCTIVE TECHNOLOGIES ALTER THE HEALING OF EXTRACTION SOCKETS?

The application of reconstructive technologies at fresh extractions sites is performed in order to improve the quality and maximize the quantity of bone for the placement and osseo-integration of a dental implant, as well as to avoid post-extraction alterations of the ridge profile that may negatively affect the aesthetic of a prosthetic rehabilitation. Three main procedures have been proposed in the literature for the above-mentioned purposes: implantation of graft materials, application of barrier membranes, and implantation/treatment with bioactive agents. Also, combinations of different technologies have been evaluated.

For each reconstructive technology, the histological and clinical findings from the most relevant studies evaluating its application at fresh extraction sites are reported below. Results from controlled studies, if any, evaluating the adjunctive effect of each technology (alone or in combination) to the spontaneous healing of extraction sockets on (1) the tissue components participating in the healing process, and (2) the extent of the dimensional alterations of the socket walls, were retrieved and included.

Graft materials

Rationale for the implantation of graft materials in fresh extraction sockets

Once positioned in the socket immediately after tooth removal, grafts materials act as solid scaffolds which help to stabilize the coagulum during the early phases of healing by impeding the interference of mechanical destabilizing factors on the maturation of the clot into mineralized tissue. A direct modulatory effect on gene expression of osteoblastic cells, leading to an increased production of proteins of the extracellular matrix, was also demonstrated for some graft materials. Ideally, the graft material should sustain the entire healing process of an extraction socket, being progressively resorbed and replaced by vital, mature bone.

Histological aspects

The wound healing process of an extraction socket grafted with a hydroxyapatite-based xenograft was evaluated in several animal studies using a dog model (Cardaropoli et al. 2005; Araújo et al. 2008, 2009, 2010; Araújo and Lindhe 2009b). Within the first days after tooth extraction and socket grafting, a fibrin network entraps the graft particles. Inflammatory cells (mainly polymorphonuclears), first, and osteoclasts, second, migrate to the surface of the particles. In this phase, the osteoclastic activity results in a slow, minimal remotion of material from the outer surface of the graft particles. After 1–2 weeks of healing, the osteoclasts are replaced by osteoblasts, starting the apposition of osteoid tissue in the collagen bundles of the provisional matrix, leading to a progressive osseo-integration of the graft particles (Araújo et al. 2010). After 2 weeks of healing, immature, newly formed trabecular bone may be observed, particularly in the lateral and apical compartments of the socket, while the central and marginal compartments are still occupied by connective tissue that entraps biomaterial particles and inflammatory cells. At this stage of healing, a disturbing effect of the graft on the healing process is evident due to lower amounts of newly formed bone in the apical and lateral compartments of the grafted sockets compared to non-grafted sockets, which, in contrast, show large amounts of woven bone (Araújo et al. 2009). In the intermediate and latest phases of healing, the presence of a biomaterial seems not to exert a detrimental effect on bone formation. At 3 months after tooth extraction and socket grafting, the presence of the graft did not affect the processes of modeling and remodeling of the socket walls and, in particular, it did not influence the amount of mineralized tissue (Araújo et al. 2008). The latest phases of healing of grafted extraction sockets were also studied in experimentally created cylindrical defects resembling tooth extraction wounds (Cardaropoli et al. 2005). After 3 months of healing, in the central and apical portions of the non-grafted defects bone marrow and mineralized bone were about 61% and 39% of the tissues, respectively. In grafted defects, the biomaterial occupied a substantial portion of the tissue volume, with 85% of the periphery of the graft particles being in direct contact with newly formed mineralized bone. Woven bone and bone marrow made up 47% and 26% of the newly formed tissue. When considering the composition of the mineralized tissue present in grafted and non-grafted sockets, similar proportions of woven bone and lamellar bone were observed (Cardaropoli et al. 2005).

The healing stages of extraction wounds grafted with a hydroxyapatite-based biomaterial were partly described also in humans (Artzi et al. 2000, 2001; Carmagnola et al. 2003; Norton et al. 2003; Farina et al. 2005; Heberer et al. 2008; Mangano et al. 2008). Marked *de novo* bone formation was reported at 6 weeks after tooth extraction and socket filling with a xenograft, despite a high inter-individual heterogeneity with respect to the amount of newly formed bone. An increasing gradient of bone density was observed from the coronal to the apical portion of the socket (Heberer et al. 2008). Two studies from the same research group evaluated the healing of extraction sockets grafted with a xenograft at 9 months (Artzi et al. 2000, 2001). The density of bony structure increased from the coronal to the apical compartments of the socket (15.9% and 63.9%, respectively). In accordance, connective tissue showed an inverse tendency, being more present in the coronal compartments (52.4%) compared to the apical compartments (9.5%) of the socket (Artzi et al. 2000). The greater proportion of the newly formed bone in the coronal area was woven-type bone, while lamellar structures were observed mainly in the apical region. More specifically, the lamellar/woven bone ratio varied from 1:12.9 in the coronal area to 1:3.8 in the mid-section area and 1:1.7 in the apical area (Artzi et al. 2001). After 9 months of healing, mineralizing activity was still evident due to the presence of osteoblasts lining the outer surface of the xenograft particles and depositing an osteoid layer (Artzi et al. 2001). Residual graft particles were present in all specimens and occupied a fraction of the total area, ranging from 26.4% to 35.1%, with the majority of the xenograft particles being in direct contact with mineralized tissue and presenting small areas of decalcification on their outer surface (Artzi et al. 2001). Although the degradation of the particles continues also in the long term, hydroxyapatite-based materials may persist in the socket for long periods of time. Mangano et al. (2008) reported that residual graft particles occupied about 38% of the total area of a socket grafted 20 years before histological sampling. All graft particles, however, were in close contact with bone and neither gaps nor fibrous tissues were present at the bone–biomaterial interface (Mangano et al. 2008).

Among the resorbable material grafted into the fresh extraction socket, polylactic-polyglycolide acid (PLGA) and calcium sulfate were the most investigated. In previous studies, polylactic acid was shown not to interfere with the healing process (Olson et al. 1982), with no histologically observable pathological tissue reactions during up to 6 months (Nair and Schug 2004). At 3 months from implantation, particles of PLGA were completely resorbed, and the sockets were filled with newly trabecular bone, highly mineralized and well structured. Control sites also showed well-structured tissue, with a slightly minor percentage of mineralized bone (Serino et al. 2008). At 6 months, bone tissue was highly mineralized, mature and well structured (Serino et al. 2003). In contrast, other studies showed that non-porous PLGA graft caused an initial decalcification of the bone surrounding the extraction sockets that was subsequently repaired along with the bone healing of the extraction sockets (Nair and Schug 2004). It is known that hydraulic degradation of the PLGA copolymers results in the release of lactic acid monomers that are oxidized to pyruvic acid. The latter eventually enters the citric acid cycle and is metabolized to yield energy, CO_2 and water. The release of organic acids from the PLGA graft may result in quantities that could not be immediately metabolized by the body which possibly resulted in an initial demineralization of the bone surrounding the graft (Nair and Schug 2004).

At 3 months after socket grafting, sockets filled with calcium sulfate showed a mean prevalence of trabecular bone of about 58% in all the compartments of the socket, with a complete resorption of the material being entirely replaced by newly formed bone (Guarnieri et al. 2005). The use of calcium sulfate in a wide post-extraction defect resulted in a complete filling of the defect with mature, dense, newly formed bone at 5 months following implantation, with a total resorption of the grafted material (Sbordone et al. 2005).

Clinical aspects

Several pre-clinical studies have evaluated the dimensional changes of post-extraction sockets grafted with deproteinized bovine bone mineral (Araújo et al. 2008, 2009; Fickl et al. 2008b, 2008c, Araújo 2009a, 2009b). Results from these studies consistently indicate that the presence of the xenograft may not inhibit the processes of modeling and remodeling that take place in the socket walls during the 2–6 months following tooth extraction. The xenograft may help to preserve the hard tissue volume and the profile of the ridge in the coronal portion of the socket, limiting, but not avoiding, the post-operative wound shrinkage (Araújo et al. 2008, 2009b; Fickl et al. 2008b, 2008c; Figs. 8.6a–j). In particular, a study by

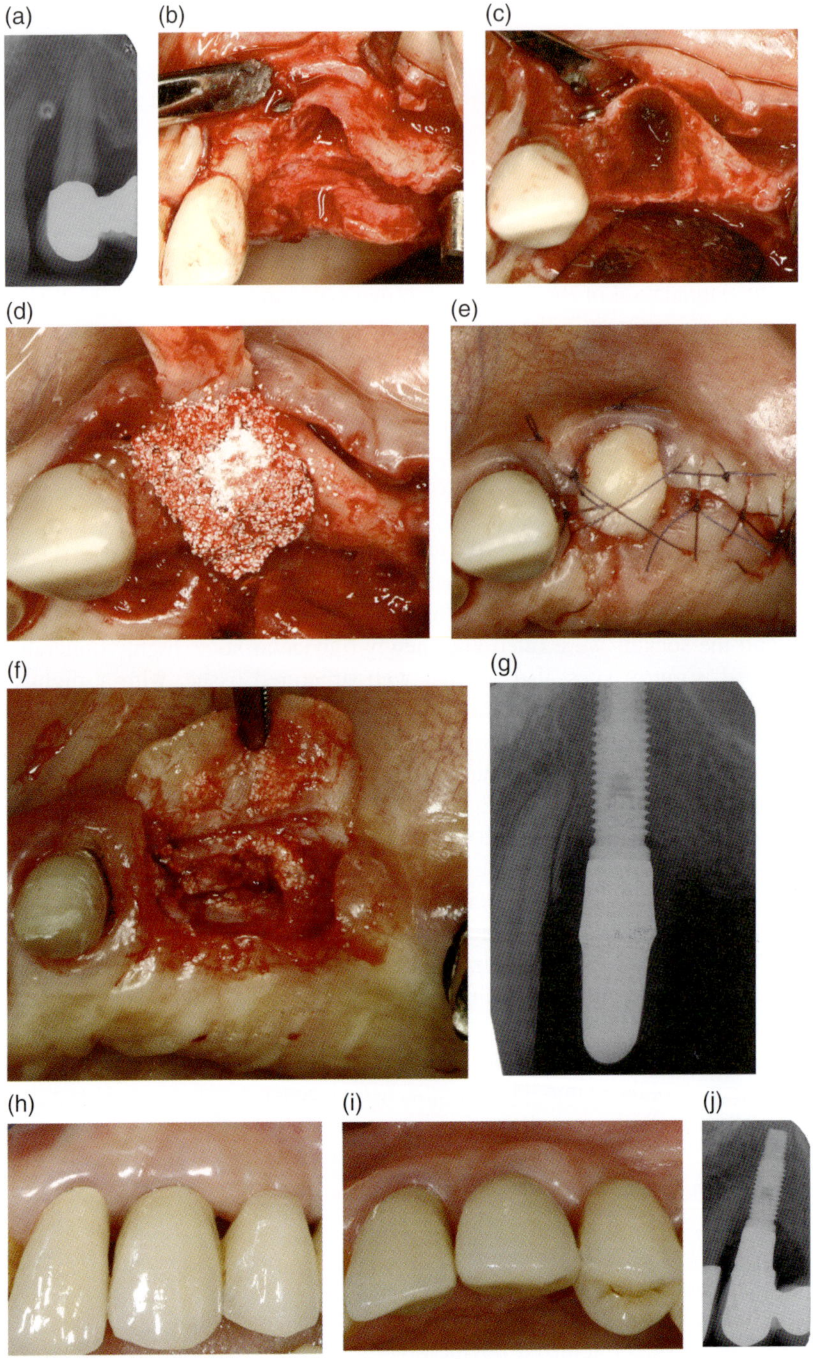

Fig. 8.6 Healing of an extraction socket grafted with a hydroxyapatite-based bone substitute. (a) A maxillary canine is candidated to extraction due to the presence of a deep intraosseous defect complicated by the persistence of a fixation pin left during a previous regenerative procedure. (b, c) After tooth extraction, the socket exhibits thin residual socket walls, particularly at the buccal aspect. (d) The socket is grafted with a hydroxyapatite-based bone substitute (Biostite, GABA Vebas, Rome, Italy). (e) A connective tissue graft is then fixed with sutures over the socket. (f, g) After 4 months, the edentulous site has vertical and horizontal dimensions sufficient for the placement of a 3.75 mm × 13 mm implant. (h, i, j) At 3 years from tooth extraction, the stability of hard and soft peri-implant tissues is maintained.

Fickl et al. (2008b) demonstrated that the incorporation of a xenograft into the extraction socket has a limited impact on the vertical resorption of the buccal crest, while it may significantly reduce the extent of horizontal centripetal contraction of the socket walls, especially at the most coronal portion of the socket (i.e. at 1 mm from the alveolar crest) (Fickl et al. 2008b). When the effect of the placement of a xenograft at the external aspect of the buccal cortical plate on the dimensional alterations of extraction sockets was investigated, a limited effect was found, indicating that overbuilding the buccal aspect in combination with socket preservation is not a suitable technique to compensate for the alterations after tooth extraction (Fickl et al. 2009a, 2009b).

Other studies evaluated the use of different biomaterials. Rothamel et al. (2008) observed that the use of a nanocrystalline hydroxyapatite paste failed to prevent the dimensional modifications of the socket at 3 and 6 months after socket grafting. Differently, an injectable bone substitute obtained by combining a polymer solution and granules of a biphasic calcium phosphate ceramic significantly limited alveolar crest resorption compared to control sockets (Boix et al. 2006). The evidence supporting the use of these materials for socket preservation procedures, however, is still limited.

In humans, the use of a xenograft was investigated in 36 maxillary anterior extraction sites. Grafted sockets showed a loss of less than 20% of the horizontal ridge dimension in 15 of 19 test sites (79%). In contrast, 12 of 17 control sockets (71%) demonstrated a loss of more than 20% in the ridge width (Nevins et al. 2006).

When sockets grafted with a PLGA were compared to control sites, the vertical dimensions of the grafted sockets were better preserved (Serino et al. 2003).

The level of evidence from human studies, in general, and randomized controlled trials, in particular, supporting the rationale for the use of biomaterials to prevent or limit the dimensional alteration of the extraction sockets, however, is still scarce.

Barrier membranes

Rationale for the application of barrier membranes at extraction sites

The enhancement of the healing process of an extraction socket by the placement of a barrier membrane is expected by two main mechanisms: (1) exclusion of the cell populations characterized by a high proliferation rate (i.e. fibroblasts and epithelial cells) from the repopulation of the wound, in order to favor the undisturbed migration and proliferation of cells of the osteoblastic lineage, and (2) providing the space, together with the socket walls, which is needed for defect filling with newly formed bone by limiting the collapse of soft tissues into the wound.

Ideally, a membrane should act as a space-providing barrier up to the formation of hard tissue into the wound, and then should be progressively resorbed in order to avoid a second surgery for its removal.

Histological aspects

Limited histological evidence is presently available with respect to the healing of post-extraction sockets covered with a membrane device.

In six patients with a residual buccal dehiscence occurring after tooth extraction, a non-resorbable (polytetrafluoroethylene) membrane was used. At 6 months after tooth extraction and concomitant membrane placement, lamellar bone with large medullary spaces was present. Increased bone density was observed at 9 months (Dies et al. 1996). Consistent results were obtained in another study evaluating the use of a high-density polytetrafluoroethylene membrane without the use of a graft material. At 12 months after surgery, large amounts of bone were observed (Hoffmann et al. 2008).

When a resorbable membrane was used, large amounts of lamellar bone and bone marrow and small proportions of woven bone were observed. Sites treated with a membrane device showed a lower mean proportion of lamellar bone and a higher proportion of woven bone when compared to non-membrane treated controls (40.1% vs 56.1% and 12.9% vs 0.5%, respectively) (Carmagnola et al. 2003).

Clinical aspects

In a study by Pinho et al. (2006), single rooted teeth were extracted and the sockets were covered with a non-resorbable titanium membrane. Membranes were removed at least 10 weeks after placement. Although a substantial bone fill of the socket was observed, a mean horizontal contraction of the socket walls was also reported (Pinho et al. 2006). When the effect of non-resorbable (e-PTFE) membrane was evaluated and compared to spontaneously healed sockets in a split-mouth study, the adjunctive use of a membrane resulted in a significant preservation of ridge dimensions at 6 months following extraction. It was also observed that this beneficial effect was absent at sites that had previously undergone membrane exposure (Lekovic et al. 1997).

In a study with a similar split-mouth design, the clinical effectiveness of a bioabsorbable membrane (PLGA) was evaluated. No membrane exposure was observed during the experimental period (6 months). At 6 months following tooth extraction, membrane-treated sites were characterized by significantly less loss of alveolar bone height, more internal socket bone fill and less horizontal resorption of the alveolar bone ridge when compared to non-membrane sites (Lekovic et al. 1998).

Bioactive agents

Rationale for the implantation of bioactive agents in fresh extraction sockets

Advances in the areas of cellular and molecular biology have allowed the elucidation of functions of several bioactive agents and their participation in the different phases of wound healing. Recent *in vitro* and *in vivo* studies have confirmed that the administration/delivery of some bioactive agents into the wound can improve the capacity of tissues to regenerate by enhancing cellular chemoattraction, differentiation and proliferation. In recent years, treatment with specific bioactive agents has also been used to influence the wound healing dynamics of fresh extraction sockets.

Histological aspects

The majority of the studies evaluating the healing of post-extraction sockets treated with bioactive agents focused on the use of bone morphogenetic proteins (BMPs). More specifically, several studies evaluated the use of recombinant human BMP-2 (rhBMP-2). In a rat model, a PLGA copolymer-coated gelatin sponge carrier was implanted with or without rhBMP-2 in the mesial root sockets after removal of maxillary first molars. The results indicated that rhBMP-2 may stimulate proliferation and differentiation of mesenchymal cells in the healing extraction wound (Matin et al. 2001). Several clinical studies tested the implantation of rhBMP-2 in fresh extraction sockets (Howell et al. 1997; Cochran et al. 2000; Matin et al. 2001; Fiorellini et al. 2005). In six patients who underwent rhBMP-2 implantation in an absorbable collagen sponge, histological evaluation of the human bone core biopsies revealed the formation of a mineralized tissue identical to the surrounding native bone (Cochran et al. 2000). The use of rhBMP-2 delivered on an absorbable collagen sponge was also compared to the collagen carrier alone as well as no treatment in a human buccal wall defect model following tooth extraction in a large sample of patients. rhBMP-2 treatment resulted in greater amounts of newly formed bone compared to both control treatments, with no difference in bone density and histological quality between newly formed bone and native bone (Fiorellini et al. 2005).

Preliminary clinical evidence suggested a beneficial effect of the use of plasma rich in growth factors of autologous origin in socket preservation procedures (Anitua 1999).

Bone repair was evaluated in extraction sockets treated with peptide 15 (P-15) in either a particulate form or a hydrogel formulation. The histologic evaluation showed enhanced bone formation and active resorption of the implant with both P-15 formulations (Hahn et al. 2003).

Clinical aspects

Limited data are presently available on the dimensional changes of post-extraction sockets conditioned with bioactive agents.

Fresh extraction sockets treated with two different doses (0.75 mg/ml or 1.50 mg/ml) of rhBMP-2 delivered on an absorbable collagen sponge showed that the amount of bone for implant placement was approximately twice as great in the rhBMP-2/ACS groups compared to no treatment or carrier alone (Fiorellini et al. 2005).

Platelet-rich plasma (PRP) was positioned in third molar extraction fresh sockets and clinical and radiographic assessments were performed at 1, 3, 5, 7, 9, 12 and 16 weeks postoperatively. The margins between the socket and surrounding bone, radiopacity of bone filling the socket and presence of trabecular bone formation were evaluated. Radiographic evidence of bone formation was already visible at 1 week only in sockets treated with PRP (Simon et al. 2004).

Combination of different reconstructive technologies

The results of controlled (pre-clinical and clinical) studies evaluating the histologic and clinical effects of the combined use of different reconstructive technologies are summarized in Tables 8.1 and 8.2, respectively. Data concerning the comparison of the combined approach versus either the spontaneous healing or each reconstructive technology when used alone have been reported. A paradigmatic case illustrating the use of a combined graft/membrane approach is reported in Figs. 8.7a–f.

Table 8.1 Studies evaluating the effect of the combination of different reconstructive technologies on the healing of extraction sockets: histological aspects. Only results of controlled (pre-clinical and clinical) studies evaluating the effects of the combined approach versus either the spontaneous healing or each reconstructive technology when used alone have been included.

Author	Year	Animal/ Human	Materials		Observation intervals (time elapsed from socket grafting)	Comparison between test treatment and spontaneous healing	Comparison between test treatment and single reconstructive technology
			Test treatment	Control treatment/s			
			GRAFT+MEMBRANE				
Becker	1996	Human	DFDBA + ePTFE membrane	DFDBA	4–13 months	—	No adjunctive effect of ePTFE membrane over DFDBA
Dies	1996	Human	DFDBA or DBBM + ePTFE membrane	DFDBA, DBBM	6–9 months	—	Graft residual particles retard/impair bone regeneration compared to ePTFE membrane alone
Smukler	1999	Human	DFDBA + ePTFE membrane	Spontaneous healing	8–23 months	No adjunctive effect of ePTFE membrane over spontaneous healing	—
Iasella	2003	Human	FDBA + collagen membrane	Spontaneous healing	4–6 months	More bone in experimental sites, but including also non-vital bone	—
Molly	2008	Human	DBBM, PLA/PGA or CC + ePTFE membrane	ePTFE membrane	6 months	—	Sites treated with DBMM + ePTFE membrane had lower percentage of viable bone compared to membrane alone, while PLA/PGA + ePTFE membrane or CC + ePTFE membrane did not
			GRAFT+BIOACTIVE AGENTS				
Brandao	2002	Animal (rat)	HA+BMPs	Spontaneous healing, HA	7–42 days	No differences in the amount of bone between HA+BMPs and spontaneous healing at 7 days. HA+BMPs resulted in a delayed healing in terms of percentage of new bone at 21 days, but not at 42 days when compared to spontaneous healing	No differences in the amount of bone between HA+BMPs and HA at 7 days. HA+BMPs resulted in a delayed healing in terms of percentage of new bone at 21 days, but not at 42 days compared to HA

Shi	2007	Animal (dog)	CS + PRP	Spontaneous healing, CS	8 weeks	CS + PRP promoted bone formation compared to spontaneous healing	The addition of PRP to CS resulted in the enhancement of bone regeneration in the early phase of healing
Neiva	2008	Human	Xenograft/P15 + collagen dressing material	Collagen dressing material	16 weeks	—	No differences in vital bone, marrow and fibrous tissue between xenograft/P15 + collagen dressing and collagen dressing alone
			GRAFT+SOFT TISSUE GRAFT				
Luczyszyn	2005	human	HA+ADM	ADM	6 months	—	Frequent presence of HA particles enclosed in fibrous connective tissue in sites treated with HA+ADM, not in ADM group
			STEM CELLS				
De Kok	2005	animal (dog)	HA/TCP+BMMSCs	Spontaneous healing, TCP	49 days	No difference in new bone formation area between HA/TCP+BMMSCs and spontaneous healing	Significantly greater new bone formation area in HA/TCP+BMMSCs compared to HA/TCP
Marei	2005	animal (rabbit)	PLA/PGA+BMMSCs	Spontaneous healing, PLA/PGA	2 weeks, 4 weeks	Evidence of active bone deposition in PLA/PGA+BMMSCs at 4 weeks, not in spontaneous healing	Evidence of active bone deposition in PLA/PGA+BMMSCs at 4 weeks, not in PLA/PGA

DFDBA: demineralized freeze-dried bone allograft; ePTFE: expanded polytetrafluoroethylene; DBBM: deproteinized bovine bone mineral; FDBA: freeze-dried bone allograft; PLA/PGA: polylactic/polyglycolic acid; CC: calcium carbonate ceramic; HA: hydroxyapatite BMP: bone morphogenetic protein; CS: calcium sulfate; PRP: platelet rich plasma; P15: peptide 15; ADM: acellular dermal matrix; TCP: tricalcium phosphate; BMMSCs: bone marrow mesenchymal stem cells.

Table 8.2 Studies evaluating the effect of the combination of different reconstructive technologies on the healing of extraction sockets: clinical aspects. Only results of controlled (pre-clinical and clinical) studies evaluating the effects of the combined approach versus either the spontaneous healing or each reconstructive technology when used alone have been included.

Author	Year	Animal/ Human	Materials		Observation intervals (time elapsed from socket grafting)	Comparison between test treatment and spontaneous healing	Comparison between test treatment and single reconstructive technology
			Test treatment	Control treatment/s			
			GRAFT+MEMBRANE				
Iasella	2003	Human	FDBA + collagen membrane	Spontaneous healing	4–6 months	1.6 mm less horizontal contraction for FDBA+collagen membrane compared to spontaneous healing; vertical gain in experimental sockets, vertical loss in control sockets (inter-group difference: 2.2 mm)	—
Pinho	2006	Human	Autologous bone + titanium membrane	Titanium membrane	6 months	—	No difference in vertical and horizontal changes between treatments
Kim	2008	Animal (dog)	DBBM + collagen membrane	Spontaneous healing, DBBM	4 months	Greater bone augmentation in DBBM+collagen membrane compared to spontaneous healing	Greater bone augmentation in DBBM+collagen membrane compared to DBBM
			GRAFT+BIOACTIVE AGENTS				
Shi	2007	Animal (dog)	CS + PRP	Spontaneous healing, CS	2 months	Significantly less reduction in ridge height in CS+PRP compared to spontaneous healing at anterior sites	No significant difference in the reduction of ridge height between CS+PRP and CS

			GRAFT+SOFT TISSUE GRAFT				
Luczyszyn	2005	Human	HA+ADM	ADM	6 months	—	Less horizontal ridge resorption in HA+ADM compared to ADM
Fickl	2008a	Animal (dog)	DBBM + free soft tissue graft	Spontaneous healing	2–4 months	Lower resorption rate of buccal and lingual crest compared to spontaneous healing	—
Fickl	2008b	Animal (dog)	DBBM + free soft tissue graft	Spontaneous healing, DBBM	4 months	No difference in vertical changes and lower horizontal (at 1 mm from the crest) resorption compared to spontaneous healing	Greater vertical changes and lower horizontal resorption (at 1 mm from the crest) compared to DBBM
Fickl	2008c	Animal (dog)	DBBM + free soft tissue graft	Spontaneous healing, DBBM	2–4 months	Lower resorption of buccal crest compared to spontaneous healing	No difference in buccal and lingual crest resorption compared to DBBM

FDBA: freeze-dried bone allograft; DBBM: deproteinized bovine bone mineral; CS: calcium sulfate; PRP: platelet rich plasma; HA: hydroxyapatite; ADM: acellular dermal matrix.

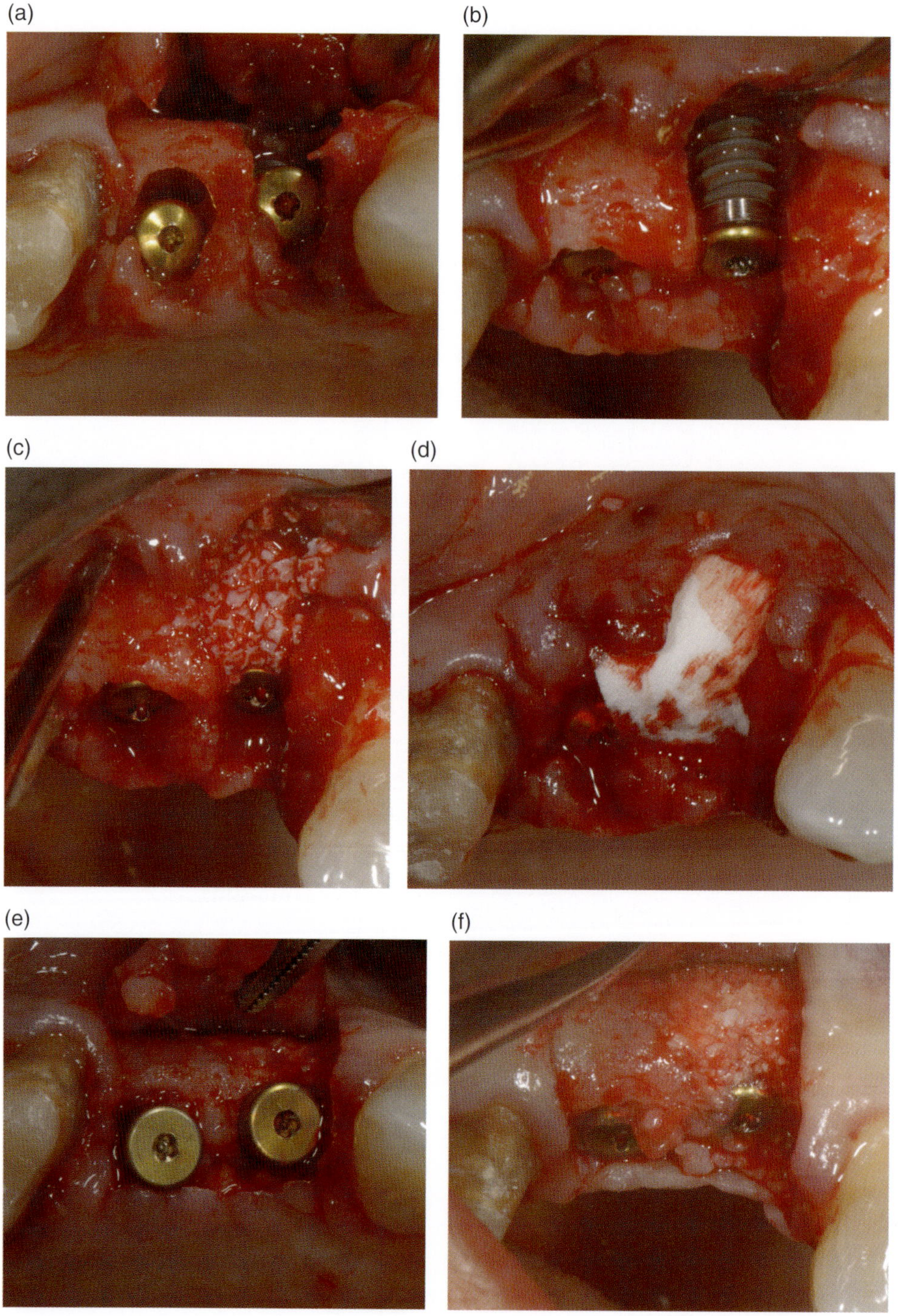

Fig. 8.7 Healing of an extraction socket with immediate implant placement and concomitant treatment with a combined graft/membrane procedure. (a) Immediate implant insertion at fresh extraction sockets of teeth 1.4 and 1.5. (b) Note the severe bone dehiscence at the buccal aspect of the first premolar site. (c, d) The dehiscence is grafted with deproteinized bovine bone mineral (Bio-Oss, Geistlich Biomaterials, Wolhusen, Switzerland) and covered with a resorbable collagen membrane. (e, f) At surgical re-entry, the buccal surface of the implant at the first premolar site is entirely covered by a newly formed hard tissue, while the bone-to-implant gap at the second premolar site has healed spontaneously.

CONCLUSIONS

In this chapter, the healing process of a tooth extraction wound was described. Factors affecting the histological aspects of the healing phase as well as the post-extraction alterations of the ridge dimensions were also considered. Additionally, the healing of an extraction socket where a dental implant has been placed immediately after tooth removal was described in detail. Finally, the histological and clinical outcomes of the application of different reconstructive technologies to the post-extraction socket were evaluated.

In summary, the available data indicate that:

1. After tooth extraction, each tissue component involved in the healing process (i.e. blood clot, granulation tissue, provisional matrix, woven and lamellar bone, and marrow) shows a well-defined tendency to change over time, leading to a progressive increase in the amount of newly formed bone.
2. A great inter-individual variability exists with respect to the dynamics of new bone formation. Thus, whereas a provisional connective tissue consistently forms within the first weeks of healing, the interval during which mineralized bone is laid down is much less predictable. The bone organization and architecture may be still not completed at 24 weeks after tooth extraction.
3. The dimensional alterations (height and width) of the extraction socket mainly occur within the first 6 months following tooth extraction; however, the edentulous ridge tends to remodel up to at least 12 months.
4. The extent of the ridge alterations following tooth extraction may be influenced by healing determinants related to the patient (e.g. smoking), site (tooth location, concomitant extraction of adjacent teeth) and treatment protocol (e.g. flap elevation, chlorhexidine administration).
5. Immediate implant placement seems not to prevent the dimensional alterations of the alveolar crest occurring after tooth extraction.
6. The healing of the post-extraction socket around immediate implants is influenced by several factors, including the adopted surgical protocol, the morphology/dimensions of the socket and the characteristics of the implant.
7. Evidence, although limited, supports the use of graft material, membranes and bioactive agents to limit the vertical and horizontal collapse of the ridge after tooth extraction.

REFERENCES

Amler, M.H. (1969). The time sequence of tissue regeneration in human extraction wounds. *Oral Surg Oral Med Oral Pathol* **27**: 309–318.

Amler, M.H., Johnson, P.L. et al. (1960). Histological and histochemical investigation of human alveolar socket healing in undisturbed extraction wounds. *J Am Dent Assoc* **61**: 32–44.

Amler, M.H., Salman, I. et al. (1964). Reticular and collagen fiber characteristics in human bone healing. *Oral Surg Oral Med Oral Pathol* **17**: 785–796.

Anitua, E. (1999). Plasma rich in growth factors: preliminary results of use in the preparation of future sites for implants. *Int J Oral Maxillofac Implants* **14**(4): 529–535.

Araújo, M.G. and Lindhe, J. (2005). Dimensional ridge alterations following tooth extraction. An experimental study in the dog. *J Clin Periodontol* **32**: 212–218.

Araújo, M.G. and Lindhe, J. (2009a). Ridge alterations following tooth extraction with and without flap elevation: an experimental study in the dog. *Clin Oral Implants Res* **20**: 545–549.

Araújo, M.G., Lindhe, J. (2009b). Ridge preservation with the use of Bio-Oss collagen: a 6-month study in the dog. *Clin Oral Implants Res* **20**: 433–440.

Araújo, M.G., Sukekava, F., et al. (2005). Ridge alterations following implant placement in fresh extraction sockets: an experimental study in the dog. *J Clin Periodontol* **32**: 645–652.

Araújo, M.G., Sukekava, F., et al. (2006a). Tissue modeling following implant placement in fresh extraction sockets. *Clin Oral Implants Res* **17**: 615–624.

Araújo, M.G., Wennstrom, J.L., et al. (2006b). Modeling of the buccal and lingual bone walls of fresh extraction sites following implant installation. *Clin Oral Implants Res* **17**: 606–614.

Araújo, M., Linder, E., et al. (2008). The influence of Bio-Oss Collagen on healing of an extraction socket: an experimental study in the dog. *Int J Periodontics Restorative Dent* **28**: 123–135.

AraújoAraújo, M., Linder, E., et al. (2009). Effect of a xenograft on early bone formation in extraction sockets: an experimental study in dog. *Clin Oral Implants Res* **20**: 1–6.

Araújo, M.G., Liljenberg, B., et al. (2010). Dynamics of Bio-Oss collagen incorporation in fresh extraction wounds: an experimental study in the dog. *Clin Oral Implants Res* **21**: 55–64.

Artzi, Z., Tal, H., et al. (2000). Porous bovine bone mineral in healing of human extraction sockets. Part 1: histomorphometric evaluations at 9 months. *J Periodontol* **71**: 1015–1023.

Artzi, Z., Tal, H., et al. (2001). Porous bovine bone mineral in healing of human extraction sockets: 2. Histochemical observations at 9 months. *J Periodontol* **72**: 152–159.

Atieh, M.A., Payne, A.G., et al. (2009). Immediate restoration/loading of immediately placed single implants: is it an effective bimodal approach? *Clin Oral Implants Res* **20**: 645–659.

Becker, W., Urist, M., et al. (1996). Clinical and histologic observations of sites implanted with intraoral autologous bone grafts or allografts. 15 human case reports. *J Periodontol* **67**(10): 1025–1033.

Blanco, J., Nunez, V., et al. (2008). Ridge alterations following immediate implant placement in the dog: flap versus flapless surgery. *J Clin Periodontol* **35**: 640–648.

Boix, D., Weiss, P., et al. (2006). Injectable bone substitute to preserve alveolar ridge resorption after tooth extraction: a study in dog. *J Mater Sci Mater Med* **17**: 1145–1152.

Botticelli, D., Berglundh, T., et al. (2004). Hard-tissue alterations following immediate implant placement in extraction sites. *J Clin Periodontol* **31**: 820–828.

Botticelli, D., Berglundh, T., et al. (2005). Bone regeneration at implants with turned or rough surfaces in self-contained defects. An experimental study in the dog. *J Clin Periodontol* **32**: 448–455.

Boyne, P.J. (1966). Osseous repair of the postextraction alveolus in man. *Oral Surg Oral Med Oral Pathol* **21**: 805–813.

Brägger, U., Schild, U., et al. (1994). Effect of chlorhexidine (0.12%) rinses on periodontal tissue healing after tooth extraction. (II). Radiographic parameters. *J Clin Periodontol* **21**: 422–430.

Brandao, A.C., Brentegani, L.G., et al. (2002). Histomorphometric analysis of rat alveolar wound healing with hydroxyapatite alone or associated to BMPs. *Braz Dent J* **13**(3): 147–154.

Caneva, M., Salata, L.A., et al. (2010). Influence of implant positioning in extraction sockets on osseointegration: histomorphometric analyses in dogs. *Clin Oral Implants Res* **21**: 43–49.

Canullo, L., Iurlaro, G., et al. (2009). Double-blind randomized controlled trial study on post-extraction immediately restored implants using the switching platform concept: soft tissue response. Preliminary report. *Clin Oral Implants Res* **20**: 414–420.

AraújoCardaropoli, G., Araújo, M., et al. (2003). Dynamics of bone tissue formation in tooth extraction sites. An experimental study in dogs. *J Clin Periodontol* **30**: 809–818.

Cardaropoli, G., Araújo, M., et al. (2005). Healing of extraction sockets and surgically produced – augmented and non-augmented – defects in the alveolar ridge. An experimental study in the dog. *J Clin Periodontol* **32**: 435–440.

Carmagnola, D., Adriaens, P., et al. (2003). Healing of human extraction sockets filled with Bio-Oss. *Clin Oral Implants Res* **14**: 137–143.

Chang, S.W., Shin, S.Y., et al. (2009). Immediate implant placement into infected and noninfected extraction sockets: a pilot study. *Oral Surg Oral Med Oral Pathol Oral Radiol Endod* **107**: 197–203.

Chen, S.T., Buser, D. (2009). Clinical and esthetic outcomes of implants placed in post-extraction sites. *Int J Oral Maxillofac Implants* **24 Suppl**: 186–217.

Chen, S.T., Wilson, T.G. Jr, et al. (2004). Immediate or early placement of implants following tooth extraction: review of biologic basis, clinical procedures, and outcomes. *Int J Oral Maxillofac Implants* **19 Suppl**: 12–25.

Chen, S.T., Darby, I.B., et al. (2009). Immediate implant placement postextraction without flap elevation. *J Periodontol* **80**: 163–172.

Claflin, R.S. (1936). Healing of disturbed and undisturbed extraction wounds. *J Am Dent Assoc* **23**: 945–959.

Cochran, D.L., Jones, A.A., et al. (2000). Evaluation of recombinant human bone morphogenetic protein-2 in oral applications including the use of endosseous implants: 3-year results of a pilot study in humans. *J Periodontol* **71**(8): 1241–1257.

Cordaro, L., Torsello, F., et al. (2009). Clinical outcome of submerged vs. non-submerged implants placed in fresh extraction sockets. *Clin Oral Implants Res* **20**: 1307–1313.

Cornelini, R. (2000). Immediate transmucosal implant placement: a report of 2 cases. *Int J Periodont Restor Dent* **20**: 199–206.

Covani, U., Cornelini, R., et al. (2003). Bucco-lingual bone remodeling around implants placed into immediate extraction sockets: a case series. *J Periodontol* **74**: 268–273.

Covani, U., Bortolaia, C., et al. (2004a). Bucco-lingual crestal bone changes after immediate and delayed implant placement. *J Periodontol* **75**: 1605–1612.

Covani, U., Barone, A., et al. (2004b). Soft tissue healing around implants placed immediately after tooth extraction without incision: a clinical report. *Int J Oral Maxillofac Implants* **19**: 549–553.

Covani, U., Cornelini, R., et al. (2007). Vertical crestal bone changes around implants placed into fresh extraction sockets. *J Periodontol* **78**: 810–815.

Crespi, R., Cappare, P., et al. (2008). Immediate versus delayed loading of dental implants placed in fresh extraction sockets in the maxillary esthetic zone: a clinical comparative study. *Int J Oral Maxillofac Implants* **23**: 753–758.

Christopher, E.R. (1942). Histological study of bone healing in relation to the extraction of teeth. *Northwest Univ Bull* **45**: 5.

De Kok, I.J., Drapeau, S.J., et al. (2005). Evaluation of mesenchymal stem cells following implantation in alveolar sockets: a canine safety study. *Int J Oral Maxillofac Implants* **20**(4): 511–518.

De Rouck, T., Collys, K., et al. (2008). Single-tooth replacement in the anterior maxilla by means of immediate implantation and provisionalization: a review. *Int J Oral Maxillofac Implants* **23**: 897–904.

de Sanctis, M., Vignoletti, F., et al. (2009). Immediate implants at fresh extraction sockets: bone healing in four different implant systems. *J Clin Periodontol* **36**: 705–711.

Dies, F., Etienne, D., et al. (1996). Bone regeneration in extraction sites after immediate placement of an e-PTFE membrane with or without a biomaterial. A report on 12 consecutive cases. *Clin Oral Implants Res* **7**(3): 277–285.

Evans, C.D. and Chen, S.T. (2008). Esthetic outcomes of immediate implant placements. *Clin Oral Implants Res* **19**: 73–80.

Evian, C.I., Rosenberg, E.S., et al. (1982). The osteogenic activity of bone removed from healing extraction sockets in humans. *J Periodontol* **53**: 81–85.

Farina, R., Scabbia, A., et al. (2005). Valutazione istologica di apatite biomimetica SINTlife® in alveoli post estrattivi umani. *Implantologia* **3**: 237–246.

Farina, R., Pramstraller, M., et al. (2011). Alveolar ridge dimensions in maxillary posterior sextants.A retrospective comparative study of dentate and edentulous sites using computerized tomography data. *Clin Oral Implants Res* **22**(10): 1138–1144.

Ferrus, J., Cecchinato, D., et al. (2010). Factors influencing ridge alterations following immediate implant placement into extraction sockets. *Clin Oral Implants Res* **21**: 22–29.

Fickl, S., Zuhr, O., et al. (2008a). Tissue alterations after tooth extraction with and without surgical trauma: a volumetric study in the beagle dog. *J Clin Periodontol* **35**: 356–363.

Fickl, S., Zuhr, O., et al. (2008b). Hard tissue alterations after socket preservation: an experimental study in the beagle dog. *Clin Oral Implants Res* **19**: 1111–1118.

Fickl, S., Zuhr, O., et al. (2008c). Dimensional changes of the alveolar ridge contour after different socket preservation techniques. J Clin Periodontol **35**: 906–913.

Fickl, S., Schneider, D., et al. (2009a). Dimensional changes of the ridge contour after socket preservation and buccal overbuilding: an animal study. *J Clin Periodontol* **36**: 442–448.

Fickl, S., Zuhr, O., et al. (2009b). Hard tissue alterations after socket preservation with additional buccal overbuilding: a study in the beagle dog. *J Clin Periodontol* **36**: 898–904.

Fiorellini, J.P., Howell, T.H., et al. (2005). Randomized study evaluating recombinant human bone morphogenetic protein-2 for extraction socket augmentation. *J Periodontol* **76**(4): 605–613.

Fujii, N., Kusakari, H., et al. (1998). A histological study on tissue responses to titanium implantation in rat maxilla: the process of epithelial regeneration and bone reaction. *J Periodontol* **69**: 485–495.

Guarnieri, R., Aldini, N.N., et al. (2005). Medial-grade calcium sulfate hemihydrate (surgiplaster) in healing of a human extraction socket–histologic observation at 3 months: a case report. *Int J Oral Maxillofac Implants* **20**: 636–641.

Guida, L., Iezzi, G., et al. (2008). Immediate placement and loading of dental implants: a human histologic case report. *J Periodontol* **79**: 575–581.

Hahn, J., Rohrer, M.D., et al. (2003). Clinical, radiographic, histologic, and histomorphometric comparison of PepGen P-15 particulate and PepGen P-15 flow in extraction sockets: a same-mouth case study. *Implant Dent* **12**(2): 170–174.

Heberer, S., Al-Chawaf, B., et al. (2008). Histomorphometric analysis of extraction sockets augmented with Bio-Oss Collagen after a 6-week healing period: a prospective study. *Clin Oral Implants Res* **19**: 1219–1225.

Heitz-Mayfield, L.J.A., Trombelli, L., et al. (2002). A systematic review of the effect of surgical debridment vs. non-surgical debridment for the treatment of chronic periodontitis. *J Clin Periodontol* **29**: 92–102.

Hoffmann, O., Bartee, B.K., et al. (2008). Alveolar bone preservation in extraction sockets using non-resorbable dPTFE membranes: a retrospective non-randomized study. *J Periodontol* **79**: 1355–1369.

Howell, T.H., Fiorellini, J., et al. (1997). A feasibility study evaluating rhBMP-2/absorbable collagen sponge device for local alveolar ridge preservation or augmentation. *Int J Periodont Restor Dent* **17**(2): 124–139.

Hsieh, Y.D., Devlin, H., et al. (1994). Early alveolar ridge osteogenesis following tooth extraction in the rat. *Arch Oral Biol* **39**: 425–428.

Huynh-Ba, G., Pjetursson, B.E., et al. (2010). Analysis of the socket bone wall dimensions in the upper maxilla in relation to immediate implant placement. *Clin Oral Implants Res* **21**: 37–42.

Iasella, J.M., Greenwell, H., et al. (2003). Ridge preservation with freeze-dried bone allograft and a collagen membrane compared to extraction alone for implant site development: a clinical and histologic study in humans. *J Periodontol* **74**(7): 990–999.

Jaffin, R., Kolesar, M., et al. (2007). The radiographic bone loss pattern adjacent to immediately placed, immediately loaded implants. *Int J Oral Maxillofac Implants* **22**: 187–194.

Johnson, K. (1969). A study of the dimensional changes occurring in the maxilla following tooth extraction. *Aust Dent J* **14**: 241–244.

Kanyama, M., Kuboki, T., et al. (2003). Connective tissue growth factor expressed in rat alveolar bone regeneration sites after tooth extraction. *Arch Oral Biol* **48**: 723–730.

Karabuda, C., Sandalli, P., et al. (1999). Histologic and histomorphometric comparison of immediately placed hydroxyapatite-coated and titanium plasma-sprayed implants: a pilot study in dogs. *Int J Oral Maxillofac Implants* **14**: 510–515.

Kim, M., Kim, J.H., et al. (2008). Effect of bone mineral with or without collagen membrane in ridge dehiscence defects following premolar extraction. *In Vivo* **22**(2): 231–236.

Kuboki, Y., Hashimoto, F., et al. (1988). Time-dependent changes of collagen crosslinks in the socket after tooth extraction in rabbits. *J Dent Res* **67**: 944–948.

Lekic, P., Rojas, J., et al. (2001). Phenotypic comparison of periodontal ligament cells in vivo and in vitro. *J Periodontal Res* **36**: 71–79.

Lekovic, V., Kenney, E.B., et al. (1997). A bone regenerative approach to alveolar ridge maintenance following tooth extraction. Report of 10 cases. *J Periodontol* **68**: 563–570.

Lekovic, V., Camargo, P.M., et al. (1998). Preservation of alveolar bone in extraction sockets using bioabsorbable membranes. *J Periodontol* **69**: 1044–1049.

Lin, W.L., McCulloch, C.A., et al. (1994). Differentiation of periodontal ligament fibroblasts into osteoblasts during socket healing after tooth extraction in the rat. *Anat Rec* **240**: 492–506.

Luczyszyn, S.M., Papalexiou, V., et al. (2005). Acellular dermal matrix and hydroxyapatite in prevention of ridge deformities after tooth extraction. *Implant Dent* **14**(2): 176–184.

Mangano, C., Piattelli, A., et al. (2008). Dense hydroxyapatite inserted into postextraction sockets: a histologic and histomorphometric 20-year case report. *J Periodontol* **79**: 929–933.

Mangos, J.F. (1941). The healing of extraction wounds. An experimental study based on microscopic and radiographic investigations. *N Zeal Dent J* **37**: 4–24.

Marei, M.K., Nouh, S.R., et al. (2005). Preservation and regeneration of alveolar bone by tissue-engineered implants. *Tissue Eng* **11**: 751–767.

Matin, K., Nakamura, H., et al. (2001). Impact of recombinant human bone morphogenetic protein-2 on residual ridge resorption after tooth extraction: an experimental study in the rat. *Int J Oral Maxillofac Implants* **16**(3): 400–411.

Molly, L., Vandromme, H., et al. (2008). Bone formation following implantation of bone biomaterials into extraction sites. *J Periodontol* **79**(6): 1108–1115.

Nair Pn, P.R., Schug, J. (2004). Observations on healing of human tooth extraction sockets implanted with bioabsorbable polylactic-polyglycolic acids (PLGA) copolymer root replicas: a clinical, radiographic, and histologic follow-up report of 8 cases. *Oral Surg Oral Med Oral Pathol Oral Radiol Endod* **97**: 559–569.

Neiva, R.F., Tsao, Y.P., et al. (2008). Effects of a putty-form hydroxyapatite matrix combined with the synthetic cell-binding peptide P-15 on alveolar ridge preservation. *J Periodontol* **79**(2): 291–299.

Nevins, M., Camelo, M., et al. (2006). A study of the fate of the buccal wall of extraction sockets of teeth with prominent roots. *Int J Periodont Restor Dent* **26**: 19–29.

Norton, M.R., Odell, E.W., et al. (2003). Efficacy of bovine bone mineral for alveolar augmentation: a human histologic study. *Clin Oral Implants Res* **14**: 775–783.

Olson, R.A., Roberts, D.L., et al. (1982). A comparative study of polylactic acid, Gelfoam, and Surgicel in healing extraction sites. *Oral Surg Oral Med Oral Pathol* **53**: 441–449.

Parr, G.R., Steflik, D.E., et al. (1993). Histomorphometric and histologic observations of bone healing around immediate implants in dogs. *Int J Oral Maxillofac Implants* **8**: 534–540.

Pieri, F., Aldini, N.N., et al. (2009). Immediate occlusal loading of immediately placed implants supporting fixed restorations in completely edentulous arches: a 1-year prospective pilot study. *J Periodontol* **80**: 411–421.

Pietrokovski, J. (1975). The bony residual ridge in man. *J Prosthet Dent* **34**: 456–462.

Pietrokovski, J. and Massler, M. (1967). Alveolar ridge resorption following tooth extraction. *J Prosthet Dent* **17**: 21–27.

Pietrokovski, J., Starinsky, R., et al. (2007). Morphologic characteristics of bony edentulous jaws. *J Prosthodont* **16**: 141–147.

Pinho, M.N., Roriz, V.L., et al. (2006). Titanium membranes in prevention of alveolar collapse after tooth extraction. *Implant Dent* **15**(1): 53–61.

Pramstraller, M., Farina, R., et al. (2011). Ridge dimensions of the edentulous posterior maxilla: a retrospective analysis of a cohort of 127 patients using computerized tomography data. *Clin Oral Implants Res* **22**(1): 54–61.

Rasmusson, L., Kahnberg, K.E., et al. (2001). Effects of implant design and surface on bone regeneration and implant stability: an experimental study in the dog mandible. *Clin Implant Dent Relat Res* **3**: 2–8.

Rimondini, L., Bruschi, G.B., et al. (2005). Tissue healing in implants immediately placed into postextraction sockets: a pilot study in a mini-pig model. *Oral Surg Oral Med Oral Pathol Oral Radiol Endod* **100**: e43–50.

Rothamel, D., Schwarz, F., et al. (2008). Dimensional ridge alterations following socket preservation using a nanocrystalline hydroxyapatite paste: a histomorphometrical study in dogs. *Int J Oral Maxillofac Surg* **37**: 741–747.

Saldanha, J. B., Casati, M.Z., et al. (2006). Smoking may affect the alveolar process dimensions and radiographic bone density in maxillary extraction sites: a prospective study in humans. *J Oral Maxillofac Surg* **64**: 1359–1365.

Sanz, M., Cecchinato, D., et al. (2010). A prospective, randomized-controlled clinical trial to evaluate bone preservation using implants with different geometry placed into extraction sockets in the maxilla. *Clin Oral Implants Res* **21**: 13–21.

Sato, H. and Takeda, Y. (2007). Proliferative activity, apoptosis, and histogenesis in the early stages of rat tooth extraction wound healing. *Cells Tissues Organs* **186**: 104–111.

Sbordone, L., Bortolaia, C., et al. (2005). Clinical and histologic analysis of calcium sulfate in treatment of a post-extraction defect: a case report. *Implant Dent* **14**: 82–87.

Schropp, L., Isidor, F. (2008a). Clinical outcome and patient satisfaction following full-flap elevation for early and delayed placement of single-tooth implants: a 5-year randomized study. *Int J Oral Maxillofac Implants* **23**: 733–743.

Schropp, L., Isidor, F. (2008b). Timing of implant placement relative to tooth extraction. *J Oral Rehabil* **35 Suppl 1**: 33–43.

Schropp, L., Wenzel, A., et al. (2003). Bone healing and soft tissue contour changes following single-tooth extraction: a clinical and radiographic 12-month prospective study. *Int J Periodont Restor Dent* **23**: 313–323.

Serino, G., Biancu, S., et al. (2003). Ridge preservation following tooth extraction using a polylactide and polyglycolide sponge as space filler: a clinical and histological study in humans. *Clin Oral Implants Res* **14**: 651–658.

Serino, G., Rao, W., et al. (2008). Polylactide and polyglycolide sponge used in human extraction sockets: bone formation following 3 months after its application. *Clin Oral Implants Res* **19**: 26–31.

Shi, B., Zhou, Y., et al. (2007). Alveolar ridge preservation prior to implant placement with surgical-grade calcium sulfate and platelet-rich plasma: a pilot study in a canine model. *Int J Oral Maxillofac Implants* **22**(4): 656–665.

Siciliano, V.I., Salvi, G.E., et al. (2009). Soft tissues healing at immediate transmucosal implants placed into molar extraction sites with buccal self-contained dehiscences. A 12-month controlled clinical trial. *Clin Oral Implants Res* **20**: 482–488.

Simon, D., Manuel, S., et al. (2004). Potential for osseous regeneration of platelet-rich plasma–a comparative study in mandibular third molar sockets. *Indian J Dent Res* **15**(4): 133–136.

Smukler, H., Landi, L., et al. (1999). Histomorphometric evaluation of extraction sockets and deficient alveolar ridges treated with allograft and barrier membrane: a pilot study. *Int J Oral Maxillofac Implants* **14**(3): 407–416.

Stafford, G.L. (2009). Are the outcomes of immediate and early single tooth implants comparable to conventionally placed implants? *Evid Based Dent* **10**: 77–78.

Tomasi, C., Sanz, M., et al. (2010). Bone dimensional variations at implants placed in fresh extraction sockets: a multilevel multivariate analysis. *Clin Oral Implants Res* **21**: 30–36.

Trombelli, L., Farina, R., et al. (2008). Modeling and remodeling of human extraction sockets. *J Clin Periodontol* **35**: 630–639.

Van der Weijden, F., Dell'Acqua, F., et al. (2009). Alveolar bone dimensional changes of post-extraction sockets in humans: a systematic review. *J Clin Periodontol* **36**: 1048–1058.

Vignoletti, F., de Sanctis, M., et al. (2009). Early healing of implants placed into fresh extraction sockets: an experimental study in the beagle dog. II: ridge alterations. *J Clin Periodontol* **36**: 688–697.

Villa, R. and Rangert, B. (2007). Immediate and early function of implants placed in extraction sockets of maxillary infected teeth: a pilot study. *J Prosthet Dent* **97(6 Suppl)**: S96–S108.

Wilson, T.G. Jr, Schenk, R., et al. (1998). Implants placed in immediate extraction sites: a report of histologic and histometric analyses of human biopsies. *Int J Oral Maxillofac Implants* **13**: 333–341.

Wood, D.L., Hoag, P.M., et al. (1972). Alveolar crest reduction following full and partial thickness flaps. *J Periodontol* **43**: 141–144.

Yoshiki, S., Langeland, K. (1968). Alkaline phosphatase activity in the osteoid matrix of healing alveolar socket. *Oral Surg Oral Med Oral Pathol* **26**: 381–389.

9 Flap Designs for Periodontal Healing

Leonardo Trombelli and Roberto Farina
Research Centre for the Study of Periodontal and Peri-implant Diseases, University of Ferrara, Ferrara, Italy

FLAP MANAGEMENT, WOUND STABILITY AND PERIODONTAL REGENERATION

Earlier studies evaluating periodontal wound healing suggest that the undisturbed maturation of a root surface-adhering fibrin clot is a prerequisite to periodontal regeneration (Linghorne and O'Connell 1950; Hiatt et al. 1968; Polson and Proye 1983). Using the supra-alveolar periodontal defect model, Wikesjö et al. (1991) showed that when fibrin clot adhesion to the root surface was experimentally impeded by topical administration of heparin, the gingival tissue/root surface interface largely healed by formation of a junctional epithelium or epithelial attachment. However, when the experimental heparin protocol was combined with a wound-stabilizing element supporting uneventful adsorption/adhesion/maturation of the compromised fibrin clot, the gingival tissue/root surface interface healed with connective tissue rather than an epithelial attachment (Wikesjö and Nilvéus 1990; Haney et al. 1993). It was moreover shown that space provision using a GTR device with or without a biomaterial filling the wound space supported regeneration of alveolar bone, both serving as wound-stabilizing elements. Overall, these observations strongly point to the significance of clinical surgical factors contributing wound stability in support of periodontal regeneration.

When considering the technical aspects of periodontal reconstructive procedures, the surgical management of the supracrestal soft tissues, including flap design and suturing technique, seems of paramount importance in affecting the successful outcome. In essence, the surgical manipulations of the soft tissues overlying the intraosseous component of an intrabony defect must reduce the chances of post-surgery infection and contamination of the blood clot and, possibly, protect the implanted biomaterial, membrane or biological agent. Even if there is an apparent tissue approximation at suturing, post-surgery shrinkage of the soft tissues during the early healing phase often results in substantial graft and/or membrane exposure and subsequent bacterial contamination of the wound, therefore jeopardizing the cascade of biologic events leading to periodontal regeneration. Moreover, when autogenous bone chips or bone-substitute particles are used, incomplete tissue coverage may lead to the immediate, partial or complete exfoliation of the implanted graft. Loss of primary closure in the interdental area often results in interdental soft tissue craters, with consequent difficulties for the therapist and the patient to perform adequate plaque control during the healing phase.

Oral Wound Healing: Cell Biology and Clinical Management, First Edition. Edited by Hannu Larjava.

Primary closure in the interdental area, where the great majority of the intraosseous lesions are located (Papapanou et al. 1988), often represents a challenge for the clinician. When conventional access flap surgery has been associated with reconstructive procedures based on GTR provision, flap dehiscence or membrane exposure may occur in 70–80% of the treated sites as a result of lack of primary closure at the interdental space (Becker et al. 1988; Selvig et al. 1993; Tonetti et al. 1993; Trombelli et al. 1997). Therefore, different surgical options in terms of flap design and related suture technique have been developed over the years, with the aim of optimizing the primary closure, thus promoting wound stability and blood clot maturation (Takei et al. 1985; Cortellini et al. 1995, 1999; Murphy 1996; Michaelides and Wilson 1996; Trombelli et al. 2007, 2008, 2009, 2010, 2011).

The purpose of this chapter is to critically revise the surgical options that have been described in the literature, outlining the technical steps as well as the indications and contraindications for each flap design when used to correct the periodontal intraosseous defect.

FLAP DESIGNS TO ACHIEVE PRIMARY CLOSURE

The increased predictability of the reconstructive procedures, at least from a clinical standpoint, can be strictly dependent upon (1) the surgical design and flap management for better survival of flap and graft coverage, and (2) suturing technique to optimize primary closure, thus ensuring the primary condition for blood clot stabilization and maturation in a biologic environment protected from biomechanical and microbiological challenge (Takei 1991). Proper flap design and incision placement is of utmost importance to achieve complete flap closure and flap-to-root seal at the time of suturing and during postsurgical healing as well as minimal or absent exposure and subsequent contamination and/or exfoliation of the grafted biomaterial or membrane. Therefore, it seems reasonable to classify flap designs according to (1) the outline of the incision which affects the preservation of the interdental supracrestal soft tissues and, thus, the predictability to ensure primary closure at the interdental space, and (2) the elevation of either a single (buccal *or* oral) or a double (buccal *and* oral) flap in relation to the surgical trauma exerted at the interproximal soft tissues.

Techniques without preservation of the interdental supracrestal soft tissues and with double flap elevation

Flap designs that are based on a split of the buccal and oral papilla without preservation of the integrity of the interdental supracrestal soft tissue include the Modified Widman flap (MWF) (Ramfjord and Nissle 1974) and the Full-Thickness Flap with internal mattress sutures (FTF) (Michaelides and Wilson 1996). MWF would help to preserve the gingival tissues on the buccal and lingual/palatal aspect; however, it would leave some interdental tissues remaining with the collar of tissues which separates the flaps from the teeth. This attached portion of the interdental tissues is then removed to expose the underlying bone crest and the exposed root surface for defect and root debridement. This unavoidably leads to a partial loss of the interdental soft tissues with an increased risk of compromising the primary closure in the interdental space.

FTF represents a modification of the MWF to approach intraosseous defects in the maxillary anterior dentition (Newell and Brunsvold 1985; Fig. 9.1). Intrasulcular incisions are made retaining all interpapillary thickness, thus resulting in 'pie-shaped' papillae rather than thin papillae as in MWF. Full-thickness mucoperiosteal flaps are elevated on both

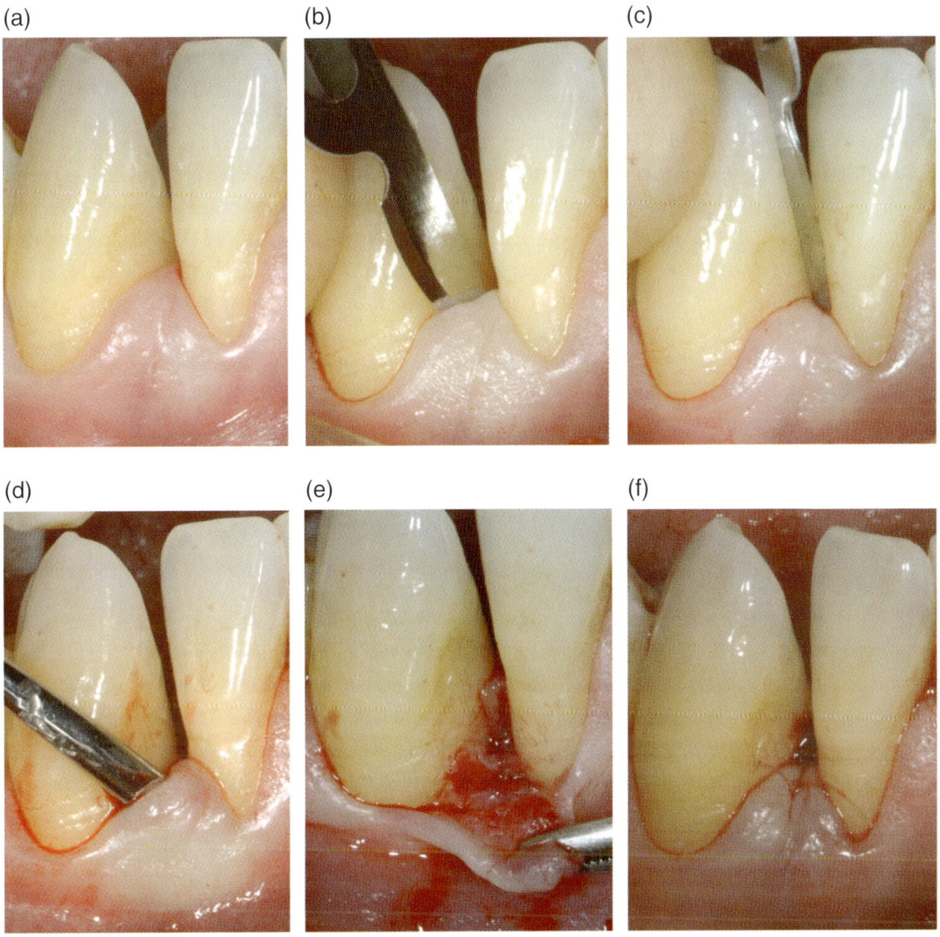

Fig. 9.1 Full-thickness flap (Michaelides and Wilson 1996). Intrasulcular incisions are made retaining all interpapillary thickness, thus resulting in 'pie-shaped' papillae (a–c). Full-thickness mucoperiosteal flaps are elevated on both buccal and lingual/palatal sides (d, e), root surface and osseous defect are debrided, then flaps are repositioned and closed by a modified vertical internal mattress suture (f).

buccal and lingual/palatal sides to get access to root surface and osseous defect. Although this technique may provide a suitable alternative approach when a narrow interdental space is present, a case-cohort study showed that FTF resulted in a relevant postsurgical incidence of loss of papilla integrity (Michaelides and Wilson 1996).

Techniques with preservation of the interdental supracrestal soft tissues and with double flap elevation

Flap designs that provide the preservation of the integrity of the interdental supracrestal soft tissue by elevating a buccal and oral flap include the Papilla Preservation Technique (PPT) introduced by Takei (Takei et al. 1985) and its subsequent surgical variants such as the Interproximal Tissue Maintenance (ITM) (Murphy 1996), the Modified Papilla Preservation Technique (MPPT) (Cortellini et al. 1995) and the Simplified Papilla Preservation Technique

(SPPT) (Cortellini et al. 1999). All these surgical techniques are characterized by the fact that no incisions are made through the interdental papilla. Either the buccal or the oral papilla is, therefore, included in the contralateral oral or buccal flap, respectively, leaving the volume of the supracrestal soft tissues intact in the interproximal area. The application of this concept as MPPT for GTR-treatment of deep intraosseous defects resulted in 73–80% of complete coverage of the membrane during the healing phase (Cortellini et al. 1995, 1996a). MPPT in association with titanium-reinforced ePTFE membrane determined a significantly greater clinical attachment gain compared to a conventional (MWF) flap approach with or without a standard ePTFE membrane (Cortellini et al. 2001). Consistently, when SPPT was used for GTR with resorbable membranes, this approach resulted in 46% to 67% of complete membrane coverage during healing (Cortellini et al. 2001).

Clinicians should always privilege the papilla preservation procedures when an adequate width of the interdental space is present. The interdental space can be regarded as 'adequate' when it is wider than 2 mm at soft tissue (papilla) level (Cortellini and Tonetti 2001) or, in the presence of a large horizontal component of the bone loss (see below), when a minimal inter-radicular width of 2.0 mm measured at the osseous crest is present (Murphy 1996). PPT, MPPT and ITM techniques place the incision line away from the bone defect, thus limiting graft or membrane exposure during postsurgical healing. In addition, MPPT includes a coronal displacement of the buccal flap, which greatly contributes to primary closure over the graft/membrane and may result in clinical attachment gain coronal to the alveolar crest (Cortellini et al. 1995). The maxillary anterior area is best suited for all these papilla preservation procedures due to excellent surgical access and wide interdental spaces. Areas of diastema as well as narrow edentulous areas are also candidate locations for these procedures. When the mesio-distal dimension of the interdental space is insufficient (i.e. $\leq$ 2 mm) to permit the displacement of the papilla in a bucco-lingual direction (or vice versa), SPPT should be preferred since it seems to facilitate primary closure of the interdental tissues over the membrane/graft compared to other procedures (Cortellini et al. 1999).

The apico-coronal dimension of the supracrestal soft tissues may also affect the selection of flap design. Bone sounding should be performed to properly assess the horizontal component of the bone loss. In essence, the greater the distance from the tip of the papilla to the underlying bone crest, the greater the amount of interdental supracrestal soft tissue that can be 'slided under' the contact area, even in the presence of a limited interdental space. In other words, when a large apico-coronal dimension of supracrestal soft tissues is present, surgical manipulation of the interdental papilla is facilitated and, therefore, techniques for interdental papilla preservation should be considered.

When approaching the selection of a papilla preservation technique, clinicians should carefully base the selection according to the area of the dentition where the intraosseous defect is present. In this respect, MPPT can be the first choice in single-rooted teeth and in lower molars without neighboring teeth. In molars with proximal teeth present, application of MPPT was shown to be technically more demanding and clinically less successful, and it did not result in the desired primary closure in almost one-third of the cases (Cortellini et al. 1995). ITM was first introduced for maxillary teeth, with thick palatal tissues and a minimal interradicular width of 2.0 mm (Murphy 1996). In the presence of narrow interdental space and/or posterior teeth SPPT is to be preferred.

The choice of a specific papilla preservation procedure is heavily affected by the morphology of the bony lesion. Bone sounding has to be accurately performed presurgically in order to assess whether the intraosseous defect only involves the interdental area or it also extends to the buccal or lingual aspect of the alveolar bone. To avoid unwanted contraction of the flap edges (with undesired tissue shrinkage and graft exposure), the incision must be placed well away from the defect site. As a general rule, if the intraosseous defect largely involves the buccal cortical plate, the interdental supracrestal tissue should remain connected with the buccal flap, and vice versa. For instance, the presence of an interproximal intraosseous defect with a large buccal extension prevents or limits the use of MPPT. When using PPT, the extension of the intraosseous defect to the palatal or buccal aspect of the interdental area will determine the position of the semilunar incison. However, in case of a palatal extension of the intraosseous defect, an ITM approach can still be suggested provided that wide and long bevelled palatal incisions, at safe distance from the bone defect margins, are performed.

Representative cases detailing the different papilla preservation techniques are illustrated in Figs. 9.2–9.5.

Techniques with preservation of the interdental supracrestal soft tissues and with a single flap elevation: the Single Flap Approach

Recently, we proposed a minimally invasive surgical procedure, the Single Flap Approach (SFA), designed for reconstructive procedures of intraosseous periodontal defects (Trombelli et al. 2007, 2008). The surgical steps of SFA are shown in Fig. 9.6. The basic principle behind SFA is the unilateral elevation of a limited mucoperiosteal flap to allow surgical access depending on the main, buccal or lingual, extension of the intraosseous defect leaving adjoining gingival tissues intact. The elevation of a limited single flap to access the intraosseous defect may pose several clinical advantages. First, it may facilitate flap repositioning and suturing; the flap can be easily stabilized to the undetached papilla, thus optimizing wound closure for primary intention healing. Moreover, by leaving a great volume of supracrestal soft tissues intact, accelerated re-establishment of the local vascular supply may occur. Wound stabilization and preservation of an intact interdental papilla may also contribute an enhanced preservation of the pre-existing gingival esthetics.

A recent randomized controlled trial evaluated the effectiveness of buccal SFA used for the surgical debridement (without any additional use of reconstructive devices or bioactive agents) of deep intraosseous defects compared to a double flap elevation associated with preservation of interdental soft tissues (SPPT or MPPT) (Trombelli et al. 2011). The results of the study showed that SFA resulted in similar, significant clinical attachment level (CAL) gain and probing pocket depth (PPD) reduction at 6 months post-surgery when compared to the double flap approach. These findings sustained the concept that the reconstructive outcome obtained with the SFA merely reflected an efficient removal of the microbial biofilm adhering to the root surface during the intra-surgical instrumentation as well as the achievement of ideal conditions for wound stability. In addition SFA and the double flap approach resulted in comparable, limited postoperative increase in gingival recession (Trombelli et al. 2011). SFA has also been successfully combined with various regenerative technologies, including bone biomaterials with or without provisions for GTR (Trombelli et al. 2007, 2008). A recent study showed that SFA combined with a hydroxyapatite (HA) biomaterial and GTR allowed substantial clinical attachment gain, limited gingival recession and generally uneventful healing in deep intraosseous periodontal defects (Trombelli et al. 2009). Comparable CAL gain and PPD reduction have also been observed when a similar minimally invasive surgical approach, based on the preservation of an intact papilla, was used in combination with an enamel matrix derivative (Cortellini and Tonetti 2009).

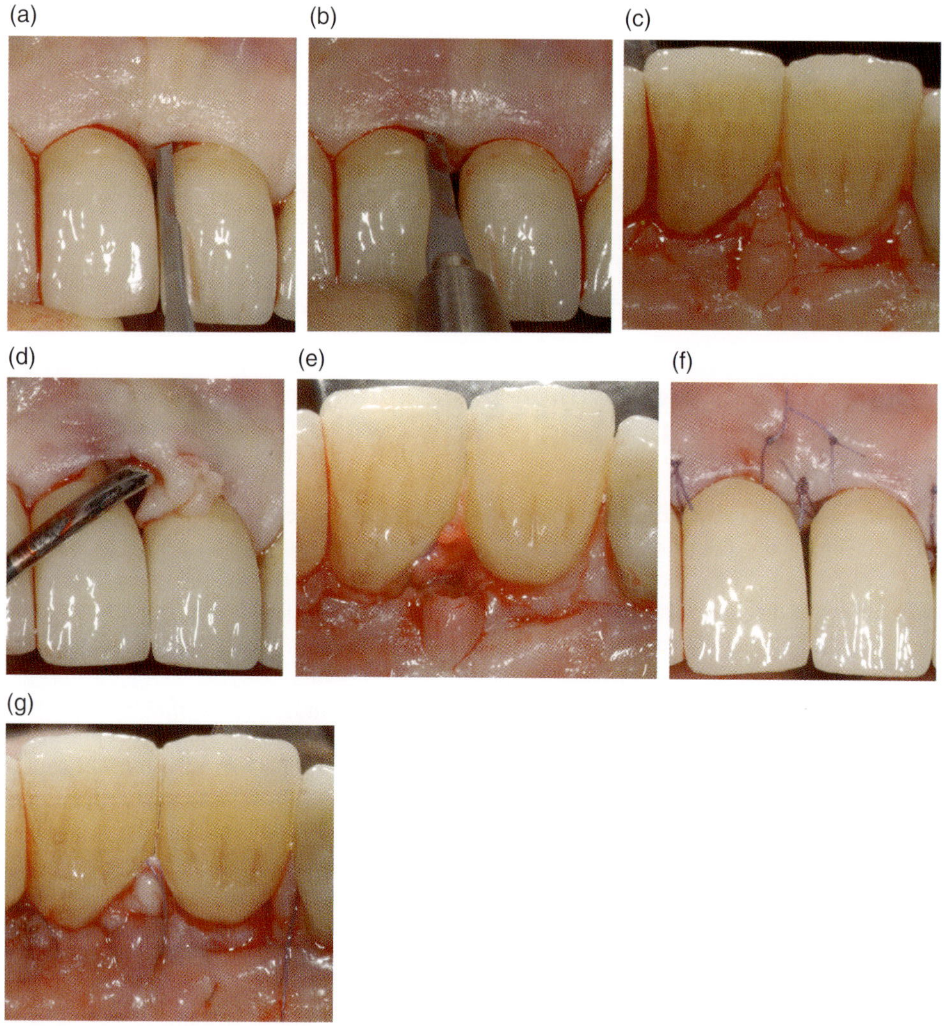

Fig. 9.2 Papilla Preservation Technique (PPT) (Takei et al. 1985). In PPT, the buccal flap is outlined with an intrasulcular incision around each tooth with no incisions being made through the interdental papilla (a, b). The lingual/palatal flap design consists of an intrasulcular incision along the lingual/palatal aspect of each tooth with a semilunar incision made across the interdental papilla. The semilunar incision starts from the line-angle of a tooth to the line-angle of the adjacent tooth, with the papillary incision line at least 5 mm apical from the gingival margin (c). The semilunar incision is made with the blade perpendicular to the outer surface of the gingiva and extends to the alveolar bone. In situations where the osseous defect has a large extension onto the palatal or lingual surface, the PPT is modified so that the semilunar incision is on the facial aspect. Then, the interdental papilla, which is made free from the underlying bone with a sharp incision, will be carefully pushed through the embrasure with a blunt instrument so that the flap may be easily reflected along with the intact papilla (d, e). Trimming of the granulation tissue from the underside of the interdental papilla should be limited or avoided to provide adequate thickness to the interdental tissue. The defect is debrided, and the root surfaces are scaled and root planed. Primary closure is achieved by internal mattress sutures, first at the base of the buccal papilla, then closing the interdental soft tissues (f, g).

(a) (b) (c) (d) (e) (f) (g) (h)

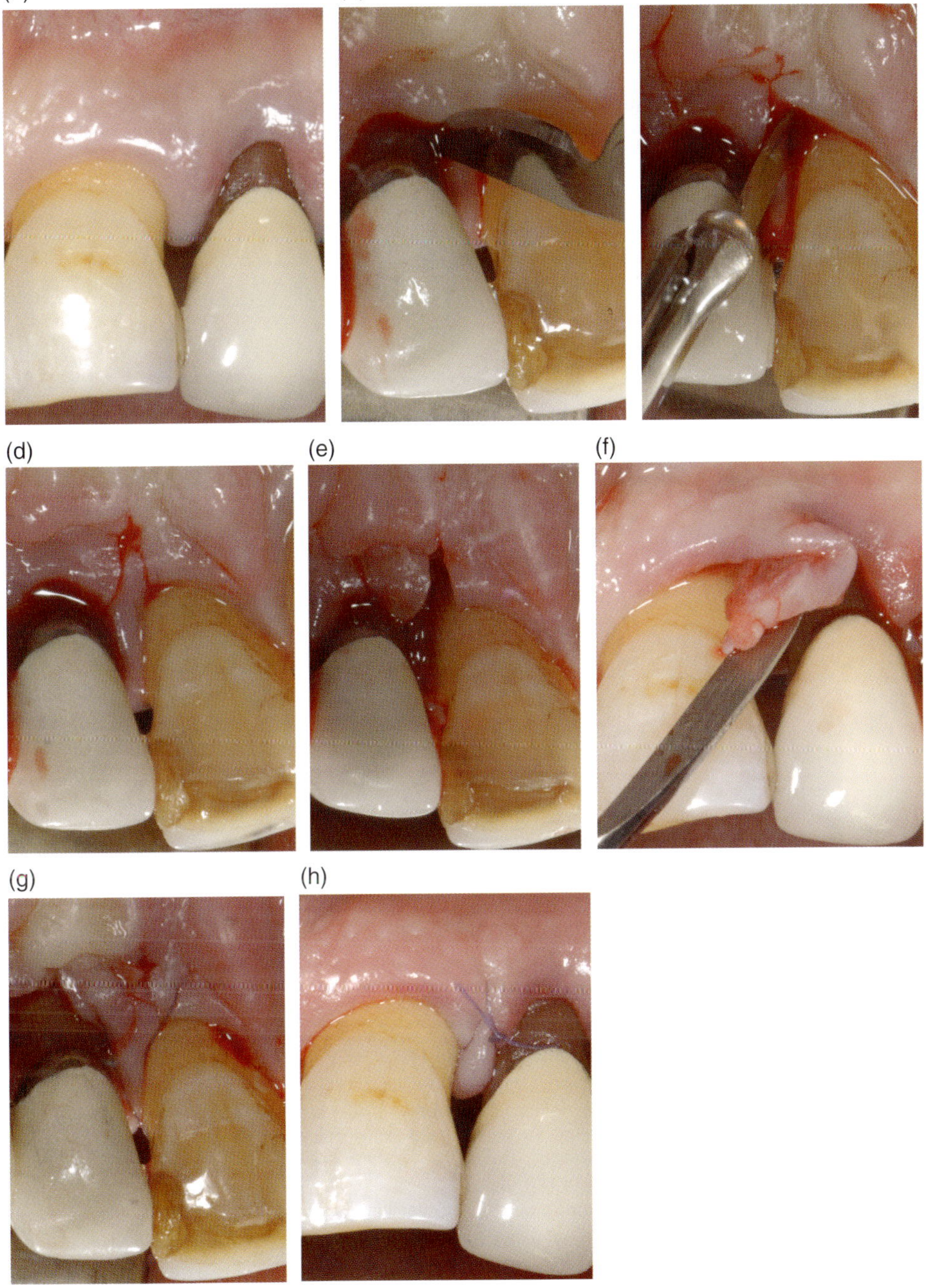

Fig. 9.3 Interproximal Tissue Maintenance (ITM) (Murphy 1996). ITM represents a modification of the PPT. Briefly, ITM involves the reflection of a triangular-shaped palatal flap (so-called papillar triangle, PT), along with the isthmus of interdental tissue, which remains contiguous with the buccal portion of the flap. This allows for the preservation of an adequate amount of interdental tissue to ensure membrane or graft protection/coverage. The surgical protocol includes an initial buccal intracrevicular incision extending one or two teeth on either side of the defect (a). Vertical releasing incisions are performed as needed. The PT is outlined by two inverse-bevelled incisions, starting from the line angles of the teeth where the interproximal osseous defect is present, and joining at a common point 7–15 mm directly apical in the palate (b–d). A full-thickness flap reflection is made, and the PT is elevated from the alveolar bone and displaced toward the buccal aspect under the contact area by means of a small periosteal elevator (e, f). After defect and root debridement, the flaps are sutured using a modified external mattress suturing technique (g, h).

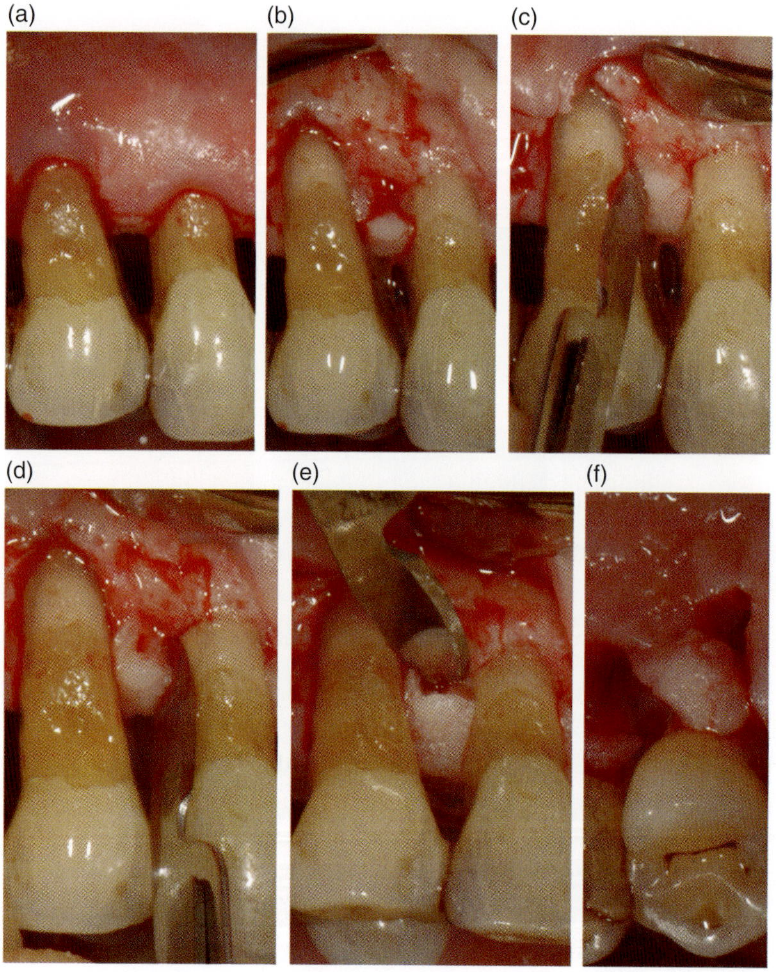

Fig. 9.4 Modified Papilla Preservation Technique (MPPT) (Cortellini et al. 1995). The MPPT procedure consists of a variation of the PPT procedure modified to allow not only the primary closure, but also the coronal positioning of the interdental tissue. A buccal and interdental primary incision to the alveolar crest, involving the two teeth neighboring the defect, is performed. An internal-bevelled, horizontal incision is then performed in the buccal gingiva of the interdental space at the base of the papilla (a). A mucoperiosteal buccal flap is elevated at the level of the buccal alveolar crest (b). The interproximal incision is continued intrasulcularly in the interdental space to reach the palatal line-angle, and extended to the palatal aspect of the defect-neighboring teeth. The base of the papilla (and the supracrestal soft tissue) is dissected from the bone crest with buccal intrasulcular and horizontal incision (c–e), and the papilla is elevated along with the palatal full-thickness flap to expose the osseous defect (f). Split-thickness incision at the base of the buccal flap is performed to allow for coronal positioning of the buccal flap without tension. After defect and root debridement, the flaps are sutured using horizontal and vertical internal mattress sutures (g, h). A horizontal internal mattress suture can be placed between the base of the palatal papilla and the buccal flap coronal to the mucogingival junction in order to coronally displace the buccal flap. Then, a second internal mattress suture (or an interrupted suture) can be placed between the most coronal portion of the palatal flap which includes the interdental papilla and the most coronal portion of the buccal flap. This suture ensures the primary closure of the buccal flap (h).

(g) (h)

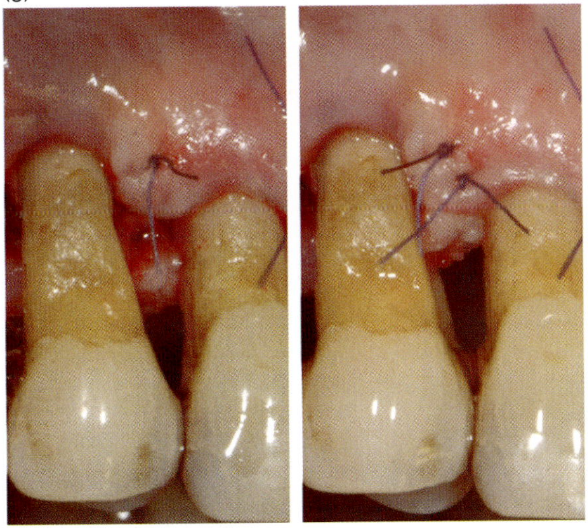

Fig. 9.4 (*Continued*).

More recently, 24 intraosseous defects were approached according to the principles of SFA using a buccal access, then randomly allocated to treatment with SFA+HA/GTR or SFA alone. Clinical outcomes assessed at 6 months post-surgery indicated that SFA with and without HA+GTR were similarly effective in the treatment of intraosseous periodontal defects (Trombelli et al. 2010). SFA supported considerable clinical improvements as a stand-alone protocol: CAL gain averaging 4.4 mm, including 11 sites showing ≥ 3 mm gain at 6 months post-surgery. Notably, no suture-line dehiscences were observed in the SFA group suggesting that a minimally invasive flap management regime may support an undisturbed maturation of the underlying fibrin clot during the early healing phase, and may be equally important to providing a robust environment from a patient-centered perspective, reducing the risk of patient-inflicted trauma to the surgical site during the early events of wound healing. Overall, these observations suggest that SFA (1) provides ample surgical access to ensure adequate subgingival instrumentation, and (2) provides conditions for primary intention healing supporting adequate wound stability allowing uneventful tissue formation and maturation.

SURGICAL TREATMENT OF PERIODONTAL INTRAOSSEOUS DEFECTS: TECHNICAL HINTS

Before undertaking a surgical reconstructive procedure, it is mandatory to instruct and motivate the patient to achieve a high level of self-performed plaque control, which should be maintained throughout the tissue maturation phase to optimize the reconstructive outcome (Nyman et al. 1977; Cortellini et al. 1996b) and reinforced during the supportive therapy to maintain the achieved attachment gain (Cortellini and Tonetti 2004). During cause-related therapy, the instrumentation of the defect to be surgically corrected should be performed by means of sonic/ultrasonic devices with small insertion tips. This will ensure proper infection control while limiting the soft tissue damage, and consequent shrinkage, in the interdental

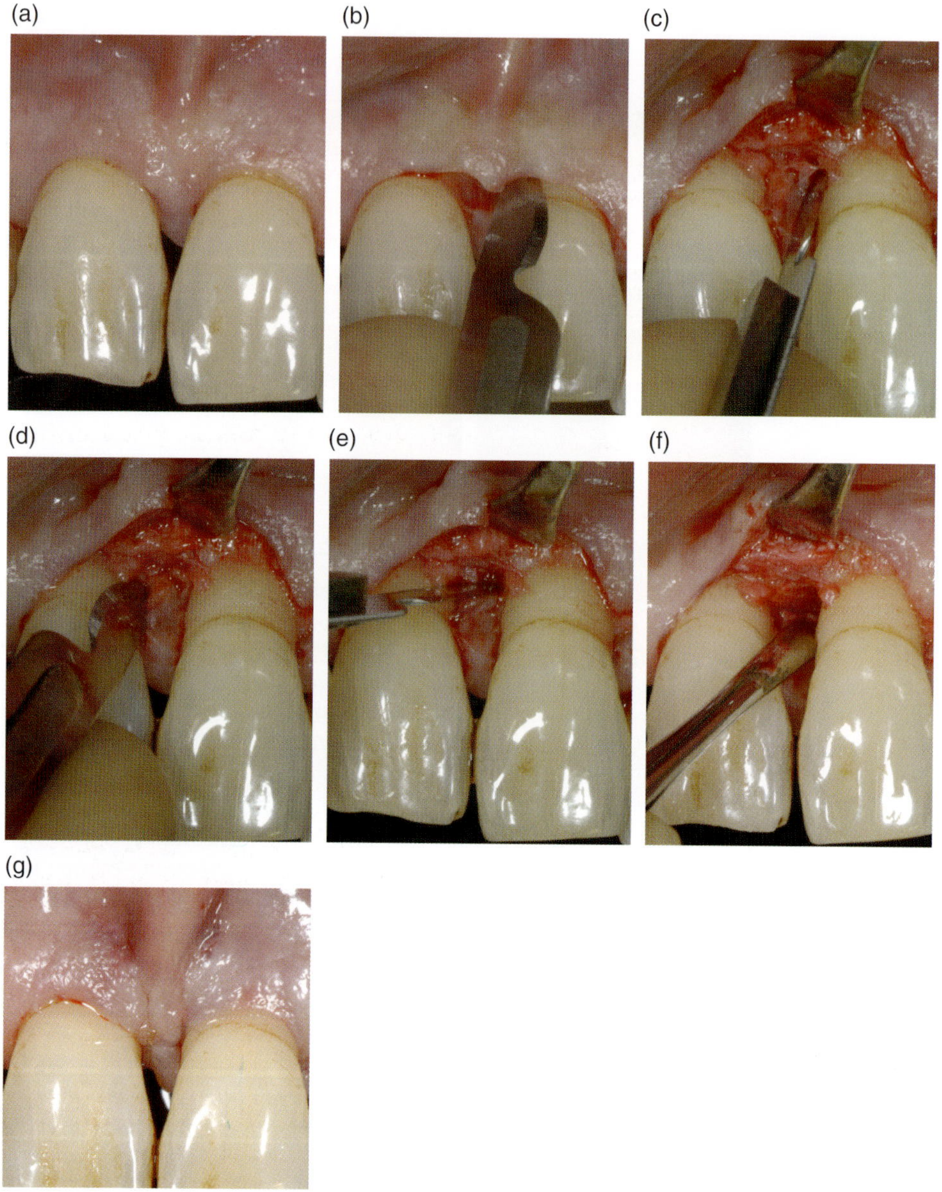

Fig. 9.5 Simplified Papilla Preservation Technique (SPPT) (Cortellini et al. 1999). SPPT has been designed to achieve and maintain the primary closure of the flaps in the presence of narrow/posterior interdental spaces, and avoid/limit the collapse of non-self-supporting barrier membranes or biomaterials into interdental bone defects (a). A first oblique buccal incision is carried out from the gingival margin at the buccal line angle of the defect tooth to reach the mid-interproximal portion of the papilla under the contact area of the adjacent tooth (b). The incision is performed by keeping the blade parallel to the long axis of the tooth in order to avoid excessive thinning of the palatal aspect of the papilla. The interdental incision is prolonged intrasulcularly on the buccal aspect of the teeth in proximity to the defect, and extended to dissect the papillae of the adjacent interdental spaces. A full-thickness buccal flap is then elevated, while the remaining (palatal) portion of the papilla above the interdental defect is carefully dissected with interdental intrasulcular incisions (c, d). To free the interdental papillary tissue left with the first buccal incision, a bucco-lingual horizontal incision is performed at the base of the papilla in close proximity to the interdental bone crest (e). Then, a full-thickness lingual/palatal flap is elevated which includes most of the supracrestal interdental tissue (f). Periosteal incision is used if tension-free primary closure is not obtained. Defect debridement and root scaling is then performed. Primary closure is achieved with a modified internal vertical mattress suture (g).

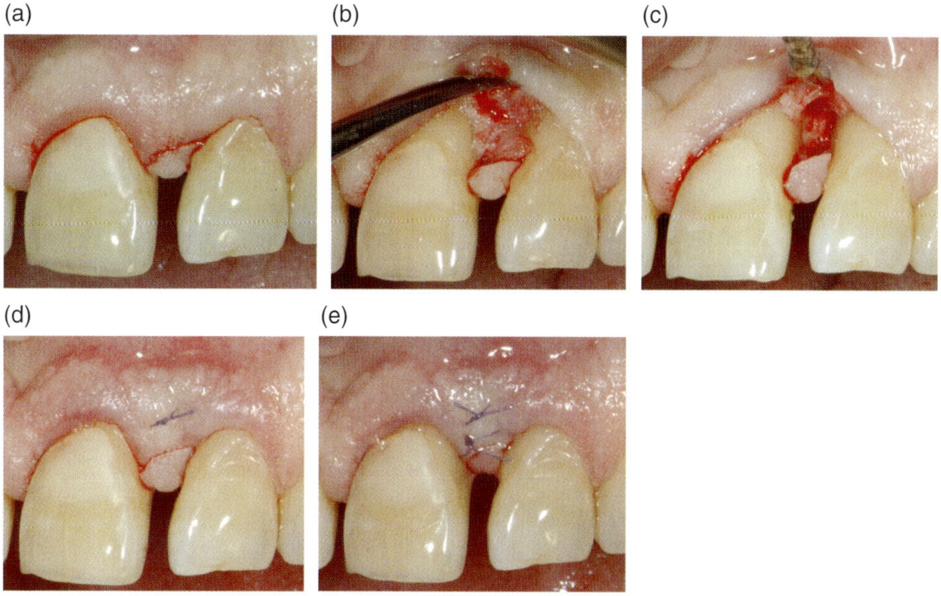

Fig. 9.6 Single Flap Approach (SFA) (Trombelli et al. 2007, 2008, 2009, 2010, 2011). SFA consists of an envelope flap (a). The mesio-distal extension of the flap is kept as limited as possible while ensuring proper access for defect debridement and graft/membrane positioning and stabilization. Sulcular incisions are performed following the gingival margin of the teeth included in the surgical area only on the side where the defect extension is prevalent (only buccal or only lingual). In the interproximal area (i.e. at the level of the interdental papilla) overlying the intraosseous defect, an oblique or horizontal incision is made following the profile of the underlying bone crest. The greater the distance from the tip of the papilla to the underlying bone crest (i.e. the greater the apico-coronal dimension of the supracrestal soft tissues), the more apical the buccal incision in the interdental area (i.e. close to the base of the papilla). This is made in order to (1) provide an adequate amount of untouched supracrestal soft tissue connected to the undetached oral papilla to ensure flap adaptation and suturing, and (2) warrant proper access to the intraosseous defect for debridement. The defect is approached by elevating a flap only on one side and leaving the opposite portion of the interdental supracrestal soft tissues undetached (b). Root and defect debridement is performed (c). Primary closure is achieved with a first horizontal internal mattress suture placed between the SFA coronal to the mucogingival junction and the base of the undetached papilla in order to provide the repositioning of the SFA (d). Then, a second horizontal internal mattress suture is placed between the most coronal portion of the SFA and the most coronal portion of the undetached papilla to ensure the primary closure of the repositioned SFA (e).

area. Maximum interdental volume of supracrestal soft tissue at the time of flap manipulation will facilitate closure for primary intention (Trombelli et al. 2002). It is recommended to delay the surgical procedure until excellent tissue tone and minimal inflammation of the supracrestal soft tissue is reached by non-surgical instrumentation. Swollen, inflamed tissues are difficult to manipulate and suture, and post-surgical shrinkage is uncontrolled. At least 3–4 weeks should elapse (after cause-related therapy) before the surgical procedure is undertaken.

When performing a surgical flap for reconstructive procedure, the use of a microsurgical approach based on specially designed instruments (surgical blades, periosteal elevators, tissue pliers, etc.) under magnifying loops or a surgical microscope is strongly recommended. Microsurgical approach in elevating, handling and suturing has been shown to increase the percentage of sites healed by primary closure (Cortellini and Tonetti 2001; Wachtel et al. 2003). Incisions should be always placed away from the grafted site in order to avoid graft exposure in the post-surgical phase due to contraction of the flap edges.

In this respect, pre-surgery bone sounding to assess the bone contour must be accurately performed on the tooth presenting the defect as well as the adjacent teeth. Provided a good access to the osseous defect is achieved, an envelope flap should be preferred, thus limiting the use of vertical/oblique releasing incisions.

When performing the intrasulcular incision in the interdental area for papilla retention approaches, attention must be paid not to undermine the isthmus of the papilla. Therefore, interdental intrasulcular incision should be carried out (1) by using a microsurgical blade, (2) by keeping the blade inclination as much parallel to the long axis of the tooth as possible, and (3) by running the blade from the sulcus beneath the contact point towards the buccal (or lingual) aspect of the tooth. When raising the flap (which is a full-thickness flap), excessive thinning of the flap should be avoided in order to ensure optimal blood supply. Split-thickness dissection should only be performed at the most apical part of the flap to release flap tension and permit coronal displacement.

Attention should be paid to minimize the reflection of the flap. Complete survival of the flap is dependent on the blood supply which also derives from the connective tissue-to-bone contact of non-reflected areas. The entire thickness of the supracrestal soft tissue in the interdental area should be maintained, because an excessive thinning of the papilla may compromise an adequate covering of the graft biomaterial or membrane. Granulation and connective tissue from the inner aspect of the flap overlying the graft or membrane should not be removed in order to warrant proper blood supply and integrity to the flap. The flap should be passively adapted in a coronal position before suturing; therefore, split-thickness dissection or periosteal fenestration at the base of the flap should be performed to release flap tension and coronally advance the flap. 5-0 to 7-0 sutures should be left in place for at least 14 days, thus providing flap adaptation and closure until a sufficient maturation of the wound may ensure resistance to mechanical disrupting forces acting on the wound margins. Sutures should be placed in the interdental area overlying the intraosseous defect coronal to the mucogingival junction (i.e. in the keratinized gingiva) to ensure proper flap stability. Flaps should be passively adapted, and sutures should not be tied too tightly and not exert excessive tension on the flap. Internal mattress sutures are placed to coronally advance the flaps without tension on the flap edges, while interrupted sutures are used to approximate wound margins.

Following the reconstructive procedure, the patient is asked to avoid mechanical oral hygiene procedures in the surgerized area for at least 4–6 weeks. Early mechanical disturbance of the healing site may be detrimental for the reconstructive outcome. Chemical plaque control is recommended along with weekly professional removal of supragingival plaque. Systemic antibiotics may be prescribed; however, there is no evidence that a post-surgery antibiotic regimen has a positive effect on the regenerative outcome (Trombelli et al. 2002). The patient should refrain or limit daily cigarette consumption since smoking has been consistently proven to impair healing response following reconstructive procedures (Tonetti et al. 1995, Trombelli et al. 1997). To optimize professional plaque control, a stringent supportive care program must be adopted with monthly recalls during the first 6 months, and every 3 months thereafter.

CONCLUSIONS

The aim of this chapter was to describe flap designs aimed at establishing favorable circumstances which may eventually enhance the clinical outcome of reconstructive procedures in periodontal intraosseous defects. The selection of a specific flap design and related suture technique must be based on the predictability to achieve optimal primary closure of the healing wound, thus creating an essential biologic prerequisite for periodontal regeneration. The surgical reconstruction of the lost attachment apparatus is a highly technique-sensitive procedure, where the choice and the technical performance of the flap design in a specific patient with a specific defect plays a key role. The clinical value to adapt the selection of the surgical approach to the anatomy of the treated area as well as the physical and biological characteristics of the regenerative materials adopted has been emphasized (Trombelli et al. 2002, 2006; Cortellini and Tonetti 2005; Trombelli 2005, 2010). Along with the use of the appropriate regenerative technology, the surgical procedures should provide conditions for primary intention healing supporting adequate wound stability allowing uneventful tissue formation and maturation. In this respect, flap design and suture technique appear of paramount importance to maximize the reconstructive potential of membrane, graft biomaterials and biological agents.

REFERENCES

Becker, W., Becker, B.E., Berg, L., et al. (1988) New attachment after treatment with root isolation procedures: report for treated Class III and Class II furcations and vertical osseous defects. *International Journal of Periodontics and Restorative Dentistry* **8**, 8–23.

Cortellini, P. and Tonetti, M.S. (2001) Microsurgical approach to periodontal regeneration. Initial evaluation in a case cohort. *Journal of Periodontology* **72**, 559–569.

Cortellini, P. and Tonetti, M.S. (2004) Long-term tooth survival following regenerative treatment of intrabony defects. *Journal of Periodontology* **75**, 672–678.

Cortellini, P. and Tonetti, M.S. (2005) Clinical performance of a regenerative strategy for intrabony defects: scientific evidence and clinical experience. *Journal of Periodontology* **76**, 341–350.

Cortellini, P. and Tonetti, M.S. (2009) Improved wound stability with a modified minimally invasive surgical technique in the regenerative treatment of isolated interdental intrabony defects. *Journal of Clinical Periodontology* **36**, 157–163.

Cortellini, P., Pini Prato, G.P. and Tonetti, M.S. (1995) The modified papilla preservation technique. A new surgical approach for interproximal regenerative procedures. *Journal of Periodontology* **66**, 261–266.

Cortellini, P., Pini Prato, G. and Tonetti, M.S. (1996a) The modified papilla preservation technique with bioresorbable barrier membranes in the treatment of intrabony defects. Case reports. *International Journal of Periodontics and Restorative Dentistry* **16**, 546–559.

Cortellini, P., Paolo, G., Prato, P. and Tonetti, M.S. (1996b) Long-term stability of clinical attachment following guided tissue regeneration and conventional therapy. *Journal of Clinical Periodontology* **23**, 106–111.

Cortellini, P., Prato, G.P. and Tonetti, M.S. (1999) The simplified papilla preservation flap. A novel surgical approach for the management of soft tissues in regenerative procedures. *International Journal of Periodontics and Restorative Dentistry* **19**, 589–599.

Cortellini, P., Tonetti, M.S., Lang, N.P., et al. (2001) The simplified papilla preservation flap in the regenerative treatment of deep intrabony defects: clinical outcomes and postoperative morbidity. *Journal of Periodontology* **72**, 1702–1712.

Haney, J.M., Nilvéus, R.E., McMillan, P.J., et al. (1993) Periodontal repair in dogs: expanded polytetrafluoroethylene barrier membranes support wound stabilization and enhance bone regeneration. *Journal of Periodontology* **64**, 883–890.

Hiatt, W.H., Stallard, R.E., Butler, E.D., et al. (1968) Repair following mucoperiosteal flap surgery with full gingival retention. *Journal of Periodontology* **39**, 11–16.

Linghorne, W.J. and O'Connell, D.C. (1950) Studies in the regeneration and reattachment of supporting structures of the teeth; soft tissue reattachment. *Journal of Dental Research* **29**, 419–428.

Michaelides, P.L. and Wilson, S.G. (1996) A comparison of papillary retention versus full-thickness flaps with internal mattress sutures in anterior periodontal surgery. *International Journal of Periodontics and Restorative Dentistry* **16**, 388–397.

Murphy, K.G. (1996) Interproximal tissue maintenance in GTR procedures: description of a surgical technique and 1-year reentry results. *International Journal of Periodontics and Restorative Dentistry* **16**, 463–477.

Newell, D.H. and Brunsvold, M.A. (1985) A modification of the "curtain technique" incorporating an internal mattress suture. *Journal of Periodontology* **56**, 484–487.

Nyman, S., Lindhe, J. and Rosling, B. (1977) Periodontal surgery in plaque-infected dentitions. *Journal of Clinical Periodontology* **4**, 240–249.

Papapanou, P.N., Wennstrom J.L. and Grondahl, K. (1988) Periodontal status in relation to age and tooth type. A cross-sectional radiographic study. *Journal of Clinical Periodontology* **15**, 469–478.

Polson, A.M. and Proye, M.P. (1983) Fibrin linkage: a precursor for new attachment. *Journal of Periodontology* **54**, 141–147.

Ramfjord, S.P. and Nissle, R.R. (1974) The modified widman flap. *Journal of Clinical Periodontology* **45**, 601–607.

Selvig, K.A., Kersten, B.G. and Wikesjo, U.M. (1993) Surgical treatment of intrabony periodontal defects using expanded polytetrafluoroethylene barrier membranes: influence of defect configuration on healing response. *Journal of Periodontology* **64**, 730–733.

Takei, H.H. (1991) Surgical techniques for reconstructive periodontics. *Dental Clinics of North America* **35**, 531–539.

Takei, H.H., Han, T.J., Carranza, F.A. Jr, et al. (1985) Flap technique for periodontal bone implants. Papilla preservation technique. *Journal of Periodontology* **56**, 204–210.

Tonetti, M.S., Pini Prato, G. and Cortellini, P. (1993) Periodontal regeneration of human intrabony defects. IV. Determinants of healing response. *Journal of Periodontology* **64**, 934–940.

Tonetti, M.S., Pini Prato, G. and Cortellini, P. (1995) Effect of cigarette smoking on periodontal healing following GTR in infrabony defects. A preliminary retrospective study. *Journal of Clinical Periodontology* **22**, 229–234.

Trombelli, L. (2005) Which reconstructive procedures are effective for treating the periodontal intraosseous defect? *Periodontology 2000* **37**, 88–105.

Trombelli, L. (2010) Flap design and suturing techniques to optimize reconstructive outcomes. In: Sculean, A. (ed.) *Periodontal Regenerative Therapy*, pp 241–258. Quintessence Publishing, New Malden, Surrey.

Trombelli, L., Kim, C.K., Zimmerman, G.J., et al. (1997) Retrospective analysis of factors related to clinical outcome of guided tissue regeneration procedures in intrabony defects. *Journal of Clinical Periodontology* **24**, 366–371.

Trombelli, L., Heitz-Mayfield, L.J., Needleman, I., et al. (2002) A systematic review of graft materials and biological agents for periodontal intraosseous defects. *Journal of Clinical Periodontology* **29 Suppl 3**, 117–135.

Trombelli, L., Annunziata, M., Belardo, S., et al. (2006) Autogenous bone graft in conjunction with enamel matrix derivative in the treatment of deep periodontal intra-osseous defects: a report of 13 consecutively treated patients. *Journal of Clinical Periodontology* **33**, 69–75.

Trombelli, L., Farina, R., Franceschetti, G., et al. (2007) Single Flap Approach in periodontal reconstructive surgery (article in Italian). *Dental Cadmos* **8**, 15–25.

Trombelli, L., Farina, R., Franceschetti, G., et al. (2008) Management of the soft tissues according to the principles of the Single Flap Approach in the treatment of periodontal intraosseous defects (article in Italian). *Dental Clinics* **3**, 1–8.

Trombelli, L., Farina, R., Franceschetti, G., et al. (2009) Single Flap Approach with buccal access in periodontal reconstructive procedures. A case series. *Journal of Periodontology* **80**, 353–60.

Trombelli, L., Simonelli, A., Pramstraller, M., et al. (2010) Single Flap Approach with and without guided tissue regeneration and a hydroxyapatite biomaterial in the management of intraosseous periodontal defects. *Journal of Periodontology* **9** (Epub ahead of print).

Trombelli, L., Simonelli, A., Schincaglia, G.P., Alessandro, C., Farina, R. (2011) Single Flap Approach for Surgical Debridement of Deep Intraosseous Defects: A Randomized Controlled Trial. *Journal of Periodontology* (Epub ahead of print).

Wachtel, H., Schenk, G., Bohm, S., et al. (2003) Microsurgical access flap and enamel matrix derivative for the treatment of periodontal intrabony defects: a controlled clinical study. *Journal of Clinical Periodontology* **30**, 496–504.

Wikesjö, U.M., Claffey, N. and Egelberg, J. (1991) Periodontal repair in dogs. Effect of heparin treatment of the root surface. *Journal of Clinical Periodontology* **18**, 60–64.

Wikesjö, U.M., Nilvéus, R. (1990) Periodontal repair in dogs: effect of wound stabilization on healing. *Journal of Periodontology* **61**, 719–724.

10 Periodontal Regeneration: Experimental Observations – Clinical Consequences

Ulf M.E. Wikesjö, Cristiano Susin, Jaebum Lee, Douglas P. Dickinson and Giuseppe Polimeni

Laboratory for Applied Periodontal & Craniofacial Regeneration, Departments of Periodontics and Oral Biology, Georgia Health Sciences University College of Dental Medicine, Augusta, Georgia, USA

INTRODUCTION

Periodontal regeneration is defined as the reproduction or reconstitution of a lost or injured part, such that the form and function of lost structures is restored (American Academy of Periodontology 2001). In consequence, periodontal regeneration requires regeneration of alveolar bone, cementum, periodontal ligament and gingiva. However, the periodontium has traditionally not been considered amendable to regeneration. Once a periodontal defect had been thoroughly debrided and the root surfaces decontaminated from biofilm (thereby exposing an alveolar landscape of valleys, ridges, craters, ravines and caves), wound healing and maturation following wound closure was expected to include some regeneration or remodeling of crestal bone, but rarely (if ever) regeneration of the periodontal attachment (i.e. extrinsic fiber cementum including a perpendicularly or obliquely oriented Sharpey's fiber attachment inserting into the newly formed alveolar bone). Indeed, histologic observations from clinical cases and non-human primate experimental models cemented a paradigm of a race among tissues circumscribing the wound in which rapid formation of a long junctional epithelium or an epithelial attachment onto the periodontally denuded root inevitably precluded any possibility for regeneration of the periodontal attachment (Caton and Greenstein 1993). However, Dr Anthony H. Melcher (1976), cataloging tissues potentially involved in periodontal wound healing/regeneration, advanced the hypothesis that tissue resources sequestered within the periodontal ligament would present with the appropriate condiment for periodontal regeneration. His hypothesis nurtured incremental advances in research and clinical application, eventually unfolding into the possibility of periodontal regeneration (Karring et al. 1993). Structural observations of periodontal wound healing/regeneration led to a clarity that has advanced a triad of clinical conditions to be met in order to unleash this innate regenerative potential: wound stability, space provision and wound closure for primary intention healing being a clinical *conditio sine*

Oral Wound Healing: Cell Biology and Clinical Management, First Edition. Edited by Hannu Larjava.

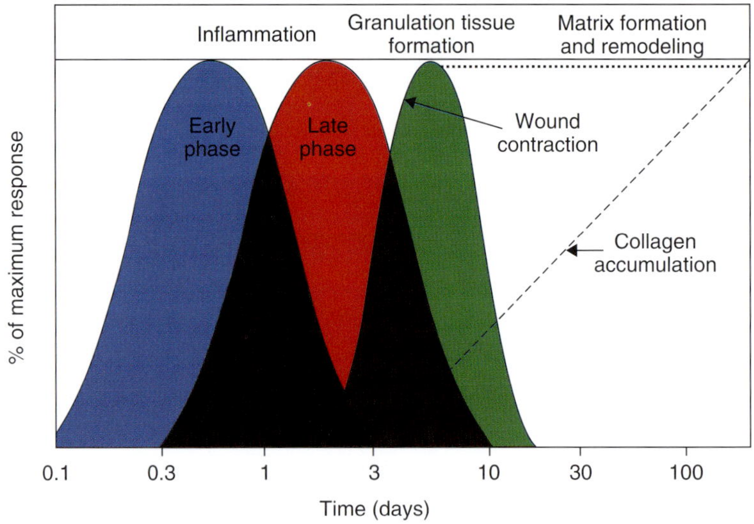

Fig. 10.1 Phases of wound healing (epidermal incisional wounds) including an early (within hours) and late (within days) phase of inflammation dominated by polymorphonuclear neutrophils and macrophages, respectively. The magnitude of wound contraction parallels the phase of granulation tissue formation. Collagen accumulation is first observed during the phase of granulation tissue formation, and continues through the phase of matrix formation and remodeling. (Redrawn with permission from Dr Richard A.F. Clark.).

qua non for periodontal regeneration (Polimeni et al. 2006). Nevertheless, a specific understanding of involved cells and the molecular cues and signals necessary to recruit and stimulate these cells is still lacking. The objective of this text is to deliberate biologic observations of periodontal wound healing/regeneration from discriminating large animal models and relate these observations to clinical measures that may enhance therapeutic outcomes.

WOUND HEALING

Wound healing is a well-orchestrated interplay among key effector cells (including neutrophils, macrophages, lymphocytes, endothelial cells and fibroblasts), soluble mediators which affect various cells and extracellular matrix synthesis, and remodeling. Although the onset of inflammation is a requisite part of healing, excessive production of inflammatory mediators can lead the wound healing process astray. Healing of incisional and excisional wounds in non-oral sites has been studied in considerable depth (Fig. 10.1) (Clark 1996). The general principles and the cellular and molecular events observed in non-oral sites also apply to wound healing following periodontal surgery. Traumatic and surgical injury causes capillary damage and hemorrhage, and as a result a fibrin clot is formed. The formation of a clot is the immediate response to any trauma. The clot has dual functions: it temporarily protects the denuded tissues, and it serves as a provisional matrix for cell migration (Clark 1996). The fibrin clot amasses all cellular components of blood (including red and white blood cells and platelets) in a matrix of fibrin, plasma fibronectin, vitronectin and thrombospondin (Martin 1997).

Clot formation is followed by an early stage of inflammation. Within hours of injury, inflammatory cells, predominantly neutrophils and monocytes, dominate the clot. These cells cleanse the wound of bacteria, effete and necrotic tissue through phagocytosis and the release of enzymes and toxic oxygen species. Within 3 days the inflammatory reaction morphs into its late phase. Macrophages migrate into the wound area and in addition to wound debridement secrete a wealth of polypeptide mediators, targeting cells involved in the wound healing process (Clark 1996; Wikesjö and Selvig 1999).

The macrophage plays an important role in granulation tissue formation. Growth factors and cytokines secreted by macrophages are involved in the proliferation and migration of fibroblasts, endothelial cells and smooth muscle cells into the wound area. The cell-rich granulation tissue next undergoes maturation and remodeling. Fibroblasts responsible for the replacement of the provisional extracellular matrix produce a new collagen-rich matrix. Approximately a week following wounding, and once the collagen matrix is synthesized, some fibroblasts undergo transformation into myofibroblasts and express α-smooth muscle actin. This transformation and synthesis is responsible for wound contraction. Endothelial cells, responsible for angiogenesis, migrate into the provisional wound matrix to form vascular tubes and loops, and as the provisional matrix matures the endothelial cells undergo programmed cell death (apoptosis) and the number of vascular units is reduced (Martin 1997; Aukhil 2000).

Epithelization of wounds is initiated within hours of injury. Epithelial cells from the basal layer proliferate and migrate through the fibrin clot and eventually the breach in the epithelium is sealed. The epithelial cells in normal gingival tissues use surface receptors known as integrins to bind to laminin in the basal lamina. In order to initiate migration the keratinocytes dissolve this attachment and start expressing integrins suitable for the wound environment (Aukhil 2000).

Maturation of the granulation tissue will lead to regeneration or repair (scar formation) of injured tissues. Whether the tissues heal by regeneration or repair depends upon the availability of necessary cells and the presence or absence of cues and signals to recruit and stimulate these cells. This summary represents an oversimplified account of the wound-healing process. Portrayed steps may considerably overlap and the time needed for completion of each stage may vary depending on local and systemic factors.

PERIODONTAL WOUND HEALING

Conceptually more complex conditions arise when a mucoperiosteal flap is apposed to an instrumented root deprived of its periodontal attachment. The wound now not only comprises opposing vascular margins and the connective tissue and epithelium of the mucogingival flap, but also the rigid, mineralized and non-vascular root surface. In addition, the periodontal wound includes tissue resources sequestered in the alveolar bone and periodontal ligament. Clot formation at the interface between the tooth and a gingival flap is initiated as blood elements are imposed onto the root surface during surgery and at wound closure in an apparently random fashion. Thus, the very initial healing event at the tooth–mucogingival flap interface is the adsorption/adhesion of plasma proteins onto the root surface (Fig. 10.2) (Wikesjö et al. 1991a). Within minutes, a fibrin clot is developed that – at least in part – is attached to the root surface. The wound may also contain voids that eventually fill with serum products, depending on wound volume and approximation of adjoining tissues. Within hours, one may observe the early phase of inflammation as inflammatory cells,

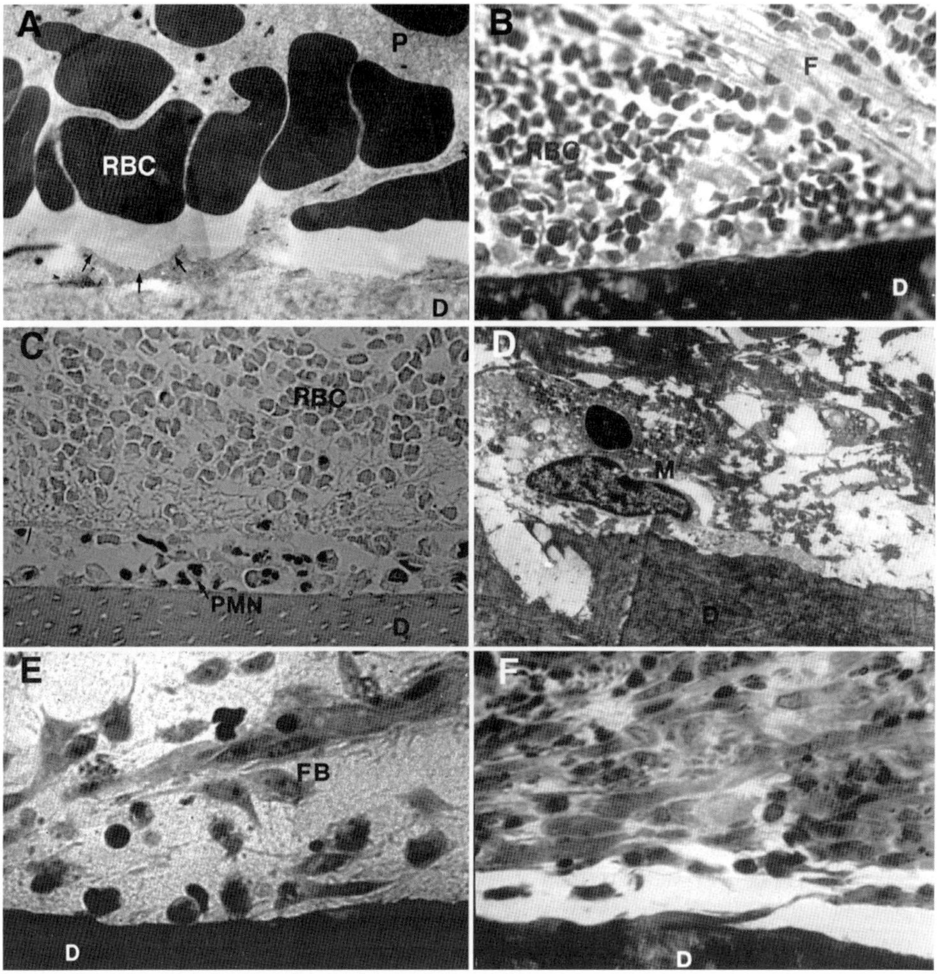

Fig. 10.2 Early healing events at the tooth–gingival flap interface: (a) Red blood cells in a granular precipitate adhering to the dentin surface shown immediately (10 minutes) upon wound closure; an artifactual split (arrows) between the red blood cells and the dentin adhering precipitate verifies the absorption/adhesion of blood elements to the dentin surface (transmission electron micrograph, × 4000). (b) Red blood cells in a fibrin network in close proximity to the root surface observed within 1 hour of wound closure (photomicrograph × 450). (c) Early phase of inflammation: red blood cell aggregates loosely interspersed in an organized fibrin network at 6 hours. The fibrin clot appears attached to the dentin surface. Numerous polymorphonuclear cells may be observed lining the dentin surface (photomicrograph × 450). (d) Late phase of inflammation at 3 days following wound closure, showing a macrophage lining the dentin surface (transmission electron micrograph, × 10,500). (e) Granulation tissue formation including fibroblasts in the maturing fibrin clot at the dentin surface at 3 days (photomicrograph, × 450). (f) Cell-rich connective tissue closely adapted to the dentin surface at 7 days following wound closure (photomicrograph, × 450). D: dentin/root surface; RBC: red blood cells; PMN: polymorphonuclear neutrophils; M: macrophage; FB: fibroblast; F: fibrin; P: plasma precipitate. (For detail see Wikesjö et al. 1991. Figures copyrighted by and modified with permission from the American Academy of Periodontology.).

predominantly neutrophils and monocytes, accumulate onto the root surface, and within 3 days the late phase of inflammation as macrophages migrate into the wound paralleled by granulation tissue formation. At 7 days, a connective tissue attachment may be observed; however, a fibrin clot at various stages of maturation may remain depending on the volume of the wound and tissue resources circumscribing the wound space. These histologic observations suggest that healing at the tooth–mucogingival flap interface does not progress much differently than that in incisional or excisional epidermal wounds, despite the fact that the tooth represents a transgingivally positioned, avascular and rigid wound margin. These observations may also suggest that the first requirement for a new connective tissue attachment or periodontal regeneration in large part rests with the unimpeded adsorption/adhesion of plasma proteins onto the root surface.

The structural observations above have concerned the adsorption, adhesion and maturation of the fibrin clot in periodontal wound healing but have not taken into account the functional integrity of the tooth–gingival flap interface. Only a few experimental studies have evaluated the functional integrity of a maturing periodontal wound. Hiatt et al. (1968) evaluated the tensile strength of the tooth–gingival flap interface following reconstructive surgery of relatively small surgical dehiscence defects over the maxillary canine teeth in dogs, and found that the tensile strength increased from approximately 200 g at day 3 to 340 g at days 5/7, to exceed 1700 g by day 14 post surgery. In other words, even relatively limited periodontal wounds might not reach functional integrity until 2 weeks post surgery! These data further reveal that wound integrity during the early healing phase rests primarily with the stabilization of the gingival tissues offered by suturing. Importantly, they also underscore the significance of passive adaptation of the mucogingival flaps and protection from potentially wound-rupturing tensile forces using strategically placed holding sutures, closing sutures to seal the wound for primary intention healing and, as deemed necessary, stabilizing sutures to neutralize wound rupturing forces. At the same time, the suture-holding strength of the mucogingival tissues as well as innate properties of suture materials must also be considered (Selvig et al. 1998; Leknes et al. 2005; Cortellini and Tonetti 2009). Traumatic effects from post-surgery procedures, including early suture removal, application/removal of surgical dressings and mechanical hygiene routines, must be reconsidered in order to allow wound maturation to reach structural integrity of the surgical site.

PERIODONTAL REGENERATION – NEW ATTACHMENT

Periodontal regeneration requires processes by which collagen fibers form and attach to an instrumented root surface. This usually functionally oriented attachment originates in a newly formed cellular/acellular mixed/extrinsic fiber cementum. Periodontal repair, on the other hand, appears to be characterized by fibrous encapsulation, sometimes referred to as 'collagen adhesion' (Stahl et al. 1972); although collagen fibrils may have a physicochemical attachment by close approximation (Selvig et al. 1995). Periodontal repair may also comprise intrinsic fiber cementum (repair cementum) and root resorption/ankylosis replacing tooth structure with connective tissue and/or bone (Wikesjö and Selvig 1999).

The biological postulates for periodontal wound healing/regeneration formulated by Dr Melcher (1976) were elucidated in a series of studies in dogs by Drs Karring, Nyman and co-workers (Karring et al. 1993). They showed that the surgically severed periodontal ligament residing on extracted teeth exhibited a potential for reattachment, whereas root surfaces exposed to simulated periodontitis conditions, deprived of the periodontal ligament and then root planed, become subject to root resorption/ankylosis when implanted into alveolar bone or covered by mucoperiosteal flaps (Karring et al. 1980; Nyman et al. 1980). Evidently, cell resources within the periodontal ligament — but not adjoining alveolar bone and gingival connective tissue — reconstituted a connective tissue attachment, in part supporting Melcher's postulates.

In subsequent studies using a non-human primate model, Karring and Nyman established that a new connective tissue attachment may form over a root surface deprived of its periodontal attachment by giving preference to cells from the periodontal ligament (Nyman et al. 1982). By creating periodontal fenestration defects over the maxillary lateral incisor and mandibular canine teeth in non-human primates, and then covering the defects with a Millipore filter (with the intent to prevent gingival connective tissue from contacting the root surface), they demonstrated the potential for regeneration of the periodontal ligament – including cementum formation and formation of a functional collagenous attachment – within a 6-month healing interval. Using the same approach and rationale, they provided the first biologic evidence that periodontal regeneration can be obtained over a periodontitis-affected root surface in humans (Nyman et al. 1982; Gottlow et al. 1986). The treatment concept generated from these studies was named guided tissue regeneration, or GTR, because it conceptually steers tissues from the periodontal ligament, and also alveolar bone, to form a regenerate in the wound space provided by an occlusive membrane while blocking contribution from the mucogingival tissues (Karring et al. 1993).

WOUND STABILITY

Early observations of periodontal wound healing may be interpreted as suggesting that a lack of mechanical integrity of the wound is a central factor representing the genesis of a long junctional epithelium or epithelial attachment (Linghorne and O'Connell 1950). Whereas surgical dehiscence defects at maxillary canine teeth in a dog model healed by formation of a new (connective tissue) attachment, identical defect sites at the mandibular canine teeth healed with formation of an epithelial attachment. Undoubtedly, local factors are responsible for the different outcomes between maxillary and mandibular sites, rather than an inclination of the junctional epithelium to selectively migrate and proliferate onto the root surface at mandibular but not maxillary sites. A plausible explanation is that the mandibular sites are subject to wound-rupturing tensile forces that compromise the fibrin seal to the root surface; this initiates epithelial migration and proliferation until an intact tooth–fibrin–gingival interface is reached.

Subsequent studies, also using a dog surgical dehiscence defect model, support the elementary role of the root surface-adhering fibrin clot in periodontal wound healing/regeneration (Hiatt et al. 1968). At 2/3 days post surgery, the fibrin clot provisional matrix in the interface between the mucogingival flap and the tooth was described: 'a very thin layer of fibrin was interposed between the margin of the flap and the tooth …'. This fibrin clot 'prevented a reattachment of the epithelium to the tooth …'. At 7 days post surgery, 'Proliferation of connective tissue along the entire cut surface of the flap was apparent. However, the fibrin had not been completely replaced …'; yet 'no evidence of down growth or increase in epithelial proliferation could be seen …'. Still other studies, using a non-human primate tooth replantation model, resonate with these seminal observations of the significance of unimpeded adsorption/adhesion and maturation

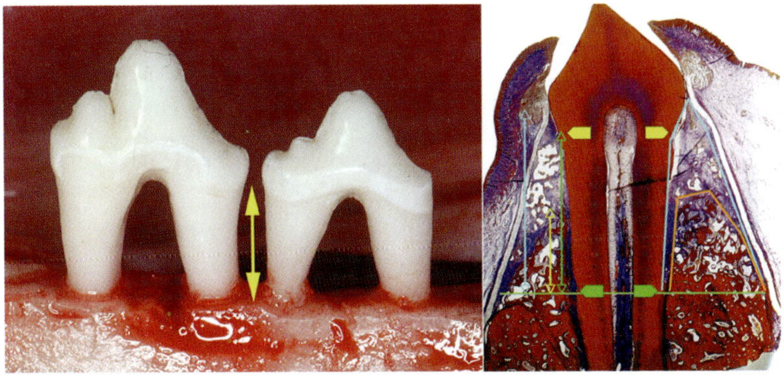

Fig. 10.3 The Critical-size, Supra-alveolar Periodontal Defect Model. The alveolar bone and periodontal attachment (including the cementum) are surgically reduced circumferentially around the 3rd and 4th mandibular premolar teeth to a level 5–6 mm from the cemento-enamel junction. The 1st molar is reduced to the level of the reduced alveolar bone and the 1st and 2nd premolars are extracted. Experimental treatments are applied immediately upon defect induction. Wound closure for primary intention healing may be transgingival (leaving the tooth structure intact) or submerged (following reduction of the clinical crowns). Examples of histometric parameters evaluated in the Critical-size, Supra-alveolar Periodontal Defect Model are shown. The green line and arrowheads represent the base of the surgically created defect and the yellow arrowheads, the cemento-enamel junction. The defect height (vertical green arrow), bone regeneration height (vertical yellow arrow), defect area (blue lines) delineated by an ePTFE membrane in this example (membrane height: vertical blue arrow) and bone regeneration area (orange lines) are shown. The white irregular 'ghost' structures within the wound area and regenerated alveolar bone represent a bone biomaterial evaluated in this example. (For detail see Wikesjö and Nilvéus 1991; Wikesjö et al. 1994; Koo et al. 2004a, 2004b. Figures copyrighted by and modified with permission from Wiley-Blackwell.).

of a fibrin clot for the establishment of a connective tissue attachment, rather than an epithelial attachment, and suggest 'Fibrin linkage: A precursor for new attachment' (Polson and Proye 1983).

Coordinated studies, using the Critical-size, Supra-alveolar, Periodontal Defect Model (Figs. 10.3 and 10.4; Wikesjö and Nilvéus 1991; Wikesjö et al. 1994; Koo et al. 2004a, 2004b), have further detailed the significance of fibrin clot formation/adsorption/adhesion/maturation to the root surface in the shaping of a connective tissue attachment rather than an epithelial attachment (Wikesjö and Nilvéus 1990; Wikesjö et al. 1991b; Haney et al. 1993). Exposed root surfaces subject to gingival flap surgery were treated with heparin prior to wound closure with the intent to compromise fibrin clot formation/adsorption/adhesion; control root surfaces were treated with sterile saline. While the experimental teeth healed with formation of a long junctional epithelium or epithelial attachment, in control sites (without heparin) the epithelium was arrested at, or immediately apical to, the cemento-enamel junction (Fig. 10.5). That is, the heparin application apparently compromised local fibrin clot formation/adsorption/adhesion either by compromising the clotting cascade, by some non-specific surface action, or by a combination of these effects. This isolated manipulation precluded maturation of the fibrin clot into a viable connective tissue attachment and instead resulted in epithelial migration and proliferation along the root surface. This was likely a consequence of exposure of the compromised fibrin clot to local factors, such as induced or physiologic wound-rupturing tensile forces acting on the mucogingival wound margins.

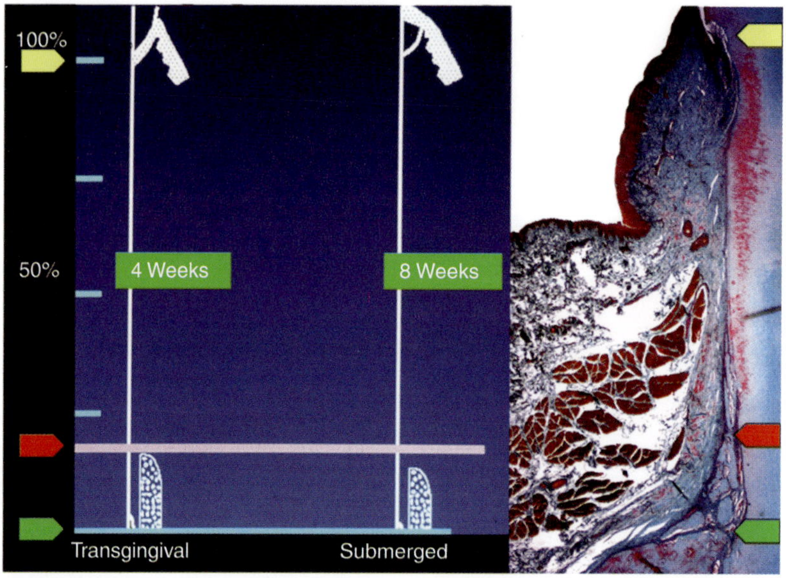

Fig. 10.4 The Critical-size, Supra-alveolar Periodontal Defect Model. The photomicrograph shows a representative section of a sham-surgery control following transgingival wound closure and a 4-week healing interval. The green arrowhead identifies the apical extension of the defect (see Fig. 10.3); the red arrowhead delineates the extent of alveolar regeneration; the yellow arrowheads show the cemento–enamel junction. The schematic illustration shows healing (expressed as percentage) of the defect height in the Model following a 4-week healing interval and transgingival wound closure and following an 8-week healing interval and submerged wound closure. Note that the epithelium is arrested at or immediately below the cemento–enamel junction in sham-surgery control sites. There is limited, if any, regeneration of the periodontal attachment as evaluated by regeneration of cementum or a cementum-like tissue extending from the apical extension of the defect. Bone regeneration is limited to less than 25% of the defect height following a 4- or 8-week healing interval, indicating that in control sites bone regeneration is exhausted within 4 weeks. These characteristics provide a discriminating critical-size model for evaluation of the clinical potential of implantable/injectable devices, biomaterials, biologics and cell constructs with or without root surface bio-modifications. Substantial regeneration in this discriminating model warrants clinical pursuit. Limited regeneration appears less deserving. (For detail see Wikesjö and Nilvéus 1991; Wikesjö et al. 1994; Koo et al. 2004a, 2004b. Figures copyrighted by and modified with permission from Wiley-Blackwell.).

In subsequent experiments, supra-alveolar periodontal defects treated with heparin to compromise fibrin clot adsorption/adhesion/maturation were implanted with either a macro-porous polylactic acid matrix or tissue occlusive expanded polytetrafluoroethylene (ePTFE) barrier membranes, with the intent to stabilize the wound and deflect any wound-rupturing tensile forces from the root surface, thereby allowing wound maturation into a connective tissue attachment (Wikesjö and Nilvéus 1990; Haney et al. 1993). This simple wound stabilizing measure was sufficient to prevent development of an epithelial attachment. In fact, the epithelium was commonly arrested at some distance coronal to the macro-porous polylactic acid devices or ePTFE membranes (Fig. 10.6). Altogether, these observations point to the critical importance of blood elements interacting with the root surface during surgery and at wound closure in order to establish an attachment that endures normal physiologic and other potentially wound-rupturing tensile forces and remains stable until the fibrin clot provisional wound matrix has matured into connective tissue attachment exhibiting structural integrity.

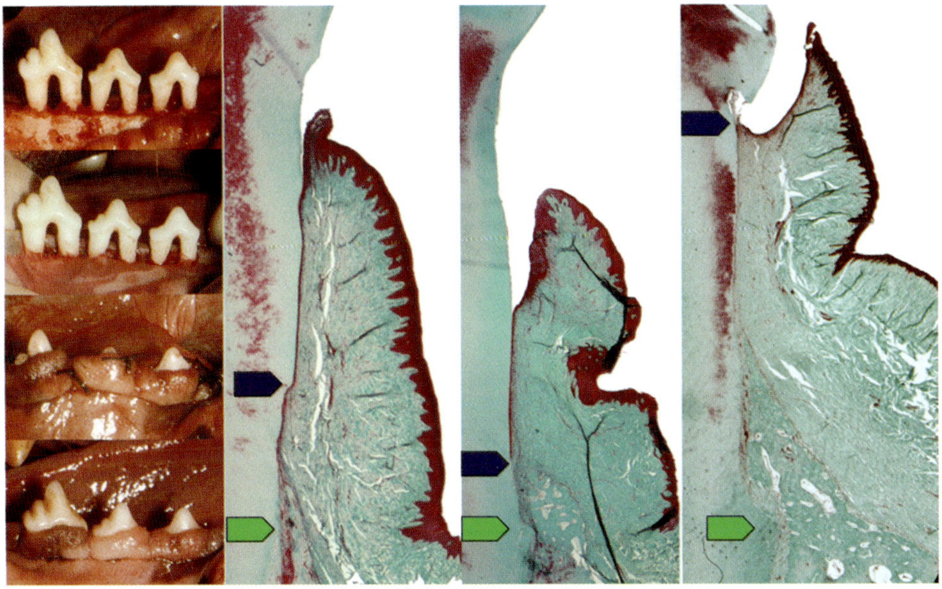

Fig. 10.5 Critical-size, 5-mm, supra-alveolar periodontal defect including coating the root surfaces with a heparin solution immediately prior to wound closure with the intent to interfere with local fibrin clot formation/adsorption/adhesion. The clinical series shows the defect; the root surfaces isolated with rubber dam for the heparin application; transgingival wound closure; and healing at 4 weeks. The left photomicrographs show sites having received the heparin coating. The green arrowheads indicate the base of the defects, the blue arrowhead the apical termination of an epithelial attachment (long junctional epithelium) formed in these sites. Apparently, the heparin coating compromised the fibrin clot in the tooth–gingival flap interface to an extent that allowed apical migration and proliferation of cells from the gingival epithelium rather than maturation into a connective tissue attachment. In contrast, the epithelium is arrested at the cemento–enamel junction in control sites (right) treated with saline, leaving the entire denuded root surface with a new connective tissue attachment. This singular manipulation aimed at interfering with coagulum formation/absorption/adhesion points to the critical importance of the provisionary matrix of the fibrin clot in periodontal wound healing and ultimately periodontal regeneration. Healing interval 4 weeks. (For detail see Wikesjö et al. 1991. Figures copyrighted by and modified with permission from Wiley-Blackwell.).

SPACE PROVISION

Defect configuration has long been considered a significant factor for clinical outcomes of periodontal wound healing/regeneration (Cortellini and Tonetti 2000). Deep, narrow intrabony defects emerge as favored candidates for regenerative procedures compared with wide shallow defects, and three-wall intrabony defects compared with two- and one-wall intrabony defects. It appears rational to assume that the relative abundance of tissue resources – bone and periodontal ligament – circumscribing the defect area in deep three-wall intrabony defects should enhance regenerative potential of these sites in comparison to that of two- and one-wall intrabony defects.

Observations of periodontal wound healing/regeneration in the Critical-size, Supra-alveolar, Periodontal Defect Model demonstrate the extensive regenerative potential of the periodontal attachment and alveolar bone using supracrestal 'zero-wall' periodontal defects (Figs. 10.7–10.11). These reports, using GTR barrier technology, all point to space-provision

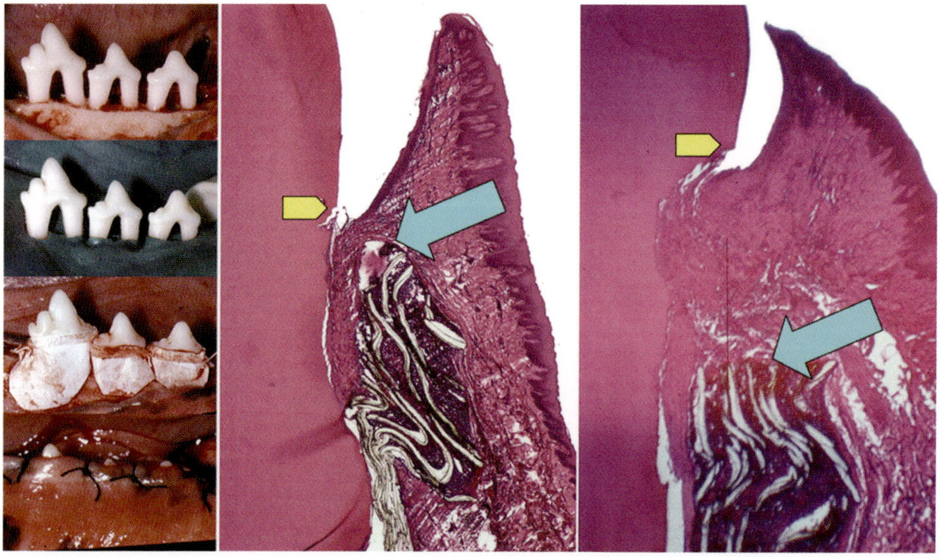

Fig. 10.6 Critical-size, 5-mm, supra-alveolar periodontal defect including coating of the root surfaces with a heparin solution immediately prior to wound closure with the intent to interfere with local fibrin clot formation/adsorption/adhesion. The clinical series shows the defect; the root surfaces isolated with rubber dam for the heparin application; placement of an ePTFE membrane with the intent to stabilize the wound; and transgingival wound closure. Control defects were coated with heparin but did not receive ePTFE membranes. The photomicrographs show the epithelium arrested at the cemento–enamel junction at some distance from the coronal extension of the ePTFE membrane (blue arrow) in heparin-coated defects. The controls (not shown) exhibited formation of an epithelial attachment (long junctional epithelium). Similar observations were made in heparin-coated defects implanted with a polylactic acid block biomaterial (data not shown; Wikesjö and Nilvéus 1990). Collectively, these observations suggest that the implanted device or biomaterial provided some stability to the heparin-compromised tooth–gingival flap interface, allowing the provisionary matrix, the fibrin clot, to mature into a connective tissue attachment rather than migration and proliferation of cells from the gingival epithelium resulting in formation of an epithelial attachment. Healing interval 4 weeks. (For detail see Haney et al. 1993. Figures copyrighted by and modified with permission from the American Academy of Periodontology.).

as one key clinical element in periodontal regenerative therapy (Haney et al. 1993; Sigurdsson et al. 1994; Trombelli et al. 1999; Wikesjö et al. 2003a, 2003b, 2003c). Haney et al. (1993) reported a significant correlation ($r = 0.997$; $p = 0.002$) between the space provided by the membrane and the newly formed bone (Fig. 10.7). Sigurdsson et al. (1994) showed that sites subject to space-provision exhibit extensive periodontal regeneration compared with control (Figs. 10.8. and 10.9). A large wound area resulted in enhanced bone regeneration although the space underneath the GTR barrier was not completely filled with bone. The newly formed bone assumed a 'physiologic' form along the root surface, much like the resident alveolar bone, with the rest of the space underneath the membrane being occupied by dense connective tissue (Figs. 10.8 and 10.9).

While GTR devices traditionally have been occlusive to separate mucogingival tissues from the wound site, cell occlusive membranes do not represent an absolute prerequisite for periodontal regeneration (Wikesjö et al. 2003a, 2003b, 2003c). Space-providing porous GTR membranes have been demonstrated as effective devices in support of periodontal regeneration, with limited post-operative complications compared to occlusive membranes (Fig. 10.10).

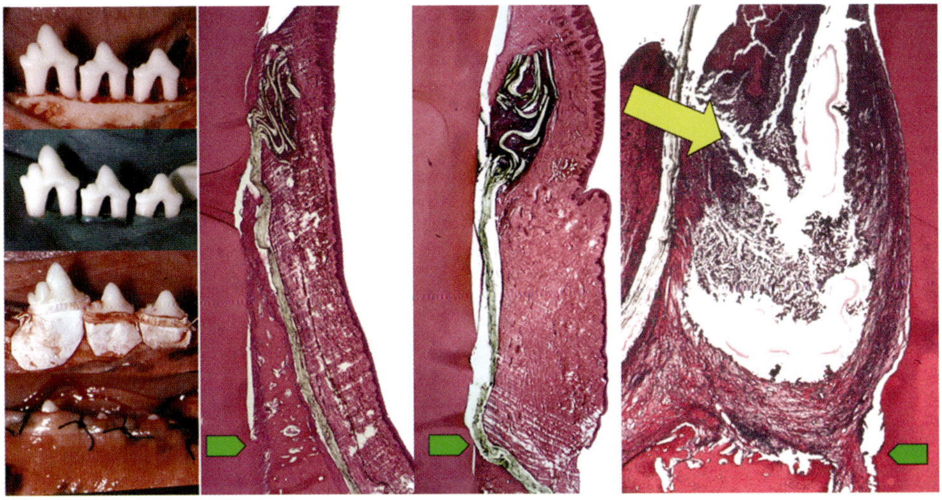

Fig. 10.7 Critical-size, 5-mm, supra-alveolar periodontal defect including coating of the root surfaces with a heparin solution immediately prior to wound closure with the intent to interfere with local fibrin clot formation/absorption/adhesion. The clinical series shows the defect; the root surfaces isolated with rubber dam for the heparin application; placement of an ePTFE membrane with the intent to stabilize the wound; and transgingival wound closure. Control defects were coated with heparin but did not receive ePTFE membranes. The left photomicrograph shows a site where the ePTFE membrane allows a space at the root surface resulting in complete fill with newly formed alveolar bone. The center photomicrograph shows a membrane collapsed or compressed onto the root surface obstructing any regeneration of periodontal structures. There was a significant correlation between the space provided by the membrane and the newly formed alveolar bone (r = 0.997; p = 0.002). The right photomicrograph (yellow arrow) shows an experimental site with wound failure, membrane exposure, infection, inflammation and necrosis. The green arrowheads delineate the apical extension of the defects. Healing interval 4 weeks. (For detail see Haney et al. 1993. Figures copyrighted by and modified with permission from the American Academy of Periodontology.).

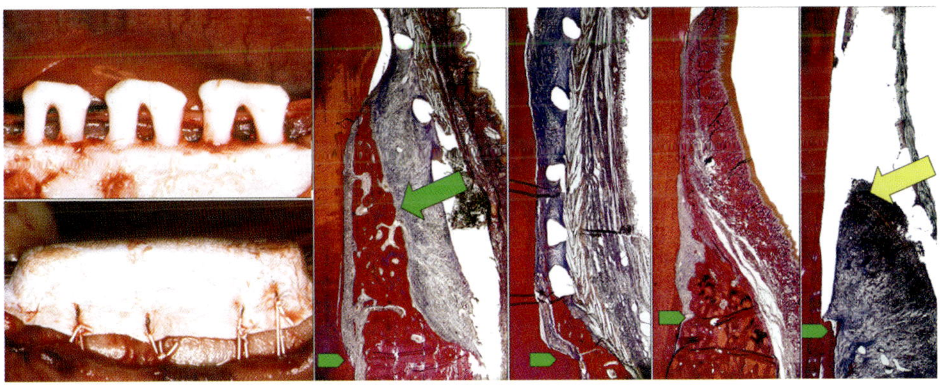

Fig. 10.8 Critical-size, 5-mm, supra-alveolar periodontal defect implanted with an occlusive, space-providing ePTFE membrane. The green arrow points to newly regenerated bone reaching from the apical aspect of the defect to the cemento–enamel junction, the ePTFE membrane provides a suitable space for periodontal regeneration, and the green arrowheads delineate the apical aspect of the supra-alveolar periodontal defect. The second photomicrograph shows the membrane collapsed or compressed onto the root with minimal regeneration as a consequence. The third photomicrograph shows a sham-surgery control also with minimal regeneration, the mucogingival flap being collapsed or compressed onto the root. Finally, the fourth photomicrograph with a yellow arrow shows a site where the membrane has been exposed to the oral cavity resulting in infection and necrosis without any regeneration of periodontal tissues. This study points to the critical importance of primary intention wound healing and unobstructed space-provision for periodontal regeneration. Healing interval 8 weeks. (For detail see Sigurdsson et al. 1994. Figures copyrighted by and modified with permission from the American Academy of Periodontology.).

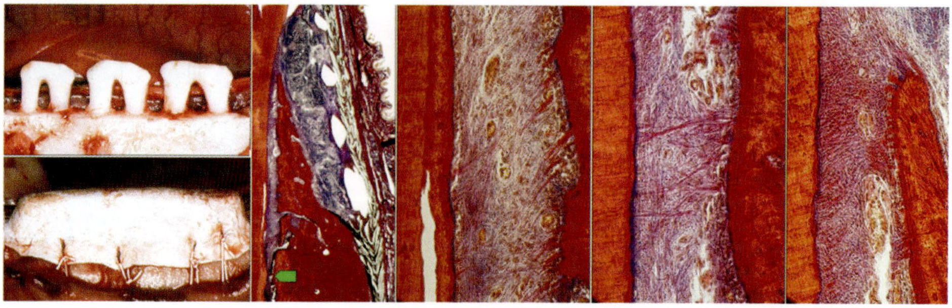

Fig. 10.9 Critical-size, 5-mm, supra-alveolar periodontal defect implanted with an occlusive, space-providing ePTFE membrane. The high magnification photomicrographs from the apical, mid and coronal aspect of the defect show regeneration of the periodontal attachment including cellular cementum, a functionally oriented periodontal ligament and alveolar bone. Note the gradual thinning of the cellular regenerated cementum in a coronal direction. Healing interval 8 weeks. (For detail see Sigurdsson et al. 1994. Figures copyrighted by and modified with permission from the American Academy of Periodontology.).

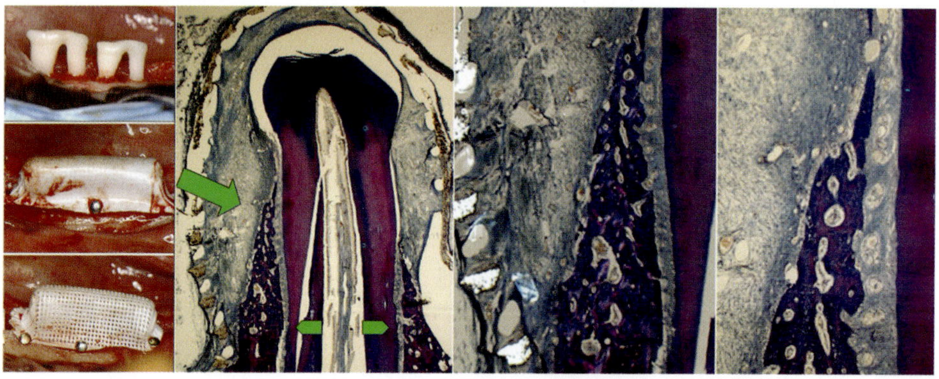

Fig. 10.10 Critical-size, 5-mm, supra-alveolar periodontal defect implanted with occlusive and macroporous, space-providing ePTFE membranes; the photomicrographs show a site implanted with the porous membrane. Note significant periodontal regeneration including a functionally oriented periodontal ligament, cellular cementum and alveolar bone approaching the cemento–enamel junction (green arrow). Similar results were found in sites implanted with the occlusive membrane, clearly suggesting that tissue occlusion is not a critical requirement for periodontal regeneration. Healing interval 8 weeks. (For detail see Wikesjö et al. 2003b. Figures copyrighted by and modified with permission from the American Academy of Periodontology.)

One clinical approach to enhance space-provision for periodontal regeneration uses bone biomaterials ('bone grafts'). A study evaluating GTR procedures including placement of a non-resorbable bone biomaterial in support of space-provision for periodontal regeneration provides clinically significant observations with general implications (Fig. 10.11) (Trombelli et al. 1999). While, as expected, a significant positive correlation was found between space-provision by the GTR membrane and alveolar regeneration ($p < 0.01$), a significant negative correlation was found between the presence of the biomaterial and alveolar regeneration ($p < 0.01$). In other words, the bone biomaterial filling the wound space actually obstructed rather than enhanced bone formation!

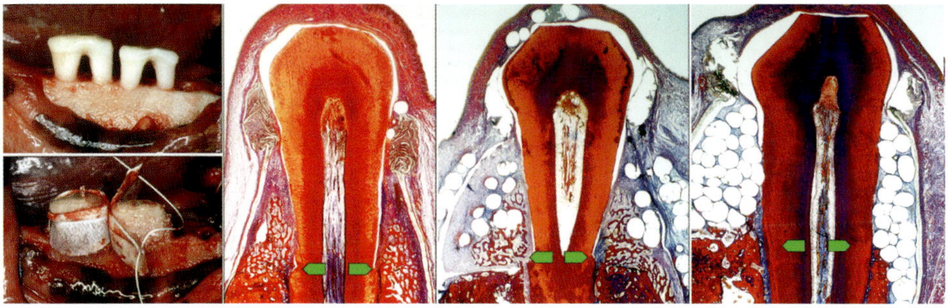

Fig. 10.11 Critical-size, 5-mm, supra-alveolar periodontal defect implanted with an occlusive ePTFE membrane and an osteoconductive biomaterial. Note significant regeneration of alveolar bone in the left photomicrograph in absence of the biomaterial. It is shown that the more biomaterial is used, the less tissue regeneration occurs, raising the question of any benefit of using slowly resorbing or non-resorbable bone biomaterials in conjunction with periodontal regenerative surgery. This study points to the critical importance of unobstructed space-provision for periodontal regeneration. Healing interval 4 weeks. (For detail see Trombelli et al. 1999. Figures copyrighted by and modified with permission from Wiley-Blackwell.).

Polimeni et al. (2004a, 2004b, 2004c, 2004d, 2005, 2009) further detailed the correlation between space-provision and the innate regenerative potential of the periodontium using the Critical-size Supra-alveolar Periodontal Defect Model and using the height of the regenerated alveolar bone along the root surface as a proxy for periodontal regeneration. The height of the regenerated alveolar bone was chosen as a proxy having displayed a high degree of concordance and a significant linear relationship with cementum and periodontal ligament regeneration, indicating that their formation occurs virtually in tandem in this defect model (Polimeni et al. 2009). Regeneration of the periodontal attachment extending just coronally of the alveolar crest in supra-alveolar periodontal defects actually suggests that the periodontal ligament may provide the leading edge for the regenerating periodontal tissues. In brief, in this experimental series, space-provision was shown to be a significant factor for periodontal regeneration in the presence and absence of provisions for GTR (Polimeni et al. 2005). When a coral-derived bone biomaterial was used in conjunction with GTR, it was shown that while the biomaterial enhanced space provision it did not enhance osteogenic bone formation (Polimeni et al. 2004a). In other words, sites of similar size without the biomaterial displayed the same regenerative potential as those with it. When the relative effectiveness of porous versus occlusive GTR barrier membranes was compared, the magnitude of regeneration was significantly enhanced at sites receiving the occlusive GTR device adjusted for the effect of wound area (Polimeni et al. 2004b). Thus, while space-provision appears a critical factor for regeneration, membrane occlusion might provide additional benefits.

The precision and detailed analysis offered in experimental studies using well-characterized model systems (as described herein) is difficult to achieve in clinical studies. However, in broad strokes, the appreciation of space-provision as a critical element for successful periodontal regenerative procedures in model systems is recapitulated in clinical studies evaluating factors affecting the healing response of intrabony defects following GTR and access flap surgery (Cortellini et al. 1995; Tonetti et al. 1996).

WOUND CLOSURE FOR PRIMARY INTENTION HEALING

Wound failure (including suture-line dehiscencies, biomaterials and membrane exposures) is a scourge of periodontal regenerative therapy utilizing GTR and also other approaches, which makes the procedure unpredictable in clinical settings (Selvig et al. 1992; Trombelli et al. 1997; Sanz et al. 2004). A GTR membrane, bone biomaterial or graft can be difficult to completely submerge by gingival tissues at wound closure, or it may exhibit a subclinical exposure or poor flap retention – even following the best techniques for wound closure – and thus becomes exposed during the healing phase. Clinical experience and histologic evaluations of periodontal wound healing in supra-alveolar periodontal defects demonstrate that GTR membranes frequently become exposed, possibly as a consequence of compromised nutritional support to the overlying gingival tissues (Sigurdsson et al. 1994; Wikesjö et al. 2003b; Sanz et al. 2004). Oral bacteria in turn colonize the exposed sites, provoking an inflammatory reaction within the regenerate underneath the membrane. In early studies, animals experiencing membrane exposures received systemic antimicrobial therapy and daily rinses with a chlorhexidine gluconate solution throughout the healing phase. Although this treatment maintains optimal gingival health in non-exposed sites, exposed sites still exhibit large inflammatory infiltrates and necrotic tissues with limited, if any, signs of periodontal regeneration in the histological evaluation (Figs. 10.7 and 10.8). In contrast, when GTR membranes were removed immediately upon exposure followed by wound closure over the exposed regenerate, the newly formed tissues matured into alveolar bone, cementum and a functionally oriented periodontal ligament, remarkably even in sites where the wound failure/membrane exposure occurred as early as 1 week post surgery (Wikesjö et al. 2003b). At sites where periodontal regeneration is allowed to progress without interference under conditions for primary intention healing, complete (or almost complete) regeneration of the periodontal attachment becomes an eminent possibility (Figs. 10.7–10.11; Sigurdsson et al. 1994; Wikesjö et al. 2003a, 2003b, 2003c). The clinical significance of these biologic observations is demonstrated in a retrospective evaluation of GTR therapy in 38 healthy patients receiving treatment of intrabony periodontal defects with a defect depth averaging 6.5 ± 1.6 mm and probing depth averaging 7.6 ± 1.5 mm (Trombelli et al. 1997). Probing bone level gain in sites without membrane exposure averaged 4.1 ± 2.3 mm in contrast to 2.2 ± 2.3 mm for sites with membrane exposure. These observations likely apply to all membrane technologies and likely also to implantable bone biomaterials, including those serving as scaffolds for biologics, and collectively demonstrate the critical significance of primary (unexposed) intention healing for periodontal regeneration.

CONCLUSIONS

Biologic evidence thus far points to the presence of cells originating from the periodontal ligament, wound stability, space-provision and primary intention healing as central biologic and clinical factors that must be afforded to a site to obtain periodontal regeneration. Only profound appreciation of these biological and clinical variables affecting the outcome of periodontal regenerative procedures will allow clinicians to proficiently manipulate them to optimize the clinical result and elevate predictability of periodontal regenerative therapy.

ACKNOWLEDGMENT

Earlier versions of this text have been published as reviews in journals and book chapters. The text is continuously subject to revisions and updating as new information becomes available in our laboratory.

REFERENCES

American Academy of Periodontology (2001) *Glossary of Periodontal Terms*, 4th edn. American Academy of Periodontology, Chicago, Illinois.

Aukhil, I. (2000) Biology of wound healing. *Periodontology* **22**, 44-50.

Caton, J.G. and Greenstein, G.G. (1993) Factors related to periodontal regeneration. *Periodontology* **1**, 9–15.

Clark, R.A.F. (1996) Wound repair. Overview and general considerations. In: Clark, R.A.F., ed. *The Molecular and Cellular Biology of Wound Repair*, 2nd edn. Plenum Press, New York, pp. 3–50.

Cortellini, P. and Tonetti, M.S. (2000) Focus on intrabony defects: guided tissue regeneration. *Periodontology* **22**, 104–132.

Cortellini, P. and Tonetti, M.S. (2009) Improved wound stability with a modified minimally invasive surgical technique in the regenerative treatment of isolated interdental intrabony defects. *Journal of Clinical Periodontology* **36**, 157–163.

Cortellini, P., Pini Prato, G. and Tonetti, M.S. (1995) Periodontal regeneration of human intrabony defects with titanium reinforced membranes. A controlled clinical trial. *Journal of Periodontology* **66**, 797–803.

Gottlow, J., Nyman, S., Lindhe, J., Karring, T. and Wennström, J. (1986) New attachment formation in the human periodontium by guided tissue regeneration. Case reports. *Journal of Clinical Periodontology* **13**, 604–616.

Haney, J.M., Nilvéus, R.E., McMillan, P.J. and Wikesjö, U.M.E. (1993) Periodontal repair in dogs: expanded polytetrafluoroethylene barrier membranes support wound stabilization and enhance bone regeneration. *Journal of Periodontology* **64**, 883–890.

Hiatt, W.H., Stallard, R.E., Butler, E.D. and Badgett, B. (1968) Repair following mucoperiosteal flap surgery with full gingival retention. *Journal of Periodontology* **39**, 11–16.

Karring, T., Nyman, S. and Lindhe, J. (1980) Healing following implantation of periodontitis affected roots into bone tissue. *Journal of Clinical Periodontology* 7(2), **96**–105.

Karring, T., Nyman, S., Gottlow, J. and Laurell, L. (1993) Development of the biological concept of guided tissue regeneration – animal and human studies. *Periodontology* **1**, 26–35.

Koo, K.-T., Polimeni, G., Albandar, J.M. and Wikesjö, U.M.E. (2004a) Periodontal repair in dogs: analysis of histometric assessments in the supraalveolar periodontal defect model. *Journal of Periodontology* **75**, 1688–1693.

Koo, K.-T., Polimeni, G., Albandar, J.M. and Wikesjö, U.M.E. (2004b) Periodontal repair in dogs: examiner reproducibility in the supraalveolar periodontal defect model. *Journal of Clinical Periodontology* **31**, 439–442.

Leknes, K.N., Selvig, K.A., Bøe, O.E. and Wikesjö, U.M.E. (2005) Tissue reactions to sutures in the presence and absence of anti-infective therapy. *Journal of Clinical Periodontology* **32**, 130–138.

Linghorne, W.J. and O'Connell, D.C. (1950) Studies in the regeneration and reattachment of supporting structures of teeth. I. Soft tissue reattachment. *Journal of Dental Research* **29**, 419–428.

Martin, P. (1997) Wound Healing – aiming for perfect skin regeneration. *Science* **276**, 75–81.

Melcher, A.H. (1976) On the repair potential of periodontal tissues. *Journal of Periodontology* **47**, 256–260.

Nyman, S., Karring, T., Lindhe, J. and Plantén, S. (1980) Healing following implantation of periodontitis-affected roots into gingival connective tissue. *Journal of Clinical Periodontology* **7**, 394–401.

Nyman, S., Gottlow, J., Karring, T. and Lindhe, J. (1982) The regenerative potential of the periodontal ligament. An experimental study in the monkey. *Journal of Clinical Periodontology* **9**, 257–265.

Polimeni, G., Koo, K.-T., Qahash, M., Xiropaidis, A.V., Albandar, J.M. and Wikesjö, U.M.E. (2004a) Prognostic factors for alveolar regeneration: effect of a space-providing biomaterial on guided tissue regeneration. *Journal of Clinical Periodontology* **31**, 725–729.

Polimeni, G., Koo, K.-T., Qahash, M., Xiropaidis, A.V., Albandar, J.M. and Wikesjö, U.M.E. (2004b) Prognostic factors for alveolar regeneration: effect of tissue occlusion on alveolar bone regeneration with guided tissue regeneration. *Journal of Clinical Periodontology* **31**, 730–735.

Polimeni, G., Koo, K.-T., Qahash, M., Xiropaidis, A.V., Albandar, J.M. and Wikesjö, U.M.E. (2004c) Prognostic factors for alveolar regeneration: bone formation at teeth and titanium implants. *Journal of Clinical Periodontology* **31**, 927–932.

Polimeni, G., Albandar, J.M. and Wikesjö, U.M.E. (2004d) Prognostic factors for alveolar regeneration: osteogenic potential of resident bone. *Journal of Clinical Periodontology* **31**, 840–844.

Polimeni, G., Albandar, J.M. and Wikesjö, U.M.E. (2005) Prognostic factors for alveolar regeneration: effect of space provision. *Journal of Clinical Periodontology* **32**, 951–954.

Polimeni, G., Xiropaidis, A.V. and Wikesjö, U.M.E. (2006) Biology and principles of periodontal wound healing/regeneration. *Periodontology* **41**, 30–47.

Polimeni, G., Susin, C. and Wikesjö, U.M.E. (2009) Regenerative potential and healing dynamics of the periodontium: a critical-size supra-alveolar periodontal defect study. *Journal of Clinical Periodontology* **36**, 258–264.

Polson, A.M. and Proye, M.P. (1983) Fibrin linkage: a precursor for new attachment. *Journal of Periodontology* **54**, 141–147.

Sanz, M., Tonetti, M.S., Zabalegui, I., et al. (2004) Treatment of intrabony defects with enamel matrix proteins or barrier membranes: results from a multicenter practice-based clinical trial. *Journal of Periodontology* **75**, 726–733.

Selvig, K.A., Kersten, B.G., Chamberlain, A.D., Wikesjö, U.M.E. and Nilvéus, R.E. (1992) Regenerative surgery of intrabony periodontal defects using ePTFE barrier membranes: scanning electron microscopic evaluation of retrieved membranes versus clinical healing. *Journal of Periodontology* **63**, 974–788.

Selvig, K.A., Sigurdsson, T.J. and Wikesjö, U.M.E. (1995) "Collagen adhesion" revisited. *International Journal of Periodontics and Restorative Dentistry* **15**, 529–537.

Selvig, K.A., Biagiotti, G.R., Leknes, K.N. and Wikesjö, U.M.E. (1998) Oral tissue reactions to suture materials. *International Journal of Periodontics and Restorative Dentistry* **18**, 474–487.

Sigurdsson, T.J., Hardwick, R., Bogle, G.C. and Wikesjö, U.M.E. (1994) Periodontal repair in dogs: space provision by reinforced ePTFE membranes enhances bone and cementum regeneration in large supraalveolar defects. *Journal of Periodontology* **65**, 350–356.

Stahl, S.S., Slavkin, H.C., Yamada, L. and Levine, S. (1972) Speculations about gingival repair. *Journal of Periodontology* **43**, 395–402.

Tonetti, M.S., Pini Prato, G. and Cortellini, P. (1996) Factors affecting the healing response of intrabony defects following guided tissue regeneration and access flap surgery. *Journal of Clinical Periodontology* **23**, 548–556.

Trombelli, L., Kim, C.K., Zimmerman, G.J. and Wikesjö, U.M.E. (1997) Retrospective analysis of factors related to clinical outcome of guided tissue regeneration procedures in intrabony defects. *Journal of Clinical Periodontology* **24**, 366–371.

Trombelli, L., Lee, M.B., Promsudthi, A., Guglielmoni, P.G. and Wikesjö, U.M.E. (1999) Periodontal repair in dogs: histologic observations of guided tissue regeneration with a prostaglandin E_1 analog/methacrylate composite. *Journal of Clinical Periodontology* **26**, 381–387.

Wikesjö, U.M.E. and Nilvéus, R. (1990) Periodontal repair in dogs: effect of wound stabilization on healing. *Journal of Periodontology* **61**, 719–724.

Wikesjö, U.M.E. and Nilvéus, R. (1991) Periodontal repair in dogs: healing patterns in large circumferential periodontal defects. *Journal of Clinical Periodontology* **18**, 49–59.

Wikesjö, U.M.E. and Selvig, K.A. (1999) Periodontal wound healing and regeneration. *Periodontology* **19**, 21–39.

Wikesjö, U.M.E., Crigger, M., Nilvéus, R. and Selvig, K.A. (1991a) Early healing events at the dentin–connective tissue interface. Light and transmission electron microscopy observations. *Journal of Periodontology* **62**, 5–14.

Wikesjö, U.M.E., Claffey, N. and Egelberg, J. (1991b) Periodontal repair in dogs: effect of heparin treatment of the root surface. *Journal of Clinical Periodontology* **18**, 60–64.

Wikesjö, U.M.E., Kean, C.J.C. and Zimmerman, G.J. (1994) Periodontal repair in dogs: supraalveolar defect models for evaluation of safety and efficacy of periodontal reconstructive therapy. *Journal of Periodontology* **65**, 1151–1157.

Wikesjö, U.M.E., Xiropaidis, A.V., Thomson, R.C., Cook, A.D., Selvig, K.A. and Hardwick, W.R. (2003a) Periodontal repair in dogs: rhBMP-2 significantly enhances bone formation under provisions for guided tissue regeneration. *Journal of Clinical Periodontology* **30**, 705–714.

Wikesjö, U.M.E., Lim, W.H., Thomson, R.C. and Hardwick, W.R. (2003b) Periodontal repair in dogs: gingival tissue occlusion, a critical requirement for guided tissue regeneration? *Journal of Clinical Periodontology* **30**, 655–664.

Wikesjö, U.M.E., Lim, W.H., Thomson, R.C., Cook, A.D., Wozney, J.M. and Hardwick, W.R. (2003c) Periodontal repair in dogs: evaluation of a bioresorbable space-providing macro-porous membrane with recombinant human bone morphogenetic protein-2. *Journal of Periodontology* **74**, 635–647.

11 Biological Agents and Cell Therapies in Periodontal Regeneration

Hannu Larjava[1], Yi Yang[1], Edward Putnins[1], Jyrki Heino[2] and Lari Häkkinen[1]

[1]Laboratory of Periodontal Biology, Department of Oral Biological and Medical Sciences, Faculty of Dentistry, University of British Columbia, Vancouver, BC, Canada

[2]Department of Biochemistry, University of Turku, Finland

INTRODUCTION

Regeneration of periodontal structures is a complex challenge for periodontal wound healing. As discussed in the previous chapter by Wikesjö et al., wound space-provision, primary stability and healing by primary intention serve as critical factors for attempts to regenerate the periodontium. Barrier membranes for space maintenance can be cumbersome to use in a clinical setting and have proven to provide only partial success in regenerative therapies. Not surprisingly, investigators and clinicians have started to search biological molecules and cell technologies that could help to either speed up or modify the healing process which depends on migration and differentiation of several different cell populations. In this chapter, we briefly review the technologies that are currently in use or in clinical trials. Readers are welcome to review in-depth publications for further details on this complex and evolving area of research.

ADJUNCT GROWTH FACTORS IN PERIODONTAL WOUND REPAIR

Over the years, a number of growth factors have been tested for periodontal regeneration. For true regeneration, four different tissues need to be regenerated, namely cementum, periodontal ligament (PDL), alveolar bone and gingiva. In addition, this regeneration must happen in an environment where bacterial biofilms and mechanical forces are constantly challenging the wound healing process. The fact that so many different tissue types in the presence of a harsh environment are involved explains the lack of progress in perfecting regeneration, regardless of whether or not growth factors, differentiation factors or stem cell therapies are employed (see below). The number of growth factors and cytokines that influence wound healing outcomes are numerous and need to act in a synchronized and

Oral Wound Healing: Cell Biology and Clinical Management, First Edition. Edited by Hannu Larjava.

Table 11.1 Agents (growth and differentiation factors, peptides and enamel matrix proteins) currently approved for clinical applications or in human trials for regeneration of periodontal defects.

Agent name	Scaffold	Product name/ company	Potential mechanisms
PDGF	ß-TCP	GEM 21S/ Osteohealth	Proliferation of fibroblasts, osteogenic cells ↑ Recruitment of pericytes/stem cells?
FGF-2	3% HPC	NA/in clinical trials	Proliferation of fibroblasts, osteogenic cells ↑ Recruitment of stem cells?
GDF-5	ß-TCP/PLGA	NA/in pilot study stage	Proliferation of fibroblasts↑, recruitment of stem cells lineage for ligament formation
P-15	ABM/HA	PepGen P-15/ Denstply	Adhesion and proliferation of fibroblasts Osteogenic differentiation, bone formation TGF-ß1 expression ↑
EMPs	PGA	Emdogain/ Strauman	Fibroblast proliferation ↑, expression of TGF-ß1, IGF-1 ↑ Reduced inflammation, increased angiogenesis Recruitment of stem cells?

PDGF, platelet derived growth factor; FGF-2, fibroblast growth factor-2; GDF-5, growth and differentiation factor-5; P-15, collagen derived peptide; EMPs, enamel matrix proteins; ß-TCP, beta-tricalcium phosphate; HPC, hydroxy propyl cellulose; ABM, anorganic bovine mineral; HA, hyaluronic acid; PGA, propylene glycol alginate.

concerted manner (see Chapter 6). Over the years, many of these growth factors have been tested in the regulation of periodontal ligament fibroblast function as well as in animal studies. At the present time, one commercial product containing growth factors is available for human use in periodontal defects [recombinant human platelet-derived growth factor-BB (rhPDGF-BB) with beta-tricalcium phosphate scaffold (ß-TCF); GEM 21S®; Osteohealth] and two others are in clinical trials [fibroblast growth factor-2 (FGF-2); growth/differentiation factor-5 (GDF-5)] (Table 11.1).

PDGF AND IGF-1 IN PERIODONTAL REGENERATION

PDGFs are polypeptide growth factors released from activated platelets during blood clotting but also expressed by most human tissues (Fredriksson et al. 2004). PDGFs are powerful cytokines that are believed to play important roles in wound healing (see below). Topical application of PDGF has been used for chronic soft tissue wounds that fail to heal. To this end, PDGF (Regranex; Systagenix Wound Management Inc.) has been approved as an adjunct therapy for the treatment of diabetic neuropathic ulcers that extend to subcutaneous tissue or beyond and have an adequate blood supply. It has been reported to increase the incidence of complete ulcer closure in this patient group (Steed 2006).

The PDGF family is composed of four polypeptide chains (A, B, C and D) that can form five disulfide-linked isoforms (AA, AB, BB, CC and DD). The first three isoforms are the most studied and display similar stimulatory effects on neural crest and mesenchymal cells, including PDL fibroblasts (Matsuda et al. 1992; Oates et al. 1993; Boyan et al. 1994; Dennison et al. 1994; Ojima et al. 2003). The rationale for using PDGF-BB for periodontal regeneration does not appear to be clear unless its biological function is explored in more depth and beyond the stimulation of cell proliferation and soft tissue healing. For example, PDGF-BB does not seem to directly stimulate bone cell differentiation. During development, however, PDGF signaling is crucial for neural crest-derived mesenchymal cells that form the bone and cartilage of the head, as illustrated with embryonic skeletal defects in the face of the PDGF or its receptor mutants (Betsholtz 2004; Andrae et al. 2008). PDGF induces osteoblast cell proliferation but inhibits their differentiation (Hock and Canalis 1994; Kubota et al. 2002). In addition, PDGF-BB signaling has no significant effect on differentiation of mesenchymal stem cell (MSCs) to osteoblasts, although proliferation is promoted (Tokunaga et al. 2008; Kumar et al. 2010). In other studies, however, cell proliferation and also expression of some osteogenic differentiation markers were stimulated in MSCs from osteoporotic bone by high doses of PDGF-BB (Pountos et al. 2010). Furthermore, chronic myeloid leukemia patients receiving PDGF receptor inhibitors (imatinibmesylate) show increased bone formation, suggesting that long-term inhibition of PDGF signaling promotes bone formation (O'Sullivan et al. 2007; Fitter et al. 2008). Therefore, it seems unlikely that PDGF-BB promotes periodontal regeneration through differentiation of cells of osteoblastic lineage. Expression of PDGFs and their receptors is stimulated, however, in bone repair (Fujii et al. 1999; Rasubala et al. 2003).

It is possible that PDGF could contribute to bone healing by recruiting pericytes, many of which are MSCs capable of differentiation to osteoblasts (Caplan and Correa 2011). This is in accordance with the observation demonstrating that mice with targeted mutations in PDGF-BB and its receptor die at late gestation due to leaking microvasculature caused by a shortage of pericytes around blood vessels (Levéen et al. 1994; Soriano 1994). Tissue-specific knockout studies have confirmed that endothelium-produced PDGF is responsible for the recruitment of pericytes and that the retention of PDGF-BB (presence of C-terminus of PDGF-BB) is crucial for pericyte–endothelial cell interaction at the sprouting endothelium (reviewed in Betsholtz 2004). Therefore locally produced PDGR-BB has been proposed to enhance blood vessel formation and MSC/pericyte recruitment that stimulates bone formation (Caplan and Correa 2011). It has been known for decades that pericytes/MSCs exist around blood vessels of the periodontium and that they are mobilized during wound repair (Gould et al. 1977; Gould 1983; also see references below). Based on the existing evidence, it can be concluded that PDGF-BB serves as a strong stimulator of mesenchymal cell proliferation, including fibroblasts and pericytes/MSCs, but it may not be sufficient for osteoblast differentiation and bone formation without additional factors/stimuli. Theoretically, therefore, the most advantageous timing for applying recombinant human PDGF-BB (rhPDGF-BB) into periodontal defects would be during early wound healing before the differentiation of MSCs to osteoblasts is initiated (see below).

In early animal studies using dogs and non-human primates, it was observed that in combination with IGF-1 or alone, PDGF could stimulate periodontal regeneration (Lynch et al. 1989, 1991; Cho et al. 1995; Giannobile et al. 1996). Also in combination with a barrier membrane, PDGF-BB appears to induce regeneration (Park et al. 1995). Although the mechanism is not entirely clear, in early wounds PDGF seems to stimulate fibroblast proliferation (Wang et al. 1994) that then leads to generation of all other tissues involved. It is possible that some of the fibroblasts observed actually represent pericytes/MSCs that can differentiate to cells capable of making cementum, PDL and alveolar bone. PDGF-BB in the carrier beta-tricalcium phosphate (ß-TCP) could also increase vascular endothelial growth factor (VEGF) release in periodontal wounds, thus promoting angiogenesis, which is crucial for regeneration (Cooke et al. 2006). However, to validate this mechanism, further experimental evidence is needed. In addition, bone remodeling marker (collagen type I telopeptide) does not correlate with the clinical efficacy dose of PDGF-BB (Sarment et al. 2006).

In the early animal studies, PDGF-BB was often used in combination with insulin-like growth factor-1 (IGF-1) (reviewed in Lee et al. 2010a). These studies led to a clinical trial in humans. Promising clinical results were observed with the combined use of PDGF-BB and

IGF-1 in one phase I/II clinical trial (Howell et al. 1997). IGF-1 and its binding proteins play critical roles in skeletal growth and development (reviewed in Yakar et al. 2010). For example, lack of IGF-1 signaling results in reduced growth and weaker bones (Yakar et al. 2010).

At the cellular level, IGF-1 stimulates osteoblast proliferation and matrix productions but does not appear to affect their differentiation (Conover 2000; Fisher et al. 2005). It also stimulates gingival and PDL fibroblast proliferation (Nishimura and Terranova 1996). In contrast, IGF-1 does not increase the proliferation of MSCs but enhances their migration (Li et al. 2007). Therefore, IGF-1 and PDGF-BB have similar functions on osteoblasts, PDL fibroblasts and MSCs. In fact, any periodontal regeneration expected from the single use of either PDGF or IGF-1 is likely dependent on recruitment of stem cells that are capable of regenerating cementum, bone and PDL.

In animal studies in which IGF-1 has been used alone, variable results have been reported, ranging from no effect on periodontal wound healing (Giannobile et al. 1996) to significant tissue regeneration (Chen et al. 2006). This variation may relate to the carriers used for growth factor delivery. The delivery vehicle of any growth factor dictates the duration, bioavailability and dose of the factor in space and time that ultimately determines cell behaviour and healing outcome. For example, when PDGF-BB is added to ß-TCP particles (0.24–1.0 mm in size), the particles start absorbing the growth factor, reaching a maximum in about 60 minutes, depending on the concentration (Bateman et al. 2005). When the PDGF-saturated ß-TCP particles are placed in animal tissues, 50% of the PDGF is released within 6 days and the remaining 50% disappears within 17 days (Bateman et al. 2005). This represents a significantly longer time than was observed with topically applied PDGF delivered in a methylcellulose gel (Lynch et al. 1991). In other studies, PDGF was almost completely released from either small or large ß-TCP particles within 3 days *in vivo* (Young et al. 2009), suggesting that in clinical use the majority of the growth factor is released within a few days to a week. Because the growth factor (PDGF-BB) and the carrier (ß-TCP) are mixed by the clinician or assisting personnel at the time of surgery, the possibility for variations from the manufacturer's protocol is increased. The operating clinician may not be aware that the concentration of the factor that is absorbed by the particles might be critical for a successful outcome, as poorly mixed product may result in faster release and higher initial dose of the factor, which affects the clinical outcome.

A high dose of PDGF-BB has been reported to be less effective than a lower dose in clinical trials (Nevins et al. 2005). Before these trials, PDGF-BB had been used in early human clinical studies in various carriers with promising clinical results (reviewed in Kaigler et al. 2011). In a phase III trial, PDGF-BB was delivered in ß-TCP carrier in two doses of 0.3 mg/ml and 1 mg/ml. Both doses were safe and produced no adverse side effects (Nevins et al. 2005). The lower dose produced enhanced clinical attachment levels at 3 and 6 months, although the difference was relatively small. Bone fill was also significantly increased in the group that received the lower dose. Interestingly, the higher dose did not improve the clinical attachment level or the bone fill amount. PDGF-BB in ß-TCP is commercially available with recommended clinical applications for intrabony and class II furcation defects as well as for the treatment of gingival recessions (GEM 21S® product information). The recommendation for its use in gingival recessions was based on case series studies documenting similar clinical results to connective tissue grafting when PDGF-BB in ß-TCP carrier is used with a collagen membrane (McGuire et al. 2009). Although some evidence points to the long-term maintenance and stability of the clinical results after using PDGF-BB in ß-TCP (Kaigler et al. 2011), only the wide clinical use of this product in the field by clinicians outside research settings will prove its usefulness for periodontal therapy.

PLATELET-RICH PLASMA IN PERIODONTAL THERAPY

PDGF is also one important factor in platelet-rich plasma (PRP) that has been advocated for periodontal regeneration. PRP is prepared in the office from the patient's own blood, typically by a two-step centrifugation, and the platelets are then activated with thrombin (reviewed in Eppley et al. 2006). PRP contains several growth factors released mainly from activated platelets, including PDGF-AB (100–300 ng/ml), significantly less PDGF-BB, high levels of transforming growth factor-ß (TGF-ß; 100–500 ng/ml) and also some IGF-1 and VEGF (Eppley et al. 2006; Kotsovilis et al. 2010). However, the concentration of these factors can vary considerably in different PRP preparations, possibly due to differences in plasma collection and processing, the efficiency of platelet activation and variations in plasma composition between different donors. Nevertheless, the concentration of total PDGF in the PRP is less than a thousand-fold compared to GEM 21S®. A large number of case studies and clinical trials have been performed using PRP in periodontal defects (reviewed in Trombelli and Farina 2008; Kotsovilis et al. 2010). Both positive and negative outcomes have been reported. For example, in two randomized controlled clinical trials with a limited number of patients and using a split-mouth approach, different outcomes were reported. In one study, PRP mixed with ß-TCP did not seem to improve the clinical outcome in intrabony defects in periodontitis patients (Harnack et al. 2009). In the other study, PRP was applied directly to the periodontal defect and then bovine bone xenograft mixed with PRP was added to fill the defect while the control sites received the xenograft only (Hanna et al. 2004). Significant clinical improvement in periodontal parameters was reported in this study. Studies using PRP have used inconsistent methods for collection and activation of PRP, different carriers for mixing it and variable application methods, which may explain the heterogeneity of the clinical outcomes. In many studies, the concentrations of growth factors in the final product were also not reported. Nor is it known how quickly the growth factors are released from various combinations of PRP and bone grafts. PRP has also been used for sinus graft procedures. It does not seem, however, to improve the clinical outcome for bone grafts in sinus lift procedures (Arora et al. 2010; Esposito et al. 2010). In summary, although promising results with PRP have been reported, more studies need to be performed to optimize PRP collection, preparation and application techniques before it can be applied more widely to clinical practice in periodontics.

FGF-2 IN PERIODONTAL REGENERATION

Recently, fibroblast growth factor-2 (FGF-2) has been reported to stimulate periodontal regeneration in a multi-centre, randomized, double-blinded and placebo-controlled study in 253 patients (Kitamura et al. 2011). The human FGF family of growth factors contains 22 members that have a wide variety of biological functions in various wound-healing related cellular processes including cell proliferation, migration, differentiation and angiogenesis (reviewed in Yun et al. 2010). FGF-2, also called basic FGF (bFGF), together with FGF-1 (acidic FGF), forms a FGF-1 subfamily of FGFs. They signal through tyrosine kinase fibroblast growth factor receptors (FGFRs). As the names of these growth factors reflect, they stimulate fibroblast proliferation. Accordingly, FGF-2 stimulates proliferation of PDL fibroblast and also gingival epithelial cells, depending on culture conditions (Takayama et al. 1997, 2002). Bone cells also express FGF-2 and store it in their extracellular matrix, from where it can be released in a bioactive form (Globus et al. 1989). In general,

FGF-2 stimulates osteoblast proliferation and non-collagen matrix synthesis (Canalis et al. 1988; Globus et al. 1988; McCarthy et al. 1989) but seems to inhibit collagen synthesis and alkaline phosphatase activity (Rodan et al. 1989; Hurley et al. 1993). Depending on the dose and duration, FGF-2 can either inhibit or stimulate osteoblast differentiation and mineralization (Fakhry et al. 2005). Although some actions of FGF-2 on bone cells *in vitro* appear inhibitory to bone formation, *in vivo* studies have demonstrated stimulation of endosteal bone formation. Intravenous administration of FGF-2 stimulates endosteal but inhibits periosteal bone formation in rats (Mayahara et al. 1993; Nakamura et al. 1995; Nagai et al. 1999). In addition, a single injection of FGF-2 improves osseous healing of experimental tibia defects and fractures and promotes mineralization of bones in osteopenic animals (Nakamura et al. 1997, 1998; Kato et al. 1998; Liang et al. 1999). Studies on FGF-2 knockout mice have further demonstrated that FGF-2 is important not only for wound healing but also for osteoblast proliferation and bone mineralization (Ortega et al. 1998; Montero et al. 2000). Because FGF-2 seems to influence mainly endosteal bone formation, it is conceivable that its actions are directed to bone marrow osteoblast precursor or mesenchymal stem cells. In addition, FGF-2 seems to be necessary for maximal induction of osteoblast differentiation by BMP-2 (Naganawa et al. 2008). FGF-2 can also directly stimulate BMP-2 expression in bone cells (Fakhry et al. 2005).

In animal models, FGF-2 appears to stimulate the regeneration of periodontal tissues, including cementum, PDL and bone (Murakami et al. 1999, 2003; Takayama et al. 2001; Shirakata et al. 2010). No ankylosis or epithelial downgrowth was observed in these studies. Two randomized human studies have evaluated the effect of FGF-2 on 2- or 3-wall periodontal defects in 74 and 253 patients, respectively (Kitamura et al. 2008, 2011). FGF-2 was mixed with 3% hydroxypropyl cellulose (HPC) and applied into the defects in three concentrations of 0.2%, 0.3% and 0.4%. Significant bone fill (mean 39–52%) was reported with all concentrations (with the optimal dose at 0.3%) over the vehicle alone group in 36 and 72 weeks (Kitamura et al. 2011). In addition, no adverse side effects were reported, suggesting that the use of FGF-2 in clinical settings is safe. It is not clear whether HPC is an optimal carrier and scaffold for FGF-2 in periodontal defects. HPC is a gel-like viscous liquid that can be expected to release the growth factor relatively quickly, producing a rapid burst of activity. In addition, HPC does not provide any 'tenting' effect that could be useful in large defects prone to gingival collapse after wound closure. FGF-2 mixed with the HPC has been compared to that absorbed into ß-TCF in an animal study which showed improved new bone and cementum formation for the FGF-2/ß-TCF group (Oi et al. 2009). This effect may relate to the slower and longer release of the growth factor from the mineral scaffold. In summary, FGF-2 may serve as a useful therapeutic agent for periodontal regeneration, but the carrier/scaffold may need to be further optimized.

GROWTH AND DIFFERENTIATION FACTOR-5 IN PERIODONTAL REGENERATION

Growth and differentiation factor-5 (GDF-5) is a member of the bone morphogenic proteins (BMPs) and related in amino acid sequence and function to GDF-6 (BMP-13) and GDF-7 (BMP-12) (reviewed in Bragdon et al. 2011). GDF-5 binds to type I BMP receptor on the cell surface and then complexes with the type II receptor to induce signaling via the Smad signaling pathway (Bragdon et al. 2011). Mice with a natural mutation in the GDF-5 gene (bp mice) show abnormalities in various tissues including cartilage, tendon, skin and bone (reviewed in Mikic 2004). Interestingly, ectopic administration of GDF-5 results in tendon and ligament formation, suggesting that it can induce precursor/stem cell differentiation towards mesenchymal cells which can form tendon/ligament (Wolfman et al. 1997). Subsequent studies have shown that GDF-5 can positively affect ligament repair (Forslund et al. 2003; Bolt et al. 2007; Dines et al. 2007). In addition to ligament repair, GDF-5 has been shown to stimulate cartilage and bone healing in a variety of animal models (reviewed in Moore et al. 2010). In craniofacial applications, GDF-5 was demonstrated to enhance bone formation, defect fill and osteointegration of titanium implants (Kuniyasu et al. 2003; Poehling et al. 2006; Simank et al. 2006; Yoshimoto et al. 2006; Gruber et al. 2008; Schwarz et al. 2008; Polimeni et al. 2009;Weng et al. 2009). Furthermore, GDF-5 applied in ß-TCF has been shown to boost bone formation in sinus elevation procedures in a mini-pig model (Gruber et al. 2008, 2009). Recently, GDF-5/ß-TCP has been used for sinus elevation procedures in a randomized human clinical pilot study with 31 patients. The osseous fill was found to be similar to autologous bone/ß-TCF mixture (Koch et al. 2010). Based on current information, GDF-5 treatment appears to be relatively safe in clinical use. More studies are needed, however, to prove if GDF-5 is an effective and safe compound to be used routinely in sinus elevations and whether it offers any advantages over BMP-2, which is available for the same application (Triplett et al. 2009).

Because GDF-5 can positively regulate ligament and bone healing, it is not surprising that it has been tested for periodontal regeneration. In addition, expression of GDF-5 has been observed in cells responsible for the development of the periodontal ligament, namely cementoblasts, osteoblasts and ligament fibroblasts (Sena et al. 2003). In cell culture, GDF-5 stimulates PDL fibroblast proliferation but does not induce osteogenic differentiation (Nakamura et al. 2003). In animal models, GDF-5 applied in either ß-TCP or PLGA carrier has been shown, however, to increase bone, cementum and periodontal ligament formation (Lee et al. 2010b; Kim et al. 2009a; Kwon et al. 2010a, 2010b; Min et al. 2011). In one-wall periodontal defects, GDF-5 showed superior results compared to PDGF-treated 'benchmark' controls (Kwon et al. 2010c). Recently, a randomized human clinical pilot study was performed on 20 patients. The treatment was reported to be safe, but its efficacy in promoting periodontal regeneration has not yet been reported (reviewed in Lee et al. 2010a). In conclusion, GDF-5 appears to be a promising differentiation factor that could support periodontal ligament healing and regeneration.

OTHER GROWTH FACTORS IN PERIODONTAL REGENERATION

Several other growth and differentiation factors have been tested for the regeneration of periodontal defects. These factors have either not shown sufficient promise (i.e. TGFß-1; BMP-2) or are still being evaluated (e.g. TGF-ß3) for periodontal regeneration. Readers are directed to recent review articles for further information (Lee et al. 2010a; Ripamonti and Klar 2010).

BIOACTIVE COLLAGEN-DERIVED PEPTIDE IN PERIODONTAL REGENERATION (PEPGEN P-15®)

A synthetic peptide derived from the type I collagen cell binding region has been developed into a commercial product recommended for intrabony periodontal osseous defects, ridge augmentations, socket preservation and sinus elevation procedures (PepGen P-15®; Dentsply). This 15-amino-acid peptide (GTPGPQGIAGQRGW corresponding to amino acids 766–780 in type I collagen alpha-1 chain) embedded in bovine inorganic xenograft (called anorganic bovine-derived bone material, ABM) has been shown to increase dermal and human periodontal ligament fibroblast adhesion and osteogenic differentiation *in vitro* (Qian and Bhatnagar 1996; Bhatnagar et al. 1999). This peptide also inhibits fibroblast adhesion to collagen (Bhatnagar et al. 1997). Interestingly, all of the known cell surface collagen receptors recognize the collagen triple helix as their ligand binding site (reviewed in Leitinger 2011). A similar domain on collagen was earlier recognized as a putative cell-binding site (Kleinman et al. 1978). It seems to require triple helical structure, however (Grab et al. 1996). It appears obvious that P-15 peptide does not contain any known sequences recognized by these receptors, although the function predicts binding by integrins or other collagen receptors.

Regardless, *in vitro* studies have demonstrated that P-15 may also promote cell survival and inhibit apoptosis (Hanks and Atkinson 2004). In addition, ABM/P-15 suspended in hydrogels such as hyaluronic acid to improve clinical delivery maintains its biological activity and supports cell adhesion and osteogenic differentiation (Nguyen et al. 2003). In this study, increased expression of osteogenic BMP-2 and -7 was observed (Nguyen et al. 2003). ABM/P-15 also seems to increase osteogenicTGF-ß1 expression in PDL fibroblasts and rat osteoblasts (Trasatti et al. 2004; Emecen et al. 2009). Other genes may also be regulated by P-15 (Carinci et al. 2004), but their regulation is likely concentration and cell-type specific. Annexin 2 has been shown to be concentrated on ABM/P-15 particles and to partially regulate alkaline phosphatase accumulation (Yuan et al. 2007). Importantly, annexin 2 has been shown to regulate alkaline phosphatase activity in lipid rafts essential for mineralization (Gillette and Nielsen-Preiss 2004). Consistent with the *in vitro* observation, ABM/P-15 has been shown to promote early bone formation in a porcine skull model (Thorwarth et al. 2005). More recently, ABM/P-15 has been tested in extracranial orthopedic models, including cancellous long bone healing in rabbits (Lindley et al. 2010) and lumbar fusion (Sherman et al. 2010). These studies support the effectiveness of ABM/P-15 in promoting bone formation to the level of gold-standard, autologous bone. In one animal study, ABM/P-15 failed to be effective, but it is unclear whether this was due to poor fixation of the femoral defects (Sarahrudi et al. 2008). In a pilot human clinical trial of 22 patients with malunion or delayed union bone fractures, ABM/P-15 showed positive results (full consolidation) in 20 patients (90% of treated patients) (Gomar et al. 2007). No controls were included in this study, however.

Positive clinical outcomes in terms of bone fill and clinical attachment level gain have been reported in studies using P-15 in patients with intrabony periodontal defects (Yukna et al. 1998, 2000, 2002; Bhongade and Tiwari 2007; Kasaj et al. 2008). These treatment outcomes are related to the peptide itself, as changing the carrier does not seem to affect the results (Vastardis et al. 2005; Matos et al. 2007). Furthermore, in animal studies, P-15, when applied with hydroxyapatite to titanium implants, may promote early osteointegration (Lutz et al. 2010). In other animal studies, ABM/P-15 has been successfully used for lateral ridge augmentations (Barboza et al. 2002). In recent pilot animal and human studies, ABM/P-15 was found to have a promising effect in sinus elevation procedures but was no better than bovine mineralized xenografts (Gelbart et al. 2005; Pettinicchio et al. 2010; El-Madany et al. 2011; Emam et al. 2011). Based on a case report, P-15 may also be useful in socket preservation procedures (Thompson et al. 2006).

In summary, ABM/P-15 is a commercially available product for grafting procedures that appears to positively support regeneration of bone and periodontal tissues. The biological mechanisms explaining how P-15 exerts its biological effects need to be better clarified.

ENAMEL MATRIX PROTEINS IN PERIODONTAL REGENERATION AND WOUND HEALING

Enamel matrix proteins (EMPs) have been used for over a decade in clinical periodontics for tissue regeneration, with multiple reports supporting significant gain of attachment (Figs. 11.1 and 11.2). Readers are encouraged to read these reports and the many reviews covering this topic (reviewed in Venezia et al. 2004; Trombelli and Farina 2008; Esposito et al. 2009). Because of extensive coverage in the published literature, these clinical studies will not be reviewed in detail in this chapter. In summary, superior results over conventional flap debridement in intrabony defects have been reported in human clinical trials, although

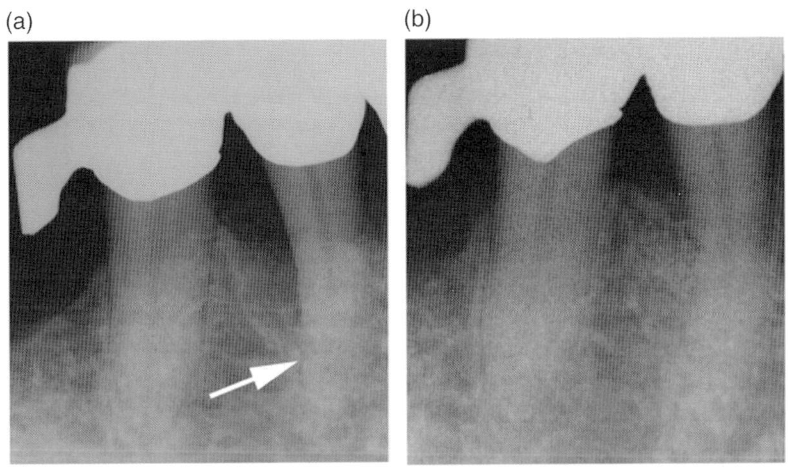

Fig. 11.1 Clinical example of bone gain obtained by application of Emdogain®. A three-wall intrabony periodontal defect distal to #44 with 10-mm probing depth (arrow) was treated with Emdogain® (a). Radiograph taken at 8 months after treatment shows excellent healing of the intrabony defect (b).

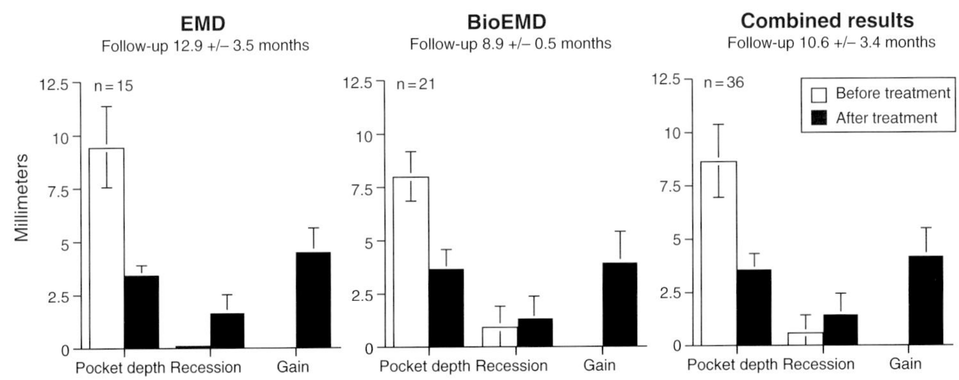

Fig. 11.2 Clinical case studies (36 cases) using Emdogain® gel alone (EMD) or in combination with bovine anorganic bone mineral (BioEMD). Significant pocket depth reduction and attachment gain was attained in both therapies at 9–13 months after treatment.

with a high degree of heterogeneity (reviewed in Venezia et al. 2004; Esposito et al. 2009). The clinical outcomes do not seem to be dependent on the additional use of barrier membranes or bone grafting materials (Trombelli and Farina 2008). EMPs have also been used in root coverage procedures. The combined use of EMPs with a connective tissue graft (CTG) does not seem to produce superior results compared to CTG alone (Rasperini et al. 2011). Significantly better results have been reported, however, with EMP-CTG procedures compared to EMP alone in Miller Class III buccal recessions (Henriques et al. 2010), although these results need to be confirmed. In a pilot study, proximal furcations also appear to respond more favourably to EMP application compared to open flap debridement, although future studies with a larger patient sample size is required to confirm these findings (Casarin et al. 2010).

Although there is extensive literature about the clinical use of EMPs in periodontics, the composition of EMP is still not fully characterized. Amelogenins comprise about 90% of EMPs, but other enamel proteins and proteolytic enzymes, protease inhibitors and TGF-ß1 may also be present (Sculean et al. 2007; Zilm and Bartold 2011). Amelogenins are well conserved in evolution, suggesting that they are crucial for biomineralization of enamel (Brookes et al. 1994). Amelogenins are rich in hydrophobic amino acids, making them insoluble in water and able to self-assemble into supramolecular nanosperes (Fincham et al. 1994). Therefore, for clinical applications, EMPs are solubilized into gel form using propylene glycolalginate (PGA) as a carrier vehicle. When applied to a clinical lesion, EMPs presumably precipitate onto the root surface where they regulate periodontal regeneration (reviewed in Hammarström 1997; Gestrelius et al. 2000). This is supported by findings from human histological studies showing that EMPs can promote the formation of cementum, PDL and bone (Sculean et al. 2003).

Although EMPs have been in clinical use for a long time, the cellular and molecular mechanisms as to how EMPs function to support periodontal regeneration are still only partially understood (Bosshardt 2008). EMPs seem to enhance the adhesion, proliferation and matrix production of fibroblasts but not epithelial cells (Gestrelius et al. 1997; Hoang et al. 2000; Kawase et al. 2000; Haase and Bartold 2001; Cattaneo et al. 2003). Attachment of human PDLFs to EMP is possibly mediated by bone sialoprotein and can be inhibited by RGD-containing peptides and with an anti-αvß3 integrin antibody (Suzuki et al. 2001). Another study suggested that ß1 integrins are important in mediating cell adhesion to EMP (van der Pauw et al. 2002). Recently, it has been demonstrated that both ß1 and αv integrins mediate PDLF adhesion to EMP (Narani et al. 2007). Interestingly, EMPs including amelogenins do not contain any known recognition sites such as RGD for integrins. It is unlikely that cell adhesion to EMPs would be only mediated by siaoloprotein contamination. It is more likely that self-aggregation of amelogenins exposes cryptic sites recognized by integrins. Consistent with this hypothesis is that amelogenins have been shown to increase binding of fibroblasts and endothelial cells via multiple integrins, including αvß3, αvß5 and αvß1 (Almqvist et al. 2010, 2011a). In addition to supporting fibroblast adhesion, several studies have shown that EMPs could stimulate the expression of TGF-ß1 and IGF-1 in PDL fibroblasts (van der Pauw et al. 2000; Lyngstadaas et al. 2001; Okubo et al. 2003; Inaba et al. 2004; Yuan et al. 2006). It is possible, therfore, that some of the clinical effects of EMPs are indirectly caused by a positive response by resident cells producing more endogenous growth factors.

Interestingly, the epithelial cell response to EMPs seems to drastically differ from that of fibroblastic cells. Unlike fibroblasts, keratinocytes cannot attach to EMP directly but need to produce their own adhesion proteins, which then mediate cell adhesion on EMP-coated surfaces (Narani et al. 2007). EMP can also bind to different extracellular matrix proteins utilized by keratinocytes, and the binding of EMPs to fibronectin or collagen may in fact reduce epithelial cell binding to these molecules (Narani et al. 2007). Thus, EMPs appear to have the ability to reduce keratinocyte adhesion to extracellular matrix and inhibit their migration. This mechanism may play a significant role in periodontal regeneration, allowing time for periodontal ligament fibroblasts (PDLFs) to gain access to the root surface prior to epithelial cells.

In periodontal lesions, EMPs must interact with the other matrix proteins such as fibronectin and type I collagen, which are major cell adhesion proteins for fibroblasts and which also play a critical role in collagen fibrillogenesis. Both fibronectin and type I collagen seem to bind to EMP, while there was no binding of type IV collagen or laminin-1 (Narani et al. 2007). This binding was dependent on EMP concentration and peaked at 100 μg/ml EMP for fibronectin and at 1 μg/ml EMP for type I collagen. Fibronectin was bound to EMP in a relatively wide concentration range, while collagen showed a very narrow binding range. This difference in binding affinity suggests that type I collagen and fibronectin bind to different molecules or molecular forms in the EMP mixture. High concentrations of EMP (>1,000 μg/ml) does not seem to promote matrix protein binding. A simple explanation could be that soluble protein aggregates which form with higher concentrations of EMP may mask the binding sites for matrix proteins. Although amelogenin isoforms comprise about 90% of this matrix (Uchida et al. 1998), there are other non-amelogenin proteins present in the enamel matrix, including tuftelin (Deutsch et al. 1991), sheathlin (Uchida et al. 1998), ameloblastin (Krebsbach et al. 1996), amelin (Fong et al. 1996), sulfated enamel proteins (Smith et al. 1995), enamelin (Fukae et al. 1996) and amelotin (Iwasaki et al. 2005). None of these proteins has been reported to bind fibronectin or type I collagen. In EMP, amelogenin and tuftelin could self-assemble (Paine et al. 1998). Furthermore, amelogenin and ameloblastin could form a heteromolecular assembly (Ravindranath et al. 2004). These assemblies could be involved in masking other protein interaction sites. Because many of the actions of EMPs are highly dependent on concentration (adhesion, migration, protein synthesis, protein binding) and EMP form (self-assembly), it is expected that some of the heterogeneity in clinical studies could result from different handling and dilution of the EMPs in the clinical defect.

Both amelogenins and EMPs have been shown to stimulate wound healing and collagen gel contraction in fibroblast culture. In addition, they promoted wound healing in a rabbit model *in vivo* by stimulating fibroblast proliferation and TGF-ß1 expression (Hoang et al. 2000; Rincon et al. 2003; Mirastchijski et al. 2004; Chong et al. 2006; Grayson et al. 2006; Rodrigues et al. 2007). Interestingly, EMPs (amelogenins) have also been reported to improve healing of chronic leg ulcers in clinical trials. These findings have led to the development of a commercial product (Xelma, Molnlycke, Gothenburg, Sweden) to treat these lesions (Vowden et al. 2007; Romanelli et al. 2008; Guest et al. 2009). It should also be kept in mind that there are many similarities between chronic wounds and periodontal lesions associated with chronic periodontal disease. Although the mechanism is not known, amelogenin has been reported to have a positive impact on fibroblast phenotype and regulate their integrin expression and proliferation (Almqvist et al. 2009, 2010). It is also possible that EMPs positively regulate new blood vessel formation and macrophage phenotype in healing wounds. EMPs including amelogenin have been shown to support angiogenesis in different models, although in low concentrations (Schlueter et al. 2007; Kauver et al. 2010; Thoma et al. 2011). In addition, EMPs do not seem to stimulate the monocyte release of pro-inflammatory cytokines (Khedmat et al. 2010). Rather, amelogenins seem to support the phenotype of macrophages associated with tissue repair (Almqvist et al. 2011b). In addition,

EMPs may limit the release of pro-inflammatory cytokines from lipopolysaccharide-exposed blood cells (Myhre et al. 2006). In animal studies, macrophages have been observed in the vicinity of roots of EMP-treated lesions (Fujishiro et al. 2008). In addition, the application of EMP seems to slightly improve initial wound healing markers of periodontal wounds (Wennström and Lindhe 2002) and reduce PDL cell gene expression of early genes involved in inflammation (Parkar and Tonetti 2004). Therefore, it appears that amelogenins in EMPs may positively regulate inflammatory cells and stimulate fibroblast function in healing wounds. It has been reported that the commercial product containing EMPs (Emdogain®, Straumann) also possess anti-microbial properties against dental plaque biofilm and periodontal pathogens (Sculean et al. 2001; Arweiler et al. 2002; Spahr et al. 2002; Newman et al. 2003; Walter et al. 2006). This anti-microbial effect is, however, largely related to the vehicle propylene glycolalginate (PGA) rather than the EMPs themselves. The combined anti-inflammatory action of amelogenins and anti-microbial properties of the vehicle may aid the healing process of chronic wounds in overcoming the chronic state.

A critical step in periodontal regeneration by EMPs is the formation of root cementum. EMPs seem to initially induce a cellular type of cementum formation (Sakallioğlu et al. 2004; Bosshardt et al. 2005). Amelogenins and their fragments that dominate in EMP seem to regulate cementoblast gene expression but not directly cementum formation (Tokiyasu et al. 2000; Viswanathan et al. 2003; Swanson et al. 2006). This is in agreement with *in vivo* findings that showed no expression of amelogenin during cementogenesis (Diekwisch 2001; Bosshardt and Nanci 2004; Janones et al. 2005). There is some preliminary evidence that EMPs could induce cementum formation on materials that do not normally support connective tissue adhesion (Craig et al. 2004). Thus, it appears that EMPs could target mainly fibroblastic cells and their differentiation rather than cementogenesis itself.

The positive effects of EMPs on bone formation have been reported in many clinical studies (radiologic bone fill, re-entry procedures). It is not clear, however, whether EMPs have indirect or direct effects on cells of osteogenic lineage. In early studies by Urist (1971), it was shown that demineralized enamel contains activity that can promote bone formation. There is some evidence that EMPs could stimulate early bone formation in different animal models of bone injuries (Kawana et al. 2001; Sawae et al. 2002; Donos et al. 2003; Yoneda et al. 2003; Cornelini et al. 2004). Effects of EMPs on osteoblastic cell lines appear to be highly cell-line specific (Schwartz et al. 2000). In some studies, EMPs seem to promote cell proliferation and ALP expression in human and rat BMSCs (Keila et al. 2004; Song et al. 2010) and also PDL fibroblasts (van der Pauw et al. 2000; Rodrigues et al. 2007) and primary mouse osteoblasts (Hägewald et al. 2004). However, other studies have suggested no direct role for EMP in promoting osteogenic differentiation (Jiang et al. 2001). Recently, EMPs were reported to stimulate proliferation of human alveolar osteoblasts but to inhibit their differentiation (Jiang et al. 2011). In addition, controversial effects of EMPs on the promotion of osteogenic differentiation of PDL and other mesenchymal cells (such as cementoblasts) have been reported (Tokiyasu et al. 2000; Hakki et al. 2001; Okubo et al. 2003). Furthermore, EMPs have been shown to increase gingival fibroblast proliferation but not osteogenic differentiation (Keila et al. 2004). Amelogenin fragments, specifically the tyrosine-rich amelogenin peptide (TRAP), may in fact decrease mineralization by cementoblast-like cells (Swanson et al. 2006). It is likely, therefore, that EMPs are more important in recruiting cells of osteoblastic lineage to the injury site rather than directly supporting bone formation. This property may be beneficial for periodontal regeneration as it may prevent ankylosis of the EMP-treated roots. An increased incidence of ankylosis has been described in periodontal sites that were treated with BMP-2 which stimulates osteoblast differentiation (Takahashi et al. 2005).

In summary, EMPs appear to have a positive effect on clinical periodontal regeneration, although results are variable. This heterogeneity in treatment outcomes may depend on EMP dose or aggregation of EMPs in the tissues. Although the exact mechanisms of actions of EMPs are still unknown, they seem to stimulate fibroblast proliferation, growth factor expression and angiogenesis and reduce inflammation.

STEM CELLS IN PERIODONTAL WOUND HEALING

As discussed above and in Chapter 10, current procedures aimed at regeneration of periodontal structures have limitations including technical problems with the insertion of barrier membranes, post-operative infections and predictability. With advancing knowledge about the regenerative potential of stem cells, stem cell therapies have been applied to healing periodontal defects in experimental settings. In the following section we, therefore, briefly discuss the potential of using stem cells in periodontal regeneration. Because this is a rapidly advancing field in regenerative medicine, we do not attempt to comprehensively cover the area but rather provide a broad overview of the potential for and challenges with this technology. Several reviews are available to help readers search the literature and find the original research papers on this topic (Morsczeck et al. 2008; Lin et al. 2009; Wu et al. 2010; Inanç and Elçin 2011).

As discussed above, many growth factor therapies for periodontal regeneration may depend on the recruitment of MSCs out of their niche around blood vessels or other sources. However, the fact that we cannot achieve complete regeneration with current treatment modalities suggests that these stem cells are not present or that we are not able to recruit them in high enough numbers, and/or that they are not appropriately induced to differentiate into the distinct cell types necessary for regeneration. To address this problem, current stem cell therapy strategies for periodontal tissue regeneration aim at delivering large numbers of stem cells into tissue defects. Differentiation of these cells into appropriate cell types is necessary for tissue regeneration and may be promoted by adding additional molecular cues that induce differentiation. Alternatively, the local tissue environment during wound healing could provide the necessary signals that lead to appropriate differentiation. In any case, key to success in this strategy is identifying putative stem cells in tissues, successfully isolating and expanding them in culture, and determining the molecular cues that guide their differentiation appropriately. In addition, appropriate methods for cell delivery into tissue defects need to be established and safety concerns addressed.

Stem cells demonstrate unique characteristics when compared to mature somatic cells. They possess an extensive self-renewal capability while maintaining their undifferentiated state. Stem cells are, however, able to differentiate in response to appropriate biological signals. Stem cells are often divided into embryonic and non-embryonic. Embryonic stem cells (ESCs) are derived from the inner cell mass of the blastocysts, whereas non-embryonic stem cells consist of hematopoietic stem cells (HSCs) and mesenchymal stem cells (MSCs) found in bone marrow (BM), skin and other tissues. In fact, BM-MSCs and tissue resident lineage-directed MSCs share many identical features (Wu et al. 2010). While ESCs can differentiate into all tissue cell types, MSCs can typically form only multiple mesenchymal connective tissues including bone, fat and cartilage. Although ESCs appear to have unlimited potential, adult stem cells have remained at the focus of research for clinical applications due to social and ethical issues related to embryonic stem cells. Embryonic stem cell-like lineages [called induced pluripotent stem cells (iPSs)] have also been created from somatic cells through overexpression of three or four key transcription factors, Oct3/4, Sox2, cMyc and Klf4 (Takahashi and Yamanaka 2006; Takahashi et al. 2007; Nakagawa et al. 2008). Recent studies have shown that iPSs can be generated from fibroblasts from various sources (reviewed in Wu and Hochedlinger 2011). Interestingly, iPSs can be generated from dental mesenchymal cells isolated from unerupted human third molar tooth germs with especially high efficiency (Oda et al. 2010). Using iPSs for periodontal regeneration would be challenging as the heterogeneous iPSs would have to be first induced for specific differentiation pathways (bone, ligament, cementum) and then purified and applied in specific scaffolds. It is also not clear how these cells will interact with the resident cells in the defect. At the present time, iPSs have not been tested in animal models for periodontal regeneration. Future use of these cells in non-life-threatening conditions such as periodontal defects will face challenges as the long-term safety remains to be clarified (Wu and Hochedlinger 2011).

In contrast to ESCs and iPSs, adult MSCs have been tested for various applications in wound repair (reviewed in Gauglitz and Jeschke 2011). For example, BM-derived MSCs expanded *in vitro* have been shown to promote healing of diabetic wounds (Falanga et al. 2007; Wu et al. 2007). This enhanced healing seems to be mediated at least partially by the promotion of angiogenesis (Wu et al. 2007). MSCs have also been used to regenerate periodontal defects (reviewed in Bartold et al. 2006). MSCs and PDL-MSCs transplanted to experimental periodontal defects appear to induce some regeneration of cementum, PDL and alveolar bone in animal models (Kawaguchi et al. 2004; Seo et al. 2004; Liu et al. 2008; Li et al. 2009; Ding et al. 2010; Yang et al. 2010). Both cell types also seem to improve bone regeneration in experimentally created acute peri-implant lesions (Kim et al. 2009b). Furthermore, allogeneic PDL-MSCs appear to possess low immunogenicity and function similarly to autologous cells (Ding et al. 2010). No human clinical trials are available demonstrating the effectiveness of treating human periodontal defects with MSCs.

Recent research has also attempted to enhance the capacity of MSCs to differentiate into desired the phenotype or to produce growth factors supportive of periodontal repair. For example, ß-TCP coated with EMPs may regulate mesenchymal stem cells and stimulate a number of genes associated with osteogenic differentiation, although not alkaline phosphatase (Mrozik et al. 2010). *In vitro* studies with BM-MSCs transfected with full-length human amelogenin genes suggest that amelogenins could regulate genes related to osteogenic differentiation (Jingchao et al. 2011). FGF-2 transfected BM-MSCs accelerated periodontal repair in furcation defects in dogs (Tan et al. 2009). In addition, BM-MSCs transfected with a BMP-2 construct were able to induce more extensive periodontal regeneration than control BM-MSCs that did not express BMP-2 in a rabbit model (Chen et al. 2008).

In summary, adult mesenchymal stem cells show promise for future therapy in regenerating lost periodontal tissues. In fact, it is probable that some existing and experimental therapies including the use of PDGF, FGF-2, GDF-5 and EMPs are based on their property to act on locally recruited or bone marrow-derived MSCs. The application of *in vitro* expanded MSCs still faces several challenges regarding their uncertain safety when applied in any regenerative therapy. Better markers to identify stem cells and better methods to expand them in cell culture are needed as the yield of stem cells isolated from tissues is currently low and the populations are phenotypically heterogenous. In addition, the current methods to expand cells in culture can cause genetic changes to the cells. Finally, the risk for malignant transformation needs to be carefully assessed for all human studies including those using MSCs for tissue repair.

CONCLUSIONS

Several therapies using growth and differentiation factors, specific peptides or enamel matrix proteins appear to have positive effects on periodontal regeneration. Although the mechanisms are not fully understood, they may share some common features such as promotion of proliferation of fibroblasts and osteogenic cells. In addition, it is likely that recruitment of local or bone marrow-derived stem cells is induced by most of these therapies. Studies showing heterogeneous clinical results may reflect patient and defect selection, the application itself or the use of scaffolds. Future studies are needed to explore whether better technologies can be developed by a combination of factors or improved scaffolds, including optimized delivery time and concentration of the active agent.

REFERENCES

Almqvist, S., Werthén, M., Johansson, A., et al. (2009) Evaluation of a near-senescent human dermal fibroblast cell line and effect of amelogenin. *Br J Dermatol,* **160**, 1163–1171.

Almqvist, S., Werthén, M., Johansson, A., et al. (2010) Amelogenin is phagocytized and induces changes in integrin configuration, gene expression and proliferation of cultured normal human dermal fibroblasts. *J Mater Sci Mater Med,* **21**, 947–954.

Almqvist, S., Kleinman, H.K., Werthén, M., et al. (2011a) Effects of amelogenins on angiogenesis-associated processes of endothelial cells. *J Wound Care* **20**(68), 70–75.

Almqvist, S., Werthen, M., Lyngstadaas, S.P., et al. (2011b) Amelogenins promote an alternatively activated macrophage phenotype *in vitro*. *Int J Nano Biomaterials*, in press.

Andrae, J., Gallini, R., Betsholtz, C. (2008) Role of platelet-derived growth factors in physiology and medicine. *Genes Dev,* **22**, 1276–1312.

Arora, N.S., Ramanayake, T., Ren, Y.-F., et al. (2010) Platelet-rich plasma in sinus augmentation procedures: a systematic literature review: Part II. *Implant Dent,* **19**, 145–157.

Arweiler, N.B., Auschill, T.M., Donos, N.M. et al. (2002) Antibacterial effect of an enamel matrix protein derivative on *in vivo* dental biofilm vitality. *Clin Oral Investig,* **6,** 205–209.

Barboza, E.P., de Souza, R.O., Caúla, A.L., et al. (2002) Bone regeneration of localized chronic alveolar defects utilizing cell binding peptide associated with anorganic bovine-derived bone mineral: a clinical and histological study. *J Periodontol* **73**, 1153–1159.

Bartold, P.M., Shi, S., Gronthos, S. (2006) Stem cells and periodontal regeneration. *Periodontol,* **40**, 164–172.

Bateman, J., Intini, G., Margarone, J., et al. (2005) Platelet-derived growth factor enhancement of two alloplastic bone matrices. *J Periodontol,* **76**, 1833–1841.

Betsholtz, C. (2004) Insight into the physiological functions of PDGF through genetic studies in mice. *Cytokine Growth Factor Rev,* **15**, 215–228.

Bhatnagar, R.S., Qian, J.J., Gough, C.A. (1997) The role in cell binding of a beta-bend within the tropical helical region in collagen alpha 1 (I) chain: structural and biological evidence for conformational tautomerism on fiber surface. *J Biomol Struct Dyn,* **14**, 547–560.

Bhatnagar, R.S., Qian, J.J., Wedrychowska, A., et al. (1999) Design of biomimetic habits for tissue engineering with P-15, a synthetic peptide analogue of collagen. *Tissue Eng,* **5**, 53–65.

Bhongade, M.L., Tiwari, I.R. (2007) A comparative evaluation of the effectiveness of an anorganic bone matrix/cell binding peptide with an open flap debridement in human infrabony defects: a clinical and radiographic study. *J Contemp Dent Pract,* **8**, 25–34.

Bolt, P., Clerk, A.N., Luu, H.H., et al. (2007) BMP-14 gene therapy increases tendon tensile strength in a rat model of Achilles tendon injury. *J Bone Joint Surg Am,* **89**, 1315–1320.

Bosshardt, D.D. (2008) Biological mediators and periodontal regeneration: a review of enamel matrix proteins at the cellular and molecular levels. *J Clin Periodontol,* **35**, 87–105.

Bosshardt, D.D., Nanci, A. (2004) Hertwig's epithelial root sheath, enamel matrix proteins, and initiation of cementogenesis in porcine teeth. *J Clin Periodontol,* **31**, 184–192.

Bosshardt, D.D., Sculean, A., Windisch, P., et al. (2005) Effects of enamel matrix proteins on tissue formation along the roots of human teeth. *J Periodontal Res*, **40**, 158–167.

Boyan, L.A., Bhargava, G., Nishimura, F., et al. (1994) Mitogenic and chemotactic responses of human periodontal ligament cells to the different isoforms of platelet-derived growth factor. *J Dent Res*, **73**, 1593–1600.

Bragdon, B., Moseychuk, O., Saldanha, S., et al. (2011) Bone morphogenetic proteins: a critical review. *Cell Signal*, **23**, 609–620.

Brookes, S.J., Bonass, W.A., Kirkham, J., et al. (1994) The human amelogenin C-terminal sequence is completely homologous to the C-terminal sequence of amelogenin in all species so far studied. *J Dent Res*, **73**, 716–717.

Canalis, E., Centrella, M., McCarthy, T. (1988) Effects of basic fibroblast growth factor on bone formation *in vitro*. *J Clin Invest*, **81**, 1572–1577.

Caplan, A.I., Correa, D. (2011) PDGF in bone formation and regeneration: new insights into a novel mechanism involving MSCs. *J Orthop Res*, **29**, 1795–803, May 25. doi: 10.1002/jor.21462 [Epub ahead of print].

Carinci, F., Pezzetti, F., Volinia, S. et al. (2004) P-15 cell-binding domain derived from collagen: analysis of MG63 osteoblastic-cell response by means of a microarray technology. *J Periodontol*, **745**, 66–83.

Casarin, R.C.V., Ribeiro, E.D.P., Nociti, F.H. Jr., et al. (2010) Enamel matrix derivative proteins for the treatment of proximal class II furcation involvements: a prospective 24-month randomized clinical trial. *J Clin Periodontol*, **37**, 1100–1109.

Cattaneo, V., Rota, C., Silvestri, M., et al. (2003) Effect of enamel matrix derivative on human periodontal fibroblasts: proliferation, morphology and root surface colonization. An *in vitro* study. *J Periodontal Res*, **38**, 568–574.

Chen, F., Zhao, Y., Wu, H., et al. (2006) Enhancement of periodontal tissue regeneration by locally controlled delivery of insulin-like growth factor-I from dextran-co-gelatin microspheres. *J Control Release*, **114**, 209–222.

Chen, Y.L., Chen, P.K., Jeng, L.B., et al. (2008) Periodontal regeneration using *ex vivo* autologous stem cells engineered to express the BMP-2 gene: an alternative to alveoplasty. *Gene Ther*, **15**, 1469–1477.

Cho, M.I., Lin, W.L., Genco, R.J. (1995) Platelet-derived growth factor-modulated guided tissue regenerative therapy. *J Periodontol*, **66**, 522–530.

Chong, C.H., Carnes, D.L., Moritz, A.J., et al. (2006) Human periodontal fibroblast response to enamel matrix derivative, amelogenin, and platelet-derived growth factor-BB. *J Periodontol*, **77**, 1242–1252.

Conover, CA. (2000) *In vitro* studies of insulin-like growth factor I and bone. *Growth Horm IGF Res*, **Suppl B**, S107–S110.

Cooke, J.W., Sarment, D.P., Whitesman, L.A. et al. (2006) Effect of rhPDGF-BB delivery on mediators of periodontal wound repair. *Tissue Eng*, **12**, 1441–1450.

Cornelini, R., Scarano, A., Piattelli, M., et al. (2004) Effect of enamel matrix derivative (Emdogain) on bone defects in rabbit tibias. *J Oral Implantol*, **30**, 69–73.

Craig, R.G., Kallur, S.P., Inoue, M., et al. (2004) Effect of enamel matrix proteins on the periodontal connective tissue-material interface after wound healing. *J Biomed Mater Res A*, **69**, 180–187.

Dennison, D.K., Vallone, D.R., Pinero, G.J., et al. (1994) Differential effect of TGF-beta 1 and PDGF on proliferation of periodontal ligament cells and gingival fibroblasts. *J Periodontol*, **65**, 641–648.

Deutsch, D., Palmon, A., Fisher, L.W., et al. (1991) Sequencing of bovine enamelin (tuftelin) a novel acidic enamel protein. *J Biol Chem*, **266**, 16021–16028.

Diekwisch, T.G. (2001) The developmental biology of cementum. *Int J Dev Biol*, **45**, 695–706.

Dines, J.S., Weber, L., Razzano, P., et al. (2007) The effect of growth differentiation factor-5 coated sutures on tendon repair in a rat model. *J Shoulder Elbow Surg*, **16**, S215–S221.

Ding, G., Liu, Y., Wang, W., et al. (2010) Allogeneic periodontal ligament stem cell therapy for periodontitis in swine. *Stem Cells*, **28**, 1829–1838.

Donos, N., Sculean, A., Glavind, L., et al. (2003) Wound healing of degree III furcation involvements following guided tissue regeneration and/or Emdogain. A histologic study. *J Clin Periodontol*, **30**, 1061–1068.

El-Madany, I., Emam, H., Sharawy, M. (2011) Comparison of cellular response to anorganic bone matrix/cell binding peptide and allogenic cranial bone after sinus augmentation in rhesus monkeys. *J Oral Implantol*, **37**, 233–245.

Emam, H., Beheiri, G., Elsalanty, M., et al. (2011) Microcomputed tomographic and histologic analysis of anorganic bone matrix coupled with cell-binding peptide suspended in sodium hyaluronate carrier after sinus augmentation: a clinical study. *Int J Oral Max Impl*, **26**, 561–570.

Emecen, P., Akman, A.C., Hakki, S.S., et al. (2009) ABM/P-15 modulates proliferation and mRNA synthesis of growth factors of periodontal ligament cells. *Acta Odontologica Scandinavica*, **67**, 65–73.

Eppley, B.L., Pietrzak, W.A., Blanton, M. (2006) Platelet-rich plasma: a review of biology and applications in plastic surgery. *Plast Reconstr Surg*, **118**, 147e–159e.

Esposito, M., Grusovin, M.G., Papanikolaou, N., et al. (2009) Enamel matrix derivative (Emdogain(R)) for periodontal tissue regeneration in intrabony defects. *Cochrane DB Syst Rev*, **7**, CD003875.

Esposito, M., Grusovin, M.G., Rees, J., et al. (2010) Effectiveness of sinus lift procedures for dental implant rehabilitation: a Cochrane systematic review. *Eur J Oral Implantol*, **3**, 7–26.

Fakhry, A., Ratisoontorn, C., Vedhachalam, C., et al. (2005) Effects of FGF-2/-9 in calvarial bone cell cultures: differentiation stage-dependent mitogenic effect, inverse regulation of BMP-2 and noggin, and enhancement of osteogenic potential. *Bone*, **36**, 254–266.

Falanga, V., Iwamoto, S., Chartier, M., et al. (2007) Autologous bone marrow-derived cultured mesenchymal stem cells delivered in a fibrin spray accelerate healing in murine and human cutaneous wounds. *Tissue Eng*, **13**, 1299–1312.

Fincham, A.G., Moradian-Oldak, J., Simmer, J.P., et al. (1994) Self-assembly of a recombinant amelogenin protein generates supramolecular structures. *J Struct Biol*, **112**, 103–109.

Fisher, M.C., Meyer, C., Garger, G., et al. (2005) Role of IGFBP2, IGF-I and IGF-II in regulating long bone growth. *Bone*, **37**, 741–750.

Fitter, S., Dewar, A.L., Kostakis, P., et al. (2008) Long-term imatinib therapy promotes bone formation in CML patients. *Blood*, **111**, 2538–2547.

Fong, C.D., Hammarström, L., Lundmark, C., et al. (1996) Expression patterns of RNAs for amelin and amelogenin in developing rat molars and incisors. *Adv Dent Res*, **10**, 195–200.

Forslund, C., Rueger, D., Aspenberg, P. (2003) A comparative dose response study of cartilage-derived morphogenetic protein (CDMP)-1,-2 and -3 for tendon healing in rats. *J Orthop Res*, **21**, 617–621.

Fredriksson, L., Li, H., Eriksson, U. (2004) The PDGF family: four gene products form five dimeric isoforms. *Cytokine Grow F R*, **15**, 197–204.

Fujii, H., Kitazawa, R., Maeda, S., et al. (1999) Expression of platelet-derived growth factor proteins and their receptor alpha and beta mRNAs during fracture healing in the normal mouse. *Histochem Cell Biol*, **112**, 131–138.

Fujishiro, N., Anan, H., Hamachi, T., et al. (2008) The role of macrophages in the periodontal regeneration using Emdogain® gel. *J Periodont Res*, **43**, 143–155.

Fukae, M., Tanabe, T., Murakami, C., et al. (1996) Primary structure of the porcine 89-kDa enamelin. *Adv Dent Res*, **10**, 111–118.

Gauglitz, G.G., Jeschke, M.G. (2011) Combined gene and stem cell therapy for cutaneous wound healing. *Mol Pharm*, June 22 [Epub ahead of print].

Gelbart, M., Friedman, R., Burlui, V., et al. (2005) Maxillary sinus augmentation using a peptide-modified graft material in three mixtures: a prospective human case series of histologic and histomorphometric results. *Implant Dent*, **14**, 185–193.

Gestrelius, S., Andersson, C., Lidström, D., et al. (1997) *In vitro* studies on periodontal ligament cells and enamel matrix derivative. *J Clin Periodontol*, **24**, 685–692.

Gestrelius, S., Lyngstadaas, S.P., Hammarström, L. (2000). Emdogain – periodontal regeneration based on biomimicry. *Clin Oral Investig*, **4**, 120–125. Review.

Giannobile, W.V., Hernandez, R.A., Finkelman, R.D., et al. (1996) Comparative effects of platelet-derived growth factor-BB and insulin-like growth factor-I, individually and in combination, on periodontal regeneration in *Macaca fascicularis*. *J Periodontal Res*, **31**, 301–312.

Gillette, J.M., Nielsen-Preiss, S.M. (2004) The role of annexin-2 in osteoblastic mineralization. *J Cell Sci*, **117**, 441–449.

Globus, R.K., Patterson-Buckendahl, P., Gospodarowicz, D. (1988) Regulation of bovine bone cell proliferation by fibroblast growth factor and transforming growth factor beta. *Endocrinology*, **123**, 98–105.

Globus, R.K., Plouet, J., Gospodarowicz, D. (1989) Cultured bovine bone cells synthesize basic fibroblast growth factor and store it in their extracellular matrix. *Endocrinology*, **124**, 1539–1547.

Gomar, F., Orozco, R., Villar, J.L., et al. (2007) P-15 small peptide bone graft substitute in the treatment of non-unions and delayed union. A pilot clinical trial. *Int Orthop*, **31**, 93–99.

Gould, T.R. (1983) Ultrastructural characteristics of progenitor cell populations in the periodontal ligament. *J Dent Res*, **62**, 878–876.

Gould, T.R., Melcher, A.H., Brunette, D.M. (1977) Location of progenitor cells in periodontal ligament of mouse molar stimulated by wounding. *Anat Rec*, **188**, 133–141.

Grab, B., Miles, A.J., Furcht, L.T., et al. (1996) Promotion of fibroblast adhesion by triple-helical peptide modules of type I collagen-derived sequences. *J Biol Chem,* **271**, 12234–12240.

Grayson, R.E., Yamakoshi, Y., Wood, E.J., et al. (2006) The effect of the amelogenin fraction of enamel matrix proteins on fibroblast-mediated collagen matrix reorganization. *Biomaterials,* **27**, 2926–2933.

Gruber, R.M., Ludwig, A., Merten, H.A., et al. (2008) Sinus floor augmentation with recombinant human growth and differentiation factor-5 (rhGDF-5): a histological and histomorphometric study in the Goettingen miniature pig. *Clin Oral Implan Res,* **19**, 522–529.

Gruber, R.M., Ludwig, A., Merten, H.A., et al. (2009) Sinus floor augmentation with recombinant human growth and differentiation-5 (rhGDF-5): a pilot study in the Goettingen miniature pig comparing autogenous bone and rhGDF-5. *Clin Oral Implan Res,* **20**, 175–182.

Guest, J.F., Nagy, E., Sladkevicius, E., et al. (2009) Modelling the relative cost-effectiveness of amelolegenin in non-haling venous leg ulcers. *J Wound Care,* **18**, 218–224.

Haase, H.R., Bartold, P.M. (2001) Enamel matrix derivative induces matrix synthesis by cultured human periodontal fibroblast cells. *J Periodontol,* **72**, 341–348.

Hägewald, S., Pischon, N., Jawor, P., et al. (2004) Effects of enamel matrix derivative on proliferation and differentiation of primary osteoblasts. *Oral Surg Oral Med Oral Pathol Oral Radiol Endod,* **98**, 243–249.

Hakki, S.S., Berry, J.E., Somerman, J.M. (2001) The effect of enamel matrix protein derivative on follicle cells *in vitro*. *J Periodontol,* **72**, 679–687.

Hammarström, L. (1997) Enamel matrix, cementum development and regeneration. *J Clin Periodontol,* **24**, 658–668.

Hanks, T., Atkinson, B.L. (2004) Comparison of cell viability on anorganic bone matrix with or without P-15 cell binding peptide. *Biomaterials,* **25**, 4831–4836.

Hanna, R., Trejo, P.M., Weltman, R.L. (2004) Treatment of intrabony defects with bovine-derived xenograft alone and in combination with platelet-rich plasma: a randomized clinical trial. *J Periodontol,* **75**, 1668–1677.

Harnack, L., Boedeker, R.H., Kurtulus, I., et al. (2009) Use of platelet-rich plasma in periodontal surgery–a prospective randomized double-blind clinical trial. *Clin Oral Invest,* **13**, 179–187.

Henriques, P.S.G., Pelegrine, A.A., Nogueira, A.A., et al. (2010) Application of subepithelial connective tissue graft with or without enamel matrix derivative for root coverage: a split-mouth randomized study. *J Oral Sci,* **52**, 463–471.

Hoang, A.M., Oates, T.W., Cochran, D.L. (2000) *In vitro* wound healing responses to enamel matrix derivative. *J Periodontol,* **71**, 1270–1277.

Hock, J.M., Canalis, E. (1994) Platelet-derived growth factor enhances bone cell replication, but not differentiated function of osteoblasts. *Endocrinology,* **134**, 1423–1428.

Howell, T.H., Fiorellini, J.P., Paquette, D.W., et al. (1997) A phase I/II clinical trial to evaluate a combination of recombinant human platelet-derived growth factor-BB and recombinant human insulin-like growth factor-1 in patients with periodontal disease. *J Periodontol,* **68**, 1186–1193.

Hurley, M.M., Abreu, C., Harrison, J.R., et al. (1993) Basic fibroblast growth factor inhibits type I collagen gene expression in osteoblastic MC3T3-E1 cells. *J Biol Chem,* **268**, 5588–5593.

Inaba, H., Kawai, S., Nakayama, K., et al. (2004) Effect of enamel matrix derivative on periodontal ligament cells *in vitro* is diminished by *Porphyromonas gingivalis*. *J Periodontol*, **75**, 858–865.

Inanç, B., Elçin, Y.M. (2011) Stem cells in tooth tissue regeneration—challenges and limitations. *Stem Cell Rev*, **7**, 683–692.

Iwasaki, K., Bajenova, E., Somogyi-Ganss, E., et al. (2005) Amelotin – a novel secreted, ameloblast-specific protein. *J Dent Res,* **84**, 1127–1132.

Janones, D.S., Massa, L.F., Arana-Chavez, V.E. (2005) Immunocytocehmical examination of the presence of amelogenin during the root development of rat molars. *Arch Oral Biol,* **50**, 527–532.

Jiang, J., Found, A.F., Safavi, K.E., et al. (2001) Effects of enamel matrix derivative on gene expression of primary osteoblasts. *Oral Surg Oral Med Oral Pathol Oral Radiol Endod,* **91**, 95–100.

Jiang, S.-Y., Shu, R., Song, Z.-C., et al. (2011) Effects of enamel matrix proteins on proliferation, differentiation and attachment of human alveolar osteoblasts. *Cell Prolif,* **44**, 372–379.

Jingchao, H., Rong, S., Zhongchen, S., et al. (2011) Human amelogenin up-regulates osteogenic gene expression in human bone marrow stroma cells. *Biochem Biophys Res Commun,* **408**, 437–441.

Kaigler, D., Avila, G., Wisner-Lynch L, et al. (2011) Platelet-derived growth factor applications in periodontal and peri-implant bone regeneration. *Expert Opin Biol Ther,* **11**, 375–385.

Kasaj, A., Röhrig, B., Reichert, C., et al. (2008) Clinical evaluation of anorganic bovine-derived hydroxyapatite matrix/cell binding peptide (P-15) in the treatment of infrabony defects. *Clin Oral Invest,* **12**, 241–247.

Kato, T., Kawaguchi, H., Hanada, K., et al. (1998) Single local injection of recombinant fibroblast growth factor-2 stimulates healing of segmental bone defects in rabbits. *J Orthop Res,* **16**, 654–659.

Kauver, A.S., Thoma, D.S., Carnes, D.L., et al. (2010) *In vivo* angiogenic activity of enamel matrix derivative. *J Periodontol,* **81**, 1196–1201.

Kawaguchi H, Hirachi A, Hasegawa N, et al. (2004) Enhancement of periodontal tissue regeneration by transplantation of bone marrow mesenchymal stem cells. *J Periodontol,* **75**, 1281–1287.

Kawana, F., Sawae, Y., Sahara, T. et al. (2001) Porcine enamel matrix derivative enhances trabecular bone regeneration during wound healing of injured rat femur. *Anat Rec,* **264**, 438–446.

Kawase, T., Okuda, K., Yoshie, H., et al. (2000) Cytostatic action of enamel matrix derivative (Emdogain) on human oral squamous cell carcinoma-derived SCC25 epithelial cells. *J Periodontal Res,* **35**, 291–300.

Keila, S., Nemcovsky, C.E., Moses, O., et al. (2004) *In vitro* effects of enamel matrix proteins on rat bone marrow cells and gingival fibroblasts. *J Dent Res,* **83**, 134.

Khedmat, S., Hadjati, J., Iravani, A., et al. (2010) Effects of enamel matrix derivative on the viability, cytokine secretion, and phagocytic activity of human monocytes. *J Endodont,* **36**, 1000–1003.

Kim, S.H., Kim, K.H., Seo, B.M., et al. (2009b) Alveolar bone regeneration by transplantation of periodontal ligament stem cells and bone marrow stem cells in a canine peri-implant defect model: a pilot study. *J Periodontol,* **80**, 1815–1823.

Kim, T.G., Wikesjö, U.M.E., Cho, K.-S., et al. (2009a) Periodontal wound healing/regeneration following implantation of recombinant human growth/differentiation factor-5 (rhGDF-5) in an absorbable collagen sponge carrier into one-wall intrabony defects in dogs: a dose-range study. *J Clin Periodontol,* **36**, 589–597.

Kitamura, M., Nakashima, K., Kowashi, Y., et al. (2008) Periodontal tissue regeneration using fibroblast growth factor-2: randomized controlled phase II clinical Trial. *PloS One,* **3**, e2611.

Kitamura, M., Akamatsu, M., Machigashira, M., et al. (2011) FGF-2 stimulates periodontal regeneration: results of a multi-center randomized clinical trial. *J Dent Res,* **90**, 35–40.

Kleinman, H.R., McGoodwin, E.B., Martin, G.R. et al. (1978) Localization of the binding site for cell attachment in the α1(1) chain of collagen. *J Biol Chem,* **253**, 5642–5646.

Koch, F.P., Becker, J., Terheyden, H. et al. (2010) A prospective, randomized pilot study on the safety and efficacy of recombinant human growth and differentiation factor-5 coated onto β-tricalcium phosphate for sinus lift augmentation. *Clin Oral Implan Res,* **21**, 1301–1308.

Kotsovilis, S., Markou, N., Pepelassi, E., et al. (2010) The adjunctive use of platelet-rich plasma in the therapy of periodontal intraosseous defects: a systematic review. *J Periodontal Res,* **45**, 428–443.

Krebsbach, H., Lee, S.K., Matsuki, C.Y., et al. (1996) Full-length sequence, localization, and chromosomal mapping of ameloblastin – a novel tooth-specific gene. *J Biol Chem,* **271**, 4431–4435.

Kubota, K., Sakikawa, C., Kasumata, M., et al. (2002) Platelet-derived growth factor BB secreated from osteoclasts acts as an osteoblastogenesis inhibitory factor. *J Bone Miner Res,* **17**, 257–265.

Kumar, A., Salimath, B.P., Stark, G.B., et al. (2010) Platelet-derived growth factor receptor signaling is not involved in osteogenic differentiation of human mesenchymal stem cells. *Tissue Eng Part A,* **16**, 983–993.

Kuniyasu, H., Hirose, Y., Ochi, M., et al. (2003) Bone augmentation using rhGDF-5 collagen composite. *Clin Oral Implants Res,* **14**, 490–499.

Kwon, D.H., Bennett, W., Herberg, S., et al. (2010a) Evaluation of an injectable rh GDF-5/PLGA construct for minimally invasive periodontal regenerative procedures: a histological study in the dog. *J Clin Periodontol,* **37**, 390–397.

Kwon, D.H., Bisch, F.C., Herold, R.W., et al. (2010b) Periodontal wound healing/regeneration following the application of rhGDF-5 in a beta-TCP/PLGA carrier in critical-size supra-alveolar periodontal defects in dogs. *J Clin Periodontol,* **37**, 667–674.

Kwon, H.-R., Wikesjö, U.M.E., Park, J-C., et al. (2010c) Growth/differentiation factor-5 significantly enhances periodontal wound healing/regeneration compared with platelet-derived growth factor-BB in dogs. *J Clin Periodontol,* **37**, 739–746.

Lee, J., Stavropoulos, A., Susin, C., et al. (2010a) Periodontal regeneration: focus on growth and differentiation factors. *Dent Clin North Am,* **54**, 93–111.

Lee, J.-S., Wikesjö, U.M.E., Jung, U.-W., et al. (2010b) Periodontal wound healing/regeneration following implantation of recombinant human growth/differentiation factor-5 in a β -tricalcium phosphate carrier into onewall intrabony defects in dogs. *J Clin Periodontol,* **37**, 382–389.

Leitinger, B. (2011) Transmembrane collagen receptors. *Annu Rev Cell Dev Biol,* **27**, 2.1–2.26.

Levéen, P., Pekny, M., Gebre-Medhin, S., et al. (1994) Mice deficient for PDGF B show renal, cardiovascular, and hematological abnormalities. *Genes Dev,* **8**, 1875–1887.

Li, H., Yan, F., Lei, L., et al. (2009) Application of autologous cryopreserved bone marrow mesenchymal stem cells for periodontal regeneration in dogs. *Cells Tissues Organs,* **190**, 94–101.

Li, Y., Yu, X.Y., Lin, S.G., et al. (2007) Insulin-like growth factor 1 enhances the migratory capacity of mesenchymal stem cells. *Biochem Bioph Res Co,* **356**, 780–784.

Liang, H., Pun, S., Wronski, T.J. (1999) Bone anabolic effects of basic fibroblast growth factor in ovariectomized rats. *Endocrinology,* **140**, 5780–5788.

Lin, N.H., Gronthos, S., Mark Bartold, P. (2009) Stem cells and future periodontal regeneration. *Periodontol,* **51**, 239–252

Lindley, E.M., Guerra, F.A., Krauser, J.T., et al. (2010) Small peptide (P-15) bone substitute efficacy in a rabbit cancellous bone model. *J Biomed Mater Res B,* **94**, 463–468.

Liu, Y., Zheng, Y., Ding, G., et al. (2008) Periodontal ligament stem cell-mediated treatment for periodontitis in miniature swine. *Stem Cells,* **26**, 1065–1073.

Lutz, R., Srour, S., Nonhoff, J., et al. (2010) Biofunctionalization of titanium implants with a biomimetic active peptide (P-15) promotes early osseointegration. *Clin Oral Implants Res,* **21**, 726–734.

Lynch, S.E., Williams, R.C., Polson, A.M., et al. (1989) A combination of platelet-derived and insulin-like growth factors enhances periodontal regeneration. *J Clin Periodontol,* **16**, 545–548.

Lynch, S.E., de Castilla, G.R., Williams, R.C., et al. (1991) The effects of short-term application of a combination of platelet-derived and insulin-like growth factors on periodontal wound healing. *J Periodontol,* **62**, 458–467.

Lyngstadaas, S.P., Lundberg, E., Ekdahl, H., et al. (2001) Autocrine growth factors in human periodontal ligament cells cultured on enamel matrix derivative. *J Clin Periodontol,* **28**, 181–188.

Matos, S.M., Guerra, F.A., Krauser, J., et al. (2007) Clinical evaluation of the combination of anorganic bovine-derived hydroxyapatite matrix/cell-binding peptide (P-15) in particulate and hydrogel form as a bone replacement graft material in human periodontal osseous defects: 6-month reentry controlled clinical study. *J Periodontol,* **78**, 1855–1863.

Matsuda, N., Lin, W.L., Kumar, N.M., et al. (1992) Mitogenic, chemotactic, and synthetic responses of rat periodontal ligament fibroblastic cells to polypeptide growth factors *in vitro*. *J Periodontol,* **63**, 515–525.

Mayahara, H., Ito, T., Nagai, H., et al. (1993) *In vivo* stimulation of endosteal bone formation by basic fibroblast growth factor in rats. *Growth Factors,* **9**, 73–80.

McCarthy, T.L., Centrella, M., Canalis, E. (1989) Effects of fibroblast growth factors on deoxyribonucleic acid and collagen synthesis in rat parietal bone cells. *Endocrinology,* **125**, 2118–2126.

McGuire, M.K., Scheyer, E.T., Schupbach, P. (2009) Growth factor-mediated treatment of recession defects: a randomized controlled trial and histologic and microcomputed tomography examination. *J Periodontol,* **80**, 550–564.

Mikic, B. (2004) Multiple effects of GDF-5 deficiency on skeletal tissues: implications for therapeutic bioengineering. *Ann Biomed Eng,* **32**, 466–476.

Min, C.-K., Wikesjö, U.M.E., Park, J.-C., et al. (2011) Wound healing/regeneration using recombinant human growth/differentiation factor-5 in an injectable poly-lactide-co-glycolide-acid composite carrier and a one-wall intra-bony defect model in dogs. *J Clin Periodontol,* **38**, 261–268.

Mirastchijski, U., Konrad, D., Lundberg, E., et al. (2004) Effect of a topical enamel matrix derivative on skin wound healing. *Wound Repair Regen,* **12**, 100–108.

Montero, A., Okada, Y., Tomita, M., et al. (2000) Disruption of the fibroblast growth factor-2 gene results in decreased bone mass and bone formation. *J Clin Invest,* **105**, 1085–1093.

Moore, Y.R., Dickinson, D.P., Wikesjö, U.M.E. (2010) Growth/differentiation factor-5: a candidate therapeutic agent for periodontal regeneration? A review of preclinical data. *J Clin Periodontol,* **37**, 288–298.

Morsczeck, C., Schmalz, G., Reichert, T.E., et al. (2008) Somatic stem cells for regenerative dentistry. *Clin Oral Investig*, **12**, 113–118.

Mrozik, K.M., Zilm, P.S., Bagley, C.J., et al. (2010) Proteomic characterization of mesenchymal stem cell-like populations derived from ovine periodontal ligament, dental pulp, and bone marrow: analysis of differentially expressed proteins. *Stem Cells Dev*, **19**, 1485–1499.

Murakami, S., Takayama, S., Ikezawa, K. et al. (1999) Regeneration of periodontal tissues by basic fibroblast growth factor. *J Periodont Res,* **34**, 425–430.

Murakami, S., Takayama, S., Kitamura, M., et al. (2003) Recombinant human basic fibroblast (bFGF) stimulates periodontal regeneration in class II furcation defects created in beagle dogs. *J Periodont Res,* **38**, 97–103.

Myhre, A.E., Lyngstadaas, S.P., Dahle, M.K., et al. (2006) Anti-inflammatory properties of enamel matrix derivative in human blood. *J Periodontal Res,* **41**, 208–213.

Nagai, H., Tsukuda, R., Yamasaki, H., et al. (1999) Systemic injection of FGF-2 stimulates endocortical bone modeling in SAMP6, a murine model of low turnover osteopenia. *J Vet Med Sci*, **61**, 869–875.

Naganawa, T., Xiao, L., Coffin, J.D., et al. (2008) Reduced expression and function of bone morphogenetic protein-2 in bones of Fgf2 null mice. *J Cell Biochem*, **103**, 1975–1988.

Nakagawa, M., Koyanagi, M., Tanabe, K., et al. (2008) Generation of induced pluripotent stem cells without Myc from mouse and human fibroblasts. *Nat Biotechnol*, **26**, 101–106.

Nakamura, K., Kawaguchi, H., Aoyama, I., et al. (1997) Stimulation of bone formation by intraosseous application of recombinant basic fibroblast growth factor in normal and ovariectomized rabbits. *J Orthoped Res*, **15**, 303–313.

Nakamura, T., Hanada, K., Tamura, M., et al. (1995) Stimulation of endosteal bone formation by systemic injections of recombinant basic fibroblast growth factor in rats. *Endocrinology*, **136**, 1276–1284.

Nakamura, T., Hara, Y., Tagawa, M., et al. (1998) Recombinant human basic fibroblast growth factor accelerates fracture healing by enhancing callus remodeling in experimental dog tibial fracture. *J Bone Miner Res*, **13**, 942–949.

Nakamura, T., Yamamoto, M., Tamura, M., et al. (2003) Effects of growth/differentiation factor-5 on human periodontal ligament. *J Periodontal* Res, **38**, 597–605.

Narani, N., Owen, G.R., Häkkinen, L., et al. (2007) Enamel matrix proteins bind to wound matrix proteins and regulate their cell-adhesive properties. *Eur J Oral Sci*, **115**, 288–295.

Nevins, M., Giannobile, W.V., McGuire, M.K., et al. (2005) Platelet-derived growth factor stimulates bone fill and rate of attachment level gain: results of a large multicenter randomized controlled trial. *J Periodontol*, **76**, 2205–2215.

Newman, S.A., Coscia, S.A., Jotwani, R., et al. (2003) Effects of enamel matrix derivative on Porphyromonas gingivalis. *J Periodontol*, **74**, 1191–1195.

Nguyen, H., Qian, J.J., Bhatnagar, R.S. (2003) Enhanced cell attachment and osteoblastic activity by P-15 peptide-coated matrix in hydrogels. *Biochem Bioph Res Co*, **311**, 179–186.

Nishimura, F., Terranova, V.P. (1996) Comparative study of the chemotactic responses of periodontal ligament cells and gingival fibroblasts to polypeptide growth factors. *J Dent Res*, **75**, 986–992.

Oates, T.W., Rouse, C.A., Cochran, D.L. (1993) Mitogenic effects of growth factors on human periodontal ligament cells *in vitro*. *J Periodontol*, **64**, 142–148.

Oda, Y., Yoshimura, Y., Ohnishi, H., et al. (2010) Induction of pluripotent stem cells from human third molar mesenchymal stromal cells. *J Biol Chem*, **285**, 29270–29278.

Oi, Y., Ota, M., Yamamoto, S., et al. (2009) Beta-tricalcium phosphate and basic fibroblast growth factor combination enhances periodontal regeneration in intrabony defects in dogs. *Dent Mater J*, **28**, 162–169.

Ojima, Y., Mizuno, M., Kuboki, Y., et al. (2003) *In vitro* effect of platelet-derived growth factor BB on collagen synthesis and proliferation of human periodontal ligament cells. *Oral Dis*, **9**, 144–151.

Okubo, K., Kobayashi, M., Takiguchi, T., et al. (2003) Participation of endogenous IGF-I and TGF-beta 1 with enamel matrix derivative-stimulated cell growth in hyuman periodontal ligament cells. *J Periodontal Res*, **38**, 1–9.

Ortega, S., Ittmann, M., Tsang, S.H. et al. (1998) Neuronal defects and delayed wound healing in mice lacking fibroblast growth factor 2. *Proc Natl Acad Sci*, **95**, 5672–5677.

O'Sullivan, S., Naot, D., Callon, K., et al. (2007) Imatinib promotes osteoblast differentiation by inhibiting PDGFR signaling and inhibits osteoclastogenesis by both direct and stromal cell-dependent mechanisms. *J Bone Miner Res*, **22**, 1679–1689.

Paine, C.T., Paine, M.L., Snead, M.L. (1998) Identification of tuftelin- and amelogenin-interacting proteins using the yeast two-hybrid system. *Connect Tissue Res*, **38**, 257–267.

Park, J.B., Matsuura, M., Han, K.Y., et al. (1995) Periodontal regeneration in class III furcation defects of beagle dogs using guided tissue regenerative therapy with platelet-derived growth factor. *J Periodontol*, **66**, 462–477.

Parkar, M.H., Tonetti, M. (2004) Gene expression profiles of periodontal ligament cells treated with enamel matrix proteins *in vitro*: analysis using cDNA arrays. *J Periodontol*, **75**, 1539–1546.

Pettinicchio, M., Traini, T., Murmura, G. et al. (2010) Histologic and histomorphometric results of three bone graft substitutes after sinus augmentation in humans. *Clin Oral Investig*, November 3 [Epub ahead of print].

Poehling, S., Pippig, S.D., Hellerbrand, K., et al. (2006) Superior effect of MD05, beta-tricalcium phosphate coated with recombinant human growth/differentiation factor -5, compared to conventional bone substitutes in the rat calvarial defect model. *J Periodontol*, **77**, 1582–1590.

Polimeni, G., Susin, C., Wikesjö, U.M.E. (2009) Regenerative potential and healing dynamics of the periodontium: a critical size supra-alveolar periodontal defect study. *J Clin Periodontol*, **36**, 258–264.

Pountos, I., Georgoli, T., Henshaw, K. et al. (2010) The effect of bone morphogenetic protein-2, bone morphogenetic protein-7, parathyroid hormone, and platelet-derived growth factor on the proliferation and osteogenic differentiation of mesenchymal stem cells derived from osteoporotic bone. *J Orthop Trauma*, **24**, 552–556.

Qian, J.J., Bhatnagar, R.S. (1996) Enhanced cell attachment to anorganic bone mineral in the presence of a synthetic peptide related to collagen. *J Biomed Mater Res*, **31**, 545–554.

Rasperini, G., Roccuzzo, M., Francetti, L., et al. (2011) Subepithelial connective tissue graft for treatment of gingival recessions with and without enamel matrix derivative: a multicenter, randomized controlled clinical trial. *Int J Periodont Rest*, **31**, 133–139.

Rasubala, L., Yoshikawa, H., Nagata, K., et al. (2003) Platelet-derived growth factor and bone morphogenetic protein in the healing of mandibular fractures in rats. *Br J Oral Maxillofac Surg*, **41**, 173–178.

Ravindranath, H.H., Chen, L.S., Zeichner-David, M., et al. (2004) Interaction between the enamel matrix proteins amelogenin and ameloblastin. *Biochem Biophys Res Commun*, **323**, 1075–1083.

Rincon, J.C., Haase, H.R., Bartold, P.M. (2003) Effect of Emdogain® on human periodontal fibroblasts in an *in vitro* wound-healing model. *J Periodontal Res*, **38**, 290–295.

Ripamonti, U., Klar, R.M. (2010) Regenerative frontiers in craniofacial reconstruction: grand challenges and opportunities for the mammalian transforming growth factor-β proteins. *Front Physiol*, **1**, 143.

Rodan, S.B., Wesolowski, G., Yoon, K., et al. (1989) Opposing effects of fibroblast growth factor and pertussis toxin on alkaline phosphatase, osteopontin, osteocalcin, and type I collagen mRNA levels in ROS 17/2.8 cells. *J Biol Chem*, **264**, 19934–19941.

Rodrigues, T.L., Marchesan, J.T., Coletta, R.D., et al. (2007) Effects of enamel matrix derivative and transforming growth factor-beta1 on human periodontal ligament fibroblasts. *J Clin Periodontol*, **34**, 514–522.

Romanelli, M., Kaha, E., Stege H., et al. (2008) Effect of amelogenin extracellular matrix protein and compression on hard-to-heal venous leg ulcers: follow-up data. *J Wound Care*, **17**, 17–18.

Sakallioğlu, U., Açikgöz, G., Ayas, B., et al. (2004) Healing of periodontal defects treated with enamel matrix proteins and root surface conditioning – an experimental study in dogs. *Biomaterials*, **25**, 1831–1840.

Sarahrudi, K., Mousavi, M., Grossschmidt, K., Sela, N., König, F., Vécsei, V., Aharinejad, S. (2008) Combination of anorganic bovine-derived hydroxyapatite with binding peptide does not enhance bone healing in a critical-sized defect in a rabbit model. *J Orthoped Res*, **26**, 759–763.

Sarment, D.P., Cooke, J.W., Miller, S.E. et al. (2006) Effect of rhPDGF-BB on bone turnover during periodontal repair. *J Clin Periodontol*, **33**, 135–144.

Sawae, Y., Sahara, T., Kawana, F., et al. (2002) Effects of enamel matrix derivative on mineralized tissue formation during wound healing in rat parietal bone defects. *J Electron Microsc (Tokyo)*, **51**, 413–423.

Schlueter, S.R., Carnes, D.L. Jr., Cochrane D.L. (2007) *In vitro* effects of enamel matrix derivative on microvascular cells. *J Periodontol*, **78**, 141–151.

Schwarz, F., Rothamel, D., Herten, M., et al. (2008) Lateral ridge augmentation using particulated or block bone substitutes biocoated with rhGDF-5 and rhBMP-2: an immunohistochemical study in dogs. *Clin Oral Implan Res*, **19**, 642–652.

Schwartz, Z., Carnes, D.L. Jr., Pulliam, R., et al. (2000) Porcine fetal enamel matrix derivative stimulates proliferation but not differentiation of pre-osteoblastic 2T9 cells, inhibits proliferation and stimulates differentiation of osteoblast-like MG63 cells, and increases proliferation and differentiation of normal human osteoblast NHOst cells. *J Periodontol*, **71**, 1287–1296.

Sculean, A., Auschill, T.M., Donos, N., et al. (2001) Effect of an enamel matrix protein derivative (Emdogain) on *ex vivo* dental plaque vitality. *J Clin Periodontol*, **28**, 1074–1078.

Sculean, A., Windisch, P., Keglevich, T., et al. (2003) Clinical and histologic evaluation of human intrabony defects treated with an enamel matrix protein derivative combined with a bovine-derived xenograft. *Int J Periodont Rest*, **23**, 47–55.

Sculean, A., Schwarz, F., Becker, J., et al. (2007) The application of an enamel matrix protein derivative (Emdogain) in regenerative periodontal therapy: a review. *Med Princ Pract*, **16**, 167–180.

Sena, K., Morotome, Y., Baba, O., et al. (2003) Gene expression of growth differentiation factors in the developing periodontium of rat molars. *J Dent Res*, **82**, 166.

Seo, B.M., Miura, M., Gronthos, S., et al. (2004) Investigation of multipotent postnatal stem cells from human periodontal ligament. *Lancet*, **364**, 149–155.

Sherman, B.P., Lindley, E.M., Turner, A.S. et al. (2010) Evaluation of ABM/P-15 versus autogenous bone in an ovine lumbar interbody fusion model. *Eur Spine J*, **19**, 2156–2163.

Shirakata, Y., Taniyama, K., Yoshimoto, T., et al. (2010) Regenerative effect of basic fibroblast growth factor on periodontal healing in two-wall intrabony defects in dogs. *J Clin Periodontol*, **37**, 374–381.

Simank, H.G., Stuber, M., Frahm, R., et al. (2006) The influence of surface coatings of dicalcium phosphate (DCPD) and growth and differentiation on factor-5 (GDF-5) on the stability of titanium implants *in vivo*. *Biomaterials*, **27**, 3988–3994.

Smith, C.E., Chen, W.Y., Issid, M. (1995) Enamel matrix protein turnover during amelogenesis: basic biochemical properties of short-lived sulfated enamel proteins. *Calcif Tissue Res*, **57**, 133–144.

Song, Z.C., Shu, R., Zhang, X.L. (2010) Cellular responses and expression profiling of human marrow stromal cells stimulated with enamel matrix proteins *in vitro*. *Cell Prolif*, **43**, 84–94.

Soriano, P. (1994) Abnormal kidney development and hematological disorders in PDGF beta-receptor mutant mice. *Genes Dev*, **8**, 1888–1896.

Spahr, A., Lyngstadaas, S.P., Boeckh, C., et al. (2002) Effect of the enamel matrix derivative Emdogain on the growth of periodontal pathogens *in vitro*. *J Clin Periodontol*, **29**, 62–72.

Steed, D.L. (2006) Clinical evaluation of recombinant human platelet-derived growth factor for the treatment of lower extremity ulcers. *Plast Reconstr Surg*, **117**, 143S–149S.

Suzuki, N., Ohyama, M., Maeno, M., et al. (2001) Attachment of human periodontal ligament cells to enamel matrix-derived protein is mediated via interaction between BSP-like molecules and integrin alpha(v)beta3. *J Periodontol*, **72**, 1520–1526.

Swanson, E.C., Fong, H.K., Foster B.L., et al. (2006) Amelogenins regulate expression of genes associated with cementoblasts *in vitro*. *Eur J Oral Sci*, **114**, 239–243.

Takahashi, D., Odajima, T., Morita, M., et al. (2005) Formation and resolution of anklyosis under application of recombinant human bone morphogenetic protein-2 (rhBMP-2) to class III furcation defects in cats. *J Periodontol Res*, **40**, 299–305.

Takahashi, K., Yamanaka, S. (2006) Induction of pluripotent stem cells from mouse embryonic and adult fibroblast cultures by defined factors. *Cell*, **126**, 663–676.

Takahashi, K., Okita, K., Nakagawa, M., et al. (2007) Induction of pluripotent stem cells from fibroblast cultures. *Nat Protoc*, **2**, 3081–3089.

Takayama, S., Murakami, S., Miki, Y., et al. (1997) Effects of basic fibroblast growth factor on human periodontal ligament cells. *J Periodontol Res*, **32**, 667–675.

Takayama, S., Murakami, S., Shimabukuro, Y., et al. (2001) Periodontal regeneration by FGF-2 (bFGF) in primate models. *J Dent Res*, **80**, 2075.

Takayama, S., Yoshida, J., Hirano, H., et al. (2002) Effects of basic fibroblast growth factor on human gingival epithelial cells. *J Periodontol*, **73**, 1467–1473.

Tan, Z., Zhao, Q., Gong, P., et al. (2009) Research on promoting periodontal regeneration with human basic fibroblast growth factor-modified bone marrow mesenchymal stromal cell gene therapy. *Cytotherapy*, **11**, 317 325.

Thoma, D.S., Villar, C.C., Carnes, D.L. et al. (2011) Angiogenic activity of an enamel matrix derivative (EMD) and EMD-derived proteins: an experimental study in mice. *J. Clin Periodontol*, **38**, 253–260.

Thompson, D.M., Rohrer, M.D., Prasad, H.S. (2006) Comparison of bone grafting materials in human extraction sockets: clinical, histologic, and histomorphometric evaluations. *Implant Dent*, **15**, 89–96.

Thorwarth, M., Schultze-Mosgau, S., Wehrhan, F. et al. (2005) Bioactivation of an anorganic bone matrix by P-15 peptide for the promotion of early bone formation. *Biomaterials*, **26**, 5648–5657.

Tokiyasu, Y., Takata, T., Saygin, E., et al. (2000) Enamel factors regulate expression of genes associated with cementoblasts. *J Periodontol*, **71**, 1829–1839.

Tokunaga, A., Oya, T., Ishii, Y. et al. (2008) PDGF receptor β is a potent regulator of mesenchymal stromal cell function. *J Bone Miner Res*, **23**, 1519–1528.

Trasatti, C., Spears, R., Gutmann, J.L., et al. (2004) Increased Tgf-β1 production by rat osteoblasts in the presence of PepGen P-15 *in vitro*. *J Endodont*, **30**, 213–217.

Triplett, R.G., Nevins, M., Marx, R.E., et al. (2009) Pivotal, randomized, parallel evaluation of recombinant human bone morphogenetic protein-2/absorbable collagen sponge and autogenous bone graft for maxillary sinus floor augmentation. *J Oral Maxillofac Surg*, **67,** 1949–1960.

Trombelli, L., Farina, R. (2008) Clinical outcomes with bioactive agents alone or in combination with grafting or guided tissue regeneration. *J Clin Periodontol*, **35**, 117–135.

Uchida, T., Murakami, C., Wakida, K., et al. (1998) Sheath proteins: synthesis degradation and fate in forming enamel. *Eur J Oral Sci*, **106**, 308–314.

Urist, M.R. (1971) Bone histogenesis and morphogenesis in implants of demineralized enamel and dentin. *J Oral Surg*, **29**, 88–102.

van der Pauw, M.T., Van den Bos, T., Everts, V., et al. (2000) Enamel matrix-derived protein stimulates attachment of periodontal ligament fibroblasts and enhances alkaline phosphatase activity and transforming growth factor beta1 release of periodontal ligament and gingival fibroblasts. *J Periodontol*, **71**, 31–43.

van der Pauw, M.T., Everts, V., Beertsen, W. (2002) Expression of integrins by human periodontal ligament and gingival fibroblasts and their involvement in fibroblast adhesion to enamel matrix-derived proteins. *J Periodontal Res*, **37**, 317–323.

Vastardis, S., Yukna, R.A., Mayer, E.T., Atkinson, B.L. (2005) Periodontol regeneration with peptide-enhanced anorganic bone matrix in particulate and putty form in dogs. *J Periodontol*, **76**, 1690–1696.

Venezia, F., Goldstein, M., Boyan, B.D., et al. (2004) The use of enamel matrix derivative in the treatment of periodontal defects: a literature review and meta-analysis. *Crit Rev Oral Biol Med*, **15**, 382–402.

Viswanathan, H.L., Berry, J.E., Foster, B.L., et al. (2003) Amelogenin: a potential regulator of cementum-associated genes. *J Periodontol*, **74**, 1423–1431.

Vowden, P., Romanelli, M., Price, P. (2007) Effect of amelogenin extracellular matrix protein and compression on hard-to-heal venous leg ulcers. *J Wound Care*, **16**, 189–195.

Walter, C., Jawor, P., Bernimoulin, J.P., et al. (2006) Moderate effect of enamel matrix derivative (Emdogain Gel) on Porphyromonas gingivalis growth *in vitro*. *Arch Oral Biol*, **51**, 171–176.

Wang, H.L., Pappert, T.D., Castelli, W.A., et al. (1994) The effect of platelet-derived growth factor on the cellular response of the periodontium: an autoradiographic study on dogs. *J Periodontol*, **65**, 429–436.

Weng, D., Poehling, S., Pippig, S., et al. (2009) The effects of recombinant human growth/differentiation factor-5 (rhGDF-5) on bone regeneration around titanium dental implants in barrier membrane-protected defects: a pilot study in the mandible of beagle dogs. *Int J Oral Max Impl*, **24**, 31–37.

Wennström, J.L., Lindhe, J. (2002) Some effects of eanmel matrix proteins on wound healing in the dento-gingival region. *J Clin Periodontol*, **29**, 9–14.

Wolfman, N.M., Hattersley, G., Cox, K. et al. (1997) Ectopic induction of tendon and ligament in rats by growth and differentiation factors 5, 6, and 7, members of the TGF-β gene family. *J Clin Invest*, **100**, 321–330.

Wu, S.M., Hochedlinger, K. (2011) Harnessing the potential of induced pluripotent stem cells for regenerative medicine. *Nat Cell Biol*, **13**, 497–505.

Wu, Y., Chen, L., Scott, P.G., Tredget, E.E. (2007) Mesenchymal stem cells enhance wound healing through differentiation and angiogenesis. *Stem Cells*, **25**, 2648–2659.

Wu, Y., Zhao, R.C., Tredget, E.E. (2010) Concise review: bone marrow-derived stem/progenitor cells in cutaneous repair and regeneration. *Stem Cells*, **28**, 905–915.

Yakar, S., Courtland, H.W., Clemmons, D. (2010) IGF-1 and bone: new discoveries from mouse models. *J Bone Miner Res*, **25**, 2543–2552. Erratum in: *J Bone Miner Res* (2011), **26**, 439.

Yang, Y., Rossi, F.M.V., Putnins, E.E. (2010) Periodontal regeneration using engineered bone marrow mesenchymal stromal cells. *Biomaterials*, **31**, 8574–8582.

Yoneda, S., Itoh, D., Kuroda, S., et al. (2003) The effects of enamel matrix derivative (EMD) on osteoblastic cells in culture and bone regeneration in a rat skull defect. *J Periodontal Res*, **38**, 333–342.

Yoshimoto, T., Yamamoto, M., Kadomatsu, H., et al. (2006) Recombinant human growth/differentiation factor-5 (rhGDF-5) induced bone formation in murine calvariae. *J Periodontal Res*, **41**, 140–147.

Young, C.S., Ladd, P.A., Browning, C.F. et al. (2009) Release, biological potency, and biochemical integrity of recombinant human platelet-derived growth factor-BB (rhPDGF-BB) combined with Augment™ Bone Graft or GEM 21S beta-tricalcium phosphate (β-TCP). *J Control Release*, **140**, 250–255.

Yuan, K., Hsu, C.W., Tsai, W.H. (2006) The induction and possible subsequent effect of human antibodies against porcine enamel matrix derivative. *J Periodontol*, **77**, 1355–1361.

Yuan, K., Huang, J.-S., Hsu, C-W., et al. (2007) A mineralization-associated membrane protein plays a role in the biological functions of the peptide-coated bovine hydroxyapatite. *J Periodontal Res*, **42**, 420–428.

Yukna, R.A., Callan, D.P., Krauser, J.T., et al. (1998) Multi-center clinical evaluation of combination anorganic bovine-derived hydroxyapatite matrix (ABM)/cell binding peptide (P-15) as a bone replacement graft material in human periodontal osseous defects. 6-month results. *J Periodontol*, **69**, 655–663.

Yukna, R.A., Krauser, J.T., Callan, D.P. et al. (2000) Multi-center clinical comparison of combination anorganic bovine-derived hydroxyapatite matrix (ABM)/cell binding peptide (P-15) and ABM in human periodontal osseous defects. 6-month results. *J Periodontol*, **71**, 1671–1679.

Yukna, R.A., Krauser, J.T., Callan, D.P. et al. (2002) Thirty-six month follow-up of 25 patients treated with combination anorganic bovine-derived hydroxyapatite matrix (ABM)/cell-binding peptide (P-15) bone replacement grafts in human infrabony defects. I. Clinical Findings. *J Periodontol* **73**, 123–128.

Yun, Y.-R., Won, J.E., Jeon, E., et al. (2010) Fibroblast growth factors: biology, function and application for tissue regeneration. *J Tissue Eng*, doi 10.4061/2010/218142.

Zilm, P.S., Bartold, P.M. (2011) Proteomic identification of proteinase inhibitors in the porcine enamel matrix derivative, EMD®. *J Periodontal Res,* **46**, 111–117.

12 Wound Healing Around Dental Implants

Cristina Cunha Villar, Guy Huynh-Ba, Michael P. Mills and David L. Cochran

Department of Periodontics, University of Texas, Health Science Center at San Antonio, San Antonio, TX, USA

INTRODUCTION

The introduction of the 'modern dental implant' to dentistry has revolutionized the approach to patient care. The edentulous patient with severely resorbed ridges for whom there were few to no viable treatment options or the patient who would require heroic and expensive dental treatment to save a single tooth now have what has become successful and predictable alternatives to care.

The international demand for dental implants has spurred the development of an implant industry with a rapidly expanding market place. Competition between dental implant manufacturers to secure larger portions of the world market has resulted in increased funding for research and development (R&D). These R&D efforts have introduced new or modified implant designs, material and surface treatments. Similar advances have also been made in soft and hard tissue site development in order to achieve enhanced function and esthetics. Technological improvements in regenerative materials, devices and surgical approaches have and will continue to contribute greatly to the delivery and success of dental implant therapy. It is therefore not only imperative to understand the normal events of healing following the creation of the *implant wound*, but also equally important to know how various implant surface preparations, designs and mechanics influence tissue and cells.

HISTORICAL DEVELOPMENT

Ever since humans have inhabited the earth, they have had to cope with dental diseases and the subsequent loss of teeth. Ancient recorded history documents the use of various materials to replace missing teeth such as teeth from other humans or animals, or those carved from animal tusks or seashells. One of the most significant archeological finds occurred in 1931 in Honduras by Dr and Mrs Wilson Popenoe. They discovered a fragment from a female Mayan mandible dating back to 600 AD, which had tooth-shaped shells implanted into the sockets of three lower incisor teeth. From a radiographic analysis of the fragment, Professor Amadeo Bobbio described the presence of dense cortical bone encapsulating two of the shell teeth. He concluded that the shell teeth must have been placed while the Mayan woman was living, and not at the time of death as had been the ancient custom (Ring 1995).

Oral Wound Healing: Cell Biology and Clinical Management, First Edition. Edited by Hannu Larjava.

A much earlier archeological team made a similar discovery in 1890 of an 800 AD skull also unearthed in Honduras. A missing lower lateral incisor tooth had been replaced by a tooth carved from stone. The presence of 'tartar' on the stone tooth suggested that it had been present for some time (Ring 1995).

In the 1800s and early 1900s, attempts to replace missing teeth in humans reported the use of various materials: allografts or autografts of human teeth; sterilized bovine incisor teeth; a tooth root made of 18-carat gold; a porcelain post encased in surface-roughened lead; a corrugated porcelain root supporting a porcelain crown; a capsule of platinum foil covered with lead and soldered with pure silver; and tubes of gold or iridium inserted into fresh extraction sites (Ring 1995). In 1913, Dr E.J. Greenfield published an article in *Dental Cosmos* in which he described the replacement of missing teeth with an 'artificial root' that he had designed and tested in several patients.

> 'This new process of implantation is no less than the making of a few circular incisions in the jaw-bone of an edentulous mouth, inserting properly prepared artificial roots of iridio-platinum, and mounting on each a base or anchorage, to which can be attached a full set of permanent, natural-appearing teeth, capable of rendering as good and efficient service as those endowed by nature at her best' (Greenfield 1913).

The surgical procedure called for the utilization of a trephine bur to prepare a circular trough in the alveolar ridge into which a wire basket-shaped root was inserted over the bony core. The presence of the core of bone and a precise fit of the basket in the trough would allow for the growth of bone through and around the wire basket. This was considered essential to the success of the implant. After a healing period of approximately 1 month, a crown could be constructed to fit on the implant platform.

In 1941, the subperiosteal implant to restore the edentulous jaw was designed by Dr Gustav Dahl of Sweden. A metal framework was constructed on a model that had been 'scraped' to simulate what the clinician thought to be the morphology of the underlying bone. This framework would then be delivered surgically and stabilized with screws placed in the bony ridge. A prosthesis could then be constructed which was retained on the transmucosal posts of the implant. Subsequent years brought several modifications to the fabrication of the subperiosteal implant which improved its poor initial success rate. Even with modern computerized tomography and CAD-CAM construction, this type of implant is rarely utilized today (Ring 1995).

Dr Leonard Linkow (1988) introduced the endosseous Vent-Plant implant in 1963 and the Blade-Vent implant in 1967 (Linkow and Rinaldi 1988). The Vent-Plant is a vented screw-shaped implant, whereas the Blade-Vent consists of a flat, usually horizontal shaped body of varying lengths and heights with a width of approximately 2–3 mm. The horizontal blade is designed to be placed in areas of limited ridge width and height and where anatomical limitations may exist such as the maxillary sinus. The Vent-Plant and Blade-Vent implants were initially designed as one-stage systems, but may now be placed as submerged or two-stage implants. In the early 1960s, these implants were constructed of chrome cobalt, stainless steel or tantalum. However, because of their biocompatibility, commercially pure titanium or titanium alloy (Ti-6Al-4V) became the primary metal construct for the Vent-Plant in 1964 and for the Blade-Vent in 1971.

The emergence of titanium as the metal of choice for dental implants is usually attributed to the early work of Dr Per Ingvar Brånemark, Swedish physician and orthopedic surgeon (Albrektsson and Zarb 1989). In the 1950s, Dr Brånemark began vital microscopic studies on the microcirculation of bone marrow and soft tissue (Branemark et al. 1985). Using small (50–100 μm diameter) observation chambers constructed of titanium and inserted into the tibia and ears of rabbits, he was able to study the revascularization and healing patterns over a period of days. At the end of the experiment, Dr Brånemark observed that the titanium chambers placed in the rabbit leg could not be retrieved without sectioning surrounding bone. Although he found this to be an interesting finding, he did not give it serious thought until he conducted vital microscopic studies of wound revascularization in the 1960s using similar titanium chambers. The chambers were placed in a human skin tube, which had been surgically created 3–6 months earlier from twin pedicle flaps on the inside of the upper arm. He found the titanium chambers were extremely well tolerated with no apparent adverse reaction at the skin–chamber interface. He thus concluded that titanium must be a highly biocompatible material that deserved further investigation into its properties for potential application in medicine and dentistry. Dr Brånemark subsequently set about obtaining research funding and putting together a team comprised of surgeons, dentists, metallurgists, bioengineers and psychiatrists.

The Brånemark Team soon began investigating the possibility of utilizing titanium structures to support dental prostheses for the rehabilitation of edentulism, especially in patients demonstrating significant atrophy of the jaws. Studies were first conducted in the dog model where various implant designs were tested for their biocompatibility and function. The experiments showed that integrated titanium screw-shaped fixtures could successfully bear the load of a prosthetic rehabilitation, i.e. a dental bridge, over 10 years without significant adverse reaction. Interestingly, at the time of the dog sacrifice, it was only at the cost of fracturing the surrounding bone that the titanium fixture could be removed. The interface between the bone and titanium was still intact; thus demonstrating just how intimate this interface was. At the light microscopic level, no perceptible gap could be observed between the bone and implant surface wherever they made contact. To describe this healing phenomenon, Brånemark coined the term *osseointegration*; a term that is universally used when referring to a successful healing outcome following dental implant placement.

In 1965, the Brånemark Team successfully treated the first edentulous patient with threaded titanium fixtures according to the principles of osseointegration. Over the next years, procedural protocols for the design, diagnosis, placement, restoration and follow-up of the dental implant were established. The clinical application and long-term success of the Brånemark dental implant system was confirmed in numerous studies. It soon emerged as the implant industry's model for most root form, endosseous dental implants used today.

Paralleling the development of machined titanium implants in the 1970s and 1980s were two other surface preparations: *titanium plasma-sprayed* (TPS) and *hydroxyapatite-coated* (HA) (Ring 1995). Both processes involved coating a titanium core with molten particles of titanium or hydroxyapatite applied under high heat and air pressure. The result was the creation of a 'rough' surface coating designed to enhance earlier osseointegration of the implant. The TPS surface was used successfully for a number of years on Straumann® hollow-cylinder and hollow screw designed implants. Later, Straumann abandoned these implant designs and developed a solid screw with a surface texture produced by sandblasting the titanium with large grit followed by acid-etching.

HA coatings were shown to stimulate a bond between bone and the implant HA-coating (Meffert et al. 1987). This direct bond between the bone and HA surface was observed under electron microscopy and coined 'Biointegration'. When compared to machined or turned titanium implants, HA coated implants demonstrated more rapid osseointegration than a machined implant, but were also associated with significant amounts of bone destruction in cases of peri-implantitis.

TITANIUM – THE METAL OF CHOICE

Today, there are several different dental implant systems and designs, nearly all of which offer a textured or roughened implant surface (Binon 2000). The differences in the nature and properties of the various types of 'rough' surfaces are primarily related to how the surfaces are prepared and processed, and whether additional surface modifications have been made. How surface roughness impacts the events of healing will be discussed later in this chapter.

Titanium or titanium alloy became the metal of choice for implantation devices in medicine and dentistry because of their biocompatibility. That titanium is corrosion resistant, provides a surface conducive to cell proliferation, differentiation and survival, and is structurally stable under function are a few of the properties that make this metal biocompatible, and thus so universally popular.

There are four types (types 1, 2, 3 and 4) of commercially pure titanium (CpTi). Each type consists of 99% pure titanium with the remaining 1% representing various impurities such as iron, oxygen, nitrogen, carbon and hydrogen. Type 1 has the fewest impurities but is considered the weakest, whereas type 4 contains the most impurities but is the strongest of the four types of CpTi. Titanium is a reactive metal forming an oxide layer on contact with air which is approximately 3–5 nm thick; it is the oxygen in this layer that the body recognizes and thus it does not react to the titanium (Steinemann 1998). Of the titanium oxides (TiO, TiO_2, TiO_3), titanium dioxide (TiO_2) is the predominant molecular form on the surface. It is the constant low solubility of the titanium dioxide layer between pH 3 and pH 12 that gives titanium excellent passivity and makes it highly stable and resistant to corrosion in body fluids. As a result, no metal ion in the titanium oxide layer will ever reach the surface or be released into the surrounding tissue where it may be toxic to cells (Steinemann 1998).

Titanium is also an allotropic metal, existing in more than one crystallographic form: alpha, beta and alpha-beta (Brunette et al. 2001). The alpha phase exists when titanium is at room temperature and the beta phase appears after titanium has solidified from a liquid form or has been heated to 1623°F. Titanium may be alloyed with other elements in order to stabilize each phase at room temperature. The alpha phase can be stabilized by aluminum, oxygen or tin and the beta phase by niobium, molybdenum, tantalum, chromium, iron and vanadium. Alpha and beta stabilizing metals may also be combined and alloyed with titanium, forming an alpha-beta phase.

An alloy used by some dental implant manufacturers to increase tensile strength as compared to commercially pure titanium alone is titanium-6% aluminum-4% vanadium (Ti-Al6-V4). However, when titanium is alloyed with other metals such as vanadium, there is the potential for a foreign body reaction. This can occur if metal ions of the alloy leach out into the surrounding tissue as a result of corrosion in body fluids (Steinemann 1998).

Most recently, Institut Straumann AG, Basel, Switzerland, has alloyed titanium with zirconium (TiZr), forming an alpha-beta phase that increases both tensile and mechanical strength in their narrowest diameter implant line (Roxolid®). In the miniature pig model, Gottlow (2010) found that dental implants made of TiZr1317 (Roxolid®, Straumann) had significantly higher removal torque values at 4 weeks than CpTi dental implants with the same hydrophilic sandblasted acid-etched surface (SLActive®) (Gottlow et al. 2010). In this same study, specially designed bone chamber implants also made of TiZr1317 showed significantly more bone area within the chamber than those made from CpTi (Gottlow et al. 2010). Results from *in vitro* (Tsucihya 1998) and *in vivo* (Ikarashi 2005) studies have also shown the TiZr alloy to be more biocompatible than pure titanium, demonstrating greater cell proliferation and differentiation and less immune cell inflammatory response, respectively (Tsuchiya 1998; Ikarashi 2005). It would appear that alloys of titanium or like metals may surpass CpTi as the primary components for dental implant construction, given their improved properties of strength and biocompatibility.

HEALING FOLLOWING IMPLANT PLACEMENT

Concurrently with the identification of titanium as the metal of choice in the field of implant dentistry, experiments were designed to provide a better understanding of the peri-implant tissue healing. In contrast with teeth that develop in synchrony with the surrounding periodontal tissues, dental implants are surgically placed directly into native or regenerated bone. This limits the number of cell types that migrate to, attach and differentiate on the implant surface during healing.

Nonetheless, soft and hard tissue healing following implant placement lead to marginal soft tissue attachment and osseointegration. Marginal soft tissue adaptation plays a key role in establishing a physical seal between the oral environment and the bone-surrounded implant (Branemark et al. 1977; Schroeder et al. 1981; Lindhe and Berglundh 1998), which in turn is expected to prevent microbial organisms and contaminated products from the oral cavity reaching the underlying bone. Limiting migration of bacteria and bacterial products along the implant surface reduces the risk for peri-implantitis and implant failure. Additionally, a stable peri-implant soft tissue attachment, in the presence of bone support, has a critical impact on the long-term esthetic outcomes of implant therapy. Along these lines, it has been suggested that the attachment between the peri-implant soft tissue and the implant surface plays an important role both in achieving and maintaining desired soft tissue contour around dental implants.

On the other hand, formation of a direct structural and functional connection between living recipient bone and titanium dioxide on the implant surfaces, without any interposed soft tissue, provides mechanical stability for implants. This allows for functional loading of implant-supported prosthesis. Based on the critical importance of soft tissue adaptation and osseointegration on the maintenance and functional stability of implant-supported prosthesis, this chapter will describe the chronological healing sequence of peri-implant soft and hard tissues following dental implant placement, as well as the nature of the interface between implants and peri-implant tissues.

PERI-IMPLANT SOFT TISSUE HEALING

Over the last two decades, several animal studies have focused on investigating the osseous healing around dental implants. However, ever since osseointegration of dental implants became a highly predictable outcome, efforts have been redirected towards achievement of esthetic outcomes. Based on this, more attention has been placed on the healing and ultra-structure architecture of the peri-implant mucosa. Following implant placement, a series of cellular and molecular events take place on the oral mucosa adjacent to the newly placed implant, leading to the formation of a peri-implant mucosa.

A recent animal study revealed that immediately following implant placement, a blood coagulum separates the oral mucosa from the implant surface and the alveolar bone

(Berglundh et al. 2007). The blood coagulum is soon infiltrated by inflammatory cells, primarily polymorphonuclear cells, and replaced by a dense fibrin network. The initial mucosal seal is established by the formation of a fibrin layer at day 4 after implant placement (Berglundh et al. 2007). Fibroblasts then invade the fibrin network and produce collagen fibers to form a connective tissue. During this process, the fibrin network is progressively replaced by a fibrous connective tissue (Berglundh et al. 2007). Two weeks following implant placement, a newly formed connective tissue rich in vascular units and fibroblasts is in close contact with the implant surface.

First signs of proliferation and migration of epithelial cells from the periphery of the soft tissue wound margins occurs after 1–2 weeks of healing (Berglundh et al. 2007). Migration and proliferation of epithelial cells lead to the formation of a junctional epithelium, which in turn further lengthens the contact interface between the implant surface and the peri-implant mucosa. Maturation of the peri-implant mucosa occurs between 6 and 12 weeks following implant placement (Berglundh et al. 2007) and is mainly characterized by formation of a mature epithelial barrier and organization and alignment of collagen fibers.

IMPLANT/PERI-IMPLANT MUCOSA INTERFACE

This sequence of healing events leads to the formation of a peri-implant mucosa. The peri-implant mucosal attachment to the implant surface is 3–4 mm high (Cochran et al. 1997; Hermann et al. 2000, 2001) and consists structurally of a junctional epithelium supported by an underlying connective tissue coronal to the alveolar bone (Steflik et al. 1990; Berglundh et al. 1991; Buser et al. 1992; Listgarten et al. 1992; Steflik et al. 1993; Abrahamsson et al. 1998, 1999, 2002). The junctional epithelium comprises the marginal 60% of the mucosal attachment, and the remaining 40% of the attachment is made of a fiber-rich connective tissue (Abrahamsson et al. 1999, 2002).

The peri-implant mucosa has many characteristics in common with the dentogingival unit adjacent to the natural tooth (Buser et al. 1992; Cochran et al. 1997; Hermann et al. 2000, 2001; Abrahamsson et al. 2001). The external surface of the peri-implant mucosa is covered by a well-keratinized oral epithelium. This oral epithelium contains several layers of cells similar to skin that form rete pegs extending into the adjacent connective tissue (Buser et al. 1992). The sulcular epithelium emerges in continuity with the oral epithelium and defines the peri-implant sulcus (Fig. 12.1). The peri-implant sulcular epithelium contains 5–15 layers of basal and suprabasal cells tightly attached to each other through desmosomes (Schupbach and Glauser 2007). Desquamation of the most coronal peri-implant sulcular epithelial cells is preceded by a decrease in desmosomal connection between these cells (Schupbach and Glauser 2007), and is likely to represent an epithelial response to the constant exposure to microbial insults. Immediately apical to the sulcular epithelium, the junctional epithelium gradually decreases in width from 15 to 1 cell layer (Schupbach and Glauser 2007). Junctional epithelial cells flatten, align parallel to the long axis of the implant surface (Buser et al. 1992; Abrahamsson et al. 1996, 1999; Fig. 12.1) and attach to the implant surface via hemidesmosomes and focal adhesions (Listgarten and Lai 1975; James 1979; Gould, et al. 1981, 1984; Pendegrass et al. 2008). Junctional epithelial attachment is likely to act as a physical barrier against microbial penetration. Moreover, epithelial attachment to the implant surface is expected to contribute to the stability of soft tissue contours around dental implants.

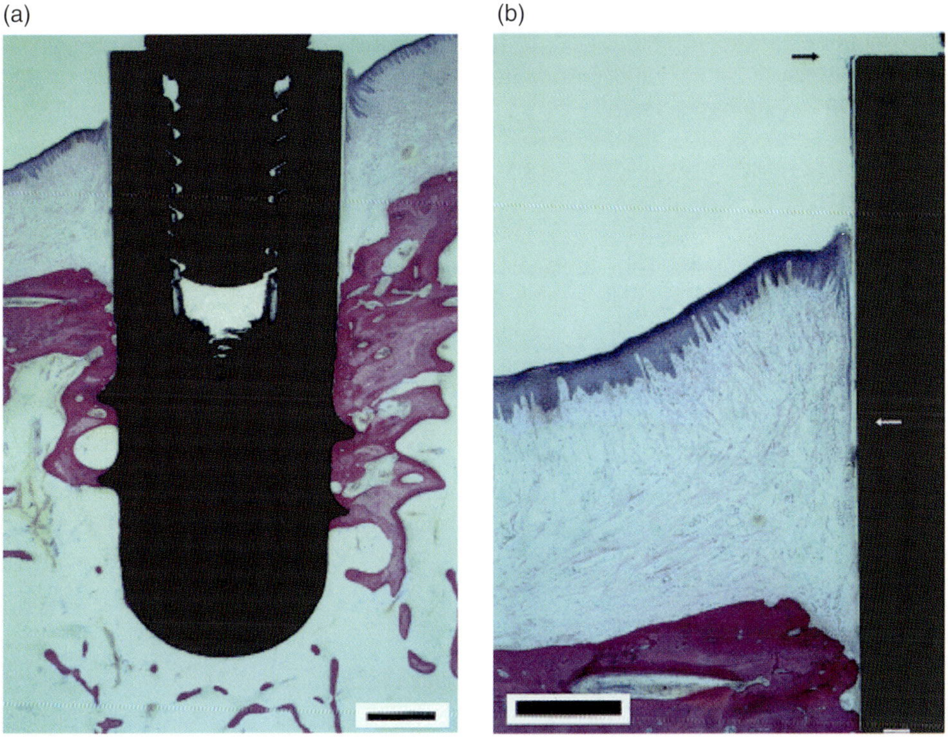

Fig. 12.1 Mesio-distal section of implant and surrounding soft and hard peri-implant tissues (a). (b) Close-up view of part a showing the left (mesial) aspect of the non-submerged implant. The white bar shows the level of the first bone-to-implant contact. The white arrow indicates the most apical cell of the junctional epithelium, and the black arrow the top of the implant. [From Hermann et al. (2006) Biologic width around one- and two-piece titanium implants. *Clin Oral Implants Res*, 12(6), by John Wiley and Sons. All rights reserved.]

The connective tissue lateral to the oral, sulcular and junctional epithelia is comprised of a dense collagenous tissue with scattered fibroblasts and inflammatory cells (Buser et al. 1992). Collagen fibers running from the alveolar crest and supra-alveolar periosteum towards the oral epithelium follow a vertical pathway. These vertically oriented fibers give rise to fine branches that run in a perpendicular orientation towards the sulcular and junctional epithelia. However, as these fine branches come close to the epithelial basement membrane, they change their orientation into a vertical direction (Buser et al. 1992). Vascular units derived from the supraperiosteal vessels form a crevicular plexus located at close proximity (50 μm) to the basal epithelial cell layers (Abrahamsson et al. 1996).

Apical to the junctional epithelium lies the zone of connective tissue attachment. This zone is divided based on its composition and proximity to the implant surface into inner and outer zones. The inner connective tissue zone is approximately 40 μm wide and lies adjacent to the implant surface (Abrahamsson et al. 2002). This zone is composed of collagen fibers (65%), fibroblasts (35%) and a small number of thin capillary-like vascular structures (0.2%) (Listgarten et al. 1992; Abrahamsson et al. 2002). Most studies have demonstrated that the collagen fibers in this zone originate from the bone crest and run a course predominantly parallel to the implant surface, either circumferentially or in an apical-coronal direction (Berglundh et al. 1991; Listgarten et al. 1991, 1992; Buser et al. 1992; Liljenberg et al. 1996; Abrahamsson et al. 1998), without inserting into the implant surface. However, evidence that collagen fibers in this zone insert to the implant surface and assume a functional orientation has also been reported in the literature (Schroeder et al. 1981; Schwarz et al. 2007a). Fibroblasts located in the inner zone of the connective tissue attachment are elongated and oriented parallel to the implant surface.

Continuous and lateral to the inner zone, the outer connective tissue zone is about 160 μm wide and presents a significantly higher collagen (86%) and vascular content (11%), but a smaller percentage of fibroblasts (15%) (Listgarten et al. 1992; Moon et al. 1999; Abrahamsson et al. 2002). Unlike the collagen fibers in the inner zone that run in a parallel orientation to the implant surface, collagen fibers in the outer zone of the connective tissue attachment run in many different directions. Moreover, the blood vessels in the outer zone are continuous with the supra-alveolar arteries and larger in size than the thin capillary-like vessels from the inner connective tissue zone.

The critical importance of the peri-implant mucosal attachment is highlighted by the fact that in sites with thin oral mucosa, bone resorption occurs during healing to allow the formation and accommodation of a stable mucosal attachment around dental implants (Abrahamsson et al. 1996, 1997, 1998; Berglundh and Lindhe 1996).

PERI-IMPLANT HARD TISSUE HEALING

Placement of a dental implant into the alveolar bone is followed by a sequence of healing events that result in the establishment of osseointegration, characterized by a direct contact between vital bone and the implant surfaces. Studies in animal models have shown that immediately after surgical placement of a dental implant, the peripheral part of the implant treads are in close contact with the recipient bone and thereby provide primary implant mechanical stability during the early phases of healing (Cochran et al. 1998). The inner parts of the threads, however, make limited or no contact with the adjacent recipient bone bed, depending on the implant design, and the space formed between the implant surface and the surrounding alveolar bone bed becomes occupied with a fibrin coagulum containing erythrocytes, polymorphonuclear neutrophils and few macrophages (Berglundh et al. 2003; Schwarz et al. 2007a). Debris of cortical and trabecular bone are often found at wound sites during early phases of healing, and represent remnant residues of the bone bed surgical preparation (Abrahamsson et al. 2004; Schwarz et al. 2007a).

The coagulum is then penetrated by vascular units and fibroblast-like cells, which in turn form a granulation tissue (Berglundh et al. 2003; Abrahamsson et al. 2004). Vascular units originate from the adjacent recipient alveolar bone and invade the provisional tissue evenly (Schwarz et al. 2007a). It has been proposed that angiogenesis precedes and positively regulates bone formation (Schmid et al. 1997; Schwarz et al. 2007b). In this context, first signs of bone formation has been demonstrated as early as 4 days after implant placement around hydrophilic implants (i.e. SLActive) that stimulate formation of a dense network of blood vessels (Schwarz et al. 2007a).

After 1 week of wound healing, bone debris/fragments devoid of viable osteocytes are still visible immediately laterally to the implant pitch threads (Slaets et al. 2007). Osteoclasts migrate to these sites and bone fragments undergo a process of osteoclastic resorption and remodeling, leading to their incorporation into newly formed woven bone (Berglundh et al.

2003). Simultaneously, blood coagulum and granulation tissue are replaced with a provisional connective tissue matrix containing massive amounts of fibroblast-like mesenchymal cells. Some of the fibroblast-like mesenchymal cells line up in a parallel orientation along the implant surface and formation of collagen fiber bundles is initiated (Abrahamsson et al. 2004; Schwarz et al. 2007a). Newly synthesized collagen fibrils are randomly distributed around sprouting vascular structures (Berglundh et al. 2003; Schwarz et al. 2007a, 2007b).

Fibroblast-like mesenchymal cells soon differentiate into osteoblasts (Colnot et al. 2007) that are able to deposit a collagen fiber matrix that mineralizes (Steflik et al. 1998). Thereby, newly formed woven bone consisting of mineralized collagen fiber matrix associated with an inorganic (hydroxylapatite) matrix is deposited within the provisional connective tissue (Steflik et al. 1998; Schwarz et al. 2007a). The newly produced woven bone trabeculae are characterized by large areas of mineralized matrix and contain numerous osteocytes located in large lacunae (Schwarz et al. 2007b). Most of the newly formed woven bone extends from the existing old lamellar bone, in a process that has been referred to as appositional bone formation or distance osteogenesis (Davies 1998), and is found in continuity with the surgical bone bed (Berglundh et al. 2003, 2007; Abrahamsson et al. 2004). In distance osteogenesis, the recipient bone bed provides osteogenic cells that secrete a collagen-containing bone matrix. This bone matrix grows, mineralizes and gradually advances towards the implant surface (Fig. 12.2a). However, some woven bone has also been found in close contact with the implant surface at a distance from the existing parent bone bed (Davies 1998; Berglundh et al. 2003; Berglundh et al. 2007; Schwarz et al. 2007b). This bone is

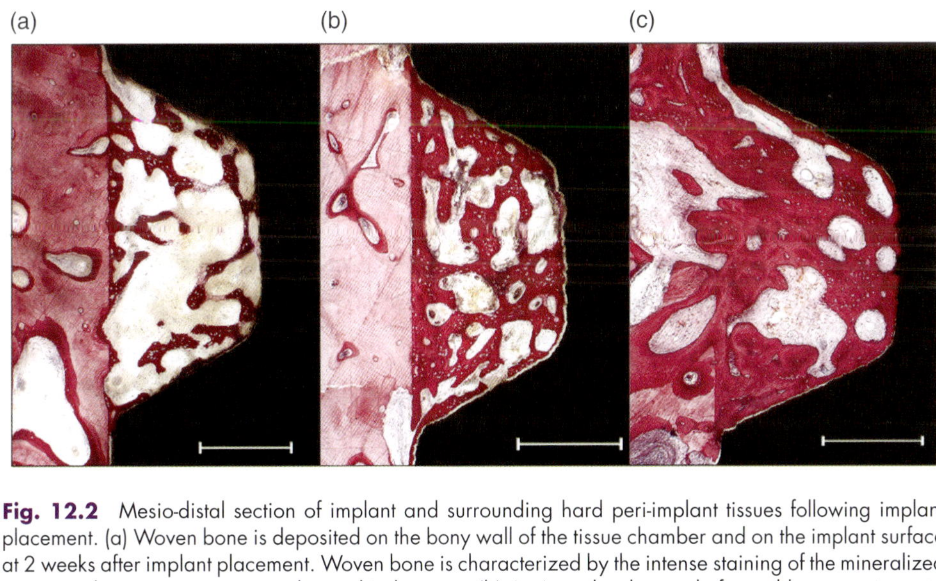

Fig. 12.2 Mesio-distal section of implant and surrounding hard peri-implant tissues following implant placement. (a) Woven bone is deposited on the bony wall of the tissue chamber and on the implant surface at 2 weeks after implant placement. Woven bone is characterized by the intense staining of the mineralized matrix and numerous osteocytes located in lacunae. (b) At 4 weeks, the newly formed bone continues to extend from the bone recipient bed to the implant surface. The density of the bone scaffold increases by the formation of new trabeculae and by deposition of more mature, parallel-fibered bone onto the primary scaffold. The gap between bone and implant surface is an artifact (bar = 500 μm). (c) Eight weeks following implant placement, mature parallel-fiber bone is found in contact with the implant surface. Remodeling has started, replacing the primary bone by secondary osteons (arrows; bar = 500 μm). [From Buser et al. (2004) Enhanced bone apposition to a chemically modified SLA titanium surface. *J Dent Res*, 83(7), by SAGE Publications Ltd. All rights reserved.]

thought to be formed by contact osteogenesis, a process by which differentiating osteogenic cells, derived from peri-vascular connective tissue cells, migrate to the implant surface, differentiate into osteoblasts and secrete a granular afibrillar organic matrix that provides nucleation sites for mineralization (Davies 1998).

Wound healing progresses with marked woven bone formation and maturation in such a way that after 4 weeks of healing, the newly formed woven bone extends from the cut of the bone bed into the implant surface (Fig. 12.2b; Berglundh et al. 2003), occupying close to 30% of this space (Abrahamsson et al. 2004; Vignoletti et al. 2009). The newly deposited woven bone is gradually remodeled and replaced over the course of 1–3 months by lamellar bone containing bone marrow adipocytes, blood vessels, collagen fibers and minute amounts of leukocytes (Fig. 12.2c; Berglundh et al. 2003; Schwarz et al. 2007a; Vignoletti et al. Sanz 2009). Osteoblasts are observed at the implant–bone interface, while osteocytes are regularly observed within the newly formed bone and extend cellular processes through canaliculi to adjacent osteocytes, vascular elements and directly to the bone–implant interface (Steflik et al. 1990, 1992). As the volume occupied by the mineralized tissue increases from the early to the late phases of healing, the volume occupied by lining osteoblasts and fibroblast-like mesenchymal cells gradually decreases (Abrahamsson et al. 2004). Moreover, increases in tissue mineralization occurring over the course of the healing are accompanied by rises in the bone-to-implant contact (Abrahamsson et al. 2004), which allows for the functional loading of implants. In this regard, it is important to note that bone does not interface the entire length of the implant and that the presence of 100% bone-to-implant contact is inconsistent with results from preclinical and clinical studies.

Bone modeling and remodeling continues at a slow rate over the first year of implant placement and contributes to higher implant resistance to shear forces (Johansson and Albrektsson 1987; Steflik et al. 1998). This continuous process of bone modeling and remodeling is regulated by the local mechanical stress, as loading regulates proliferation and differentiation of osteoblasts and the bone healing process (Carter and Giori 1991; Frost 2000).

Although these preclinical studies performed in dogs have unveiled the sequence of healing events that take place after implant placement, direct clinical application of these data is limited, as the turnover rate of bone remodeling in dogs is approximately four times faster than in humans (Draper 1994). Along this line, a recent clinical study has confirmed previously described healing events but suggested that the rate of osseointegration in humans is slower than in animals (Lang et al. 2011). Finally, although the general sequence of healing events is not affected by implant surface topographies, the rate of hard tissue healing and osseointegration can be influenced by implant topography and chemistry (for review see Albrektsson et al. 2008; Wennerberg and Albrektsson 2009).

FROM HEALING TO CLINICAL APPLICATION

The healing events described in the previous sections allow the formation of a stable interface between the hard and soft tissues and the dental implants, which in turn allows the clinician to load dental implants with prosthetic devices to restore esthetic and function for partially and fully edentulous patient. While it was advocated that a 6- to 9-month unloaded healing period was necessary (Branemark et al. 1977) to allow the implant to successfully withstand functional loading, immediate loading can be performed under specific clinical circumstances (Weber et al. 2009). These two extreme situations have yet in common the fact that stability has to be achieved and maintained during the dynamic process of healing to allow the intimate contact between the bone and the titanium surface to develop.

Many tests have been developed to assess the biomechanical properties of the implant–bone interface to better characterize the stability of implants as it relates to successful osseointegration and ultimately successful function (Albrektsson et al. 1981; Sennerby and Roos 1998). Moreover the ability to measure and monitor the stability of implants could ultimately and potentially allow such tests, if validated, to have a prognostic value of the healing process (Aparicio et al. 2006; Molly 2006).

IMPLANT STABILITY TESTING

Testing methods can be categorized as destructive methods and non-destructive methods.

Destructive methods

These include histological evaluation of the bone–implant interface with the determination of the bone-to-implant contact (BIC), torque removal tests, push-out and pull-out tests. These methods are useful for preclinical stages but are of limited value for clinical applications since they allow the evaluation at only one given time point and since the bone–implant interface is no longer intact thereafter (Berzins et al. 1997).

Schroeder developed the technique to allow the histological evaluation of an intact implant–bone interface, bringing to light the histological evidence of osseointegration (Schroeder et al. 1976). The BIC value has been used in many preclinical studies to characterize the quality of osseointegration (Schroeder et al. 1981; Sennerby et al. 1992; Ericsson et al. 1994; Gottlander et al. 1997).

New surfaces developed to improve the quality and quantity of contact and to also allow shorter time for the development of this bone–implant interface were evaluated using the BIC value as the main outcome (Buser et al. 1991, 2004; Gotfredsen et al. 1995; Wennerberg et al. 1995; Berglundh et al. 2003). In these studies, animals were sacrificed at different time points to establish a sequence in the healing process leading to osseointegration.

Since it has been shown that bone apposition on the implant surface led to increased stability (Meredith 1998) it is not unexpected that BIC values correlate well with removal torque test values. Consequently removal torque tests have been used as another mean to evaluate implant stability (Johansson and Albrektsson 1987; Carlsson et al. 1988; Tjellstrom et al. 1988; Johansson et al. 1991; Wennerberg et al. 1995; Sullivan et al. 1996; Branemark et al. 1998).

Clinically the reverse torque test is of little value because of the pass/fail nature of the test. Let us assume that an implant has been placed and is in the process of integrating. A solid osseointegration most likely would happen if the healing is left undisturbed. However, if the reversal torque test is applied before an adequate degree of osseointegration has occurred in order to withstand the torque applied, the implant can demonstrate lack of rotational stability, which eventually would lead to implant failure. Ivanoff et al. (1997) showed that a bone–implant interface that has been disrupted by removal torque testing could successfully re-osseointegrate if allowed to heal for an additional period. However, predictability of re-integration has yet to be established. Therefore, removal torque testing in clinical settings cannot be recommended as a mean to test the quality of the osseointegration (Atsumi et al. 2007; Sennerby and Meredith 2008).

Pull-out and push-out testing (Branemark and Skalak 1998) has also been used to quantify the bone–implant interfacial strength (Wong et al. 1995; Branemark et al. 1998). Again, due to the destructive nature of these tests the indication remains in the preclinical setting.

Based on these tests, preclinical trials have demonstrated, along with histological evidence, the importance of surface topology. Indeed, surface roughness is a determining factor for improved bone–implant contact and mechanical properties (Thomas and Cook 1985; Wong et al. 1995).

Overall, the use of preclinical destructive biomechanical testing has allowed the shift from initially smooth polished implant surfaces to roughened implant surfaces. The superiority demonstrated in preclinical data, i.e. *in vivo* animal models, has later been confirmed in clinical trials (for review see Cochran 1999), demonstrating the utility of such, yet destructive, testing methods.

Non-destructive methods

For clinical application, non-destructive methods of determining implant stability have been sought. They allow the assessment of the bone–implant interface without causing damage. Moreover, these methods can be repeated over time with minimal or no destructive influence. Ideally, these methods would include both a diagnostic and a prognostic value, enabling the clinician to objectively quantify the degree of primary stability at the time of implant placement and to monitor the stability over time. The ultimate goal would be to discriminate failing implants from those without complication during the early stage of healing as well as in the long term (Aparicio et al. 2006; Molly 2006; Chang et al. 2010).

Non-destructive methods that have been suggested to assess implant stability include insertion torque, Periotest® and resonance frequency analysis (RFA) measurements.

The idea that insertion torque measurement may have some prognostic value for implant stability is based on the fact that primary stability is associated with good implant integration (Lioubavina-Hack et al. 2006). Higher insertion torque presupposes adequate implant stability at the time of implant placement and may translate into improved implant osseintegration and function.

Insertion torque values have been recorded during implant placement in different trials. These studies have demonstrated that insertion torque correlated well with the quality of the bone (Johansson et al. 2004; O'Sullivan et al. 2004) and with removal torque values (Ueda et al. 1991).

In terms of prognostic value, an association between implant failure rate and implant insertion torque has been shown in implants loaded immediately. Such correlation was not found in delayed loaded implants (Friberg et al. 1999, 2003; Calandriello et al. 2003; Johansson et al. 2004; Ottoni et al. 2005). Thus, the prognostic value of insertion torque measurements has yet to be demonstrated (Molly 2006; Neukam and Flemmig 2006). Along with this line, the assumption that increased insertion torque may be of advantage for uneventful healing has been challenged since it was shown that implant placement in dense bone, i.e. with increased insertion torque values [type 1 according to Lekholm and Zarb's bone quality classification (Lekholm and Zarb 1985)], can lead to increased implant failure rate compared to that in less dense bone, i.e. types 2 and 3 (Truhlar et al. 1994).

Overheating of the bone at the time of implant bed preparation and excessive insertion torque forces, leading to compression, ischemia and ultimately bone necrosis, have been suggested to explain unfavorable implant outcomes (Eriksson et al. 1984; Truhlar et al. 1994; Piattelli et al. 1998; Misch 2007; Bashutski et al. 2009). Accordingly, an optimum torque seems required to allow osseointegration of a placed implant by assuring enough primary stability and yet, at the same time, not excessively compressive to jeopardize the early stage of healing. The thresholds of the torque value below and beyond which negative outcomes can be expected have yet to be defined. Moreover, insertion torque measurement is a conservative method to evaluate the stability of the implant–bone interface at the time of insertion, but it cannot be repeated over time, hampering the ability to monitor implant stability longitudinally. Therefore, these different limitations restrict the clinical use of insertion torque measurements to predict the survival outcome of implant therapy.

The Periotest® (Medizintechnik Gulden, Modautal, Germany) was originally developed and marketed (in 1986) to objectively measure tooth mobility. In brief, the instrument is in the form of a handpiece which contains a tapping head. The latter is accelerated by a propulsion coil. When it comes out of the handpiece, the tapping head will impact the tooth and will be decelerated. According to the tooth mobility, the percussion signal will be more or less rapidly damped. Accordingly, the greater the stability of the periodontium the greater damping effect and deceleration the tapping head will have. The time during which the tapping head is in contact with the tooth is a function of the damping effect and is then converted into a Periotest value, i.e. PTV (Lukas and Schulte 1990; Schulte and Lukas 1992). PTV scale ranges from −8 to 50 with corresponding increased tooth mobility.

Typically, low PTVs, i.e. between −5 and +5, have been reported for osseointegrated implants (Olive and Aparicio 1990; Schulte and Lukas 1993; Morris et al. 2003). It is interesting to note that the accepted normal range for osseointegrated implant represents only a very small part of the broader scale (−5 to +80), which was originally designed to assess tooth mobility. Therefore, the sensitivity of Periotest to measure implant mobility is limited (Meredith 1998; Aparicio et al. 2006;Atsumi et al. 2007).

Multiple studies have shown that PTV depends on many parameters, including the vertical distance from the striking point to the first bone to implant contact (Derhami et al. 1995; Meredith 1998; Haas et al. 1999; Faulkner et al. 2001), the implant length (van Steenberghe et al. 1995; Haas et al. 1999) and the angulation of the handpiece in relation to the implant (Meredith 1998; Faulkner et al. 2001).

PTVs have also been shown to vary according to the position of the implant – mandibular or maxillary, anterior or posterior – suggesting that PTVs correlate with bone quality. Accordingly, significantly lower PTVs are often recorded for in implants placed in the mandible as compared to implants placed in the maxilla (Buser et al. 1990; Haas et al. 1995; Salonen et al. 1997; Truhlar et al. 1997; Drago 2000). Of interest, PTVs were shown to rise with increased healing time following implant placement (Haas et al. 1995; Mericske-Stern et al. 1995; Tawse-Smith et al. 2001; Naert et al. 2004) reflecting the increased stiffness following bone apposition and remodeling during the healing process.

Due to these variables, a single measurement cannot adequately reflect the quality of osseointegration and, additionally, the reproducibility of PTV measurements is low. While negative PTVs reflect stability of the implant and high and positive value loss of stability, no threshold value allows the discrimination between successful or failing implants (Olive and Aparicio 1990). The prognostic ability of the Periotest would reside in accurately identifying implants that are at risk for loss of stability. However, this ability has yet to be demonstrated (Drago 2000; Verhoeven et al. 2000; Faulkner et al. 2001; Aparicio et al. 2006; Becker and Gansky 2007).

Importantly, although the Periotest is considered as a non-destructive testing method, the safety for primary stability testing at time of implant placement has been recently questioned since it has been demonstrated histologically that repeated PTV measurements could lead to irreversible damage of the bone–implant interface, especially in low quality bone (Seong et al. 2009).

Another non-invasive way to measure implant stability, known as resonance frequency analysis (RFA), was first described by Meredith and coworkers in 1994 (Meredith et al. 1994). The principle of this stability measurement originally relies on an attached transducer screwed onto the implant. The transducer comprises a beam and two piezoceramic elements attached to it. The transducer is vibrated by one of the piezoceramic elements with a sinusoidal signal and the response is measured by the second. The frequency of the sine wave applied varies typically from 5 to 15 kHz. When the first resonance frequency of the system including the transducer, the implant and its bone interface is reached, the second piezoceramic records a peak in the response signal.

The first generation of RFA instrumentation had many disadvantages including a large bulk of material and a time-consuming record measurement (over 1 minute). However, the newer generation of RFA instrumentation comprises a small metal rod (a peg) which is screwed onto the implant to be tested. The tip of the peg comprises a magnet that is excited by magnetic pulse delivered wirelessly by a handheld computer. The magnetic pulses cause the peg to resonate at certain frequencies which are recorded by the handheld device. The measurement of this resonance frequency is a function of the stiffness of the implant–bone system, and therefore its use to assess implant stability was suggested (Meredith et al. 1996, 1997; Sennerby and Meredith 2008). While RFA measurements were first expressed in kiloHertz, the actual dedicated scale for implant stability measurement is now expressed in Implant Stability Quotient (ISQ) units and ranges from 1 to 100.

While the striking point is determined by the operator, and is therefore variable, for the Periotest, this variability does not exist for the RFA since the transducer is attached directly to the implant. Moreover, the transducer vibration frequency is in the sonic range and the amplitude very small and, hence, the stress applied to the bone–implant interface is negligible and unlikely to damage the interface (Meredith et al. 1996). Furthermore, unlike the Periotest, the sensitivity of measurement is directed to a very small range of motion. Therefore, RFA represents an improved alternative to Periotest for measurement of implant stability.

It has been shown experimentally and clinically that RFA measurements do not vary with the overall implant length (Meredith et al. 1996; Balleri et al. 2002; Bischof et al. 2004) but do vary with the effective implant length, meaning the length between the transducer and the first bone to implant contact (Meredith et al. 1997; Friberg et al. 1999; Sennerby et al. 2005; Lachmann et al. 2006; Turkyilmaz et al. 2006). The ability to translate these findings in a clinical setting, as a diagnostic tool to detect early peri-implant bone loss, remains however questionable (Lachmann et al. 2006).

Implant stability has been measured over time in many clinical trials using RFA (Friberg et al. 1999; Barewal et al. 2003; Glauser et al. 2004; Nedir et al. 2004; Sjostrom et al. 2005; Huwiler et al. 2007; Fischer et al. 2009). Collectively, these studies have reported ISQ values associated with successfully integrated implants varying between 49 and 70. Conversely, ISQ values measured before implant failure varied between 39 and 68. Even though these wide ranges may be attributed to differences in study design, implant surface used and loading protocols, the literature suggests that there is no defined threshold, allowing the clinician to discriminate between an implant that will successfully ossointegrate and a failing implant.

Of interest, RFA variation following implant placement has been shown to follow a specific pattern (Barewal et al. 2003). In this study, 26 acid-etched, sandblasted surface implants were placed in the posterior sites of 20 patients. The RFA was recorded at nine

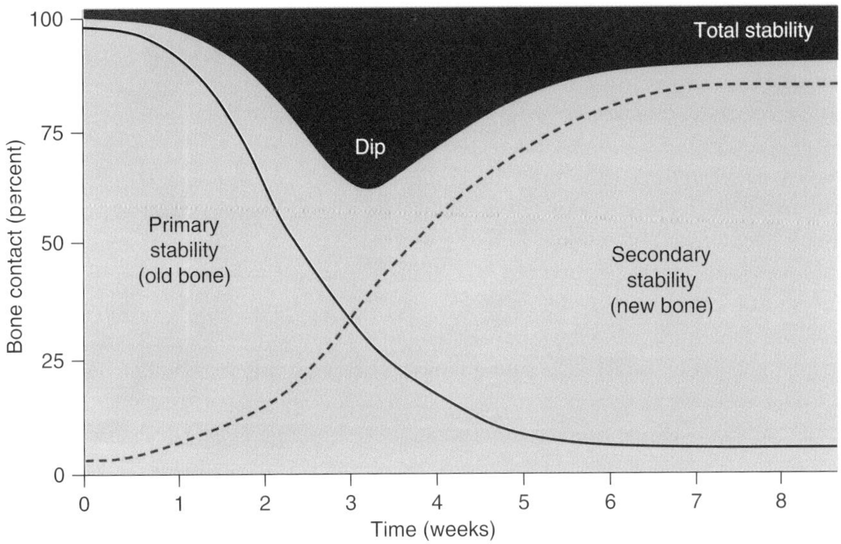

Fig. 12.3 Changes in total stability of the implant is a function of the combined changes of primary stability, created at the time of implant placement, and secondary stability created by deposition of new bone. From Raghavendra et al. (2005) Early wound healing around osseous dental implants: a review of the literature. *Int J Oral Maxillofac Implants*, 20(3), by Quintessence Publishing Co. Ltd. All rights reserved.]

different intervals between implant placement and 10-week follow-up. Interestingly, irrespective of the bone type described by Lekholm and Zarb (1985), the lowest mean stability measurement was at 3 weeks after implant placement. Then, the RFA measurements increased to reach the baseline (implant placement) values at around 4–5 weeks and, in some cases, further increased to reach a plateau at 8 weeks. All the 26 implants were successfully ossointegrated. The pattern of RFA measurements changing over time was interpreted as resulting from the primary and secondary bone contact. The overall stability was first determined by the press-fit of the implant against the cut native bone or so-called primary bone contact. Due to this compression, the native bone showed signs of necrosis and resorption, resulting in decreased primary bone contact. Concurrently, the secondary bone contact characterized by bone modeling and remodeling started on the osteoconductive surface of the implant (Cochran et al. 1998). Through this process woven bone is turned into lamellar bone and the overall stability of the implant increased until week 8. Therefore, at implant placement, the overall stability was defined solely by the primary bone contact, while at 8 weeks it was mainly defined by the secondary bone contact. The two processes were dynamic and resulted in the lowest RFA value at around 3 weeks (Raghavendra et al. 2005; Fig. 12.3). From this longitudinal analysis of RFA values, the clinical application of RFA analysis resides in the fact that if one achieves an RFA value similar or greater than the RFA at the time of implant placement, then one can assume that the implant has successfully osseointegrated.

Overall, obtaining and maintenance of high RFA values are indicative of successful implant stability outcome. However, the ability of RFA to predict implant failure or success remains to be demonstrated and the normative range of values representing implant stability have yet to be identified before RFA clinical guidelines can be formulated (Sennerby and Meredith 2008).

WOUND HEALING AND LOADING PROTOCOLS

Among the principles described by Brånemark and coworkers for predictable osseointegration, a non-loading period of 3–6 months in the mandible and 6–9 months in the maxilla were empirically advocated as determined by clinical experience (Branemark et al. 1977). As a corollary, premature loading was considered to put the implant at risk for a fibrous tissue encapsulation followed by clinical failure (Adell et al. 1981; Branemark et al. 1985). This ascertainment was further supported by animal experimental models in which loading implants during early healing phases led to fibrous encapsulation of the implants (Brunski et al. 1979; Akagawa et al. 1986). However, more recent animal studies and clinical trials have challenged these findings and have advocated early loading to stimulate bone apposition on the implant surface (Evans et al. 1996; Piattelli et al. 1997, 1993; Testori et al. 2001).

In order to reconcile these apparent contradictory findings, it was determined that it was not the loading per se that would be responsible for the loss of osseointegration and fibrous tissue encapsulation but rather an excessive micro-motion at the bone–implant interface during the healing following implant placement (Szmukler-Moncler et al. 2000). Animal experiments have suggested that the tolerated micro-motion compatible with osseointegration amounts to 50–100 μm (Pilliar et al. 1986; Brunski et al. 2000; Vandamme et al. 2007). The preclinical data and the different proof of principle trials using implants with more osteoconductive surfaces compared to machined or turned surfaces have led to loading protocols challenging the 3- to 6-month healing period advocated by Brånemark and coworkers.

One set of definitions used for different loading protocols was established by the 2003 International Team for Implantology (ITI) Consensus Conference, Gstaad, Switzerland (Cochran et al. 2004):

- Immediate loading: a restoration placed in occlusion with the opposing dentition within 48 hours of implant placement.
- Early loading: a restoration placed in contact with the opposing dentition at least 48 hours after implant placement but not later than 3 months afterward.
- Conventional loading: the prosthesis is attached in a second procedure after a healing period of 3–6 months.
- Delayed loading: the prosthesis is attached in a second procedure that takes place sometime later than the conventional healing period of 3–6 months.

While the first attempt to immediately load dental implants with overdentures goes back to 1979 (Ledermann 1979), the results of a larger multi-center trial involving 484 patients treated in four different countries were reported in 1986. After a mean follow-up of 2.7 years, a cumulative implant success rate of 88.0% to 96.1% (depending on the center) was reported (Babbush et al. 1986). Another multi-center trial involving 226 patients reported a success rate of 96.9% [according to Albrektsson's criteria for success (Albrektsson et al. 1986)] for immediately loaded implants after a mean observation time of 6.4 years (range 2–13 years) (Chiapasco et al. 1997).

The placement of four implants in the interforaminal region, splinted with a bar and loaded immediately (within 2 days of implant placement) has been reproduced in many different studies with similar survival and success rates. These rates compared well with those of four implants, splinted together and loaded with a delayed protocol, i.e. 4–8 months after implant placement (Gatti et al. 2000; Chiapasco et al. 2001; Romeo et al. 2002; Chiapasco and Gatti 2003).

The rationale of this method was to splint the implants together with a rigid bar so that the level of micro-motion would be maintained below the threshold mentioned earlier and, therefore, be compatible with osseointegration despite the immediate loading. Moreover, cross-arch stabilization and dense bone encountered in the interforaminal region further supported this rationale. More recent studies have looked at the potential of using fewer implants for immediate loading of mandibular overdentures (Stricker et al. 2004; Marzola et al. 2007; Stephan et al. 2007). Even though the results of these studies are encouraging, they have to be looked at as pilot studies considering the small patient number (between 10 and 26)) and the short follow-up period (1–2 years). Therefore, the use of less than four implants to stabilize a mandibular overdenture with an immediate loading protocol needs to be further documented before it can be recommended as an accepted treatment protocol (Gallucci et al. 2009).

The rigid splinting concept that underlies the immediate loading protocols of implant-retained mandibular overdentures can also be achieved through a fixed restoration. Immediate loading of implant-supported fixed prostheses in the edentulous mandible and the maxilla has been reported by several authors [for review see Gallucci et al. 2009)]. These studies reported an implant survival rate of between 98.0% and 100% and between 95.4 and 100% for the mandible and the maxilla, respectively. The follow-up period varied between 1 and 3 years, encompassing a total of 333 patients and 1831 implants.

Besides rigid splinting, implant surface development has played a major role in challenging the 3- to 6-month undisturbed healing period concept. The clinical application of surface development has allowed shorter healing times for dental implants even in cases of implant-supported single crowns and short-span fixed partial dentures. In these cases there is no or little possibility to decrease micro-motions through splinting, and yet many studies have shown that early loading was achievable with good clinical and radiographic outcomes (Salvi et al. 2004; Achilli et al. 2007; Cochran et al. 2007; Cooper et al. 2007; Roccuzzo et al. 2008; Weber et al. 2009).

Taken altogether, biological understanding of hard and soft tissue healing around implants, development of new implant surfaces and designs, and understanding of biomechanical principles have allowed extension of clinical indications for implant therapy. Furthermore these changes have allowed for increasing predictability and better implant success and survival.

CONCLUSIONS

Dental implants have become a part of routine dentistry. Bone healing around modern implants follows an established sequence of events and results in predictable osseointegration. In clinical studies, bone formation can be seen as early as 7 days after implant placement. In a healing bone wound, fibroblast-like osteogenic progenitor cells differentiate into osteoblasts and start to deposit woven bone directly onto the dental implant surface, particularly in those cases where the surface has been made more osteoconductive. Moreover, woven bone also gradually grows towards the implant surface from the host's bone. Thus, initial bone to implant contact at time of implant placement (primary contact) will gradually decrease and new bone on the implant surface and on the cut native bone (secondary contact) will increase during the following 1–3 months of healing. As woven bone is replaced by lamellar bone, the quality of the bone increases, which, in turn, allows for stronger support of the implant.

As a clinical application, RFA has suggested that implant stability is initially decreased up to 3 weeks due to bone remodeling (loss of primary bone contact), followed by an increase in bone support (increase in secondary bone contact) to the baseline stability at 4–5 weeks and then reaches a plateau in 8 weeks. Regardless of this remodeling, studies have shown that implants can be successfully loaded immediately after placement in certain indications, although with somewhat reduced survival rates. Development of new implant surfaces has played a critical role in expanding these clinical loading protocols.

Soft tissue healing around implants has become a focus of attention because it plays a central role in esthetic outcomes. Healing of the per-implant soft tissue follows similar principles as gingival healing around a tooth after surgical procedures. A fibrin clot serves as a provisional matrix allowing epithelial and fibroblast migration towards the implant surface. Epithelial and connective tissue contact to the implant or abutment surface is established within 1–2 weeks and further maturation follows up to at least 12 weeks. While the established interface presents many similarities to the gingival epithelium interface around a tooth, the main difference is represented by the orientation of collagen fiber bundles, which instead of attaching to the neck of the implant like a Sharpey's fiber into the cementum of a tooth, run parallel and circumferentially around the implant. Future studies are needed to develop better implant designs and surfaces that improve the soft tissue healing for more predictable esthetical outcomes.

REFERENCES

Abrahamsson, I., Berglundh, T. and Lindhe, J. (1997) The mucosal barrier following abutment dis/reconnection. An experimental study in dogs. *J Clin Periodontol* **24**: 568–572.

Abrahamsson, I., Berglundh, T., Glantz, P.O. and Lindhe, J. (1998) The mucosal attachment at different abutments. An experimental study in dogs. *J Clin Periodontol* **25**: 721–727.

Abrahamsson, I., Berglundh, T., Linder, E., Lang, N.P. and Lindhe, J. (2004) Early bone formation adjacent to rough and turned endosseous implant surfaces. An experimental study in the dog. *Clin Oral Implants Res* **15**: 381–392.

Abrahamsson, I., Berglundh, T., Moon, I.S. and Lindhe, J. (1999) Peri-implant tissues at submerged and non-submerged titanium implants. *J Clin Periodontol* **26**: 600–607.

Abrahamsson, I., Berglundh, T., Wennstrom, J. and Lindhe, J. (1996) The peri-implant hard and soft tissues at different implant systems. A comparative study in the dog. *Clin Oral Implants Res* **7**: 212–219.

Abrahamsson, I., Zitzmann, N.U., Berglundh, T., Linder, E., Wennerberg, A. and Lindhe, J. (2002) The mucosal attachment to titanium implants with different surface characteristics: an experimental study in dogs. *J Clin Periodontol* **29**: 448–455.

Abrahamsson, I., Zitzmann, N.U., Berglundh, T., Wennerberg, A. and Lindhe, J. (2001) Bone and soft tissue integration to titanium implants with different surface topography: an experimental study in the dog. *Int J Oral Maxillofac Implants* **16**: 323–332.

Achilli, A., Tura, F. and Euwe, E. (2007) Immediate/early function with tapered implants supporting maxillary and mandibular posterior fixed partial dentures: preliminary results of a prospective multicenter study. *J Prosthet Dent* **97**: S52–58.

Adell, R., Lekholm, U., Rockler, B. and Branemark, P.I. (1981) A 15-year study of osseointegrated implants in the treatment of the edentulous jaw. *Int J Oral Surg* **10**: 387–416.

Akagawa, Y., Hashimoto, M., Kondo, N., Satomi, K., Takata, T. and Tsuru, H. (1986) Initial bone-implant interfaces of submergible and supramergible endosseous single-crystal sapphire implants. *J Prosthet Dent* **55**: 96–100.

Albrektsson, T., Zarb, G., Worthington, P. and Eriksson, A.R. (1986) The long-term efficacy of currently used dental implants: a review and proposed criteria of success. *Int J Oral Maxillofac Implants* **1**: 11–25.

Albrektsson, T. and Zarb, G.A. (1989) *The Branemark Osseointegrated Implant*, pp. 21–23. Quintessence Publishing, Chicago.

Albrektsson, T., Branemark, P.I., Hansson, H.A. and Lindstrom, J. (1981) Osseointegrated titanium implants. Requirements for ensuring a long-lasting, direct bone-to-implant anchorage in man. *Acta Orthop Scand* **52**: 155–170.

Albrektsson, T., Sennerby, L. and Wennerberg, A. (2008) State of the art of oral implants. *Periodontol* **47**: 15–26.

Aparicio, C., Lang, N.P. and Rangert, B. (2006) Validity and clinical significance of biomechanical testing of implant/bone interface. *Clin Oral Implants Res* 17 Suppl **2**: 2–7.

Atsumi, M., Park, S.H. and Wang, H.L. (2007) Methods used to assess implant stability: current status. *Int J Oral Maxillofac Implants* **22**: 743–754.

Babbush, C.A., Kent, J.N. and Misiek, D.J. (1986) Titanium plasma-sprayed (tps) screw implants for the reconstruction of the edentulous mandible. *J Oral Maxillofac Surg* **44**: 274–282.

Balleri, P., Cozzolino, A., Ghelli, L., Momicchioli, G. and Varriale, A. (2002) Stability measurements of osseointegrated implants using osstell in partially edentulous jaws after 1 year of loading: a pilot study. *Clin Implant Dent Relat Res* **4**: 128–132.

Barewal, R.M., Oates, T.W., Meredith, N. and Cochran, D.L. (2003) Resonance frequency measurement of implant stability in vivo on implants with a sandblasted and acid-etched surface. *Int J Oral Maxillofac Implants* **18**: 641–651.

Bashutski, J.D., D'Silva, N.J. and Wang, H.L. (2009) Implant compression necrosis: current understanding and case report. *J Periodontol* **80**: 700–704.

Becker, W. and Gansky, S.A. (2007) Periotest comes with many false alarms for predicting early implant loss. *J Evid Based Dent Pract* **7**: 125–126.

Berglundh, T. and Lindhe, J. (1996) Dimension of the periimplant mucosa. Biological width revisited. *J Clin Periodontol* **23**: 971–973.

Berglundh, T., Abrahamsson, I., Albouy, J.P. and Lindhe, J. (2007) Bone healing at implants with a fluoride-modified surface: an experimental study in dogs. *Clin Oral Implants Res* **18**: 147–152.

Berglundh, T., Abrahamsson, I., Lang, N.P. and Lindhe, J. (2003) De novo alveolar bone formation adjacent to endosseous implants. *Clin Oral Implants Res* **14**: 251–262.

Berglundh, T., Abrahamsson, I., Welander, M., Lang, N.P. and Lindhe, J. (2007) Morphogenesis of the peri-implant mucosa: an experimental study in dogs. *Clin Oral Implants Res* **18**: 1–8.

Berglundh, T., Lindhe, J., Ericsson, I., Marinello, C.P., Liljenberg, B. and Thomsen, P. (1991) The soft tissue barrier at implants and teeth. *Clin Oral Implants Res* **2**: 81–90.

Berzins, A., Shah, B., Weinans, H. and Sumner, D.R. (1997) Nondestructive measurements of implant-bone interface shear modulus and effects of implant geometry in pull-out tests. *J Biomed Mater Res* **34**: 337–340.

Binon, P.P. (2000) Implants and components: entering the new millennium. *Int J Oral Maxillofac Implants* **15**: 76–94.

Bischof, M., Nedir, R., Szmukler-Moncler, S., Bernard, J.P. and Samson, J. (2004) Implant stability measurement of delayed and immediately loaded implants during healing. *Clin Oral Implants Res* **15**: 529–539.

Branemark, P., Zarb, G. and Albrektsson, T. (1985) *Tissue Integrated Prostheses: Osseointegration in Clinical Dentistry*. Quintessence Publishing, Chicago.

Branemark, P.I., Hansson, B.O., Adell, R., et al. (1977) Osseointegrated implants in the treatment of the edentulous jaw. Experience from a 10-year period. *Scand J Plast Reconstr Surg* Suppl **16**: 1–132.

Branemark, R. and Skalak, R. (1998) An in-vivo method for biomechanical characterization of bone-anchored implants. *Med Eng Phys* **20**: 216–219.

Branemark, R., Ohrnell, L.O., Skalak, R., Carlsson, L. and Branemark, P.I. (1998) Biomechanical characterization of osseointegration: an experimental in vivo investigation in the beagle dog. *J Orthop Res* **16**: 61–69.

Brunette, D., Tengvall, P., Textor, M. and Thomsen, P. (2001) *Titanium in Medicine*. Springer, Berlin Heidelberg New York.

Brunski, J.B., Moccia, A.F., Jr., Pollack, S.R., Korostoff, E. and Trachtenberg, D.I. (1979) The influence of functional use of endosseous dental implants on the tissue-implant interface. I. Histological aspects. *J Dent Res* **58**: 1953–1969.

Brunski, J.B., Puleo, D.A. and Nanci, A. (2000) Biomaterials and biomechanics of oral and maxillofacial implants: current status and future developments. *Int J Oral Maxillofac Implants* **15**: 15–46.

Buser, D., Broggini, N., Wieland, M., et al. (2004) Enhanced bone apposition to a chemically modified sla titanium surface. *J Dent Res* **83**: 529–533.

Buser, D., Schenk, R.K., Steinemann, S., Fiorellini, J.P., Fox, C.H. and Stich, H. (1991) Influence of surface characteristics on bone integration of titanium implants. A histomorphometric study in miniature pigs. *J Biomed Mater Res* **25**: 889–902.

Buser, D., Weber, H.P. and Lang, N.P. (1990) Tissue integration of non-submerged implants. 1-year results of a prospective study with 100 ITI hollow-cylinder and hollow-screw implants. *Clin Oral Implants Res* **1**: 33–40.

Buser, D., Weber, H.P., Donath, K., Fiorellini, J.P., Paquette, D.W. and Williams, R.C. (1992) Soft tissue reactions to non-submerged unloaded titanium implants in beagle dogs. *J Periodontol* **63**: 225–235.

Calandriello, R., Tomatis, M., Vallone, R., Rangert, B. and Gottlow, J. (2003) Immediate occlusal loading of single lower molars using branemark system wide-platform tiunite implants: an interim report of a prospective open-ended clinical multicenter study. *Clin Implant Dent Relat Res* 5 Suppl **1**: 74–80.

Carlsson, L., Rostlund, T., Albrektsson, B. and Albrektsson, T. (1988) Removal torques for polished and rough titanium implants. *Int J Oral Maxillofac Implants* **3**: 21–24.

Carter, D. and Giori, N.E. (1991) Effect of mechanical stress on tissue differentiation in the bony implant bed. In: J. Davies, ed. *The Bone-Biomaterial Interface*, p. 367. University of Toronto Press, Toronto.

Chang, P.C., Lang, N.P. and Giannobile, W.V. (2010) Evaluation of functional dynamics during osseointegration and regeneration associated with oral implants. *Clin Oral Implants Res* **21**: 1–12.

Chiapasco, M. and Gatti, C. (2003) Implant-retained mandibular overdentures with immediate loading: a 3- to 8-year prospective study on 328 implants. *Clin Implant Dent Relat Res* **5**: 29–38.

Chiapasco, M., Abati, S., Romeo, E. and Vogel, G. (2001) Implant-retained mandibular overdentures with branemark system mkii implants: a prospective comparative study between delayed and immediate loading. *Int J Oral Maxillofac Implants* **16**: 537–546.

Chiapasco, M., Gatti, C., Rossi, E., Haefliger, W. and Markwalder, T.H. (1997) Implant-retained mandibular overdentures with immediate loading. A retrospective multicenter study on 226 consecutive cases. *Clin Oral Implants Res* **8**: 48–57.

Cochran, D., Oates, T., Morton, D., Jones, A., Buser, D. and Peters, F. (2007) Clinical field trial examining an implant with a sand-blasted, acid-etched surface. *J Periodontol* **78**: 974–982.

Cochran, D.L., Morton, D. and Weber, H.P. (2004) Consensus statements and recommended clinical procedures regarding loading protocols for endosseous dental implants. *Int J Oral Maxillofac Implants* 19 Suppl: 109–113.

Cochran, D.L. (1999) A comparison of endosseous dental implant surfaces. *J Periodontol* 70: 1523–1539.

Cochran, D.L., Hermann, J.S., Schenk, R.K., Higginbottom, F.L. and Buser, D. (1997) Biologic width around titanium implants. A histometric analysis of the implanto-gingival junction around unloaded and loaded nonsubmerged implants in the canine mandible. *J Periodontol* **68**: 186–198.

Cochran, D.L., Schenk, R.K., Lussi, A., Higginbottom, F.L. and Buser, D. (1998) Bone response to unloaded and loaded titanium implants with a sandblasted and acid-etched surface: a histometric study in the canine mandible. *J Biomed Mater Res* **40**: 1–11.

Colnot, C., Romero, D.M., Huang, S., et al. (2007) Molecular analysis of healing at a bone-implant interface. *J Dent Res* **86**: 862–867.

Cooper, L.F., Ellner, S., Moriarty, J., et al. (2007) Three-year evaluation of single-tooth implants restored 3 weeks after 1-stage surgery. *Int J Oral Maxillofac Implants* **22**: 791–800.

Davies, J.E. (1998) Mechanisms of endosseous integration. Int J Prosthodont **11**: 391–401.

Derhami, K., Wolfaardt, J.F., Faulkner, G. and Grace, M. (1995) Assessment of the periotest device in baseline mobility measurements of craniofacial implants. *Int J Oral Maxillofac Implants* **10**: 221–229.

Drago, C.J. (2000) A prospective study to assess osseointegration of dental endosseous implants with the periotest instrument. *Int J Oral Maxillofac Implants* **15**: 389–395.

Draper, H. (1994) *Bone Loss in Animals. Advances in Nutritional Research*. Plenum Press, New York.

Ericsson, I., Johansson, C.B., Bystedt, H. and Norton, M.R. (1994) A histomorphometric evaluation of bone-to-implant contact on machine-prepared and roughened titanium dental implants. A pilot study in the dog. *Clin Oral Implants Res* **5**: 202–206.

Eriksson, A.R., Albrektsson, T. and Albrektsson, B. (1984) Heat caused by drilling cortical bone. Temperature measured in vivo in patients and animals. *Acta Orthop Scand* **55**: 629–631.

Evans, G.H., Mendez, A.J. and Caudill, R.F. (1996) Loaded and nonloaded titanium versus hydroxyapatite-coated threaded implants in the canine mandible. *Int J Oral Maxillofac Implants* **11**: 360–371.

Faulkner, M.G., Giannitsios, D., Lipsett, A.W. and Wolfaardt, J.F. (2001) The use and abuse of the periotest for 2-piece implant/abutment systems. *Int J Oral Maxillofac Implants* **16**: 486–494.

Friberg, B., Jisander, S., Widmark, G., et al. (2003) One-year prospective three-center study comparing the outcome of a 'soft bone implant' (prototype mk iv) and the standard branemark implant. *Clin Implant Dent Relat Res* **5**: 71–77.

Friberg, B., Sennerby, L., Grondahl, K., Bergstrom, C., Back, T. and Lekholm, U. (1999) On cutting torque measurements during implant placement: a 3-year clinical prospective study. *Clin Implant Dent Relat Res* **1**: 75–83.

Fischer, K., Backstrom, M. and Sennerby, L. (2009) Immediate and early loading of oxidized tapered implants in the partially edentulous maxilla: a 1-year prospective clinical, radiographic, and resonance frequency analysis study. *Clin Implant Dent Relat Res* **11**: 69–80.

Friberg, B., Sennerby, L., Linden, B., Grondahl, K. and Lekholm, U. (1999) Stability measurements of one-stage branemark implants during healing in mandibles. A clinical resonance frequency analysis study. *Int J Oral Maxillofac Surg* **28**: 266–272.

Friberg, B., Sennerby, L., Meredith, N. and Lekholm, U. (1999) A comparison between cutting torque and resonance frequency measurements of maxillary implants. A 20-month clinical study. *Int J Oral Maxillofac Surg* **28**: 297–303.

Frost, H.M. (2000) The Utah paradigm of skeletal physiology: an overview of its insights for bone, cartilage and collagenous tissue organs. *J Bone Miner Metab* **18**: 305–316.

Gallucci, G.O., Morton, D. and Weber, H.P. (2009) Loading protocols for dental implants in edentulous patients. *Int J Oral Maxillofac Implants* 24 Suppl: 132–146.

Gatti, C., Haefliger, W. and Chiapasco, M. (2000) Implant-retained mandibular overdentures with immediate loading: a prospective study of ITI implants. *Int J Oral Maxillofac Implants* **15**: 383–388.

Glauser, R., Sennerby, L., Meredith, N., et al. (2004) Resonance frequency analysis of implants subjected to immediate or early functional occlusal loading. Successful vs. failing implants. *Clin Oral Implants Res* **15**: 428–434.

Gotfredsen, K., Wennerberg, A., Johansson, C., Skovgaard, L.T. and Hjorting-Hansen, E. (1995) Anchorage of tio2-blasted, ha coated, and machined implants: an experimental study with rabbits. *J Biomed Mater Res* **29**: 1223–1231.

Gottlander, M., Johansson, C.B. and Albrektsson, T. (1997) Short- and long-term animal studies with a plasma-sprayed calcium phosphate-coated implant. *Clin Oral Implants Res* **8**: 345–351.

Gottlow, J., Dard, M., Kjellson, F., Obrecht, M. and Sennerby, L. (2010) Evaluation of a new titanium-zirconium dental implant: a biomechanical and histological comparative study in the mini pig. *Clin Implant Dent Relat Res*, June [Epub ahead of print].

Gould, T.R., Brunette, D.M. and Westbury, L. (1981) The attachment mechanism of epithelial cells to titanium in vitro. *J Periodontal Res* **16**: 611–616.

Gould, T.R., Westbury, L. and Brunette, D.M. (1984) Ultrastructural study of the attachment of human gingiva to titanium in vivo. *J Prosthet Dent* **52**: 418–420.

Greenfield, E. (1913) Implantation of artificial crown and bridge abutments. *Dental Cosmos* 55: 364–369.

Haas, R., Bernhart, T., Dortbudak, O. and Mailath, G. (1999) Experimental study of the damping behaviour of imz implants. *J Oral Rehabil* **26**: 19–24.

Hermann, J.S., Buser, D., Schenk, R.K., Higginbottom, F.L. and Cochran, D.L. (2000) Biologic width around titanium implants. A physiologically formed and stable dimension over time. *Clin Oral Implants Res* **11**: 1–11.

Haas, R., Saba, M., Mensdorff-Pouilly, N. and Mailath, G. (1995) Examination of the damping behavior of imz implants. *Int J Oral Maxillofac Implants* **10**: 410–414.

Hermann, J.S., Buser, D., Schenk, R.K., Schoolfield, J.D. and Cochran, D.L. (2001) Biologic width around one- and two-piece titanium implants. *Clin Oral Implants Res* **12**: 559–571.

Ikarashi, J., Obayashi E., Oi H., et al. (2005) Improved biocompatibility of titanium-zirconium (ti-zr) alloy: tissue reaction and sensitization to ti-zr alloy compared with pure ti and zr in rat implantation study. *Mater Trans* **46**: 7.

Ivanoff, C.J., Sennerby, L. and Lekholm, U. (1997) Reintegration of mobilized titanium implants. An experimental study in rabbit tibia. *Int J Oral Maxillofac Surg* **26**: 310–315.

James, R.A. (1979) The support system and pergingival mechanisms surrounding oral implants. *Biomater Med Devices Artif Organs* **7**: 147–153.

Johansson, B., Back, T. and Hirsch, J.M. (2004) Cutting torque measurements in conjunction with implant placement in grafted and nongrafted maxillas as an objective evaluation of bone density: a possible method for identifying early implant failures? *Clin Implant Dent Relat Res* **6**: 9–15.

Johansson, C. and Albrektsson, T. (1987) Integration of screw implants in the rabbit: a 1-year follow-up of removal torque of titanium implants. *Int J Oral Maxillofac Implants* **2**: 69–75.

Johansson, C.B., Sennerby, L. and Albrektsson, T. (1991) A removal torque and histomorphometric study of bone tissue reactions to commercially pure titanium and vitallium implants. *Int J Oral Maxillofac Implants* **6**: 437–441.

Lang, N.P., Salvi, G.E., Huynh-Ba, G., Ivanovski, S., Donos, N. and Bosshardt, D.D. (2011) Early osseointegration to hydrophilic and hydrophobic implant surfaces in humans. *Clinical Oral Implants Research* **22(4)**: 349–356.

Lachmann, S., Laval, J.Y., Jager, B., et al. (2006) Resonance frequency analysis and damping capacity assessment. Part 2: Peri-implant bone loss follow-up. An in vitro study with the periotest and osstell instruments. *Clin Oral Implants Res* **17**: 80–84.

Ledermann, P. (1979) Bar-prosthetic management of the edentulous mandible by means of plasma-coated implantation with titanium screws. *Dtsch Zahnarztl Z* **34**: 907–911.

Lekholm, U. and Zarb, G. (1985) Patient selection and preparation. In: P. Branemark, G. Zarb and T. Albrektsson, eds. *Tissue-Integrated Prostheses: Osseointegration in Clinical Dentistry*, pp. 199–209. Quintessence Publishing, Chicago.

Liljenberg, B., Gualini, F., Berglundh, T., Tonetti, M. and Lindhe, J. (1996) Some characteristics of the ridge mucosa before and after implant installation. A prospective study in humans. *J Clin Periodontol* **23**: 1008–1013.

Lindhe, J. and Berglundh, T. (1998) The interface between the mucosa and the implant. *Periodontol* **17**: 47–54.

Linkow, L.I. and Rinaldi, A.W. (1988) Evolution of the vent-plant osseointegrated compatible implant system. *Int J Oral Maxillofac Implants* **3**: 109–122.

Lioubavina-Hack, N., Lang, N.P. and Karring, T. (2006) Significance of primary stability for osseointegration of dental implants. *Clin Oral Implants Res* **17**: 244–250.

Listgarten, M.A. and Lai, C.H. (1975) Ultrastructure of the intact interface between an endosseous epoxy resin dental implant and the host tissues. *J Biol Buccale* **3**: 13–28.

Listgarten, M.A., Buser, D., Steinemann, S.G., Donath, K., Lang, N.P. and Weber, H.P. (1992) Light and transmission electron microscopy of the intact interfaces between non-submerged titanium-coated epoxy resin implants and bone or gingiva. *J Dent Res* **71**: 364–371.

Listgarten, M.A., Lang, N.P., Schroeder, H.E. and Schroeder, A. (1991) Periodontal tissues and their counterparts around endosseous implants.] *Clin Oral Implants Res* **2**: 1–19.

Lukas, D. and Schulte, W. (1990) Periotest – a dynamic procedure for the diagnosis of the human periodontium. *Clin Phys Physiol Meas* **11**: 65–75.

Marzola, R., Scotti, R., Fazi, G. and Schincaglia, G.P. (2007) Immediate loading of two implants supporting a ball attachment-retained mandibular overdenture: a prospective clinical study. *Clin Implant Dent Relat Res* **9**: 136–143.

Meffert, R.M., Block, M.S. and Kent, J.N. (1987) What is osseointegration? *Int J Periodont Restor Dent* **7**: 9–21.

Meredith, N. (1998) Assessment of implant stability as a prognostic determinant. *Int J Prosthodont* **11**: 491–501.

Meredith, N., Alleyne, D. and Cawley, P. (1996) Quantitative determination of the stability of the implant-tissue interface using resonance frequency analysis. *Clin Oral Implants Res* **7**: 261–267.

Meredith, N., Book, K., Friberg, B., Jemt, T. and Sennerby, L. (1997) Resonance frequency measurements of implant stability in vivo. A cross-sectional and longitudinal study of resonance frequency measurements on implants in the edentulous and partially dentate maxilla. *Clin Oral Implants Res* **8**: 226–233.

Meredith, N., Cawley, P. and Alleyne, D. (1994) The application of modal vibration analysis to study bone healing in vivo. *J Dent Res* **73**: 793.

Mericske-Stern, R., Milani, D., Mericske, E. and Olah, A. (1995) Periotest measurements and osseointegration of mandibular ITI implants supporting overdentures. A one-year longitudinal study. *Clin Oral Implants Res* **6**: 73–82.

Misch, C. (2007) *Contemporary Implant Dentistry*, 3rd edn. Elsevier Health Sciences, Missouri.

Molly, L. (2006) Bone density and primary stability in implant therapy. *Clin Oral Implants Res* **17** Suppl 2: 124–135.

Moon, I.S., Berglundh, T., Abrahamsson, I., Linder, E. and Lindhe, J. (1999) The barrier between the keratinized mucosa and the dental implant. An experimental study in the dog. *J Clin Periodontol* **26**: 658–663.

Morris, H.E., Ochi, S., Crum, P., Orenstein, I. and Plezia, R. (2003) Bone density: its influence on implant stability after uncovering. *J Oral Implantol* **29**: 263–269.

Naert, I., Alsaadi, G., van Steenberghe, D. and Quirynen, M. (2004) A 10-year randomized clinical trial on the influence of splinted and unsplinted oral implants retaining mandibular overdentures: peri-implant outcome. *Int J Oral Maxillofac Implants* **19**: 695–702.

Nedir, R., Bischof, M., Szmukler-Moncler, S., Bernard, J.P. and Samson, J. (2004) Predicting osseointegration by means of implant primary stability. *Clin Oral Implants Res* **15**: 520–528.

Neukam, F.W. and Flemmig, T.F. (2006) Local and systemic conditions potentially compromising osseointegration. Consensus report of working group 3. *Clin Oral Implants Res* 17 Suppl **2**: 160–162.

O'Sullivan, D., Sennerby, L., Jagger, D. and Meredith, N. (2004) A comparison of two methods of enhancing implant primary stability. *Clin Implant Dent Relat Res* **6**: 48–57.

Ottoni, J.M., Oliveira, Z.F., Mansini, R. and Cabral, A.M. (2005) Correlation between placement torque and survival of single-tooth implants. *Int J Oral Maxillofac Implants* **20**: 769–776.

Olive, J. and Aparicio, C. (1990) Periotest method as a measure of osseointegrated oral implant stability. *Int J Oral Maxillofac Implants* **5**: 390–400.

Pendegrass, C.J., Gordon, D., Middleton, C.A., Sun, S.N. and Blunn, G.W. (2008) Sealing the skin barrier around transcutaneous implants: in vitro study of keratinocyte proliferation and adhesion in response to surface modifications of titanium alloy. *J Bone Joint Surg Br* **90**: 114–121.

Piattelli, A., Scarano, A., Balleri, P. and Favero, G.A. (1998) Clinical and histologic evaluation of an active 'implant periapical lesion': a case report. *Int J Oral Maxillofac Implants* **13**: 713–716.

Piattelli, A., Paolantonio, M., Corigliano, M. and Scarano, A. (1997) Immediate loading of titanium plasma-sprayed screw-shaped implants in man: a clinical and histological report of two cases. *J Periodontol* **68**: 591–597.

Piattelli, A., Ruggeri, A., Franchi, M., Romasco, N. and Trisi, P. (1993) An histologic and histomorphometric study of bone reactions to unloaded and loaded non-submerged single implants in monkeys: a pilot study. *J Oral Implantol* **19**: 314–320.

Pilliar, R.M., Lee, J.M. and Maniatopoulos, C. (1986) Observations on the effect of movement on bone ingrowth into porous-surfaced implants. *Clin Orthop Relat Res* July(**208**): 108–113.

Raghavendra, S., Wood, M.C. and Taylor, T.D. (2005) Early wound healing around endosseous implants: a review of the literature. *Int J Oral Maxillofac Implants* **20**: 425–431.

Ring, M.E. (1995) A thousand years of dental implants: a definitive history – part 1. *Compend Contin Educ Dent* **16**: 1060, 1062, 1064 passim.

Ring, M.E. (1995) A thousand years of dental implants: a definitive history – part 2. *Compend Contin Educ Dent* **16**: 1132, 1134, 1136 passim.

Roccuzzo, M., Aglietta, M., Bunino, M. and Bonino, L. (2008) Early loading of sandblasted and acid-etched implants: a randomized-controlled double-blind split-mouth study. Five-year results. *Clin Oral Implants Res* **19**: 148–152.

Romeo, E., Chiapasco, M., Lazza, A.,et al. (2002) Implant-retained mandibular overdentures with ITI implants. *Clin Oral Implants Res* **13**: 495–501.

Salonen, M.A., Raustia, A.M., Kainulainen, V. and Oikarinen, K.S. (1997) Factors related to periotest values in endosseal implants: a 9-year follow-up. *J Clin Periodontol* **24**: 272–277.

Salvi, G.E., Gallini, G. and Lang, N.P. (2004) Early loading (2 or 6 weeks) of sandblasted and acid-etched (sla) ITI implants in the posterior mandible. A 1-year randomized controlled clinical trial. *Clin Oral Implants Res* **15**: 142–149.

Schmid, J., Wallkamm, B., Hammerle, C.H., Gogolewski, S. and Lang, N.P. (1997) The significance of angiogenesis in guided bone regeneration. A case report of a rabbit experiment. *Clin Oral Implants Res* **8**: 244–248.

Schroeder, A., Pohler, O. and Sutter, F. (1976) Tissue reaction to an implant of a titanium hollow cylinder with a titanium surface spray layer. *SSO Schweiz Monatsschr Zahnheilkd* **86**: 713–727.

Schroeder, A., van der Zypen, E., Stich, H. and Sutter, F. (1981) The reactions of bone, connective tissue, and epithelium to endosteal implants with titanium-sprayed surfaces. *J Maxillofac Surg* **9**: 15–25.

Schupbach, P. and Glauser, R. (2007) The defense architecture of the human periimplant mucosa: a histological study. *J Prosthet Dent* **97**: S15–25.

Schulte, W. and Lukas, D. (1992) The periotest method. *Int Dent J* **42**: 433–440.

Schulte, W. and Lukas, D. (1993) Periotest to monitor osseointegration and to check the occlusion in oral implantology. *J Oral Implantol* **19**: 23–32.

Schwarz, F., Ferrari, D., Herten, M., et al. (2007a) Effects of surface hydrophilicity and microtopography on early stages of soft and hard tissue integration at non-submerged titanium implants: an immunohistochemical study in dogs. *J Periodontol* **78**: 2171–2184.

Schwarz, F., Herten, M., Sager, M., Wieland, M., Dard, M. and Becker, J. (2007b) Histological and immunohistochemical analysis of initial and early osseous integration at chemically modified and conventional sla titanium implants: preliminary results of a pilot study in dogs. *Clin Oral Implants Res* **18**: 481–488.

Sennerby, L. and Meredith, N. (2008) Implant stability measurements using resonance frequency analysis: biological and biomechanical aspects and clinical implications. *Periodontol* **47**: 51–66.

Sennerby, L. and Roos, J. (1998) Surgical determinants of clinical success of osseointegrated oral implants: a review of the literature. *Int J Prosthodont* **11**: 408–420.

Sennerby, L., Thomsen, P. and Ericson, L.E. (1992) A morphometric and biomechanic comparison of titanium implants inserted in rabbit cortical and cancellous bone. *Int J Oral Maxillofac Implants* **7**: 62–71.

Sennerby, L., Persson, L.G., Berglundh, T., Wennerberg, A. and Lindhe, J. (2005) Implant stability during initiation and resolution of experimental periimplantitis: an experimental study in the dog. *Clin Implant Dent Relat Res* **7**: 136–140.

Seong, W.J., Conrad, H.J. and Hinrichs, J.E. (2009) Potential damage to bone-implant interface when measuring initial implant stability. *J Periodontol* **80**: 1868–1874.

Sjostrom, M., Lundgren, S., Nilson, H. and Sennerby, L. (2005) Monitoring of implant stability in grafted bone using resonance frequency analysis. A clinical study from implant placement to 6 months of loading. *Int J Oral Maxillofac Surg* **34**: 45–51.

Slaets, E., Carmeliet, G., Naert, I. and Duyck, J. (2007) Early trabecular bone healing around titanium implants: a histologic study in rabbits. *J Periodontol* **78**: 510–517.

Steflik, D.E., Corpe, R.S., Lake, F.T., et al. (1998) Ultrastructural analyses of the attachment (bonding) zone between bone and implanted biomaterials. *J Biomed Mater Res* **39**: 611–620.

Steflik, D.E., Hanes, P.J., Sisk, A.L., et al. (1992) Transmission electron microscopic and high voltage electron microscopic observations of the bone and osteocyte activity adjacent to unloaded dental implants placed in dogs. *J Periodontol* **63**: 443–452.

Steflik, D.E., McKinney, R.V., Sisk, A.L., Koth, D.L., Singh, B.B. and Parr, G.R. (1990) Ultrastructural investigations of the bone and fibrous connective tissue interface with endosteal dental implants. *Scanning Microsc* **4**: 1039–1047; discussion on 1047–1038.

Steflik, D.E., Parr, G.R., Sisk, A.L., Hanes, P.J. and Lake, F.T. (1992) Electron microscopy of bone response to titanium cylindrical screw-type endosseous dental implants. *Int J Oral Maxillofac Implants* **7**: 497–507.

Steflik, D.E., Sisk, A.L., Parr, G.A., Lake, F.T. and Hanes, P.J. (1993) Experimental studies of the implant-tissue interface. *J Oral Implantol* **19**: 90–94; discussion 136–137.

Steinemann, S.G. (1998) Titanium – the material of choice? *Periodontol* **17**: 7–21.

Stephan, G., Vidot, F., Noharet, R. and Mariani, P. (2007) Implant-retained mandibular overdentures: a comparative pilot study of immediate loading versus delayed loading after two years. *J Prosthet Dent* **97**: S138–145.

Stricker, A., Gutwald, R., Schmelzeisen, R. and Gellrich, N.G. (2004) Immediate loading of 2 interforaminal dental implants supporting an overdenture: clinical and radiographic results after 24 months. *Int J Oral Maxillofac Implants* **19**: 868–872.

Sullivan, D.Y., Sherwood, R.L., Collins, T.A. and Krogh, P.H. (1996) The reverse-torque test: a clinical report. *Int J Oral Maxillofac Implants* **11**: 179–185.

Szmukler-Moncler, S., Piattelli, A., Favero, G.A. and Dubruille, J.H. (2000) Considerations preliminary to the application of early and immediate loading protocols in dental implantology. *Clin Oral Implants Res* **11**: 12–25.

Tawse-Smith, A., Perio, C., Payne, A.G., Kumara, R. and Thomson, W.M. (2001) One-stage operative procedure using two different implant systems: a prospective study on implant overdentures in the edentulous mandible. *Clin Implant Dent Relat Res* **3**: 185–193.

Testori, T., Szmukler-Moncler, S., Francetti, L., et al. (2001) Immediate loading of osseotite implants: a case report and histologic analysis after 4 months of occlusal loading. *Int J Periodontics Restorative Dent* **21**: 451–459.

Tjellstrom, A., Jacobsson, M. and Albrektsson, T. (1988) Removal torque of osseointegrated craniofacial implants: a clinical study. *Int J Oral Maxillofac Implants* **3**: 287–289.

Truhlar, R.S., Lauciello, F., Morris, H.F. and Ochi, S. (1997) The influence of bone quality on periotest values of endosseous dental implants at stage II surgery. *J Oral Maxillofac Surg* **55**: 55–61.

Truhlar, R.S., Morris, H.F., Ochi, S. and Winkler, S. (1994) Second-stage failures related to bone quality in patients receiving endosseous dental implants: DICRG interim report no. 7. Dental Implant Clinical Research Group. *Implant Dent* **3**: 252–255.

Tsuchiya, T., Nakamura, A., Ohshima, Y., et al. (1998) Chondrogenic cellular responses to titanium and zirconium alloys in vitro. *Tissue Eng* **4**: 197–192–194.

Turkyilmaz, I., Sennerby, L., Tumer, C., Yenigul, M. and Avci, M. (2006) Stability and marginal bone level measurements of unsplinted implants used for mandibular overdentures: a 1-year randomized prospective clinical study comparing early and conventional loading protocols. *Clin Oral Implants Res* **17**: 501–505.

Thomas, K.A. and Cook, S.D. (1985) An evaluation of variables influencing implant fixation by direct bone apposition. *J Biomed Mater Res* **19**: 875–901.

Ueda, M., Matsuki, M., Jacobsson, M. and Tjellstrom, A. (1991) Relationship between insertion torque and removal torque analyzed in fresh temporal bone. *Int J Oral Maxillofac Implants* **6**: 442–447.

Van Steenberghe, D., Tricio, J., Naert, I. and Nys, M. (1995) Damping characteristics of bone-to-implant interfaces. A clinical study with the periotest device. *Clin Oral Implants Res* **6**: 31–39.

Vandamme, K., Naert, I., Geris, L., Vander Sloten, J., Puers, R. and Duyck, J. (2007) The effect of micro-motion on the tissue response around immediately loaded roughened titanium implants in the rabbit. *Eur J Oral Sci* **115**: 21–29.

Verhoeven, J.W., Cune, M.S. and de Putter, C. (2000) Reliability of some clinical parameters of evaluation in implant dentistry. *J Oral Rehabil* **27**: 211–216.

Vignoletti, F., Johansson, C., Albrektsson, T., De Sanctis, M., San Roman, F. and Sanz, M. (2009) Early healing of implants placed into fresh extraction sockets: an experimental study in the beagle dog. De novo bone formation. *J Clin Periodontol* **36**: 265–277.

Weber, H.P., Morton, D., Gallucci, G.O., Roccuzzo, M., Cordaro, L. and Grutter, L. (2009) Consensus statements and recommended clinical procedures regarding loading protocols. *Int J Oral Maxillofac Implants* 24 Suppl: 180–183.

Wennerberg, A. and Albrektsson, T. (2009) Effects of titanium surface topography on bone integration: a systematic review. *Clin Oral Implants Res* 20 Suppl **4**: 172–184.

Wennerberg, A., Albrektsson, T., Andersson, B. and Krol, J.J. (1995) A histomorphometric and removal torque study of screw-shaped titanium implants with three different surface topographies. *Clin Oral Implants Res* **6**: 24–30.

Wong, M., Eulenberger, J., Schenk, R. and Hunziker, E. (1995) Effect of surface topology on the osseointegration of implant materials in trabecular bone. *J Biomed Mater Res* **29**: 1567–1575.

13 The Pulp Healing Process: From Generation to Regeneration*

Stéphane Simon, Anthony J. Smith, Philip J. Lumley, Paul R. Cooper and Ariane Berdal

[1]INSERM, centre de recherche des Cordeliers, Paris;
[2]Département de Sciences Biologiques, Université Pierre et Marie Curie-Paris 6, Paris;
[3]Université Paris Descartes, Paris;
[4]Team 5-Molecular oral Physiopathology, Université Paris Diderot, Paris, France;
[5]Oral Biology, School of Dentistry, University of Birmingham, Birmingham, UK.

Dentistry has not escaped the exciting new therapeutic advances of regenerative medicine. The accumulating knowledge about dental stem cells, differentiation, and the signaling cascades of tooth development and morphogenesis has enabled the implementation of dental biomimetics. This domain offers novel approaches to oral restoration, such as whole tooth organ bioengineering and targeted regeneration of specific dental and periodontal tissues, including bone, as recently achieved in rodent models in several laboratories. These procedures have resulted in successful growth of a tooth and its periodontium with appropriate functional properties, including vascularisation, innervation and responses to biomechanical forces (Ikeda et al. 2009). However, the length of time required to perform tooth bioengineering has hampered the application of these procedures to the clinical setting. Nevertheless, there are several strategies that can be used to regenerate specific parts of the dental-bone complex that have been destroyed by oral disease.

Recent advances in biotechnology have opened opportunities for development of applications in the maintenance of pulp vitality, reactionary dentinogenesis and revascularization of the infected canal. The present chapter provides an overview of the management of pulp repair and regeneration as accessible and preferred alternatives to classical endodontics in which the whole pulp is removed and replaced by inert materials.

FROM GENERATION TO REGENERATION

Odontoblasts are actively secreting cells during primary dentinogenesis but become largely quiescent during secondary dentinogenesis. Under physiological conditions of normal aging, there is a gradual reduction in the size of both the pulp chamber and the canal, which

* Stéphane Simon, Laboratoire de Physiopathologie Orale Moléculaire, INSERM, UMR S 872, Escalier B, 15–21 rue de l'Ecole de Médecine, 75006 Paris, France.

Oral Wound Healing: Cell Biology and Clinical Management, First Edition. Edited by Hannu Larjava.

explains why the teeth of elderly persons show diminution of the root canal system compared to the teeth of younger individuals. Under pathological conditions, odontoblasts can upregulate their secretion again in response to an injurious challenge, resulting in secretion of tertiary reactionary dentine at rates similar to those of primary dentine formation. This reactionary dentine is usually only secreted focally at sites of injury and therefore shows only limited distribution.

It is probable that the processes involved in pulp repair (reactionary and reparative dentinogenesis) recapitulate those of physiological dentinogenesis, although regulation of odontoblast secretory behavior may differ in tertiary dentinogenesis (Tziafas et al. 2000, Smith & Lesot 2001).

Traditionally, after completion of root formation, secondary dentinogenesis is regarded as proceeding at a much slower rate than primary dentinogenesis, gradually reducing the size of the pulp chamber and root canal system over many years. When obliteration of the pulpal space occurs, it appears that dentinogenesis is still very active, implying dysregulation of the normal physiological control of odontoblast cells during secondary dentinogenesis.

The switch from primary to secondary cell behavior is still poorly understood. However, the continuity of the dentinal tubule strongly indicates that the same cells are secreting dentine, but at a different rate. Morphological evidence also provides the basis of our understanding of the downregulation of odontoblast secretion during secondary dentinogenesis.

Recently published data suggest that there is a change in the gene expression profile of odontoblasts from primary to secondary dentinogenesis (Simon et al. 2009), and it is hypothesised that this change may be reversible, as odontoblast secretion is seen to be upregulated during reactionary dentinogenesis (Simon et al. 2010).

Pulp capping – the procedure of placing a dedicated material over exposed pulp to induce the formation of a barrier of reparative dentine so as to allow the pulp cells to express their dentinogenic potential – is still a controversial treatment in endodontics. The indication for and the effectiveness of therapeutics directed at maintaining pulp vitality are difficult to establish, and recommendations are often based on rather limited scientific evidence. Pulp capping is traditionally recommended on young teeth only, due to the greater reparative potential of younger pulp tissue, its better blood supply and higher cell density; however, retrospective studies show clearly that the age of the patient should not be considered a limiting factor in decisions on treatment options (Al-Hiyasat et al. 2006, Barthel et al. 2000, Haskell et al. 1978).

The dentine–pulp complex

Dentine is a mineralized connective tissue made of various types of collagen such as collagen type I (the major collagenous constituent), and of non-collagenous proteins (proteoglycans, glycoproteins, dentin phosphoprotein, and so on), including dentin sialo-protein (DSP) and dentin phospho-protein (DPP), considered as being the most specific to dental tissues. Nevertheless, these proteins have also been found in other mineralized tissues, such as bone, but at significantly lower concentrations than in dentine (Goldberg & Smith 2004).

The non-collagenous proteins initiate and control mineralization of the extracellular matrix (ECM) in the area termed the 'mineralization front' (Butler 1998), and then ensure the transformation of predentine into dentine.

Dentine is a permeable tissue that is traversed by tubular structures called dentinal tubules, which contain dentinal fluid and the odontoblast processes. The extent of these odontoblast processes in the tubules remains controversial, as some authors claim that the processes extend from the pulp chamber to the enamel dentine junction (EDJ) or cemental dentine junction (CDJ) (Maniatopoulos & Smith 1983, Sigal et al. 1984, Sigal et al. 1985), whereas other authors suggest that the processes are limited to the internal third of the tubules only (Thomas & Carella 1984, Thomas & Carella 1983, Garberoglio & Brannström 1976, Pashley 2002). Dentinal permeability is an unavoidable factor that must be considered during therapeutic procedures in dentistry. Surgical intervention of teeth will inevitably cause some damage to the pulp; the responding defence processes are numerous and complex and their interplay is not yet fully understood. Nevertheless, they are the basis of the healing process, and postsurgical pain is sometimes encountered after even conservative treatment. Therefore, it is necessary to understand the defence processes occurring in the tooth in order to manage post-treatment discomfort optimally and facilitate the regenerative process.

Pulpal hydrodynamic theory (Brannström 1963) probably provides our best understanding of pulpal pain. On the basis of histological and physiological observations, Brannström (1963) proposed that dentinal sensitivity is closely associated with very fast and brief movements of dentinal fluid inside the tubules, which may trigger responses within the vascular and neural structures at the pulpal level. Since Brannström's (1963) seminal publication, recent findings suggest the possible existence of sensory properties for the odontoblast and its role in sensory transmission of stimuli to the tooth (Okumura et al. 2005, Allard et al. 2006).

Three types of dentine

Three types of dentine are commonly described (Goldberg & Smith 2004):

Primary dentine is the earliest secreted tissue and gives rise to the overall morphology of the crown and the root. It 'patterns' the tooth organ. The mantle dentine is the most external layer of the primary dentine. As the very first layer secreted as the odontoblast layer it is not well structured. The thickness of mantel dentine is about 10 µm and the tissue is atubular.

Secondary dentine is the second tissue to be secreted during tooth development. Continuous secretion of this tissue is responsible for the progressively asymmetrical loss of endodontic volume improperly called 'calcification'. This biological process explains the differences in canal volume between a young and an older tooth. Secondary dentine is physiologically secreted and not pathologic. Histologically, primary and secondary dentines are identical (Baume 1980). Only their rate of secretion differs: 4 µm/day for primary dentine and 0.4 µm/day for secondary dentine (Nanci 2003, Schour & Poncher 1937, Ziskin et al. 1949). The interface between primary and secondary dentine is sometimes demarcated by a subtle calciotraumatic line.

Tertiary dentine is secreted in response to external stimuli (e.g. caries). The function of tertiary dentine is to protect the underlying pulp. Secretion of tertiary dentine in response to moderate stress is referred to as 'reactionary detinogenesis', in which the odontoblast layer is preserved. In more stressful disease circumstances, odontoblast survival may be compromised; in such cases the healing process is more complex and entails 'reparative dentinogenesis' (Fig. 13.1).

Understanding the clear distinction between secondary (physiological) and tertiary (healing) dentine is essential, though they are often confused when reported in the literature.

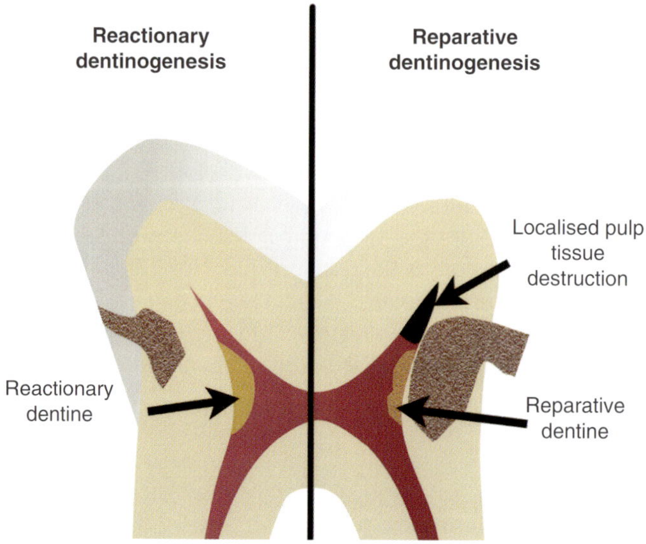

Fig. 13.1 The two types of tertiary dentonigenesis.

The odontoblast: a key cell for regenerative endodontics

Odontoblasts are highly differentiated, post-mitotic cells that are organized at the periphery of the pulp as a cellular palisade. The presence of all the elements of the secretory/mineralization machinery in these cells underscores their intense activity, notably during primary dentinogenesis. At a later stage of secondary dentinogenesis the cells return to a quiescent state, with a reduced number of cytoplasmic organelles (Jones & Boyde 1984). The odontoblasts of the palisade are interconnected by cellular junctions, such as gap junctions, thereby forming a permeability barrier; the gap junctions also allow for intracellular communication, which may be involved in regulating the pulp healing process (Magloire et al. 2004).

Odontoblasts synthesize the components of the predentine (collagen, glycoproteins and other non-collagenous proteins) and are responsible for its mineralization. Like all other cells of the dental pulp, odontoblasts are derived from neural crest mesenchymal cells and their differentiation is under the control of the internal dental epithelium (IDE). Differentiation is initiated at each cusp tip and is carried out according to a specific temporo-spatial pattern. In the mouse, the first differentiated odontoblasts appear on the 18th day of embryonic development, on the top of the main cusp of the first lower molar. The differentiation process gradually extends to the apical area and leads to the formation of a gradient of differentiation (Ruch et al. 1995).

From preodontoblast to functional odontoblast

In the early stages of tooth development, undifferentiated cells derived from the cranial neural crest migrate to the first branchial arch. The oral epithelium plays a key role in the initial patterning of the tooth, by controlling cellular commitment as well as the morphology of the tooth germs (incisor, molar, etc.).

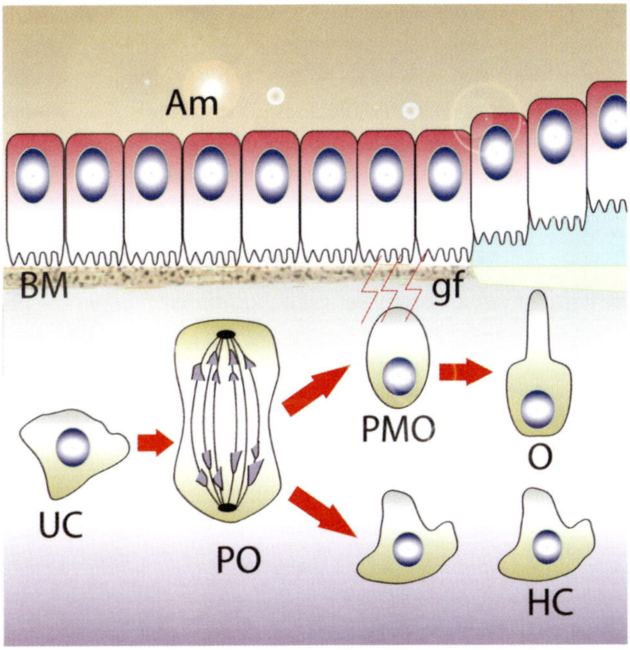

Fig. 13.2 Odontoblast differentiation process. One undifferentiated ectomesenchymal cell (UC) differentiates in preodontobalst (PO). During the last mitosis, under the control of epithelial cells (pre-améloblasts) (Am) by signaling molecules (gf) going through the basal membrane (BM), this cell divides into a post-mitotic odontoblast (PMO) and another daughter cell which is not in contact with the epithelial cells any more, and reaches the subodontoblast Höhl's layer (HC). The post-mitotic odontoblast finally differentiates into secreting odontoblast (O).

Final differentiation of preodontoblasts into odontoblasts occurs after a specific number of cell divisions (Ruch et al. 1995). All of the cells of the dental papilla have the potential to differentiate into odontoblasts; however, only those in contact with the basal membrane at the interface with the IDE undergo terminal differentiation. This consideration has implications for the healing process, in which other signaling processes are responsible for induction of odontoblast-like cell differentiation.

In mice, the preodontoblasts, located near the basal membrane (BM), undergo 14 to 15 mitoses before leaving the cell division cycle; however, in humans the number of cell divisions necessary for this process has not yet been determined. During the final division, the mitotic spindle, originally parallel to the BM, realigns to be perpendicular to this membrane (Osman & Ruch 1976). After the final mitosis, only the cell in contact with the BM is able to enter into the terminal differentiation process, while the other daughter cell (not in contact with the BM) becomes a part of Höhl's cell layer (Fig. 13.2).

Cytological modifications and odontoblast differentiation

Differentiation induces nuclear polarization and cell elongation, implying important cytological changes. The cisternae of the rough endoplasmic reticulum and the Golgi apparatus are orientated parallel to the long axis of the cell and are localized in its distal area where the cellular process will initiate elongation. The cell body of the differentiated secretory odontoblast is approximately 50–60 μm long.

Functional odontoblasts are connected by many intercellular junctions; gap junctions ensure rapid transport of ions and small molecules between cells. These junctions are present along the cytoplasmic membrane of the body of the cell, creating cell contact between odontoblasts themselves and between odontoblasts and cells in the sub-odontoblast layer (Sasaki et al. 1982). Other intercellular junctions, such as desmosomes, enable a mechanical cohesion between the odontoblasts, creating a true histological barrier. These junctions are located in the area of the cell body and the process junction (Kagayama et al. 1995). This distal junction creates a physical barrier between the compartment of the predentine and the odontoblast cell-body.

Immature odontoblasts are small and ovoid in shape, having a high nuclear/cytoplasmic ratio, a rudimentary granular endoplasmic reticulum and few Golgi cisternae. Cellular modifications appear when the cells reach the secretory phase (Goldberg & Smith 2004). Matrix vesicles were initially identified in cartilage of long bone (Bernard 1969), and then later were described in the dentine–pulp complex (Katchburian & Severs 1982). Theses vesicles are located in the ECM adjacent to the odontoblasts during mantle dentine formation. They disappear once mantle dentine formation is completed and the distal process has started to elongate.

At the ultrastructural level, these vesicles appear as extracellular spherical structures, and contain amorphous material more or less electron-dense and surrounded by a membrane. As in bone and cartilage, the membrane of these vesicles is made of three layers and contains various enzymes, especially phosphatases, involved in the mineralization process. The vesicles are the initial sites of mineralization in the mantle dentine and are also found in cartilage and bone.

Ultrastructural modifications have also been shown in the secretory cells during primary, secondary and tertiary dentonogenesis related to their functional activity (Couve 1986). Active cells appear elongated, with basal nuclei. They contain many organelles with numerous vesicles, extensive endoplasmic reticulum and a well-developed Golgi complex located between the nucleus and the distal region of the cell. Rough endoplasmic reticulum is also extensive. Morphologically, quiescent cells are stubby, cuboidal and show only limited cytoplasm and a more haematoxophilic nucleus. Organelle numbers decrease and this is related to the lower activity of the cells (Nanci 2003).

Regulation of odontoblast differentiation

During development, odontoblast differentiation is controlled by reciprocal interactions between the IDE and the dental papilla. The ECM and the BM play a critical role in this regulation, serving as a reservoir of paracrine and autocrine factors.

Only a specific dental BM is able to induce differentiation of odontoblasts; the pre-odontoblasts can respond to epigenetic signals only after having undergone a fixed number of cell divisions. Moreover, to fulfil its role, the BM is subject to modifications, regulated by the IDE. These changes are fundamental for the regulation of tooth development.

The main components of the BM are collagen IV, fibronectin, laminin (Lesot et al. 1981), nidogen, tenascin, hyaluronic acid and proteoglycans, including heparan sulfate (Thesleff et al. 1981).

Growth factors

Various growth factors and their receptors have been shown to be present at the enamel organ–dental papilla interface by immunohistochemistry and *in situ* hybridization during tooth development and have been implicated in odontoblast differentiation:

- Growth hormone (GH) plays a paracrine and/or autocrine role in dental development (Zhang et al. 1997).
- Insulin-like growth factor (IGF)-1 and -2 (Joseph et al. 1996, Cassidy et al. 1997, Begue-Kirn et al. 1994).
- Transforming growth factor-β1 (TGF-β1, -β2 and -β3 (D'Souza et al. 1990, Thesleff & Vaahtokari 1992) and bone morphogenetic protein (BMP)-2, -4 and -6 (Vainio et al. 1993) are necessary for the proper polarization and differentiation of odontoblasts (Begue-Kirn et al. 1994). Notably in adult pulp, TGFβ-1 plays an important role in the regulation of the inflammatory response and tissue regenerative processes.

The sequestration of these growth factors in the dentine matrix and their subsequent fossilization during the mineralization process appear to be key to the pulp healing process, where their release from the matrix may be responsible for various signaling events. Their precise localization in the dentine (Smith et al. 1998) and the full scope of their roles remain to be elucidated.

Transcription factors

A second level of regulation exists during dental development mediated through transcription factors. Notably, Msx1 is expressed in polarized pre-odontoblasts and Msx2 is present in mature odontoblasts (Begue-Kirn et al. 1994). Msx1 protein and transcripts have been identified in the pulp mesenchyme at early stages of tooth development and their concentrations decreased at the bell stage (Coudert et al. 2005). Msx1 sense RNA is mainly expressed in the dental pulp of the mouse at the 15th day of tooth development.

Expression of these transcription factors is under the control of growth factors, which can ultimately have broad-ranging effects. Significantly, BMP-4 upregulates Msx1 and Msx2 expression. In turn, transcription factors regulate further growth factor expression; for example, Msx1 upregulates BMP-4 synthesis in the mesenchyme and Msx2 regulates Runx2 and osteocalcin gene expression during odontogenesis (Bidder et al. 1998, Blin-Wakkach et al. 2001).

Growth factors and transcription factors are thus central to the cascade of molecular and cellular events during tooth development and are responsible for many of the temporo-spatial morphological changes observed in the developing tooth germ.

Other cells of the dental pulp

The second layer of the pulp is a dense zone of cells (the 'cell-rich layer of *Höhl*', separated from the odontoblasts by an acellular layer called the 'cell-free zone of *Weil*'). During tooth development, as mentioned above, the cellular differentiation process requires a minimum number of mitoses of the odontoblast progenitor cells before they are competent to differentiate into odontoblasts. The final mitosis has important spatial implications because it occurs perpendicularly to the dental BM, resulting in two daughter cells: the one adjacent to the BM receives the inductive signal to differentiate into an odontoblast, whereas the other cell does not and contributes to the Höhl layer instead (Ruch et al. 1995). This layer has long been considered as a potential reservoir of cells, containing incompletely differentiated cells that could be involved in the healing process for reparative dentinogenesis (Fitzgerald 1979).

The capillary and nerve plexi that exist between both layers are significant; only a few nerve fibres accompany the cytoplasmic extensions into the dentinal tubules and then only for a short distance (Carda & Peydro 2006). Capillaries are closely associated with the odontoblast palisade and provide these cells with the necessary nutrients for their mineralizing/synthetic activities.

Dental pulp stem cells

The growing interest in stem cells by the scientific community is also a key area in dental research. The description of dental pulp stem cells (DPSC) (Gronthos et al. 2000) inside the pulp parenchyma demonstrated that the dental organ provides a 'niche' environment for replacement cells. Another population of stem cells has also been reported in the pulp of deciduous teeth. These cells, or SHED (stem cells from human exfoliated deciduous teeth) (Miura et al. 2003), are singularly interesting because they are relatively easy to collect when the deciduous tooth is shed and replaced by the permanent successor.

More recently, a further group of mesenchymal stem cells has been reported in the apical papilla of human immature teeth. These pluripotent cells have been termed stem cells of apical papilla (SCAP) (Huang et al. 2008). Because they may be bone marrow-derived cells, SCAPs have potential for osteogenic and dentinogenic differentiation. Growth factor receptor genes are similar on SCAPs and DPSCs. SCAPs also express neurogenic factors such as nestin and neurofilament M when stimulated with neurogenic medium (Sonoyama et al. 2008).

The presence of stem cells in the dental pulp offers exciting possibilities for their exploitation in regenerative medicine, both for dental and other diseases. These cells are easier to collect than are cells from bone marrow, which is currently one of the main sources of postnatal stem cells. Furthermore, the dental pulp appears to be a promising reservoir of multipotent cells, and as such offers significant potential for use in various dental and non-dental biotechnological applications. In the case of regenerative dentistry, the presence of a population of stem/progenitor cells in the dental pulp provides a local source of cells for generating new 'odontoblast-like' cells for both natural pulp wound healing or regeneration and direct pulp capping after injury to the tooth. It is still unclear whether these stem cells derive from the dental papilla or migrate to the pulp through the vasculature. An important focus of future studies will be to characterize more precisely these stem cells and their potential so as to enable their most effective application in new regenerative therapies.

The discovery of stem cells in the dental pulp represents a significant advancement for dentistry. Although many questions remain unanswered, the identification of 'postnatal' stem cells in the tooth provides a new platform for development of exciting biological approaches for vital pulp therapy.

Pulpal responses to injury

During injury to the tooth (caries, trauma or wear), a cascade of pulpal responses is initiated. Depending on the nature of the injury (whether it is brief or prolonged, or of low or high intensity), the scope of the pulpal responses will likely differ. Injury of weak or moderate intensity will often be resolved by a brief inflammatory response followed by reactionary dentinogenesis. With a more severe injury, odontoblast death will occur (e.g. deep caries or severe trauma), and as long as inflammation does not become uncontrolled, differentiation of a new generation of odontoblast-like cells may occur, leading to dentine bridge formation at the sites of exposure; this process is termed reparative dentinogenesis (Cooper et al. 2010).

Reactionary versus reparative dentinogenesis: two different pathways

Reactionary and reparative dentinogenesis are two very different pathways for pulp repair (Fig 13.3). The description above of the two types of tertiary dentinogenesis highlights the need for different therapeutic strategies for pulp healing depending on which pathway is involved. Clinically, the choice of regenerative endodontic therapeutic approaches will necessarily be based on the extent of pulpal disease and, particularly, on odontoblast survival.

Translation of biological knowledge into the clinical setting can be achieved simply by adoption of a more biological thought process during treatment planning; however, it is not always that easy. For instance, the importance of tooth structure on biological events can be fairly readily appreciated, such as in the thickness of the residual dentine separating a cavity from the pulp, which can be an important factor in pulp protection.

In deeper cavities, where the thickness of the cavity floor is less than 0.5 mm, the number and the length of the 'opened' tubules is such that the communication with the pulp is possibly comparable to that of an actual cavity exposure (Smith 2002). Also, clinically it can be very difficult, if not impossible, to know both the inflammatory status of the pulp as well as the cytological state of the odontoblasts because pulpal histology does not necessarily correlate well with clinical presentation; this makes it very difficult to design an effective treatment plan in such situations, and there is an urgent need for more reliable means of diagnosis of the activity of carious lesions and the level of pulpal inflammation. Whereas thermal or electrical tests provide information on the innervation of the pulp, there is a need for tests that evaluate the vasculature and, in particular, the effects thereon of any inflammation that may be present. Unfortunately, the hard tissue shell enclosing the pulp constrains use of techniques such as laser Doppler scanning or scintography, which provide valuable information in other medical specialities.

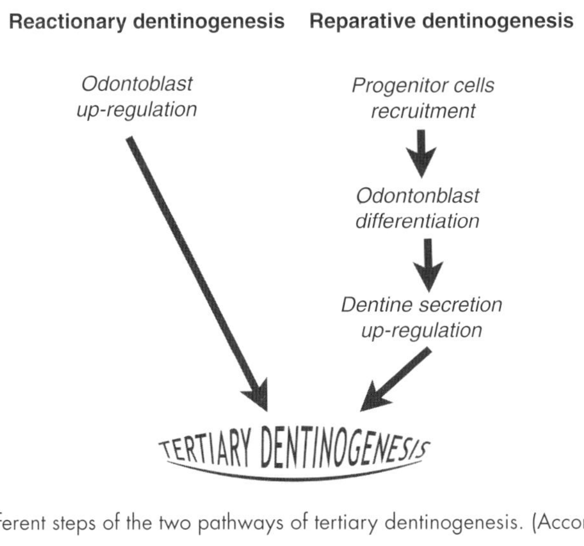

Fig. 13.3 The different steps of the two pathways of tertiary dentinogenesis. (According to Smith (55).)

Reactionary dentinogenesis

Although the rate of dentine secretion is clearly reduced in the adult, the metabolic activity of the odontoblasts can be upregulated in response to injury. Following injury, odontoblasts are released from their quiescent state and their secretory activity is subsequently upregulated, resulting in deposition of reactionary dentine. Because the same cells are responsible for secretion, it can be postulated that the molecular control processes that cause downregulation of odontoblast activity during the change from primary to secondary dentinogenesis may be reversed to stimulate the odontoblasts again during tertiary dentinogenesis. It is important to consider the nature of the signaling process between the injurious agent and the odontoblasts. Bacteria and their toxins are key candidates in the direct stimulation of odontoblasts during caries formation (Durand et al. 2006). Also, lipopolysaccharides and other bacterial toxins initiate intrapulpal inflammatory processes, but other signaling processes may also be critical in the overall balance of pulpal cell responses leading to healing and tissue regeneration (Tziafas et al. 2000, Choi et al. 2009, Magloire et al. 1992, Smith et al. 2008, Botero et al. 2006). For example, authors reported recently that tumor necrosis factor (TNF)-alpha stimulates differentiation of dental pulp cells towards an odontoblastic phenotype via p38 phosphorylation of the MAP kinase pathway (Paula-Silva et al. 2009).

Dentine contains trace amounts of very potent bio-active molecules, including cytokines and growth factors, which are sequestrated within the matrix during the mineralization process and become essentially fossilized therein. During the decay process, demineralization of the tissue is accompanied by the release of these molecules (Smith 2003) (Fig 13.4). In this pool of substances, many growth factors can be found, especially those of the TGF-β family (Cassidy et al. 1997, Smith et al. 1998). These growth factors are extremely potent and have a variety of cell signaling properties which enable them to act at very low concentrations. Once liberated, these factors traverse the tubules to the pulp and induce various cellular responses, including activation of the odontoblasts (Smith et al. 1995).

The members of the TGF-β family present in the dentine may be solubilized by plaque bacterial acids during caries (Smith et al. 1998, Smith et al. 1995) or by restorative treatments. These molecules could be responsible for the stimulation of odontoblast activity. The

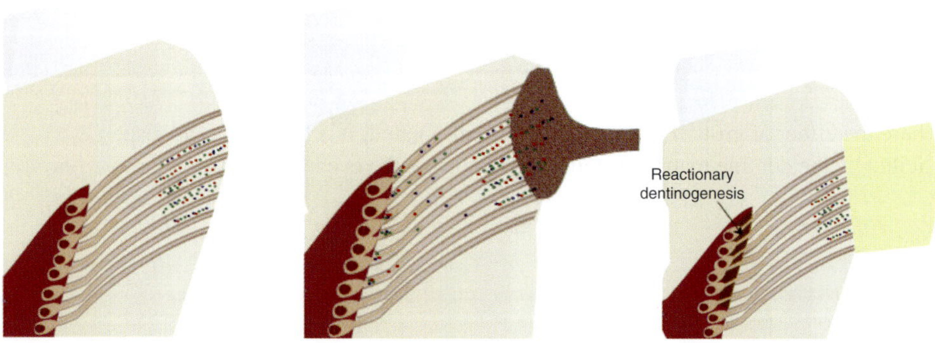

Fig. 13.4 Non-collagenous proteins, including growth factors, are fossilized in the matrix of the dentine during the physiological process of mineralization. After dissolution of the mineral matrix, these molecules are released and can reach and reactivate the quiescent odontoblasts through the dentinal tubules. These molecules should play an important role in the signaling pathway during the reactionary dentinogenesis process.

organic components secreted in response to injury give rise to the dentine matrix termed 'reactionary', corresponding to an increase in matrix secretion by the stimulated odontoblasts.

AT THE MOLECULAR LEVEL

By comparing the published data on dentine secretion rates (Schour & Poncher 1937, Hoffman & Schour 1940) and differential gene expression patterns between primary and secondary odontobalsts (Simon 2009), it can be concluded that the functional status of the odontoblast evolves, and the lower level of deposition by the cell observed during secondary dentinogenesis is associated with important changes in its transcriptome. In future studies, it would be interesting to compare the gene expression patterns reported here with those of odontoblasts or odontoblast-like cells taking part in tertiary dentinogenesis, in which secretory activity becomes upregulated again (Smith & Lesot 2001, Wennberg et al. 1982).

One of the unique features of the odontoblast is that it may be reactivated after injury and secrete reactionary dentine at similar rates to primary dentine. As similarities have been described between development and the healing process (Tziafas et al. 2000, Smith & Lesot 2001), we secondly sought to investigate the variation in protein secretory processes concomitant with the switch from early-stage to late-stage odontoblasts to examine whether key pathways could be identified which might regulate the switch from secondary to tertiary dentinogenesis. The MAPK/ERK pathway is a signal transduction pathway that couples intracellular responses to the binding of growth factors to cell surface receptors. This pathway is complex and includes many signaling mediators. It is also well established that the MAPK signaling pathway is involved in cellular differentiation.

Notably, the role of TGF-β1 is well established in odontoblast differentiation during primary development and in tertiary dentinogenesis (Smith & Lesot 2001, Unterbrink et al. 2002, D'Souza et al. 1998, D'Souza et al. 1992), and, significantly, recent publications indicate that TGF-β1 may regulate the MAPK pathway (Zhao et al. 2004, Ning et al. 2002).

Stimulation of odontoblast-like cells by several growth factors, as an *in vitro* model of tertiary dentinogenesis, or with *Streptococcus mutans*, as an *in vitro* model of caries, caused an increase in p38 phosphorylation and its nuclear translocation (Simon et al. 2010). TNF-α, adrenomedullin (ADM) and TGF-β1 produced similar patterns of p38 activation, whereas isolated dentine matrix proteins appeared to induce a different pattern. The cocktail of growth factors in the preparation of isolated dentine matrix proteins appeared to have a weaker but more enduring effect on cells than did the growth factors or bacterial stimulants alone. The effect of these dentine matrix proteins on p38 protein persisted past the point where the effect of growth factors alone had culminated. It is likely that the response profile elicited by the dentine matrix proteins better mirrors the events occurring in carious disease, in which dentine matrix components are released in combination. In view of the fact that tissue regeneration is a balance between inflammation and repair (Cooper et al. 2010), the comparatively weaker effect of dentine matrix proteins may serve the biological role of protecting the dental pulp by preventing pulpal inflammation.

Bacterial contamination of the pulp is usually described as the most important factor in pulp disease. In our experiments, when cells were stimulated with *Streptococcus mutans*, only half of the activated p38 protein was translocated. Based on this observation, we hypothesize that bacteria might stimulate the cytoplasmic pathway better, whereas growth factors might directly induce transcription. It should be noted that bacteria alone were not able to induce odontoblast activation, but that they produce a synergistic effect when combined with growth factors. It is thus critical when evaluating the healing and toxic effects of various agents that they be tested both alone and in combination. Further study is needed to determine the effect of a range of concentrations of dentine matrix proteins and other agents on odontoblast activation to allow the development of a more accurate and reliable *in vitro* model of the carious disease process.

Understanding cellular behavior in response to carious disease may allow the development of new approaches in regenerative dentistry that utilize biological and pharmacological control of cell behavior, much as p38 phosphorylation is currently exploited as a target of anti-inflammatory drugs. Better understanding of the regulation of the p38 pathway during tertiary dentinogenesis might also allow the development of new therapies, in particular for novel pharmaceuticals which facilitate bonding systems to better control the healing process and enhance the secretory activity of odontoblasts.

The role of the MAPK pathway therefore warrants further investigation to try to better understand its role during the odontoblast maturation process and its possible involvement in the reactivation of odontoblast secretory activity during tertiary dentinogenesis. Characterization of such key pathways involved in odontoblast secretion may provide exciting targets for development of novel regenerative therapies. Finally, a growing body of information suggesting similarities between pulp cells and bone cells may help us to better understand the physiology and pathology of the mineralized tissues of the body and allow more insightful comparison of data derived from bone and dental studies.

Reparative dentinogenesis and pulp capping

Odontoblasts are the only cells that secrete dentine. However, if they become damaged, formation of a dentine bridge at sites of pulpal exposure is still possible, provided that new odontoblast-like cells are 'available' in the area. Conventionally, wound healing involves cell migration from the edge of the injury, and through cell division the superficial cells advance to the centre of the injury, regenerating and repairing the tissue and allowing its reorganization.

Following pulp exposure, and after placement of an appropriate material, a dentine bridge is formed in a few weeks by new odontoblast-like cells. The origin of these secreting cells has not been firmly established. Several authors assert that the reparative processes are likely to be the same as those involved in tooth development (Smith & Lesot 2001, Mitsiadis & Rahiotis 2004). Nevertheless, the true origin of the progenitors is still unclear, and a possible migration origin from outside the tooth via the vasculature cannot be excluded.

Currently, a lack of trust in pulp capping frequently motivates many practitioners to remove the pulp of the tooth rather than attempt to maintain its viability.

Pulp capping

Many factors intervene in the prognosis of a pulp capping treatment (Murray et al. 2002, Murray et al. 2003); lack of inflammation, infection control and biocompatibility of the material used are reported to be the key factors for improving the clinical outcome (Mjor 2002, Ward 2002).

As it has also been established that an inflammatory response occurs in pulp tissue as soon as a caries reaches the dentine (even at a superficial layer), it appears that treatment of non-inflamed dental pulp would be an unlikely event, except after pulp exposure due to trauma. Pulp exposure often occurs after trauma, and as the pulp is generally free of inflammation, pulp capping in such situations represents a good approach for treatment. However, it is important to consider management of such cases in the context of the biological behavior of the pulp, especially in immature teeth which are still developing.

The ultimate goal of pulp capping with a dedicated material is to induce the formation of a barrier of reparative dentine between the pulp and the material of obturation, by allowing the pulp cells to express their dentinogenic potential (Schroder 1985). In 1965, Kakehashi demonstrated the systematic formation of a dentine bridge after pulp exposure in laboratory 'germ-free' animals (Kakehashi et al. 1965). His study highlighted that the ability of the pulp to heal depends on its environment, and can occur in the absence of bacterial infection (Cotton 1974).

Over the years, many materials have been used for pulp capping, with calcium hydroxide having long been considered the gold standard. Indeed, a search of PubMed (search keywords: calcium hydroxide and pulp capping) revealed more than 650 references (July 2009). Characterized by a very basic pH (Faraco & Holland 2001), calcium hydroxide no longer seems to be the ideal material for the following reasons:

- The induced dentine bridge is inconsistent and porous (Cox et al. 1996).
- Calcium hydroxide does not adhere to the dentinal walls.
- The sealing ability of calcium hydroxide is quite poor.
- The material has poor antibacterial properties.

Because of its high basicity, calcium hydroxide in direct contact with the pulp locally destroys a layer of pulp tissue, and thus creates an uncontrolled necrotic zone; this necrotic layer induces an inflammatory reaction which persists in time, or leads to formation of intrapulpal calcifications (Seltzer & Bender 2002).

Currently, there is considerable research focus directed towards identification of other materials able to induce the formation of a well-formed dentine bridge (Tarim et al. 1998); however, thus far, results remain inconsistent. Other approaches, including protection of the pulp with a hybrid layer of new adhesive systems, have also been studied (Cox et al. 1998).

The introduction of mineral trioxide aggregate (MTA) (Abedi et al. 1996, Pitt Ford et al. 1996, Torabinejad & Chivian 1999) has perhaps challenged the position of calcium hydroxide as the gold standard pulp capping material. Although our understanding of its composition and biological effects is limited, recent data suggest a better quality of the dentine bridge compared to that obtained with calcium hydroxide (Nair et al. 2008). Moreover, cells in direct contact with the dentine bridge express protein markers of odontoblasts (Simon et al. 2008). In a recent randomized prospective study on human teeth, Nair et al. concluded that, clinically, MTA is more appropriate than calcium hydroxide and should be considered as the new gold standard (Nair et al. 2008).

Several *in vivo* studies have shown that MTA induces the creation of a dentine bridge of good quality, with an effective hermetic seal, which can merge with the dentinal walls at the edge of the defect (Simon et al. 2008). The superior quality of the dentine bridge obtained with MTA versus calcium hydroxide has been recently demonstrated in a randomized clinical trial (Nair et al. 2008).

In spite of the lack of published information from the manufacturer on the composition of MTA, recent data suggest that Portland cement resembles the active ingredient of this material and exhibits similar properties (Abdullah et al. 2002, Estrela et al. 2000, Funteas et al. 2003, Holland et al. 2001, Saidon et al. 2003).

Pulp Capping and pulp repair
In most injury situations, pulp exposure is inevitably associated with an inflammatory response, and the following steps ensue (Cooper et al. 2010) :

- Haemostasis and formation of a blood clot.
- Inflammatory response.
- Cell proliferation and/or recruitment.
- Tissue remodeling.

The healing process in connective tissues is always characterized by these successive steps. Failure to resolve the inflammatory process leads to chronic inflammation and eventually to pulp necrosis. Pulp tissue adjacent to an exposure is characterized by the presence of necrotic debris, of blood clot formation and of a cellular response involving significant infiltration of neutrophils. Yamamura characterized the chronology of the healing process in the dog after pulp capping with calcium hydroxide (Yamamura 1985) as follows: exudative phase (3–5 days), proliferative phase (3–7 days), formation of osteodentine (5–14 days), formation of tubular dentine (14 days and more). After 3–6 days, the inflammatory layer is replaced by granulation tissue. This tissue is arranged along the wound and contains many fibroblasts and newly formed blood capillaries (Fitzgerald 1979). New ECM and nodules of mineralization are seen during healing (Schroder & Granath 1972). The first mineral deposits are found in matrix vesicles, indicating significant similarities between reparative dentinogenesis and the formation of mantle dentine (Hayashi 1982). At 11 days, the newly formed matrix surrounds cuboidal cells, and a few cells exhibit the first features of odontoblast differentiation (Mjor et al. 1991). At 14 days, cells are reorganized in a palisade of cells similar to that seen in primary or secondary dentine (Mjor et al. 1991). At 1 month, the dentine bridge and a necrotic layer associated with an inflammatory response in the adjacent pulp tissue can be seen (Fitzgerald 1979). At the ultrastructural level, 'tunnel defects' are clearly visible in the dentine bridges of 89% of the cases studied (Cox et al. 1996).

Reparative dentinogenesis is a complex process comprising a cascade of biological processes.

Interactions of pulpal cells with growth factors, cytokines and other molecular mediators during the healing process are at the origin of each of the three steps of the reparative process:

1. Recruitment of progenitor cells.
2. Cellular differentiation.
3. Upregulation of cell synthetic and secretory activity.

Progenitor cells of the 'second generation' odontoblasts
Reparative dentinogenesis during pulp healing requires progenitor cell recruitment and differentiation of these cells into odontoblast-like cells. The newly formed odontoblast-like cells result from the proliferation and differentiation of a population of stem/progenitor cells, probably residing within dental pulp (Ruch 1998). Fitzgerald et al. (1990) studied the migration and proliferation of cells in the pulp after capping with calcium hydroxide in the monkey. They stressed that the migration of cells occurred from the central pulp tissue to the pulp/material interface. They also showed that two DNA replications were necessary before the migration of these cells and their differentiation occurred.

Despite our substantial knowledge of tooth development, our understanding of these stem/progenitor cells is still limited. Pulp cells cultured under certain conditions can differentiate into cells with an odontoblast-like phenotype and have the capacity to form nodules of mineralization *in vitro* (Couble et al. 2000), although it is unclear whether all pulp cells or just a subpopulation can exhibit this behavior. More is known of the multipotent cells of bone marrow (BMSCs) and their potential to differentiate into osteoblasts, chondrocytes, adipocytes, myocytes and neuronal cells (Bennett et al. 1991, Krebsbach et al. 1997, Ferrari et al. 1998, Azizi et al. 1998, Pittenger et al. 1999). In the pulp, the origin of replacement odontoblast-like cells has not yet been clearly identified. For a long time, the cell-rich layer of Höhl was regarded as a reservoir of progenitor cells, although several origins for these stem/progenitor cells have now been proposed, including a local origin in the pulp mesenchyme and a remote one derived from the bone marrow. Pericytes in the pulp have also been proposed as candidate repair cells, although whether such cells originate from within the pulp or are transported there through the vasculature is unclear (Yamamura 1985, Shi & Gronthos 2003, Lovschall et al. 2007).

Pluripotent cells have been described in the dental pulp (Gronthos et al. 2000, Gronthos et al. 2002). These cells, called dental pulp stem cells (DPSCs), are able to form dentin-like tissue after ectopic transplantation; they can also differentiate into fat cells or neuronal cells. These DPSCs are probably progenitor cells and able to undergo self-renewal.

To date, involvement of DPSCs in the pulp healing process has not been definitively demonstrated. The definitive characterization of the origin of the cells responsible for the healing process in pulp would allow elucidation of their specific behaviour in the repair process, and help to inform the most appropriate treatment after pulp exposure.

Pulp healing and growth factors

During dentine degradation in carious injury several cytokines, including growth factors, are released from the dentine and likely also from the pulp ECM (Smith 2002, Smith et al. 2008, McLachlan et al. 2005, McLachlan et al. 2004). These cytokines play a key role in the regulation of progenitor cell recruitment, cell proliferation and differentiation of new dentine secreting cells. Members of the TGF-β family have clearly been identified as having roles in dental tissue healing events (Rutherford et al. 1993, Cassidy et al. 1997, Nakashima 1994, Rutherford et al. 1994, Baker et al. 2009). The differentiation of new odontoblast-like cells has also been reported after pulp capping with basic fibroblast growth factor (bFGF), TGF-β1 (Lovschall et al. 2001) and BMP-7 (Jepsen et al. 1997).

Direct application of growth factors to pulp tissue offers an interesting therapeutic approach; however, it is important that we first derive a clear understanding of the biological and molecular processes involved in their action before attempting to develop a reliable, reproducible and efficacious new clinical therapy based on their use (Tziafas et al. 2000).

It is with this new knowledge and an understanding of these processes that new therapeutic strategies can be developed to promote pulp vitality and healing.

Contrary to many of the studies reported with calcium hydroxide (Schroder & Granath 1972, Fitzgerald et al. 1990, Horsted et al. 1981), neither a necrotic layer nor a persistent inflammatory zone is noticed when MTA is used as the pulp capping material. Continuous bridge formation is generally observed, in good continuity with the dentine of the walls of the cavity, and with a discontinuity between the bridge and the dentinal wall (Simon et al. 2008, Holland et al. 2001, Aeinehchi et al. 2003, Dominguez et al. 2003, Asgary et al. 2006, Nair et al. 2007).

CONCLUSION

Research on pulp regeneration is growing and provides exciting possibilities for greater biological approaches to endodontics in the future. However, for significant progress to be made in translation to the clinic we need a much deeper understanding of the molecular control of odontoblast secretion and the physiological cues responsible for regulation of odontoblast behavior. Pulpectomy represents a radical treatment for non-necrotic pulp, but pulpotomy or pulp capping are only likely to find broader use if we can extend our knowledge of pulp regenerative processes. Such developments will likely bring significant progress to the area of vital pulp therapy.

Differentiation and genetic regulation of cells are also interesting to investigate during reparative dentinogenesis, as differentiation is one step of the complex system for pulp repair when the odontoblast layer had been destroyed. Nevertheless, more results are needed for understanding the complete healing process.

A key point in the repair process is the balance between infection, inflammation and tissue healing. Therefore, a full understanding of the healing process will require more data on pulp inflammation, including its clinical quantification. With these new tools, new diagnostic models and devices could be designed, and both true indications and contraindications of such new procedures would then be able to be described, with reproducible results and reliable prognosis. Then, pulp capping or other clinical strategies such as pulpotomy could be considered as alternative therapies to root canal treatment when pulp vitality is maintained.

REFERENCES

Abdullah D, Ford TR, Papaioannou S, Nicholson J, McDonald F (2002) An evaluation of accelerated portland cement as a restorative material. *Biomaterials* **23**: 4001–10.

Abedi H, Torabinejad M, Pitt Ford TR (1996) The use of mineral trioxide aggregate cement (MTA) as a pulp capping material (abstract). *J Endod* **22**: 199.

Aeinehchi M, Eslami B, Ghanbariha M, Saffar AS (2003) Mineral trioxide aggregate (MTA) and calcium hydroxide as pulp-capping agents in human teeth: a preliminary report. *Int Endod J* **36**: 225–31.

Al-Hiyasat AS, Barrieshi-Nusair KM, Al-Omari MA (2006) The radiographic outcomes of direct pulp-capping procedures performed by dental students: a retrospective study. *J Am Dent Assoc* **137**: 1699–705.

Allard B, Magloire H, Couble ML, Maurin JC, Bleicher F (2006) Voltage-gated sodium channels confer excitability to human odontoblasts: possible role in tooth pain transmission. *J Biol Chem* **281**: 29002–10.

Asgary S, Parirokh M, Eghbal MJ, Ghoddusi J, Eskandarizadeh A (2006) SEM evaluation of neodentinal bridging after direct pulp protection with mineral trioxide aggregate. *Aust Endod J* **32**: 26–30.

Azizi SA, Stokes D, Augelli BJ, DiGirolamo C, Prockop DJ (1998) Engraftment and migration of human bone marrow stromal cells implanted in the brains of albino rats – similarities to astrocyte grafts. *Proc Natl Acad Sci USA* **95**: 3908–13.

Baker SM, Sugars RV, Wendel M, et al. (2009) TGF-beta/extracellular matrix interactions in dentin matrix: a role in regulating sequestration and protection of bioactivity. *Calcif Tissue Int* **85**: 66–74.

Barthel CR, Rosenkranz B, Leuenberg A, Roulet JF (2000) Pulp capping of carious exposures: treatment outcome after 5 and 10 years: a retrospective study. *J Endod* **26**: 525–8.

Baume LJ (1980) Definitions and classifications of the pulpodentinal tissues. In: Meyers HM, ed. *The Biology of Pulp and Dentine*.S. Karger, Basel, pp. 60–62.

Begue-Kirn C, Smith AJ, Loriot M, Kupferle C, Ruch JV, Lesot H (1994) Comparative analysis of TGF beta, BMPS, IGF1, MSXS, fibronectin, osteonectin and bone sialoprotein gene expression during normal and in vitro-induced odontoblast differentiation. *Int J Dev Biol* **38**: 405–20.

Bennett JH, Joyner CJ, Triffitt JT, Owen ME (1991) Adipocytic cells cultured from marrow have osteogenic potential. *J Cell Sci* **99** (Pt 1): 131–9.

Bernard GW (1969) The ultrastructural interface of bone crystals and organic matrix in woven and lamellar endochondral bone. *J Dent Res* **48**: 781–8.

Bidder M, Latifi T, Towler DA (1998) Reciprocal temporospatial patterns of MSX2 and osteocalcin gene expression during murine odontogenesis. *J Bone Miner Res* **13**: 609–19.

Blin-Wakkach C, Lezot F, Ghoul-Mazgar S, et al. (2001) Endogenous MSX1 antisense transcript: in vivo and in vitro evidences, structure, and potential involvement in skeleton development in mammals. *Proc Natl Acad Sci USA* **98**: 7336–41.

Botero TM, Shelburne CE, Holland GR, Hanks CT, Nor JE (2006) TLR4 mediates LPS-induced VEGF expression in odontoblasts. *J Endod* **32**: 951–5.

Brannström M (1963) A hydrodynamic mechanism in the transmission of pain producing stimuli through the dentin. In: Anderson DJ, ed. *Sensory Mechanisms in Dentine*. Macmillian, New York, pp. 73–9.

Butler WT (1998) Dentin matrix proteins. *Eur J Oral Sci* **106** (Suppl 1): 204–10.

Carda C, Peydro A (2006) Ultrastructural patterns of human dentinal tubules, odontoblasts processes and nerve fibres. *Tissue Cell* **38**: 141–50.

Cassidy N, Fahey M, Prime SS, Smith AJ (1997) Comparative analysis of transforming growth factor-beta isoforms 1–3 in human and rabbit dentine matrices. *Arch Oral Biol* **42**: 219–23.

Choi BD, Jeong SJ, Wang G, et al. (2009) Temporal induction of secretory leukocyte protease inhibitor (SLPI) in odontoblasts by lipopolysaccharide and wound infection. *J Endod* **35**: 997–1002.

Cooper PR, Takahashi Y, Graham LW, Simon S, Imazato S, Smith AJ (2010) Inflammation-regeneration interplay in the dentine-pulp complex. *J Dent* **38** (9): 687–97.

Cotton WR (1974) Bacterial contamination as a factor in healing of pulp exposures. *Oral Surg Oral Med Oral Pathol* **38**: 441–50.

Couble ML, Farges JC, Bleicher F, Perrat-Mabillon B, Boudeulle M, Magloire H (2000) Odontoblast differentiation of human dental pulp cells in explant cultures. *Calcif Tissue Int* **66**: 129–38.

Coudert AE, Pibouin L, Vi-Fane B, et al. (2005) Expression and regulation of the MSX1 natural antisense transcript during development. *Nucleic Acids Res* **33**: 5208–18.

Couve E (1986) Ultrastructural changes during the life cycle of human odontoblasts. *Arch Oral Biol* **31**: 643–51.

Cox CF, Hafez AA, Akimoto N, Otsuki M, Suzuki S, Tarim B (1998) Biocompatibility of primer, adhesive and resin composite systems on non-exposed and exposed pulps of non-human primate teeth. *Am J Dent* **11** (Spec No): S55–63.

Cox CF, Subay RK, Ostro E, Suzuki S, Suzuki SH (1996) Tunnel defects in dentin bridges: their formation following direct pulp capping. *Oper Dent* **21**: 4–11.

Dominguez MS, Witherspoon DE, Gutmann JL, Opperman LA (2003) Histological and scanning electron microscopy assessment of various vital pulp-therapy materials. *J Endod* **29**: 324–33.

D'Souza RN, Cavender A, Dickinson D, Roberts A, Letterio J (1998) TGF-beta1 is essential for the homeostasis of the dentin-pulp complex. *Eur J Oral Sci* **106** (Suppl 1): 185–91.

D'Souza RN, Flanders K, Butler WT (1992) Colocalization of TGF-beta 1 and extracellular matrix proteins during rat tooth development. *Proc Finn Dent Soc* **88** (Suppl 1): 419–26.

D'Souza RN, Happonen RP, Ritter NM, Butler WT (1990) Temporal and spatial patterns of transforming growth factor-beta 1 expression in developing rat molars. *Arch Oral Biol* **35**: 957–65.

Durand SH, Flacher V, Romeas A, et al. (2006) Lipoteichoic acid increases TLR and functional chemokine expression while reducing dentin formation in in vitro differentiated human odontoblasts. *J Immunol* **176**: 2880–7.

Estrela C, Bammann LL, Estrela CR, Silva RS, Pecora JD (2000) Antimicrobial and chemical study of MTA, portland cement, calcium hydroxide paste, sealapex and dycal. *Braz Dent J* **11**: 3–9.

Faraco IM, Jr, Holland R (2001) Response of the pulp of dogs to capping with mineral trioxide aggregate or a calcium hydroxide cement. *Dent Traumatol* **17**: 163–6.

Ferrari G, Cusella-De Angelis G, Coletta M, et al. (1998) Muscle regeneration by bone marrow-derived myogenic progenitors. *Science* **279**: 1528–30.

Fitzgerald M (1979) Cellular mechanisms of dentinal bridge repair using 3H-thylidine. *J Dent Res* **58**: 2198–206.

Fitzgerald M, Chiego DJ, Jr, Heys DR (1990) Autoradiographic analysis of odontoblast replacement following pulp exposure in primate teeth. *Arch Oral Biol* **35**: 707–15.

Funteas UR, Wallace JA, Fochtman EW (2003) A comparative analysis of mineral trioxide aggregate and portland cement. *Aust Endod J* **29**: 43–4.

Garberoglio R, Brannstrom M (1976) Scanning electron microscopic investigation of human dentinal tubules. *Arch Oral Biol* **21**: 355–62.

Goldberg M, Smith AJ (2004) Cells and extracellular matrices of dentin and pulp: a biological basis for repair and tissue engineering. *Crit Rev Oral Biol Med* **15**: 13–27.

Gronthos S, Brahim J, Li W, et al. (2002) Stem cell properties of human dental pulp stem cells. *J Dent Res* **81**: 531–5.

Gronthos S, Mankani M, Brahim J, Robey PG, Shi S (2000) Postnatal human dental pulp stem cells (DPSCs) in vitro and in vivo. *Proc Natl Acad Sci USA* **97**: 13625–30.

Haskell EW, Stanley HR, Chellemi J, Stringfellow H (1978) Direct pulp capping treatment: a long-term follow-up. *J Am Dent Assoc* **97**: 607–12.

Hayashi Y (1982) Ultrastructure of initial calcification in wound healing following pulpotomy. *J Oral Pathol* **11**: 174–80.

Hoffman MM, Schour I (1940) Quantitative studies in the development of of the rat molar, I. The growth pattern of the primary and secondary dentin (from birth to 500 days of age). *Anat Rec* **78**: 238–52.

Holland R, de Souza V, Murata SS, et al. (2001) Healing process of dog dental pulp after pulpotomy and pulp covering with mineral trioxide aggregate or Portland cement. *Braz Dent J* **12**: 109–13.

Horsted P, El Attar K, Langeland K (1981) Capping of monkey pulps with dycal and a Ca-eugenol cement. *Oral Surg Oral Med Oral Pathol* **52**: 531–53.

Huang GT, Sonoyama W, Liu Y, Liu H, Wang S, Shi S (2008) The hidden treasure in apical papilla: the potential role in pulp/dentin regeneration and bioroot engineering. *J Endod* **34**: 645–51.

Ikeda E, Morita R, Nakao K,, et al. (2009) Fully functional bioengineered tooth replacement as an organ replacement therapy. *Proc Natl Acad Sci USA* **106**: 13475–80.

Jepsen S, Albers HK, Fleiner B, Tucker M, Rueger D (1997) Recombinant human osteogenic protein-1 induces dentin formation: an experimental study in miniature swine. *J Endod* **23**: 378–82.

Jones S, Boyde A (1984) In: Linde A, ed. *Dentin and Dentinigenesis*. CRC Press, Boca Raton, pp. 81–134.

Joseph BK, Savage NW, Daley TJ, Young WG (1996) In situ hybridization evidence for a paracrine/autocrine role for insulin-like growth factor-I in tooth development. *Growth Factors* **13**: 11–7.

Kagayama M, Akita H, Sasano Y (1995) Immunohistochemical localization of connexin 43 in the developing tooth germ of rat. *Anat Embryol (Berl)* **191**: 561–8.

Kakehashi S, Stanley HR, Fitzgerald RJ (1965) The effects of surgical exposures of dental pulps in germ-free and conventional laboratory rats. *Oral Surg Oral Med Oral Pathol* **20**: 340–9.

Katchburian E, Severs NJ (1982) Membranes of matrix-vesicles in early developing dentine. A freeze fracture study. *Cell Biol Int Rep* **6**: 941–50.

Krebsbach PH, Kuznetsov SA, Satomura K, Emmons RV, Rowe DW, Robey PG (1997) Bone formation in vivo: comparison of osteogenesis by transplanted mouse and human marrow stromal fibroblasts. *Transplantation* **63**: 1059–69.

Lesot H, Osman M, Ruch JV (1981) Immunofluorescent localization of collagens, fibronectin, and laminin during terminal differentiation of odontoblasts. *Dev Biol* **82**: 371–81.

Lovschall H, Fejerskov O, Flyvbjerg A (2001) Pulp-capping with recombinant human insulin-like growth factor I (RHIGF-I) in rat molars. *Adv Dent Res* **15**: 108–12.

Lovschall H, Mitsiadis TA, Poulsen K, Jensen KH, Kjeldsen AL (2007) Coexpression of notch3 and RGS5 in the pericyte-vascular smooth muscle cell axis in response to pulp injury. *Int J Dev Biol* **51**: 715–21.

Magloire H, Bouvier M, Joffre A (1992) Odontoblast response under carious lesions. *Proc Finn Dent Soc* **88** (Suppl 1): 257–74.

Magloire H, Couble ML, Romeas A, Bleicher F (2004) Odontoblast primary cilia: facts and hypotheses. *Cell Biol Int* **28**: 93–9.

Maniatopoulos C, Smith DC (1983) A scanning electron microscopic study of the odontoblast process in human coronal dentine. *Arch Oral Biol* **28**: 701–10.

McLachlan JL, Sloan AJ, Smith AJ, Landini G, Cooper PR (2004) S100 and cytokine expression in caries. *Infect Immun* **72**: 4102–8.

McLachlan JL, Smith AJ, Bujalska IJ, Cooper PR (2005) Gene expression profiling of pulpal tissue reveals the molecular complexity of dental caries. *Biochim Biophys Acta* **1741**: 271–81.

Mitsiadis TA, Rahiotis C (2004) Parallels between tooth development and repair: conserved molecular mechanisms following carious and dental injury. *J Dent Res* **83**: 896–902.

Miura M, Gronthos S, Zhao M, et al. (2003) Shed: stem cells from human exfoliated deciduous teeth. *Proc Natl Acad Sci USA* **100**: 5807–12.

Mjor IA (2002) Pulp-dentin biology in restorative dentistry. Part 7: The exposed pulp. *Quintessence Int* **33**: 113–35.

Mjor IA, Dahl E, Cox CF (1991) Healing of pulp exposures: an ultrastructural study. *J Oral Pathol Med* **20**: 496–501.

Murray PE, Hafez AA, Smith AJ, Windsor LJ, Cox CF (2003) Histomorphogenetic analysis of odontoblast-like cell numbers and dentin bridge secretory activity following pulp exposure. *Int Endod J* **36** (2): 106–16.

Murray PE, Hafez AA, Windsor LJ, Smith AJ, Cox CF (2002) Comparison of pulp responses following restoration of exposed and non-exposed cavities. *J Dent* **30**: 213–22.

Nair PN, Duncan HF, Pitt Ford TR, Luder HU (2007) Histological, ultrastructural and quantitative investigations on the response of healthy human pulps to experimental capping with mineral trioxide aggregate: a randomized controlled trial. *Int Endod J* **41** (2): 128–50.

Nair PN, Duncan HF, Pitt Ford TR, Luder HU (2008) Histological, ultrastructural and quantitative investigations on the response of healthy human pulps to experimental capping with mineral trioxide aggregate: a randomized controlled trial. *Int Endod J* **41**: 128–50.

Nakashima M (1994) Induction of dentin formation on canine amputated pulp by recombinant human bone morphogenetic proteins (BMP)-2 and -4. *J Dent Res* **73**: 1515–22.

Nanci A (2003) Dentin–pulp complex. In: Nanci A, ed. *Ten Cate's Oral Histology: Development Structure, and Function*, 6th edn. Mosby, Saint Louis, pp. 192–239.

Ning W, Song R, Li C, et al. (2002) TGF-beta1 stimulates HO-1 via the p38 mitogen-activated protein kinase in a549 pulmonary epithelial cells. *Am J Physiol Lung Cell Mol Physiol* **283**: L1094–102.

Okumura R, Shima K, Muramatsu T, et al. (2005) The odontoblast as a sensory receptor cell? The expression of trpv1 (vr-1) channels. *Arch Histol Cytol* **68**: 251–7.

Osman A, Ruch JV (1976) Topographic distribution of mitosis in the lower incisor and 1st molar in the mouse embryo. *J Biol Buccale* **4**: 331–48.

Pashley DH (2002) Pulpodentin complex. In: Hargreaves KM, Goodis HE, eds *Seltzer and Bender's Dental Pulp*. Quintessence, Illinois, pp. 63–93.

Paula-Silva FW, Ghosh A, Silva LA, Kapila YL (2009) TNF-alpha promotes an odontoblastic phenotype in dental pulp cells. *J Dent Res* **88**: 339–44.

Pittenger MF, Mackay AM, Beck SC, et al. (1999) Multilineage potential of adult human mesenchymal stem cells. *Science* **284**: 143–7.

Pitt Ford TR, Torabinejad M, Abedi H, Bakland LK, Kariyawasam SP (1996) Using mineral trioxide aggregate as pulp capping material. *J Am Dent Assoc* **127**.

Ruch JV (1998) Odontoblast commitment and differentiation. *Biochem Cell Biol* **76**: 923–38.

Ruch JV, Lesot H, Begue-Kirn C (1995) Odontoblast differentiation. *Int J Dev Biol* **39**: 51–68.

Rutherford RB, Spangberg L, Tucker M, Rueger D, Charette M (1994) The time-course of the induction of reparative dentine formation in monkeys by recombinant human osteogenic protein-1. *Arch Oral Biol* **39**: 833–8.

Rutherford RB, Wahle J, Tucker M, Rueger D, Charette M (1993) Induction of reparative dentine formation in monkeys by recombinant human osteogenic protein-1. *Arch Oral Biol* **38**: 571–6.

Saidon J, He J, Zhu Q, Safavi K, Spangberg LS (2003) Cell and tissue reactions to mineral trioxide aggregate and portland cement. *Oral Surg Oral Med Oral Pathol Oral Radiol Endod* **95**: 483–9.

Sasaki T, Nakagawa K, Higashi S (1982) Ultrastructure of odontoblasts in kitten tooth germs as revealed by freeze-fracture. *Arch Oral Biol* **27**: 897–904.

Schour I, Poncher HG (1937) The rate of apposition of human enamel and dentin as measured by the effects of acute fluorosis. *Am J Dis Child* **54**: 757–76.

Schroder U (1985) Effects of calcium hydroxide-containing pulp-capping agents on pulp cell migration, proliferation, and differentiation. *J Dent Res* **64** (Spec No): 541–8.

Schroder U, Granath LE (1972) Scanning electron microscopy of hard tissue barrier following experimental pulpotomy of intact human teeth and capping with calcium hydroxide. *Odontol Rev* **23**: 211–20.

Seltzer S, Bender I (2002) *The Dental Pulp*, 5th edn. Quintessence, Chicago.

Shi S, Gronthos S (2003) Perivascular niche of postnatal mesenchymal stem cells in human bone marrow and dental pulp. *J Bone Miner Res* **18**: 696–704.

Sigal MJ, Aubin JE, Ten Cate AR (1985) An immunocytochemical study of the human odontoblast process using antibodies against tubulin, actin, and vimentin. *J Dent Res* **64**: 1348–55.

Sigal MJ, Aubin JE, Ten Cate AR, Pitaru S (1984) The odontoblast process extends to the dentinoenamel junction: an immunocytochemical study of rat dentine. *J Histochem Cytochem* **32**: 872–7.

Simon S, Cooper P, Smith A, Picard B, Ifi CN, Berdal A (2008) Evaluation of a new laboratory model for pulp healing: preliminary study. *Int Endod J* **41**: 781–90.

Simon S, Smith AJ, Berdal A, Lumley PJ, Cooper PR (2010) The map kinase pathway is involved in odontoblast stimulation via p38 phosphorylation. *J Endod* **36**: 256–9.

Simon S, Smith AJ, Lumley PJ, et al. (2009) Molecular characterisation of young and mature odontoblasts. *Bone* **45**: 693–703.

Smith AJ (2002) Dentin formation and repair. In: Hargreaves KM Goodis HA, eds *Seltzer and Bender's Dental Pulp*. Quintessence, Illinois, pp. 41–62.

Smith AJ (2002) Pulpal responses to caries and dental repair. *Caries Res* **36**: 223–32.

Smith AJ (2003) Vitality of the dentin-pulp complex in health and disease: growth factors as key mediators. *J Dent Educ* **67**: 678–89.

Smith AJ, Lesot H (2001) Induction and regulation of crown dentinogenesis: embryonic events as a template for dental tissue repair? *Crit Rev Oral Biol Med* **12**: 425–37.

Smith AJ, Lumley PJ, Tomson PL, Cooper PR (2008) Dental regeneration and materials: a partnership. *Clin Oral Investig* **12**: 103–8.

Smith AJ, Matthews JB, Hall RC (1998) Transforming growth factor-beta1 (TGF-beta1) in dentine matrix. Ligand activation and receptor expression. *Eur J Oral Sci* **106** (Suppl 1): 179–84.

Smith AJ, Tobias RS, Cassidy N, Begue-Kirn C, Ruch JV, Lesot H (1995) Influence of substrate nature and immobilization of implanted dentin matrix components during induction of reparative dentinogenesis. *Connect Tissue Res* **32**: 291–6.

Sonoyama W, Liu Y, Yamaza T, et al. (2008) Characterization of the apical papilla and its residing stem cells from human immature permanent teeth: a pilot study. *J Endod* **34**: 166–71.

Tarim B, Hafez AA, Suzuki SH, Suzuki S, Cox CF (1998) Biocompatibility of optibond and XR-bond adhesive systems in nonhuman primate teeth. *Int J Periodontics Restorative Dent* **18**: 86–99.

Thesleff I, Barrach HJ, Foidart JM, Vaheri A, Pratt RM, Martin GR (1981) Changes in the distribution of type IV collagen, laminin, proteoglycan, and fibronectin during mouse tooth development. *Dev Biol* **81**: 182–92.

Thesleff I, Vaahtokari A (1992) The role of growth factors in determination and differentiation of the odontoblastic cell lineage. *Proc Finn Dent Soc* **88** (Suppl 1): 357–68.

Thomas HF, Carella P (1983) A scanning electron microscope study of dentinal tubules from un-erupted human teeth. *Arch Oral Biol* **28**: 1125–30.

Thomas HF, Carella P (1984) Correlation of scanning and transmission electron microscopy of human dentinal tubules. *Arch Oral Biol* **29**: 641–6.

Torabinejad M, Chivian N (1999) Clinical applications of mineral trioxide aggregate. *J Endod* **25**: 197–205.

Tziafas D, Smith AJ, Lesot H (2000) Designing new treatment strategies in vital pulp therapy. *J Dent* **28**: 77–92.

Unterbrink A, O'Sullivan M, Chen S, MacDougall M (2002) TGF beta-1 downregulates DMP-1 and DSPP in odontoblasts. *Connect Tissue Res* **43**: 354–8.

Vainio S, Karavanova I, Jowett A, Thesleff I (1993) Identification of BMP-4 as a signal mediating secondary induction between epithelial and mesenchymal tissues during early tooth development. *Cell* **75**: 45–58.

Ward J (2002) Vital pulp therapy in cariously exposed permanent teeth and its limitations. *Aust Endod J* **28**: 29–37.

Wennberg A, Mjor IA, Heide S (1982) Rate of formation of regular and irregular secondary dentin in monkey teeth. *Oral Surg Oral Med Oral Pathol* **54**: 232–7.

Yamamura T (1985) Differentiation of pulpal cells and inductive influences of various matrices with reference to pulpal wound healing. *J Dent Res* **64 (Spec No)**: 530–40.

Zhang CZ, Li H, Young WG, Bartold PM, Chen C, Waters MJ (1997) Evidence for a local action of growth hormone in embryonic tooth development in the rat. *Growth Factors* **14**: 131–43.

Zhao Q, Chen N, Wang WM, Lu J, Dai BB (2004) Effect of transforming growth factor-beta on activity of connective tissue growth factor gene promoter in mouse NIH/3T3 fibroblasts. *Acta Pharmacol Sin* **25**: 485–9.

Ziskin DE, Applebaum E, Gorlin RJ (1949) The effect of hypophysectoy upon the permanent dentition of rhesus monkey. *J Dent Res* **28**: 48–54.

14 Dermal Wound Healing and Burn Wounds

Anthony Papp

Medical Director BC Professional Firefighters' Burn, Plastic and Trauma Unit, Vancouver General Hospital, Vancouver, BC, Canada

INTRODUCTION

In the United States 2.2 million people are burned every year, leading to 60,000 hospital admissions and 5,500 deaths. The burn-related death rate has steadily decreased since 1975 with both increased survival rates but also with the decrease of absolute number of patients being burned. The most important prognostic factors in burn morbidity and mortality are the total body surface area burned (TBSA), age of patient and the presence of inhalation injury. Increased survival is mainly due to the following factors: early and more aggressive surgical management of deep burns, advances in preventing and treating infections and improved nutrition. The LA_{50} for patients 2–40 years old is relatively constant at 70–90%, but is 60% for patients less than 2 years and 30% for patients more than 70 years. Infection and its complications are still the leading causes of burn mortality.

BURN INJURY

Thermal energy or heat is a manifestation of random molecular kinetic energy. This energy is transferred from high-energy molecules to those of lower energy during contact via a process referred to as conduction. The effect of heat on a cell depends on the temperature to which the cell is heated as well as the time period for which the temperature is sustained. Protein denaturation begins at temperatures 40–44°C when cell functions get weaker, leading to increased intracellular sodium concentrations and cellular swelling. If the contact time is long enough, ongoing protein destruction leads to protein coagulation and eventually to cell death. As a part of the damage process, oxygen-free radicals are produced, promoting further cell membrane damage.

The extent of tissue destruction caused by heat depends not only on the temperature and the exposure time, but also on the thickness of skin, age of patient and vascularity of the injured area. Injury to thinner skin (e.g. thinner dermis) leads to deeper tissue injury more easily than injury to areas with thick skin.

Thermal injury causes graded tissue injury radiating from the point of injury. Following burn injury, necrosis occurs at the centre of the injury and becomes progressively less severe at the periphery, both on the lateral and deep edges of the burn. Jackson (1953) described the

Oral Wound Healing: Cell Biology and Clinical Management, First Edition. Edited by Hannu Larjava.

three zones of burn injury, which still remains our conceptual understanding of the burn wound. The zone of coagulation is the centre of the burn injury where cells are killed immediately and the surrounding extracellular matrix proteins are denaturated. Circulation ceases immediately. Surrounding this is the zone of stasis where the heat-injured tissue is characterized by decreased tissue perfusion due to vascular stasis and microvascular injury. This tissue is at risk, but is potentially salvageable and is therefore of great interest in burn wound research. The zone of stasis continues to be metabolically active for 24–48 hours. Eventually circulation ceases and part of this area dies. Impaired blood flow is due to platelet microthrombi formation, neutrophil adherence to vessel walls, fibrin deposition, endothelial swelling and vasoconstriction (Boykin et al. 1979).

Impairment of blood flow ensues within a couple of hours in more severely burned areas and is delayed for up to 16–24 hours in less severe regions (Zawacki 1974). The goal of both resuscitation and wound care is to preserve tissue perfusion and prevent irreversible damage to the tissue. The risk for conversion to non-viable tissue increases with the presence of hypoperfusion, edema, ischemia, dessication and infection. The zone of hyperemia surrounds the zone of stasis and is characterized by viable cells and vasodilation due to vasoactive mediators produced in the course of inflammatory response showing no apparent structural damage to the dermis. The redness caused by the vasodilation in the periphery of the burn wound is often mistakenly diagnosed as infection or cellulitis.

As mentioned, limiting the progression of injury in the zone of stasis is of great academic and clinical interest. For centuries, rapid cooling of the burn remains the gold standard for limiting tissue injury after burning. The optimal temperature and time of cooling remains unclear, but recent literature (Cuttle et al. 2008; Rajan et al. 2009) has showed best results with a water temperature of 15°C for 20 minutes being efficient starting as long as 60 minutes post injury.

Due to the ongoing tissue destruction in the zone of stasis burn depth progresses over the first 48 hours post injury. This is due to additive effects of inadequate tissue perfusion, free radical damage and systemic alterations in the cytokine milieu of burn patients, leading to protein denaturation and necrosis (Singh et al. 2007).

SKIN ANATOMY

Epidermis

Epidermis is the avascular outer layer of skin (Fig. 14.1). The total thickness of human epidermis varies from 50 to 120 μm (Meyer et al. 1978). In the five layers of epidermis cells undergo division and differentiation during their lifetime. Cell division takes place in the deepest part of the epidermis called the basal cell layer, while the differentiation occurs in the overlaying layers. The stratum spinosum is the layer above the basal cell layer consisting of keratinocytes responsible for the production of fibrous keratin protein, e.g. keratinization. Superficially to this is the stratum granulosum, a four- to five-cell-layered structure where cells gradually lose their form, become flattened and finally the nucleus and intracytoplasmic organelles degenerate. In the next layer, stratum lucidum, the cell is prepared to move into its final sublayer with the addition of melanin granules. This layer is easily seen only in thick skin. The stratum corneum is constructed of dead cells and it forms the outermost layer of skin (Kessel 1998). This part represents about 25% of the total thickness of the epidermis with 15–100 layers of large, flat cells filled with keratin. This provides a semipermeable

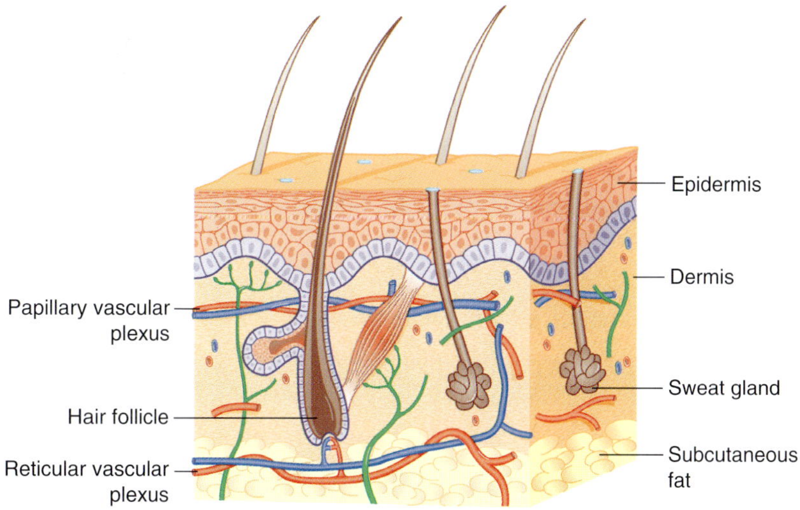

Fig. 14.1 Skin anatomy.

physical barrier against the outer environment. Epidermis also consists of melanocytes in the basal cell layer producing pigment and protecting skin from the ultraviolet radiation, Langerhans cells as a part of the immunologic defense function of skin and Merkel cells which are believed to be involved with the sensation of fine touch.

Dermis

The interface between the epidermis and dermis is called the basement membrane. Dermal thickness varies from <1 mm on the eyelids to >5 mm on the posterior trunk (Heimbach et al. 1992). It is mainly composed of collagen and elastic fibers, glycosaminoglycan and tissue water. The cells in the dermis are mostly fibroblasts, but also macrophages, mast cells, platelets and endothelial cells are found. Collagen and elastin represent approximately 75% and 4% of the dry weight of the dermis, respectively.

In the superficial papillary dermis the collagen fibers are fine structured and loosely packed, while in the deeper reticular dermis they are thick and densely arranged (Pasyk et al. 1989). Papillary dermis contains anchoring rete pegs against the epidermal rete ridges and is the most biologically active part of the dermis. The reticular dermis is responsible for durability and anchoring of the skin appendages. Elastic fibers are mainly located in the reticular dermis.

Skin vasculature

Blood circulation through skin serves two functions: nutrition of the skin and regulation of the body temperature by conduction of heat from the internal structures of the body to the skin, where it is lost by exchange with the external environment. The cutaneous circulation comprises two types of vessels: the nutritive vessels and the vascular structures concerned with heat regulation. The latter includes an extensive subcutaneous venous plexus which can hold large quantities of blood and arteriovenous anastomoses. At ordinary skin temperature the amount of blood flowing through the skin is about 10 times higher than is required for the nutrition of the skin. There are two main vascular plexuses in the dermis. The superficial papillary dermis is highly vascularized with 60–75 capillary loops/mm^2 (Hopewell 1990). The capillary density is 12–14 times that of the deeply situated reticular dermis. The diameter of the blood vessels in the papillary region is typically 10–20 μm and about 50 μm in the reticular dermis. In the papillary dermis the endothelial cells of the arterioles are covered typically with one or two layers of smooth muscle whereas there are four to five layers in the reticular dermis.

Skin appendages and subcutaneous fat

In humans, the skin appendages include hair, nails and several types of secretory glands. Together, the skin and the skin appendages are known as the integumentary system of the body. An adult human has 1.6–4.0 million sweat glands. Most of them are eccrine sweat glands which are found all over the surface of the body, being most numerous on the palms and soles. They originate deep in the dermis and connect to the surface of the skin by a coiled duct. The cells in the base of the gland secrete sweat. The apocrine sweat glands are less numerous and are located around the areolae, genital area and armpits. They are also situated deep in the dermis, but open into hair follicles. Their function remains unclear.

Sebaceous glands are most numerous in the face, scalp and upper trunk and are absent from the palms and soles. Most of them open into hair follicles also. The secreted substance called sebum helps to keep the hair and skin from drying.

The subcutaneous layer lies between the dermis and the underlying muscle fascia covering muscle. It contains groups of adipocytes which are separated by fibrous septa. It serves three functions: to insulate the body from cold, to absorb trauma and to act as storage for the body's reserve fuel.

BURN DEPTH

Burn depth has historically been classified into three categories since 1607 by Hildanus. This is still mostly accurate even though today the categorization is more detailed (Fig. 14.2).

Histology has been considered the gold standard for burn depth determination, although it has several concerns (Heimbach et al. 1992). The timing of the biopsy is controversial as burn depth is known to progress during the first few days (Converse et al. 1965; Hinshaw 1968; Zawacki 1974; Kaufman et al. 1990; Brans et al. 1994; Nanney et al. 1996; Schomacker et al. 1997; Watts et al. 2001). Burn sites might not be uniform in depth, making the site of the biopsy questionable. Biopsy leaves a permanent scar, is expensive and time consuming and requires an experienced histopathologist to make the analysis. Also, the subjective nature of the evaluation is troublesome.

The only reliable criterion differentiating a partial thickness burn from a full thickness burn is the presence or absence of surviving viable epithelial elements in the injured area (Hinshaw 1968). The nature of the skin appendages can be the most informative aspect to the observer. In addition, it is very important to evaluate blood vessels and their contents in determining the viability of burned tissue (Kahn et al. 1979; Watts et al. 2001; Papp et al. 2004). Blood vessels are found in every histological section from skin, but follicles are few. The identification of the depth of vascular or follicular necrosis is easiest to achieve and may be of more clinical relevance than other elements (Singer et al. 2000).

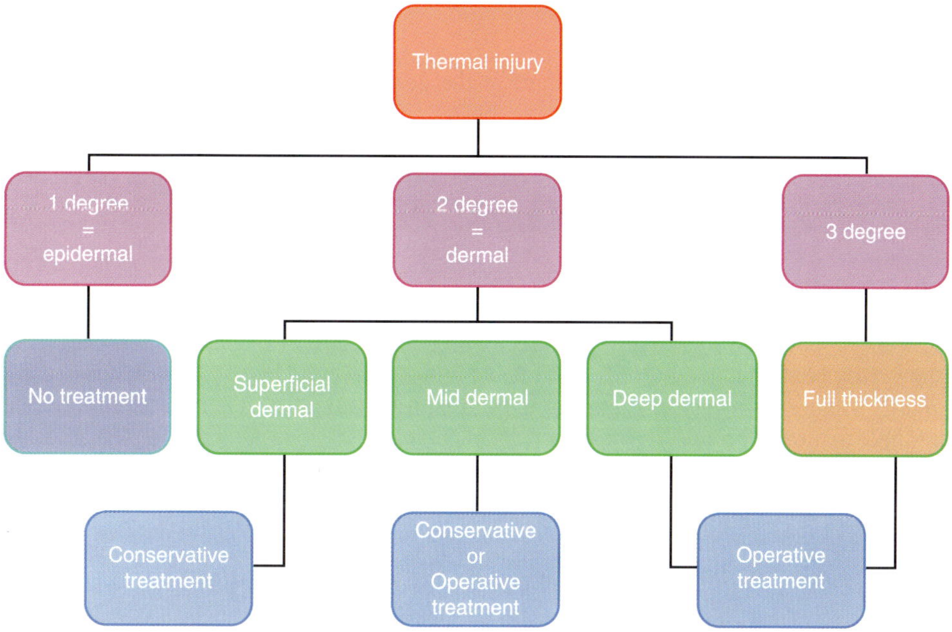

Fig. 14.2 Burn depth and treatment classification.

There is a progression of burn depth until 48–72 hours post injury. Its basis seems to be the development of edema and vascular occlusion due to vasoconstriction and thrombosis (Papp et al. 2004). The most superficial burns don't seem to progress in depth. Also, the development of microvascular injury in the dermis involves the pro-inflammatory cytokines IL-1, TNF-alpha and IL-6 and may result from reactive oxygen metabolites generated by neutrophils accumulating in the burn wound (Ravage et al. 1998). Additionally, apoptosis seems to play a role in deep partial thickness burn depth progression (Gravante et al. 2007). Due to this 'conversion' of burn depth, it is crucial to repeat the clinical assessment of burn depth to make the final burn depth determination on day 2–3 post burn. This is also the time when treatment plans should be determined, conservative vs. operative treatment.

Epidermal burns

Burns where the destruction of tissue is limited to the epidermis are called epidermal or first degree burns. The injury is similar to a sun burn. These burns are very benign with clinical findings of erythema and epidermal sloughing after 1–4 days. These burns heal without treatment in a few days with no scarring by regenerating keratinocytes. The systemic effects of these burns are non-existent and therefore these burns are not actually included in the TBSA burned estimation.

Dermal burns

Dermal burns, the so-called second degree burns, are complicated as there are actually three degrees of second degree burns which all have different healing capacities, treatment modalities and risks for scarring.

Superficial dermal burns

These burns involve the superficial third of the dermis down into the papillary vascular plexus. Clinical signs show typically late blistering and following blister removal a red, shiny, moist and painful wound bed with a good capillary refill. As most dermal elements and skin appendages are spared, the healing capacity is excellent. These burns heal conservatively with proper wound care within 14 days without scarring.

Mid-dermal burns

Tissue destruction in these burns extends to the middle third of the dermis. Clinical signs show early blistering and initially painful and moist red wound beds. Spontaneous healing time is usually 3–4 weeks. These are the most difficult ones to diagnose and they have multiple treatment options: conservative management until 3 weeks with late skin grafting to unhealed areas, early debridement and wound coverage with allograft, xenograft, amniotic membrane, artificial skin or a wound dressing or early excision and skin grafting. Many burn centers prefer early debridements and biological dressings to shorten the time for epithelialization and therefore minimize scarring.

Deep dermal burns

Deep dermal burns extend down to the reticular dermis located in the deepest third of the dermis. These are often characterized by immediate blistering and spontaneous early blister deroofing and the wound surface appears mottled pink and white. The wound does not usually blanch under pressure and is less painful than more superficial burns. Due to the destruction of most dermal elements, spontaneous healing capacity is poor, prolonging the healing time up to 6 weeks or even longer. Therefore these burns are considered 'deep burns' and should be treated with early excision and skin grafting.

Full thickness burns

Deep third degree burns extend through all the layers of the skin down to the subcutaneous fat or deeper. They are charred, insensate, dry and leathery, may be of different colors, have visible thrombosed vessels and are usually painless with no capillary refill (Fig. 14.3). Some of these burns may be red in color and may easily be confused with a more superficial injury. The distinctive difference is that these burns do not blanch under pressure. The spontaneous healing capacity is non-existent and these burns should be treated with early excision and skin grafting procedures.

WOUND HEALING

Deep full thickness burns require surgery for healing. The more superficial ones heal through epithelialization. Sources of epithelial cells are the skin appendages, such as hair follicles, sweat and sebaceous glands (Fig. 14.1) and the non-burned skin surrounding the burn. The lining of these appendages has keratinocytes that migrate towards the wound bed forming

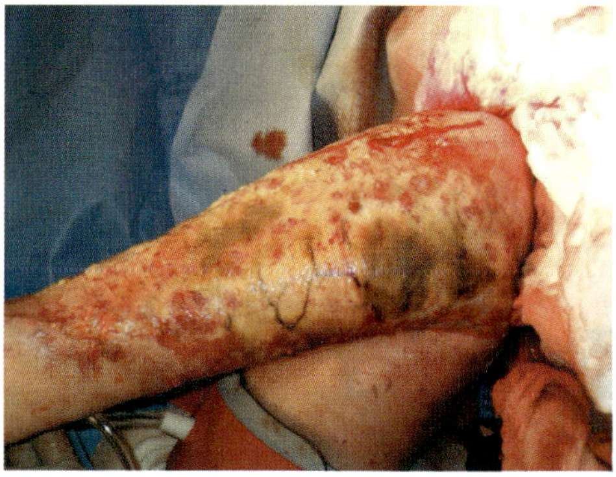

Fig. 14.3 Deep full thickness burn with visible thrombosed vessels.

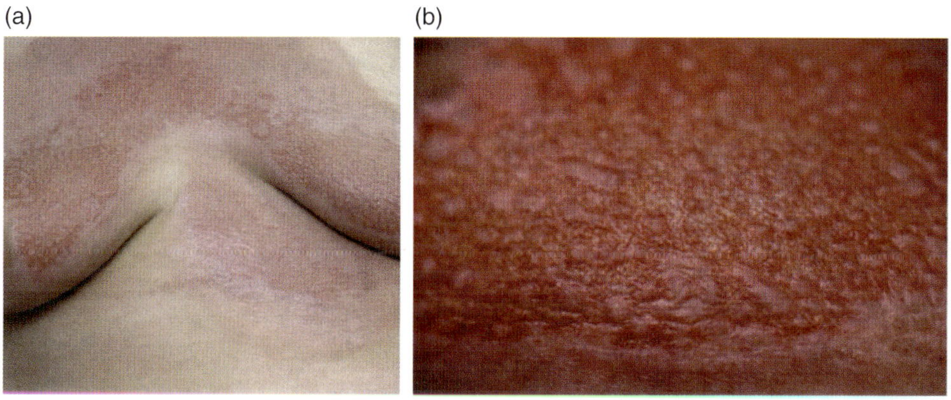

Fig. 14.4 **(a)** Partially healed superficial burn on a chest. **(b)** White epithelial buds within the burn showing partial epithelialization.

epithelial buds (Fig. 14.4a and b), which eventually cover the wound surface. The deeper the burn is, the fewer skin appendages remain viable, thus prolonging the healing time and increasing the risk for both hypertrophic scarring and scar contractures. The epithelialization process is very complex including desmosomes, hemidesmosomes, integrins, keratins, growth factors, cytokines and chemokines, eicosanoins, oxygen tension and matrix metalloproteinases (Raja et al. 2007).

The wound healing in burn wounds differs from other wounds. Different wounds have significant levels of TNF-alpha, IL-6, monocyte chemoattractant protein (MCA)-1 and keratinocyte-derived chemokine (CK). However, the concentrations of KC and IL-6 have been found to be 3 and 50-fold higher in burn wounds, respectively (Schwacha et al. 2010). The immediate appearance of platelets in wounds and the ability of platelets to release growth factors suggest that platelets are an important trigger of the tissue repair process. However, even though platelets may influence wound inflammation, they do not significantly affect the proliferative aspects of repair, including wound closure, angiogenesis and collagen synthesis (Szpaderska et al. 2003).

The role of myofibroblasts in burn wound healing is controversial. Adding myofibroblasts to a healing wound has resulted in disorganized epidermis formation and reduction of the expression of basement membrane constituents (Moulin et al. 2000). New evidence shows that fibroblasts and myofibroblasts can be recruited both locally and from bone marrow. The bone marrow-derived myofibroblasts contribute to not only promotion of granulation tissue formation but also enhancement of the dermal–epidermal interaction after thermal injury, being located beneath the regenerating epidermis (Yamaguchi 2007). As many as half of the fibroblast population and a small percentage of keratinocytes are bone marrow derived, showing that bone marrow plays an important role in providing not only cells for inflammation but also dermal and epidermal cells during burn wound healing (Rea et al. 2009). Topical fibroblast growth factor has shown beneficial effects in shortening the healing time for dermal burns (Akita et al. 2008).

TREATMENT

As a general rule, superficial burns are treated conservatively and deep burns surgically. The goal is to have the burn wound epithelialized within 3 weeks to minimize scarring. The risk of creating a hypertrophic scar is 10–15% in burns that heal in 14 days but up to 80% in those that take longer than 3–weeks to heal.

Conservative treatment

Conservative treatment of burn wounds has several objectives: to support epithelialization, obtain and maintain optimal moisture balance in the wound bed, prevent infection and protect from sheering forces. Having a dressing on a wound also has a debriding effect.

Previously, silver sulfadiazine cream was the most commonly used way to treat a burn wound. Silver has antimicrobial properties that reduce the risk of infection. A 5-mm layer of cream is laid on the wound after debriding it. The cream is then covered with an absorbent dressing. Ideally the cream is replaced every 12 hours, but most commonly this is done once a day.

Currently different modern silver-containing wound dressings are most commonly used to treat partial thickness burns. There are multiple different dressing types including hydrocolloids, foams, hydrofibers, polyethylene mesh and polyester dressings. All dressings have silver as $Ag^{\pm}$, the ionic, metallic form of silver that kills bacteria. Some dressings contain silver as nanocrystalline particles with $Ag^{\pm}$ and Ag^{0}, the non-charged silver ion which has anti-inflammatory properties (Nadworny et al. 2008). As every dressing change drops the temperature of the wound bed, thus compromising healing, and is a mechanical trauma for the wound bed the modern wound dressings enable infrequent dressing changes providing optimal circumstances for wound healing (Fig. 14.5a and b).

The use of biological dressings is considered conservative treatment even though this often requires some degree of wound debridement first. Biological dressings entail allograft (cadaveric skin), xenograft (most often pig skin), artificial skins and amniotic membrane. The principle is to apply the biological dressing on the wound to which it will adhere when the wound bed is viable and non-infected. As re-epithelialization occurs the

(a) (b)

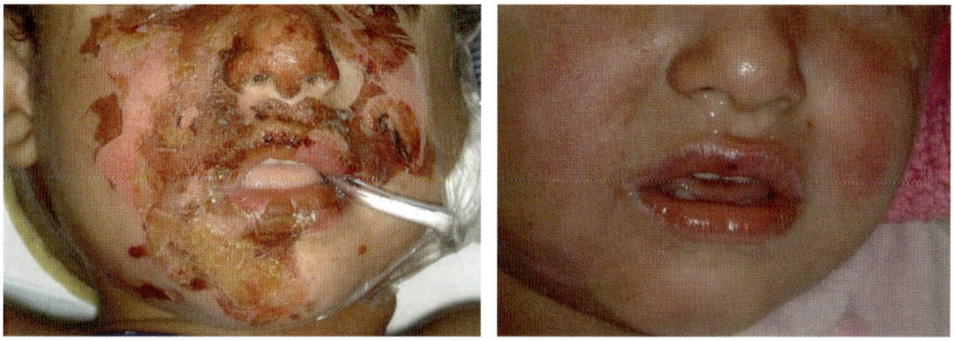

Fig. 14.5a and b Partial thickness facial burn healed with nanocrystalline silver dressings in 2 weeks.

dressing will start to lift off, typically within 10–14 days. The downsides of using biological dressings are the high costs of the products and the possible need to use the operating room and sedation for the application. The benefits include non-existing wound care and faster epithelialization times with subsequently less scarring.

Surgical treatment

Surgical excision and reconstruction procedures should be planned as soon as the diagnosis of a deep burn is done. In experienced hands this can be carried out as early as on the day of injury, but usually 48–72 hours post injury to allow burn depth progression to finish its course. Surgery includes excising the burned tissue with hand-held dermatomes such as the Cobbett, Weck, Humby, Cambell, Watson, Cambell or Goulian knives down to healthy tissue.

The depth of excision is not always easy to assess as bleeding can be evident in non-healthy tissue also. Tangential excision means excising burned tissue tangentially until the healthy tissue plane is obtained. When performing a fascial excision an incision is done with a regular blade around the burn down to the fascia and dissection is carried out at the level of the fascia. The former gives a better esthetic outcome, but the extent of the excision per surgery is limited to 30–40% of TBSA burned due to bleeding, whereas up to 80% TBSA can be excised fascially in one operation.

As soon as the correct healthy tissue plane has been reached hemostasis is obtained with saline with epinephrine compresses and cautery. Following this the defect is reconstructed. The reconstructive options are: split or full thickness skin grafts harvested from the non-burned areas of the patient, artificial skin, local or distant skin flaps or free flaps. Split thickness skin grafts are used over exposed soft tissue, such as dermis, fascia or muscle. Full thickness grafts are used over areas that are prone to contract, specifically palms and often around the eyes. Flaps are used when a bone, tendon, joint or vessels are exposed.

Split thickness skin grafts can be used as meshed or non-meshed (sheet grafts) (Fig. 14.6a and b). Meshing results in a net-like skin graft which allows drainage (seroma or blood) from the wound bed to be absorbed into the absorbent dressing. The meshing pattern is visible for the rest of the patient's life as the graft contains dermis but the holes fill in with

(a) (b)

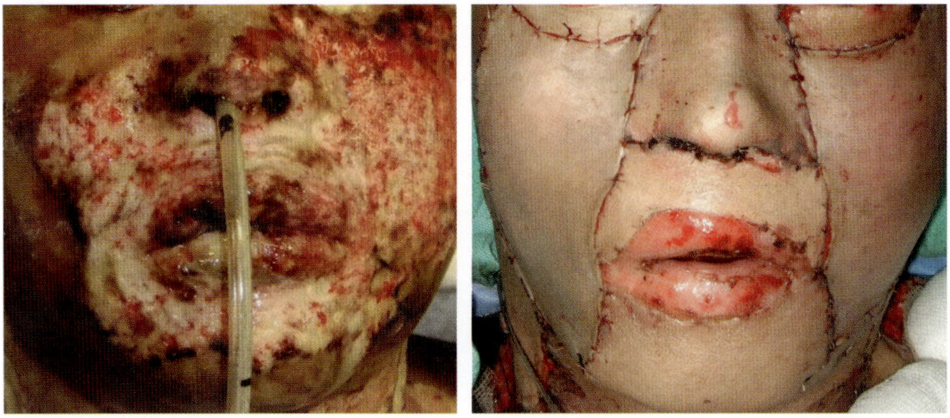

Fig. 14.6a and b Full thickness facial burn reconstructed with thick split thickness sheet grafts.

epidermis only. Sheet grafts are always used on faces and hands due to better cosmetic appearance. They can be used anywhere in the body, but they have a bigger failure rate due to the likelihood of fluid collection under the graft postoperatively.

SPECIAL FEATURES IN PERIORAL BURNS

Facial burns are always devastating as the face has such an integral role in daily communication and emotions. Deep burns always leave visible scars which may have a detrimental effect on daily living. Therefore it is of utmost importance to treat deep facial burns in a burn centre, where the greatest knowledge in treating these burns exists.

Facial burns are common in scalding accidents, explosion and electrical injuries and flame burns where the patient's shirt catches fire. In small children putting an electrical wire in the mouth is a common way or receiving intraoral or commissural burns.

Basic burn surgery principles apply when treating facial burns. However, these burns have special characteristics, including the high risk for contractions leading to eyelid ectropium, microstomia and nostril deformities. Therefore thick non-meshed split thickness or full thickness grafts are preferred (Fig. 14.6a and b). Immediately after burn excision it is often advisable to reconstruct the skin defect initially with allograft to 'test' the adequacy of the level of excision prior to final reconstruction.

Superficial intraoral burns are very common with scalding injuries from hot drinks. The healing potential of these minor burns on the oral mucosa is good and they seldom require any treatment. However, deep intraoral burns are extremely rare and challenging to treat. Most deep oral burns involve the oral commissure (Fig. 14.7). This is difficult to treat due to the three-dimensional complex structure involving the lip, muscle and intraoral mucosa in a triangular shape with various tension forces. Despite aggressive and well-planned surgery, these still often result in commissural contractures. These contractures may be treated with aggressive physiotherapy and splinting in the early phase, but severe cases require surgery, such as scar releases, z-plasties and oral mucosal flaps (Fig. 14.8a and b).

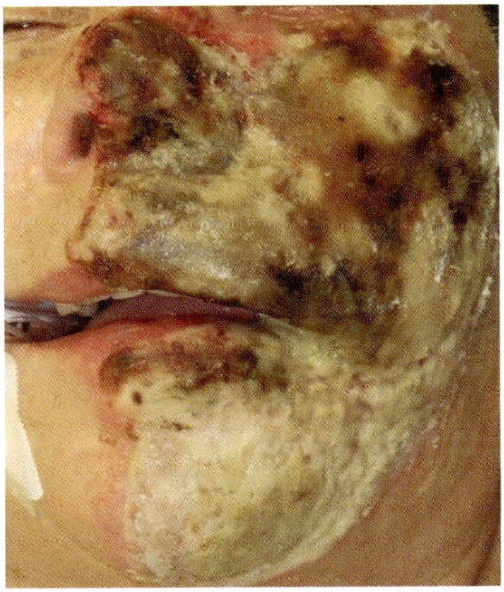

Fig. 14.7 Full thickness contact burn on face involving the left oral commissure.

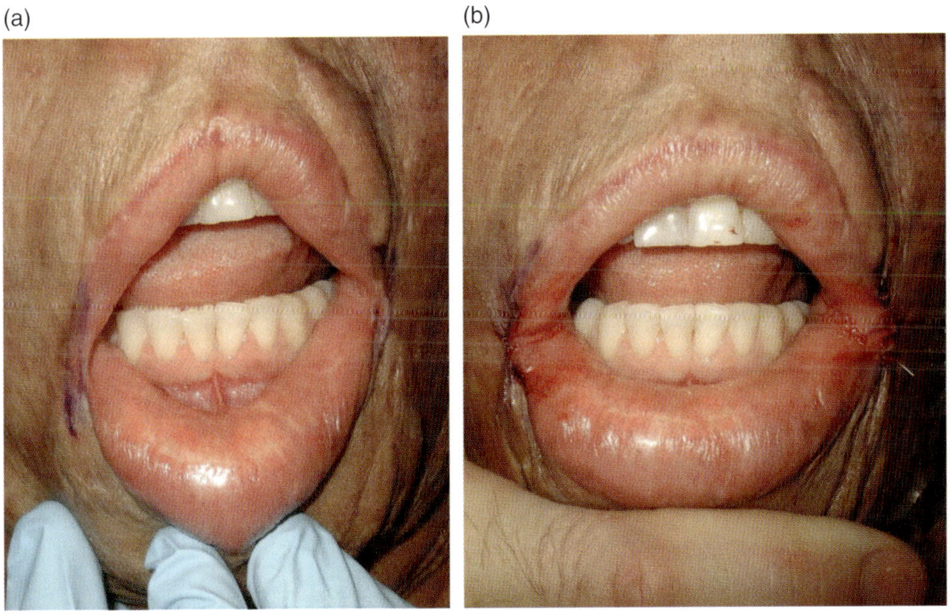

Fig. 14.8 **(a)** Burn scar contractures in bilateral oral comissures. **(b)** Contractures reconstructed with oral mucosal flaps.

CONCLUSIONS

Over the last three decades, advances in surgical management, infection control and improved nutrition have increased survival rates of burn patients. Despite these advances, burn injuries still result in significant mortality and morbidity. Outcome of the treatment depends on the surface area exposed and the depth of the injury, which tends to increase up to 72 hours after injury. This can make clinical treatment planning challenging. Superficial burns are treated conservatively and often heal with regeneration of the skin with no scars. Deep wounds are treated with early excision and skin grafting, aiming at complete wound closure within 3 weeks to avoid hypertrophic scarring which can affect function, esthetics and cause psychological disturbances. Deep facial wounds can be especially devastating in this respect. Superficial intraoral wounds heal usually without any treatment. Deep intraoral wounds are rare but difficult to treat because of complex anatomical structures and often result in commissural contractures. Treatment of hypertrophic scars remains problematic although various treatment modalities have been advocated to produce improved results. Future studies should be aimed at improved clinical decision-making and surgical and non-surgical options that can prevent hypertrophic scarring in deep and large burn wounds.

REFERENCES

Akita S, Akino K, Imaizumi T, Hirano A (2008). Basic fibroblast growth factor accelerates and improves second-degree burn wound healing. *Wound Repair Genen* 16(5):635–41.

Boykin JV, Eriksson E, Pittman RN (1979). Microcirculation of scald burn: an in vivo experimental study of the hairless mouse ear. *Burns* 6:335–8.

Brans T, Dutrieux R, Hoekstra M, Kreis R, duPont J (1994). Histopathological evaluation of scalds and contact burns in the pig model. *Burns* 20(1):48–51.

Converse J, Platt J, Ballantyne D (1965). An experimental evaluation of a histochemical diagnosis of burn depth. *J Surg Res* 5(12):547–51.

Cuttle L, Kempf M, Kravchuk O, et al. (2008). The optimal temperature of first aid treatment for partial thickness burn injuries. *Wound Repair Regen* 16(5):626–34.

Gravante G, Palmieri M, Esposito G, et al. (2007). Apoptotic death in deep partial thickness burns vs normal skin of burned patients. *J Surg Res* 141(2):141–5.

Heimbach D, Engrav L, Grube B, Marvin J (1992). Burn depth: a review. *World J Surg* 16:10–5.

Hildanus FG (1607). *De Combustionibus*. Carolus Uttenhove, Basle.

Hinshaw J (1968). Early changes in the depth of burns. *Ann N Y Acad Sci* 150:548–53.

Hopewell JW (1990). The skin: its structure and response to ionizing radiation. *Int J Radiat Biol* 23:85–95.

Jackson DM (1953). The diagnosis of the depth of burning. *Br J Surg* 40:588–96.

Kahn A, McGrady V, Rosen V (1979). Burn wound biopsy. Multiple uses in patient management. *Scand J Plast Reconstr Surg* 13:53–6.

Kaufman T, Lusthaus S, Sagher U, Wexler M (1990). Deep partial skin thickness burns: a reproducible animal model to study burn wound healing. *Burns* 16:13–6.

Kessel R (1998) The integument. In: *Basic Medical Histology: The Biology of Cells, Tissues and Organs*, pp. 338–45. Oxford University Press, New York.

Meyer W, Schwarz R, Neurand K (1978). The skin of domestic animals as a model for the human skin, with special reference to the domestic pig. *Curr Probl Dermatol* 7:39–52.

Moulin V, Auger F, Garrel D, Germail L (2000). Role of wound healing myofibroblasts on re-epithelialization of human skin. *Burns* 26(1):3–12.

Nadworny PL, Wang J, Tredget EE, Burrell RE (2008). Anti-inflammatory activity of nanocrystalline silver in a porcine contact dermatitis model. *Nanomedicine* 4(3):241–51.

Nanney L, Wenczak B, Lynch J (1996). Progressive burn injury documented with vimentin immunostaining. *J Burn Care Rehabil* 17(5):191–8.

Papp A, Kiraly K, Härmä M, Lahtinen T, Uusaro A, Alhava E (2004). The progression of burn depth in experimental burns. A histological and methodological study. *Burns* 30(7): 683–9.

Pasyk K, Thomas S, Hassett C, Cherry G, Faller R (1989). Regional differences in capillary density of the normal human dermis. *Plast Reconstr Surg* 83:939–45.

Raja K, Sivamani K, Garcia M, Isseroff R (2007). Wound re-epithelialization: modulating keratinocyte migration in wound healing. *Front Biosci* 12:2849–68.

Rajan V, Bartlett N, Harvey J, et al. (2009). Delayed cooling of an acute scald contact burn injury in a porcine model: is it worthwhile? *J Burn Care Res* 30(4):729–34.

Ravage ZB, Gomez HF, Czermak BJ, Watkins SA, Till GO (1998). Mediators of microvascular injury in dermal burn wounds. *Inflammation* 22(6):619–29.

Rea S, Giles N, Webb S, et al. (2009). Bone marrow-derived cells in the healing burn wound – more than just inflammation. *Burns* 35(3):356–64.

Schomacker K, Torri A, Sandison D, Sheridan R, Nishioka N (1997). Biodistribution of indocyanine green in a porcine burn model: light and fluorescence microscopy. *J Trauma* 43(5):813–9.

Schwacha M, Thobe B, Daniel T, Hubbard W (2010). Impact of thermal injury on wound infiltration and the dermal inflammatory response. *J Surg Research* 158(1):112–20.

Singer A, Berruti L, Thode H, McClain S (2000). Standardized burn model using a multiparametric histologic analysis of burn depth. *Acad Emerg Med* 7(1):1–6.

Singh V, Devgan L, Bhat S, Milner SM (2007). The pathogenesis of burn wound conversion. *Ann Plast Surg* 59(1):109–15. Review.

Szpaderska A, Egozi E, Gamelli R, DiPietro L (2003). The effect of thrombocytopenia on dermal wound healing. *J Invest Dermatol* 120(6):1130–7.

Watts A, Tyler M, Perry M, Roberts A, McGrouther D (2001). Burn depth and its histological measurement. *Burns* 27:154–60.

Yamaguchi R, Takami Y, Tamaguchi Y, Shimazaki S (2007). Bone marrow-derived myofibroblasts recruited to the upper dermis appear beneath regenerating epidermis after deep dermal burn injury. *Wound Repair Regen* 15(1):87–93.

Zawacki B (1974). Reversal of capillary stasis and prevention of necrosis in burns. *Ann Surg* 180(1):98–102.

15 Healing of Large Dentofacial Defects

George K.B. Sándor[1,2], Robert P. Carmichael[3,4,5], Leena P. Ylikontiola[6,7], Ahmed Jan[8], Marc G. DuVal[9] and Cameron M.L. Clokie[5]

[1]Regea Institute for Regenerative Medicine, Institute of Biomedical Technology, University of Tampere, Tampere, Finland
[2]University of Oulu, Oulu, Finland
[3]Bloorview Kids Rehab, Toronto, Canada
[4]Ontario Cleft Lip and Palate Program, Toronto, Canada
[5]University of Toronto, Canada
[6]Institute of Dentistry, University of Oulu, Oulu, Finland
[7]Oulu University Hospital, Oulu, Finland
[8]Department of Oral and Maxillofacial Surgery and Anesthesia, University of Toronto, Toronto, Canada
[9]Graduate Program in Oral and Maxillofacial Surgery and Anaesthesia, University of Toronto, Toronto, Canada

INTRODUCTION

Dentofacial defects are defined as missing areas of tissue including defects of either or both the jaws, cranium, face and neck with missing adjacent soft tissue and bony components. There are numerous causes of dentofacial defects. Congenital bony defects in the craniofacial and maxillofacial skeleton arise as a result of areas of failed development such as in cleft lip and palate patients (Carmichael and Sándor 2008; Fig. 15.1). Ablative surgery may produce bony defects (Sándor et al. 2008) when segments of bones are resected to treat tumors (Fig. 15.2). Trauma may result in large bony defects when tissue may have been traumatically avulsed (Sándor and Carmichael 2008). Such combined mucosal, osseous and even cartilaginous defects can be reconstructed using flaps and bone grafts, or hopefully in the future with bone graft substitutes or even tissue engineered constructs (Sándor and Suuronen 2008). The healing of such wounds always relies on the vascularity of the surrounding tissues (Fok et al. 2008).

The reconstruction of a specific defect must follow sound and logical surgical principles. The authors employ the concept of the reconstructive surgical ladder (Sándor et al. 2010), in which techniques of step-wise increasing complexity are used with a strong preference for the simplest possible procedure at the outset. The missing tissues are identified including

Oral Wound Healing: Cell Biology and Clinical Management, First Edition. Edited by Hannu Larjava.

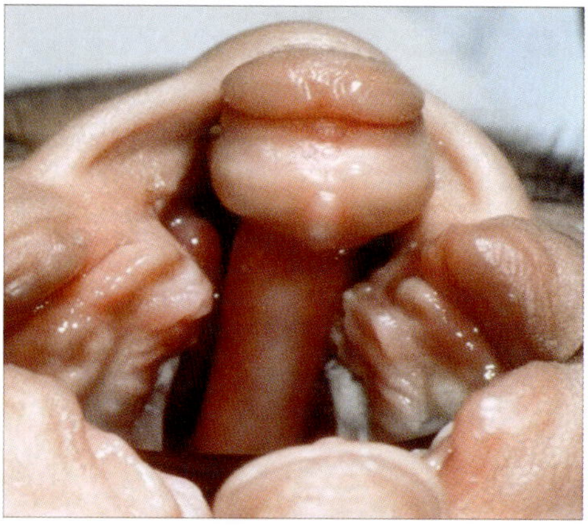

Fig. 15.1 Bilateral complete cleft lip and palate deformity with missing bone, cartilage, mucosa and skin.

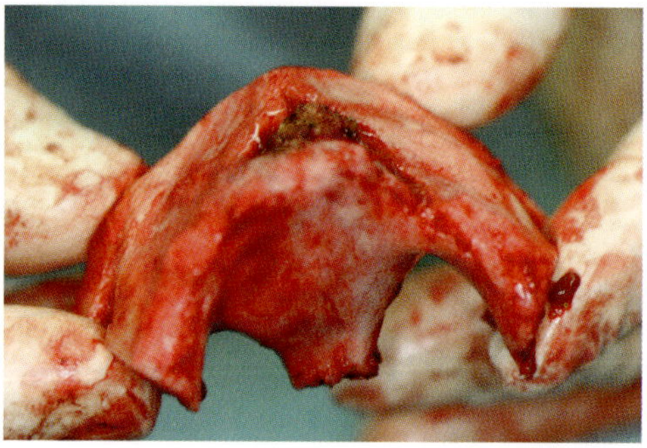

Fig. 15.2 Tumor resection specimen encompassing 11 tooth segment leaving a large mandibular dentofacial defect.

mucosa, muscle, bone, cartilage, nerve, blood vessels and skin. Then plans are made to replace missing tissue elements with similar or like tissue. In the mouth, for example, one would always aim to replace missing palatal mucosa with attached mucosa rather than unattached alveolar mucosa.

Then flaps containing the missing tissue elements are planned with the following hierarchy, using the simplest reconstructive ladder technique first:

1. Local soft tissue grafts (free gingival grafts)
2. Local flaps (buccal advancement flaps)
3. Regional flaps (tongue flaps)
4. Intra-oral harvested bone grafts (chin, ramus, zygoma)
5. Extra-oral harvested bone grafts (iliac crest, tibia)
6. Distant pedicled flaps (deltopectoral, sternocleidomastoid, pectoralis flaps)
7. Distant microvascular flaps (fibula, iliac crest, latisimus dorsi, rectus abdominis).

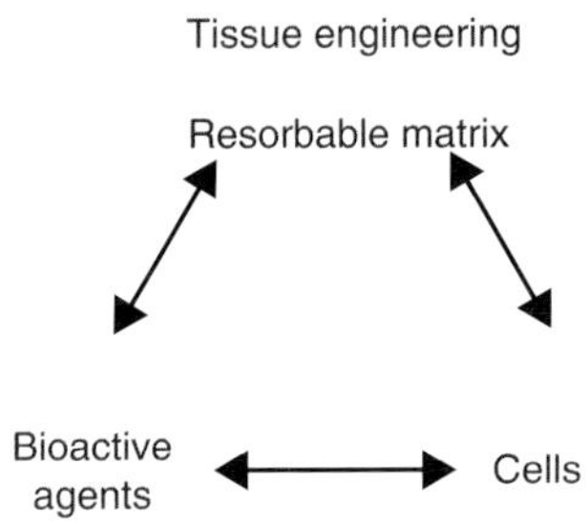

Fig. 15.3 The tissue engineering triad representing the interplay between scaffolds or biomaterials, stem cells and signaling molecules or growth factors.

THE NEED FOR BONE

Reconstruction of osseous defects in the oral and maxillofacial region represents one of the most challenging tasks to the reconstructive surgeon and encompasses the model of tissue engineering (Fig. 15.3). While significant advances have been made with bone substitutes, autogenous bone remains the gold standard in the reconstruction of bone defects (Sándor et al. 2101). To understand bone reconstruction, the surgeon must first understand bone healing (Sándor et al. 2101) and the healing of the surrounding soft tissues.

BONE HEALING

Inflammation, wound healing, vasculogenesis and bone healing are all delicately intertwined. Three types of bone healing are described: primary, secondary and gap healing. The difference between the three is dependent on the size of the osseous defect and the rigidity of fixation. The three bone healing models give information about the differences between bone regeneration within non-grafted as well as grafted defects.

Primary bone healing

Primary bone healing without callus formation occurs when the bone ends are in direct contact and rigidly fixated, or anatomically reduced and are compressed together by bone plates (Sándor et al. 2101). This process was initially described in 1949 after studying long bone fractures that were treated by rigid fixation with plating (Danis 1949). These fractures failed to show callus formation. Osteoclasts were seen to begin cutting away cores on either side in the area of compression, progressing towards the fracture at a rate of 50–80 μm per day. Cutting cores were 200 μm wide which provided space for vessel ingrowth, osteoblastic proliferation and new bone formation (Simmons 1980).

Secondary bone healing

Fractures treated without rigid fixation heal with secondary bone healing. A good example of non-rigid fixation is the wiring of fractured jaws together in maxillomandibular or intermaxillary fixation. The initial injury elicits an inflammatory response and activation of the complement cascade. Damage to surrounding blood vessels initiates cellular extravasation and cell signaling. Chemotactic factors (C5a, leukotriene B4) attract monocytes and macrophages (Marx et al. 1998). Activated macrophages release fibroblast growth factor (FGF) which stimulates endothelial cells to release plasminogen activator and procollagenase. Growth factors such as platelet derived growth factor (PDGF), transforming growth factor- β1 (TGF-β1) and – β2 are released from the alpha granules of degranulating platelets early in wound healing and are chemotactic stimulants for PMNs, lymphocytes, monocytes and macrophages. The blood clot acts as a hemostatic plug and contains the growth factors at the injured site and provides an environment for cell signaling. The injured tissue is normally hypoxic with oxygen partial pressures of 5–10 mmHg as well as being acidotic (pH 4–6). Acidosis and hypoxia are required for PMN and macrophage stimulation (Marx et al. 1998). A proliferation phase begins with the healing by day 3 and can last up to 40 days after fracture occurrence. A reparative phase follows with the appearance of new blood vessels, collagen and cells. Osteoprogenitor cells are then stimulated to proliferate and differentiate into active chondroblasts and osteoblasts, laying down large amounts of extracellular matrices forming a bridging callus. Chondroblasts lay down amorphous chondroitin sulfate matrices, then become chondrocytes, which eventually hypertrophy and die, leaving empty lacunae in a calcified matrix. These empty spaces (lacunae) allow for vascular ingrowth resulting in a higher oxygen tension and normalized pH, which in turn favor differentiation of osteoblasts. The cartilage is then removed by osteoclasts while osteoblasts lay down immature woven bone. Mobility at the regenerate site will disrupt the blood supply and result in cartilage and fibrous tissue predominance.

Gap osseous healing and bone grafts

Larger defects heal by gap healing and may require bone grafts to allow the bony wound to regenerate bone rather than produce a fibrous union. Three processes are involved in the healing of bone grafts: osteogenesis, osteoinduction and osteoconduction (Burchadt 1983).

1 Osteogenesis is defined as the formation of new bone from osteocompetent cells contained within the bone graft.
2 Osteoinduction is defined as bone formation from primitive mesenchymal cells in the recipient bed, which have been stimulated to differentiate into bone forming cells by inductive proteins within the graft.
3 Osteoconduction is defined as ingrowth of capillaries and osteoprogenitor cells from the recipient bed into and around the grafted material.

Growth factors

Growth factors important in bone healing include the bone morphogenetic proteins (BMPs). The BMP subfamily of TGF-β is made of seven conserved cysteine residues at the mature carboxy terminal (Wozney et al. 1999). BMPs are low molecular weight proteins (19–30 kDa) with a pH of 4.9–5.1 (Moghadam et al. 2001). BMPs stimulate mesenchymal stem cells to differentiate into osteoblasts during development and bone healing (Ducy et al. 1997; Schmitt et al. 1999). BMPs are present in most tissues and play an important role in remodeling of the adult skeleton. When osteoclasts resorb bone matrix, BMP is released (Hu et al. 2009a), initiating recruitment and differentiation of stem cell precursors to form osteoblasts and ultimately new bone (Dragoo et al. 2003).

BMP-7, also known as osteogenic protein 1 (OP-1), was first used to treat a mandibular segmental defect by Moghadam and colleagues in 2001 (Moghadam et al. 2001). BMP-7 was used to aid the healing of a maxillary Lefort I osteotomy by Warnke in 2003 (Warnke 2003). It is now approved for human use in maxillary sinus elevation procedures as well as in extraction socket preservation techniques. The recombinant human form is derived from a Chinese hamster ovary cell line. Both laboratory and human studies show data with superior results in regenerating critical-sized defects (Moghadam et al. 2001, 2004). Clokie and Sándor were first to report the use of OP-1 in human post-resection defects. They documented 10 cases of post-resection mandibular defects successfully reconstructed with BMP-7 (OP-1) in demineralized bone matrix (DBM) suspended in a reverse phase copolymer medium. Uneventful postoperative courses were reported with dental rehabilitation achieved 1 year post reconstruction (Moghadam et al. 2001; Clokie and Sándor 2008).

Blood supply and the soft tissue envelope

Formation of a new blood supply is critical to wound healing (Bauer et al. 2005). This is demonstrated most clearly in pathologic states where healing is compromised by diabetes, poor vascular supply, radiation, bisphosphonate exposure and where the normal healing process becomes pathologic, such as in instances of heterotopic bone formation in response to surgery or trauma (Du Val et al. 2007). The need for the re-establishment of nutrient and oxygen supply to support regeneration and repair of the wound exceeds the maintenance needs of the tissue that will ultimately form. Vascular endothelial growth factor (VEGF) is involved in the recruitment, survival and activity of endothelial cells, osteoblasts and osteoclasts in wound healing (Midy and Plouet 1994; Niida et al. 1999; Deckers and Karperien 2000; Engsig et al. 2000; Street et al. 2000; Ferrara et al. 2003; Bauer et al. 2005).

Soft tissue wound healing is required to support bone healing. It has been well described and is characterized by four phases:

1. Coagulation (immediate to 1 hour)
2. Inflammatory (1 hour to 4 days)
3. Proliferative (3–21 days)
4. Remodeling (21 days onward).

Coagulation is characterized by endothelial damage and platelet activation resulting in a fibrin clot. Platelets release angiogenic cytokines including platelet-derived growth factor (PDGF) and TGF-β.

Vasculoendothelial growth factor (VEGF) effects

VEGF is also released by monocytes, damaged keratinocytes, endothelial cells and especially active macrophages in the wound (Sheikh et al. 2000; Byrne et al. 2005). VEGF acts on nearby capillaries to induce vascular leakage, supporting inflammation in physiologic and pathologic conditions by enhancing vascular permeability (Midy and Plouet 1994). VEGF also attracts neutrophils and monocytes required for wound healing and likely also facilitates the formation of granulation tissue. The inflammatory phase is characterized by leukocyte migration, initially neutrophils to kill bacteria and then monocytes. VEGF release also increases local leukocyte rolling (a more than threefold increase) and adhesion (a more than fourfold increase) in addition to increasing vascular permeability further facilitating inflammatory processes. Monocytes differentiate into macrophages and, in addition to their role in phagocytosis, become important in releasing cytokines important in subsequent healing and granulation tissue formation. VEGF is known to play a role in the regulation of initiation and growth of new vascular structures (Midy and Plouet 1994) as well as being necessary for endochondral ossification (Midy and Plouet 1994). Endothelial cells activated by VEGF initiate angiogenesis locally. Endothelial progenitors in bone marrow are also recruited to the wound for vasculogenesis. Together both processes supply the neovascularization required for granulation tissue formation (Byrne et al. 2005), though angiogenesis dominates the process (Bauer et al. 2005).

The absence of VEGF inhibits angiogenesis in wound healing, impairs the recruitment of cells necessary for normal bone development and interferes with necessary cell to cell cytokine cross-talk due to the absence of developing vasculature. VEGF is a key player in bone repair and regeneration for similar reasons (Street et al. 2000). The potent angiogenic activity of the blood clot that forms immediately after fracture has been attributed to VEGF (Street et al. 2000). The importance of VEGF in fracture healing has been demonstrated in mice and rabbits; when VEGF is inhibited it causes a reduction in blood flow and results in disruption of the fracture repair and non-union. While the role of VEGF remains to be completely understood, VEGF is clearly necessary for healing and bone repair through modulation of angiogenesis and new vessel formation (Street et al. 2000).

In addition to stimulating and regulating angiogenesis, VEGF influences osteoblast differentiation and is involved in mineralization of fracture callus (Schilephake 2002; Barr et al. 2008). Different growth factors influence wound and bone healing in a manner that is both distinct and synergistically interconnected (Barr et al. 2008). VEGF is required in order for other factors to function, as is the case with BMP-2 and FGF-2 induced angiogenesis (Yeh and Lee 1999). Inhibition of VEGF blocks BMP-7 induction of osteoblast differentiation and BMP-4-induced bone formation (Yeh and Lee 1999).

Angiogenesis

Angiogenesis is important not only in soft tissue healing but also for bone tissue differentiation, bone formation, maintenance and remodeling. Bone repair follows four sequential steps:

1 Establishment of a thrombus
2 Formation of the soft callus
3 Formation of the hard callus, followed by
4 Bony remodeling.

The first step in angiogenesis involves the formation of a platelet- and leukocyte-rich blood clot around the site of fracture or bony defect. Activated platelets promote chemotaxis of leukocytes to assist in clearing debris. Both platelets and leukocytes release several growth factors which will ultimately favor the formation of granulation tissue rich in immature vessels which forms in and around the wound. These growth factors include: tumor necrosis factors (TNF), BMPs, FGF, insulin-like growth factor (IGF), PDGF, TGF and VEGF (Tatsuyama et al. 2000; Hu et al. 2009b). Neovessels (Street et al. 2000) and fibroblasts proliferate, forming immature fibrous tissue that is responsible for forming the early soft callus. The callus undergoes further maturation to form the hard callus and is eventually replaced by lamellar bone. Immature woven bone formed by osteoprogenitor cells will eventually undergo remodeling. Bone remodeling follows the maturation of the newly formed bone, characterized by maturation and re-organization as the fracture or defect gains tensile strength. Each step in bone healing involves the migration, proliferation, differentiation and activation of local and distant cells, and this process is closely regulated (Tatsuyama et al. 2000; Mandracchia et al. 2001). Osteoprogenitor cells respond to the presence of the growth factors including BMPs, FGF, IGF, PDGF, TGF and VEGF (Tatsuyama et al. 2000; Mandracchia et al. 2001). Bone is an excellent source of most of these growth factors, which are released after remodeling or trauma, and this is responsible in part for the success of autogenous grafting compared to alternative sources of graft material (Canalis et al. 1988). Growth factors modulate the healing response and mediate the remodeling process. VEGF increases angiogenesis at the graft or fracture site, providing greater oxygen and nutrient supply and thus enhancing differentiation of perivascular and mesenchymal stem cells into osteoblasts (Barr et al. 2008). BMPs are potent inducers of osteogenesis and are expressed during the bone deposition stage, though this is dependent on the formation of neovessels (Canalis et al. 1988).

It has been reported that a process not unlike embryonic vasculogenesis may play a role in coalescence of vessel progenitors (Sipola et al. 2007). VEGF-D, an isoform, and VEGFR-3 (VEGF receptor-3) are important in osteoblast maturation, with VEGF-D and VEGFR-3 acting downstream from VEGF in osteogenesis (Tarkka et al. 2003; Sipola et al. 2007). Rat studies have revealed VEGF splice variants VEGF121 and VEGF165, corresponding to human VEGF splice variants VEGF121 and VEGF165. These are expressed during fracture healing. VEGF is most strongly expressed in bone fracture callus at the early phase of healing, decreasing significantly by day 5 (Tarkka et al. 2003). The role of VEGF beyond 5 days in healing of the bony wound is not known. Angiogenic growth factors may mediate interaction between endothelial cells, osteoblasts and chondrocytes, all of which secrete endogenous VEGF (Tarkka et al. 2003). As healing progresses, the fibroblast dominates wound healing through the proliferative phase, forming collagen and scar tissue. Several factors assist in tipping the balance from repair to regeneration (Tarkka et al. 2003), favoring the formation of immature bone rather than fibrous tissue. For example, in a rabbit calvarial defect model, the addition of VEGF to DBM favors regeneration of the critical sized bony wounds compared to mainly repair in DBM or void controls (Emad 2006). Moreover, treatment of rabbit mandibular defects with supraphysiologic doses of exogenous human recombinant VEGF165 results in increased angiogenesis and bone regeneration (Kleinheinz 2005).

Bony wound healing, be it a fracture, a graft or a defect, requires stability and adequate blood supply. Bony wound healing relies on osteogenic progenitors from adjacent and distant bone marrow. Bone possesses limited potential for regeneration, yet this potential can be enhanced (Fok et al. 2008; Jan et al. 2006, 2009, 2010). The periosteum is a key source of blood supply and, when it remains intact, demonstrates the extensive microvasculature needed for bone healing and regeneration (Bourque et al. 1992; Glowacki 1998). Bone adjacent to a defect has limited capability for neovascularization and osteogenesis. The periosteum and, in the case of cranial defects even dura, stimulates bone formation and neovascularization (Bourque et al. 1992).

Augmented angiogenesis in bony wounds and bone grafting application may improve graft survival, minimize resorption, hopefully reduce reliance on autogenous graft, reduce the amount of autogenous graft required for a given defect or ultimately enable entirely bio-engineered grafts. Moreover, the ability to promote neo-angiogenesis could potentially prove very useful in the treatment and prevention of osteoradionecrosis and bisphosphonate related necrosis.

Efforts to use angiogenic growth factors for treatment of chronic wounds have met with limited success. To date only PDGF has been approved by the US Food and Drug Administration (FDA) for use as a topical cytokine wound ointment. PDGF is active in all phases of the healing process and has been highly effective as an adjunct measure in the treatment of chronic wounds of the foot (Bauer et al. 2005). Success is limited by the adequately perfused granulation tissue bed.

Attempts to improve bony and chronic wound healing have been the focus of much attention. Hyperbaric oxygen (HBO) improves the ability of macrophages to phagocytose bacteria, especially since hypoxic tissue impairs the oxidative function of macrophages (Bourque et al. 1992). Moreover, macrophages release higher levels of angiogenic cytokines in response to HBO (Bourque et al. 1992). Another approach under investigation is the administration of VEGF gene therapy to locally increase neovacularization (Tarkka et al. 2003). However, results have been unpredictable, and disorganized vascular tissue and hematomas have resulted instead of normal angiogenesis or vasculogenesis due, in part, to overexpression of VEGF (Tarkka et al. 2003).

VEGF has been shown to increase blood vessel formation, mineral density and bone fill in rat calvarial defects (Fok et al. 2008) and rabbit mandibular defects. VEGF has also been shown to increase bone formation and improve demineralized bone allograft consolidation (Kleinheinz 2005). Most studies using VEGF in bony wounds and fractures involve local infusions of VEGF (Street et al. 2000; Kleinheinz 2005). While such infusions are effective, they are not a practical or convenient long-term modes of delivery. Instead, delivery of VEGF incorporated into an implantable membrane or another allogenic scaffold material, possibly combined with other important growth factors, is a preferable and more viable mode of delivery which is directed at the target site with sustained exposure.

Since VEGF does not appear to drive osteoprogenitor cell differentiation, a combination therapy with BMPs may be ultimately required (Sándor and Suuronen 2008). Once combined with grafting materials, VEGF would be released initially to promote vascularization to the site followed by the release of BMP to promote osteoprogenitor cell differentiation and bone fill. This would exploit the synergy between bone formation and angiogenesis by the manufacturing bone grafting materials that promote angiogenesis in the early stages of injury, such as a tooth extraction, followed by treatment with bone growth factors, such as BMP, to stimulate osteoprogenitor cells to differentiate in the later stages. This type of combined treatment might lead to optimal wound healing.

It is clear that endogenous VEGF is required for normal bone fracture healing, remodeling, and osteoblast and osteoclast activity (Street et al. 2000). In addition, the autocrine activity of VEGF in osteoblasts adjacent to cortical defects has been demonstrated. Exogenous VEGF given by a pump over 48 hours until day 7 increases early vascularization and bone healing in bone fracture healing and bone defect healing (Street et al. 2000; Kleinheinz 2005). The angiogenic role of VEGF has been studied separately in soft tissue porcine bladder models, and VEGF has been shown to improve neovascularization of porcine bladder constructs at VEGF doses of which are 1000 times less than in studies which demonstrate effects on bone fracture and bone defect healing.

This may be largely explained by the fact that most studies on bone have used recombinant human VEGF165 (rhVEGF165), whereas recombinant human VEGF121 (rhVEGF121) has been used in many of the soft tissue studies. It is difficult to compare studies as the dose and mode of delivery of VEGF varies. Furthermore, it is not known if bone healing and angiogenesis have differing VEGF requirements. It is safe to say, however, that VEGF seems to be important in the paradigm of bone healing (Broussard 2003; Fok et al. 2008; Beaumont et al. 2010).

SURGICAL MANEUVERS TO INDUCE AND PROMOTE HEALING OF LARGE DEFECTS

Periosteal healing

Manipulating the periosteum is one method that surgeons have learned which induces bone regeneration. Periosteal stretching occurs naturally in periosteal new bone formation under pathologically stretched periosteum, in osteomyelitis for example. The periosteum is a key source of blood supply and when it remains intact it demonstrates an extensive microvasculature which is necessary for bone healing and regeneration (Bourque et al. 1992; Glowacki 1998). Bone adjacent to a defect has a limited capability for neovascularization and osteogenesis. The periosteum and, in the case of cranial defects even dura, stimulates bone formation and neovascularization (Bourque et al. 1992).

There are sites where periosteal bone regeneration can occur predictably in young children. The fibula or ribs are examples that may totally regenerate when a graft has been harvested in a child and the periosteum is maintained. The mandible has also been known to regenerate in a child when it has been resected and the periosteal sleeve was left intact. These same principles of periosteal stretching and defect maintenance are important in sinus lifting, guided bone regeneration with membranes (Humber et al. 2010) and distraction osteogenesis. Defects that are not maintained result in a periosteum that sags or collapses and there alveolar ridges become non-ideal in form.

Tent pole procedures

The value of re-establishing the continuity of a mandibular defect in tumor reconstruction with a bone graft and rigid fixation hardware is undeniable, but reconstructions like these should be considered interim if they are not functionally loaded. If they do not restore chewing function, the bone grafts tend to undergo progressive disuse atrophy, and the absence of teeth permits overeruption of the opposing dentition. The authors have observed atrophy of non-vascularized grafts and, surprisingly, vascularized fibular reconstructions of the mandible as well. Atrophy of vascularized grafts has been documented in growing children (Fenton et al. 2007) and has been observed in adult patients by these authors.

The soft tissue matrix expansion (STME) or tent pole procedure was originally described to manage severe alveolar atrophy secondary to long-standing mandibular edentulism (Figs. 15.4a–4i) by stretching the periosteum surrounding the part of the atrophic mandible to be reconstructed with dental implants (Marx et al. 2002; Kainulainen et al. 2003; McGuire et al. 2003; Kudbya et al. 2006; Carmichael et al. 2008; Sándor et al. 2008). The technique was adapted to arrest atrophy of a vascularized fibula used to reconstruct an ablative defect

(a)

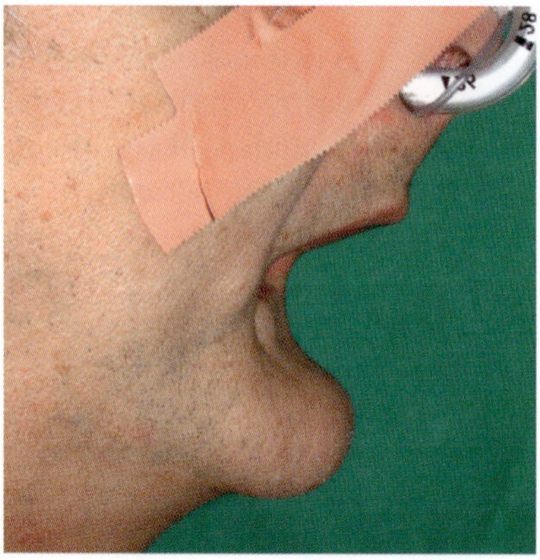

Fig. 15.4a Edentulous male with severe mandibular alveolar atrophy and limited lower lip support.

(b)

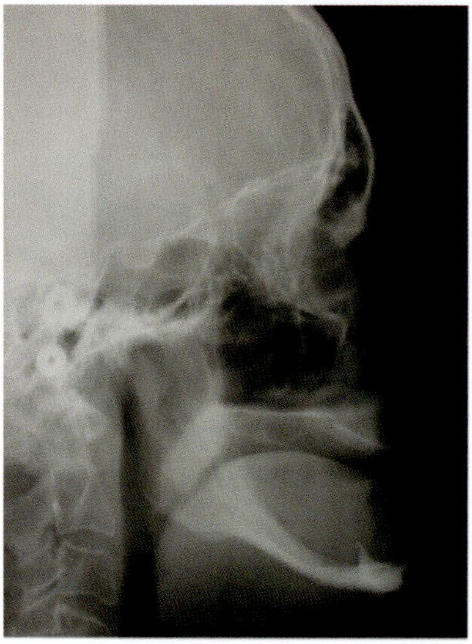

Fig. 15.4b Lateral cephalogram showing 4 mm of mandibular ridge height.

(c)

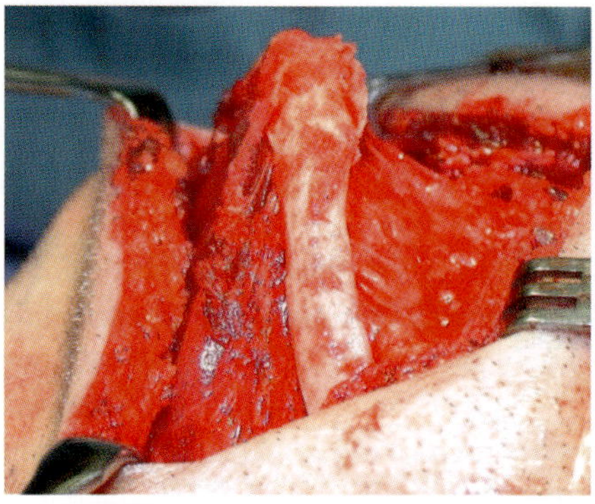

Fig. 15.4c Anterior aspect of mandible exposed through an extraoral submental skin incision. There is no intraoral incision and the periosteum overlying the superior aspect of the mandibular ridge is peeled off and kept intact.

(d)

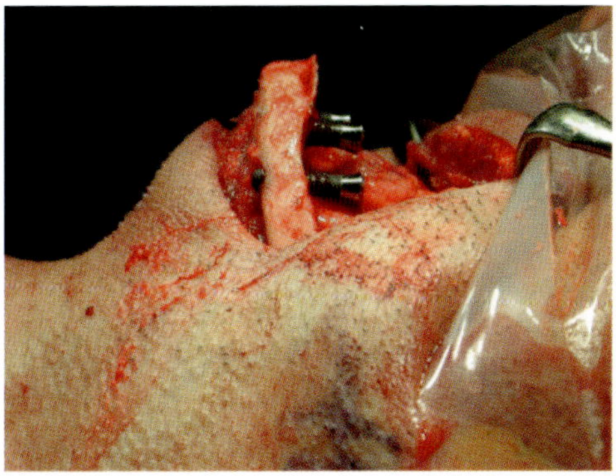

Fig. 15.4d Implants have been inserted into the basal bone of the mandible with the apical one third of each implant engaging the mandibular bone.

(e)

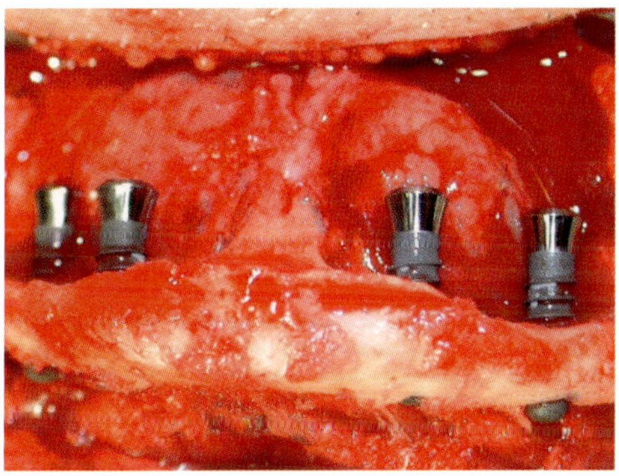

Fig. 15.4e Anterior view of the mandibular implants with healing screws attached. The exposed parts of the implants will tent up the overlying periosteum like tent poles. The exposed parts of the implants will be covered with cancellous bone obtained from the posterior iliac crest.

(f)

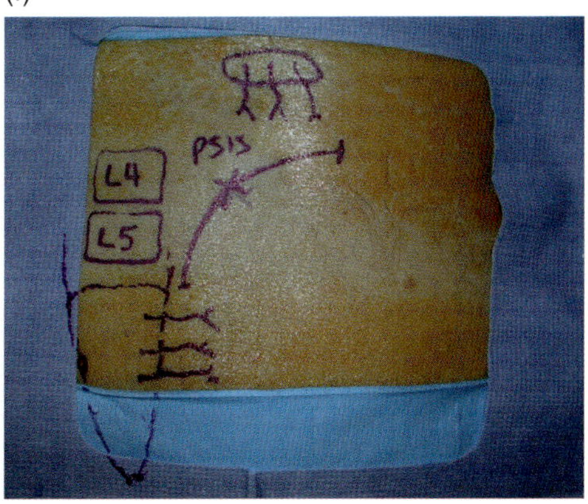

Fig. 15.4f Posterior iliac crest donor site.

(g)

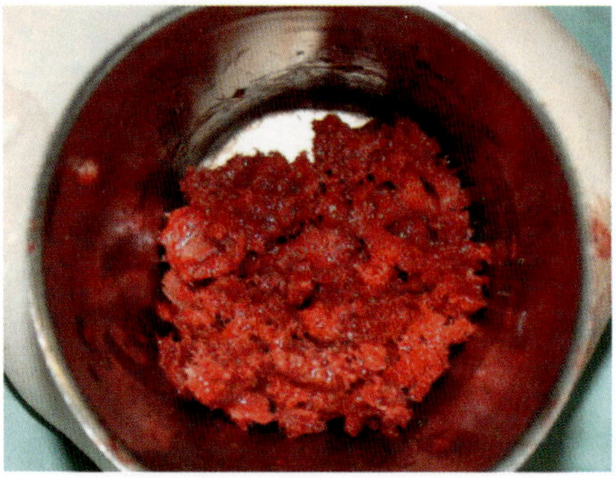

Fig. 15.4g Cancellous bone harvested from posterior iliac crest.

(h)

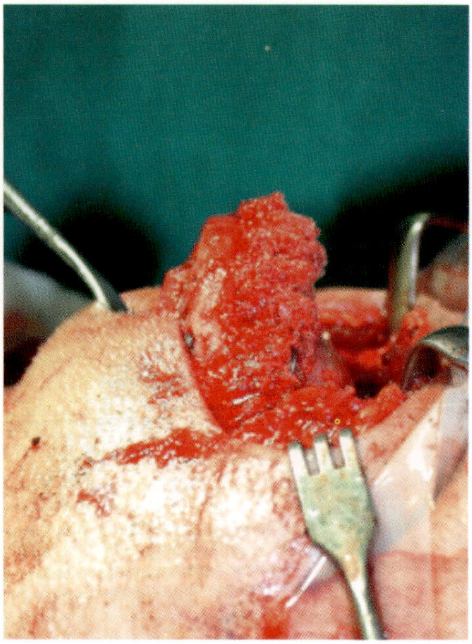

Fig. 15.4h Exposed parts of dental implants covered by cancellous bone graft. Periosteum closed overtop will act like a natural membrane allowing bone graft healing beneath with no exposure of grafted material to oral environment.

(i)

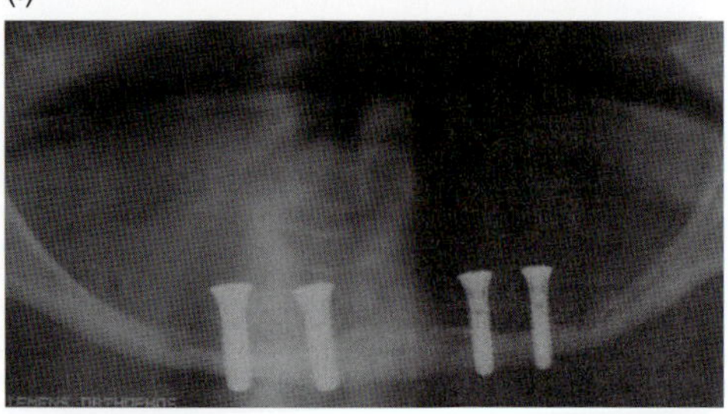

Fig. 15.4i Post-operative orthopantomogram showing recently placed dental implants in atrophic mandibular ridge with healing bone graft.

resulting from resection of a malignant tumor of the parasymphysis of the mandible in a growing child (Fenton et al. 2007). The authors have further adapted the STME technique to treat an ablative defect of the lateral aspect of the mandible reconstructed initially with a vascularized fibular graft. The following reconstruction of a large mandibular dentofacial defect illustrates the principles of this technique (Figs. 15.5a–s).

Sinus lifting/lateral ridge augmentation

Acute periosteal stretching

Sinus-augmentation procedures are well-accepted techniques to treat the loss of vertical bone height (VBH) in the posterior maxilla and are performed in two ways: an osteotome sinus floor elevation technique (Jensen 1999; Figs. 15.6a–e) and a lateral window technique

(a)

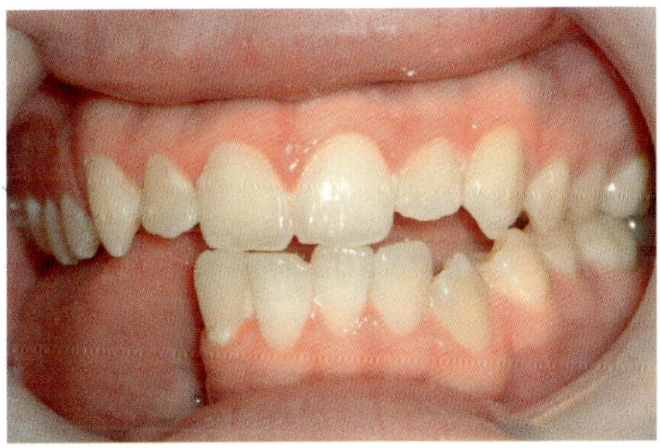

Fig. 15.5a Anterior view of teeth on presentation. Note pre existing class III malocclusion and anterior edge-to-edge relationship.

(b)

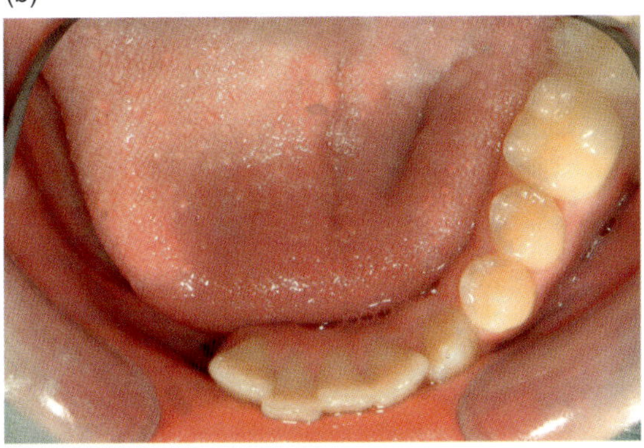

Fig. 15.5b Occlusal view of mandibular arch. Note absence of right lateral segment of mandible.

(c)

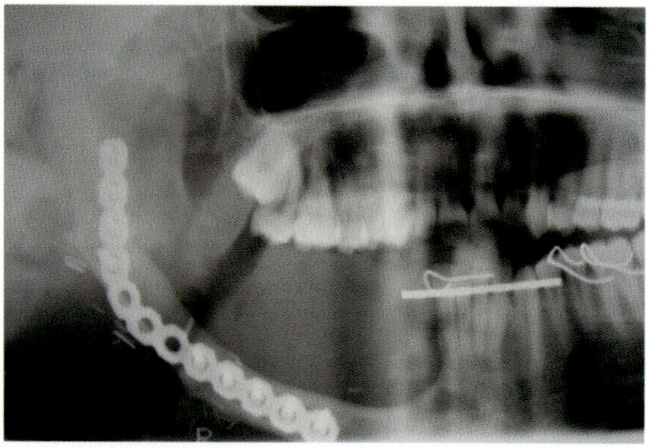

Fig. 15.5c Panoramic tomograph on presentation showing right side of mandible reconstructed with vascularized fibular graft. Note the lack of vertical height of the graft and the potential crown-implant ratio.

(d)

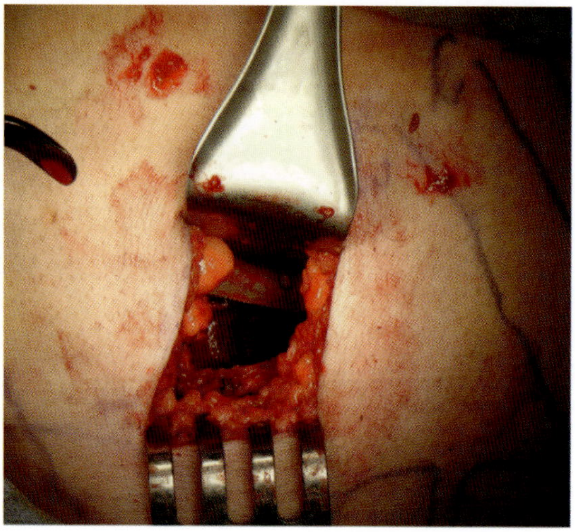

Fig. 15.5d Posterior iliac crest exposed.

(e)

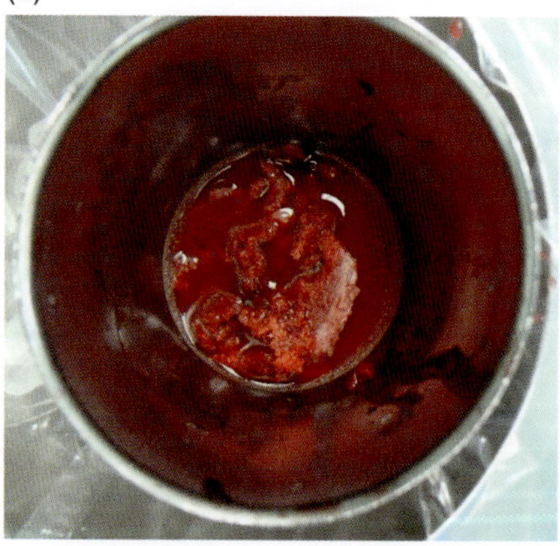

Fig. 15.5e Posterior iliac crest graft stored in saline on ice.

(f)

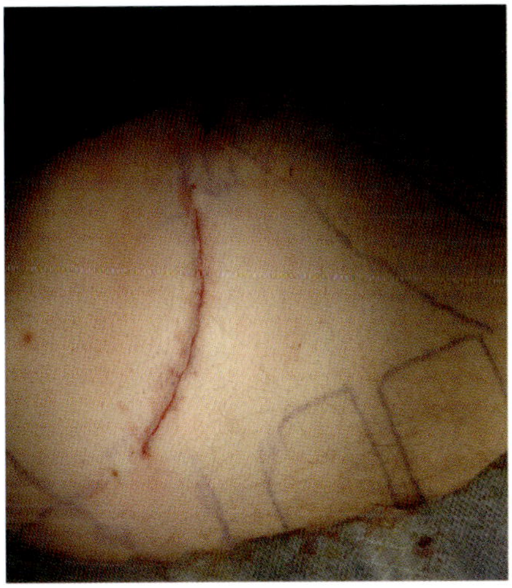

Fig. 15.5f Closure of donor site incision.

(g)

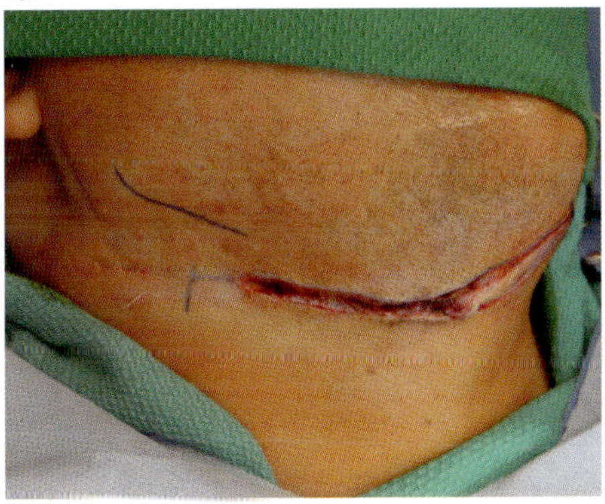

Fig. 15.5g Right submandibular incision through the pre-existing scar.

(h)

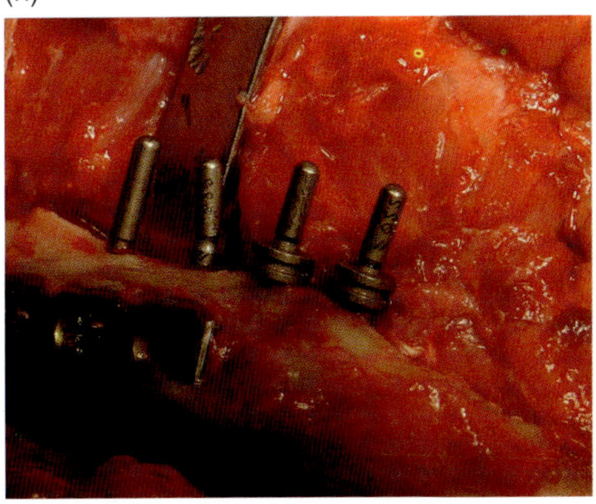

Fig. 15.5h Implant osteotomy preparation with submandibular soft tissue retracted upwards over the mandible. Note suctioning of bone particles from drilling site under irrigation.

(i)

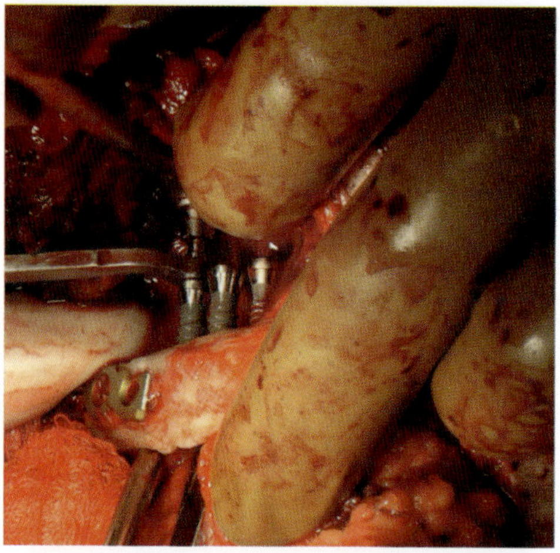

Fig. 15.5i Implants are inserted into basal bone up to junction of apical and middle thirds.

(j)

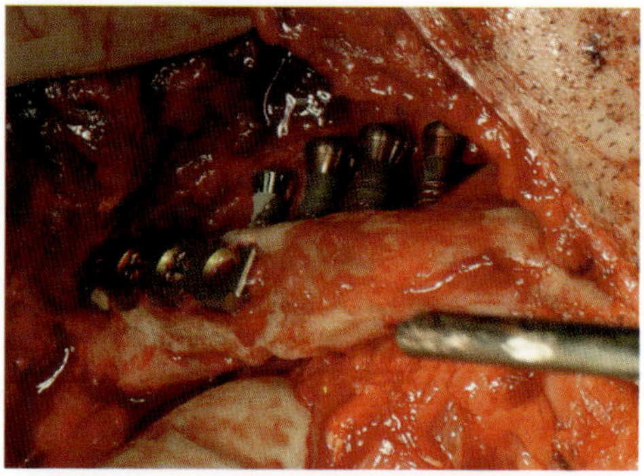

Fig. 15.5j Periosteum propped up by implants and healing caps.

(k)

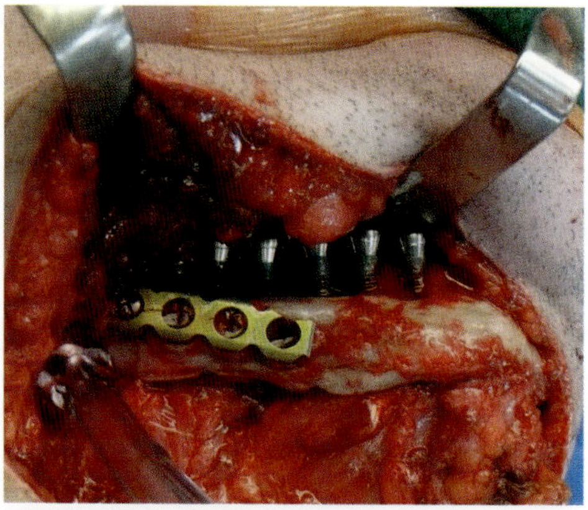

Fig. 15.5k Five standard SLA RN (Straumann Sand-Blasted Large Grit Acid Etched Regular Neck) dental implants with healing caps in fibular reconstruction.

(l)

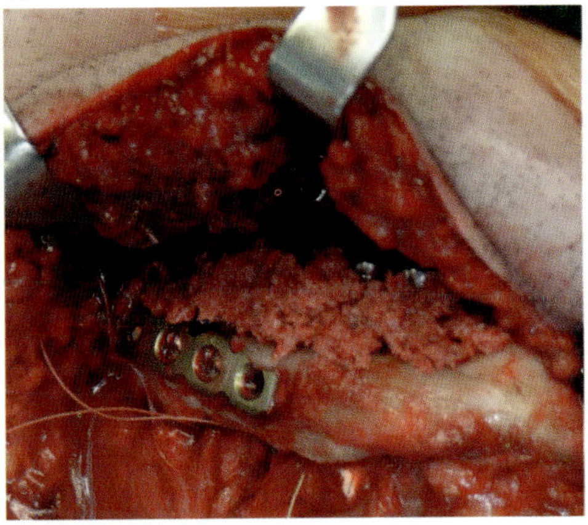

Fig. 15.5l Cancellous bone particles from the posterior iliac crest and implant osteotomies packed around dental implants in space created under propped up periosteum.

(m)

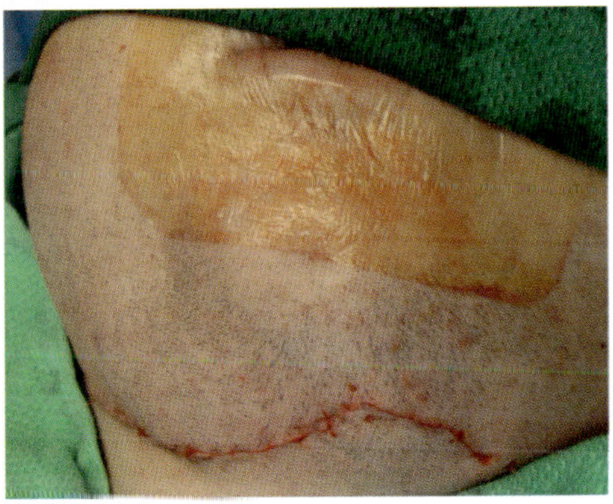

Fig. 15.5m Closure of the submandibular incision.

(n)

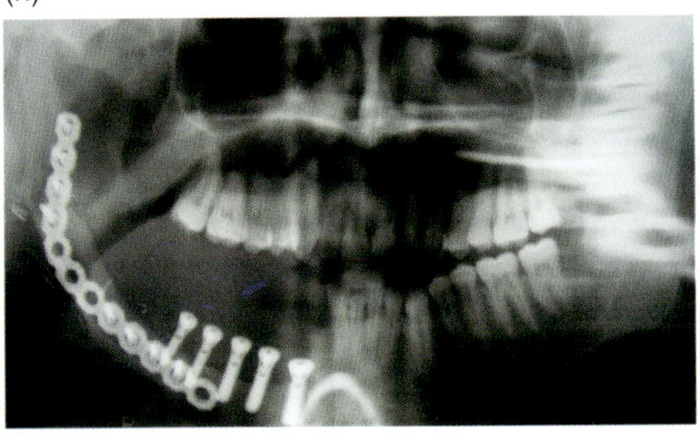

Fig. 15.5n Immediate post-operative panoramic tomograph showing implants and bone graft.

(o)

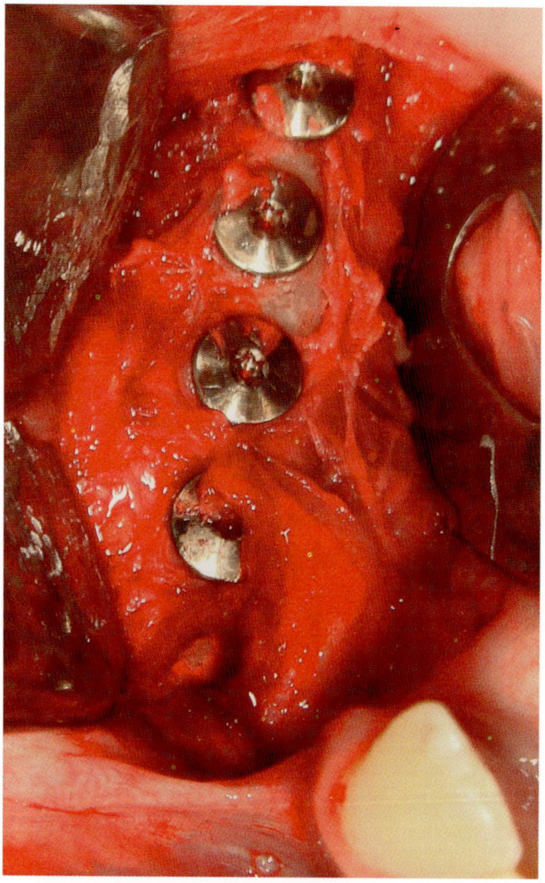

Fig. 15.5o Exposure of 2-mm healing caps through a crestal incision of the mucoperiosteum.

(p)

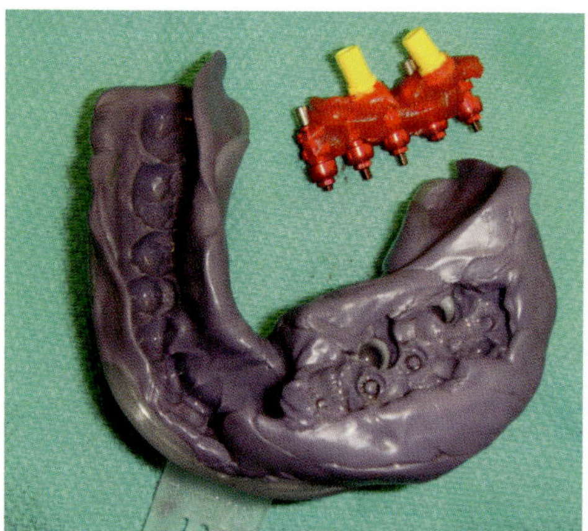

Fig. 15.5p Polyether impression and component assembly removed from mouth. Note the plastic impression caps embedded in impression.

(q)

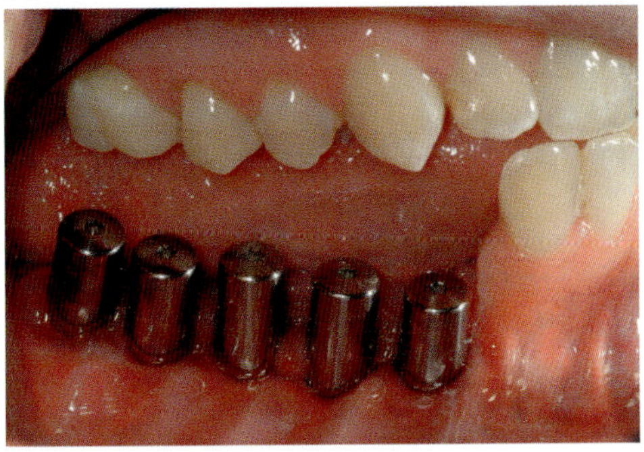

Fig. 15.5q Implants are sealed with 15-mm healing caps.

(r)

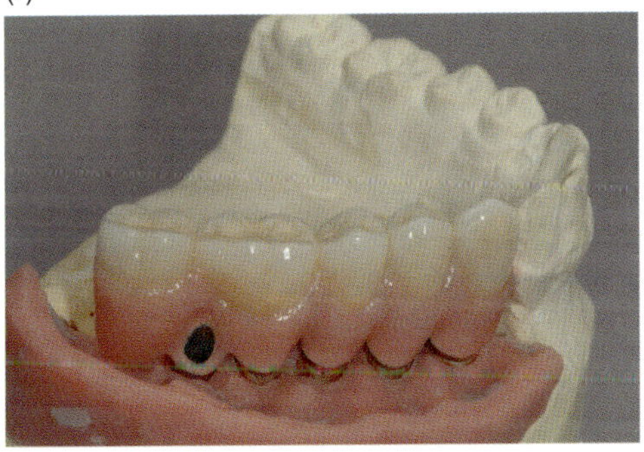

Fig. 15.5r Completed bridge on master cast, buccal view.

(s)

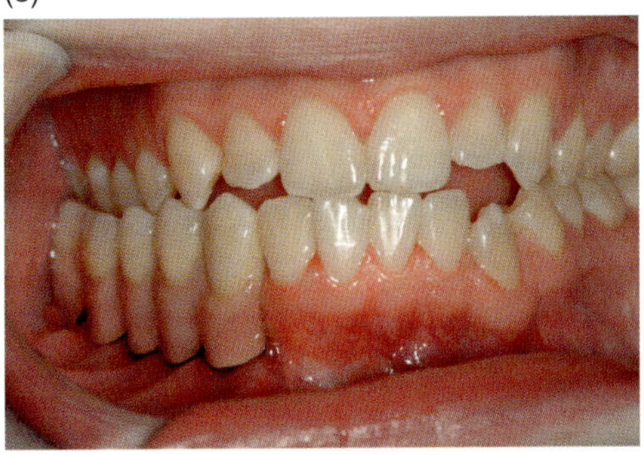

Fig. 15.5s Completed bridge in mouth, front view.

(a)

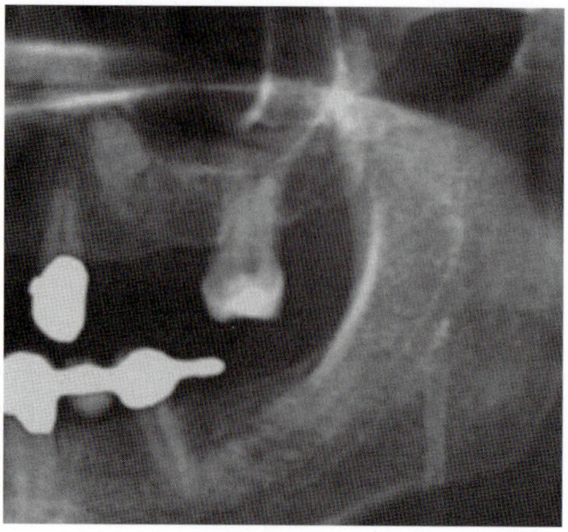

Fig. 15.6a Radiographc appearance of left maxillary sinus before implant placement using osteotome technique.

(b)

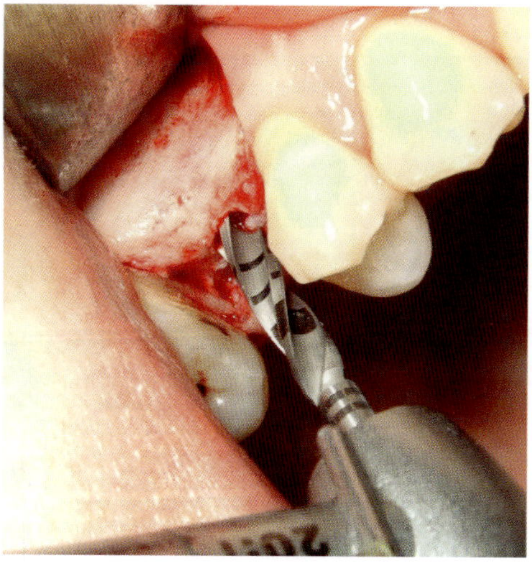

Fig. 15.6b Implant osteotomy site prepared to allow entry of sinus elevator.

(c)

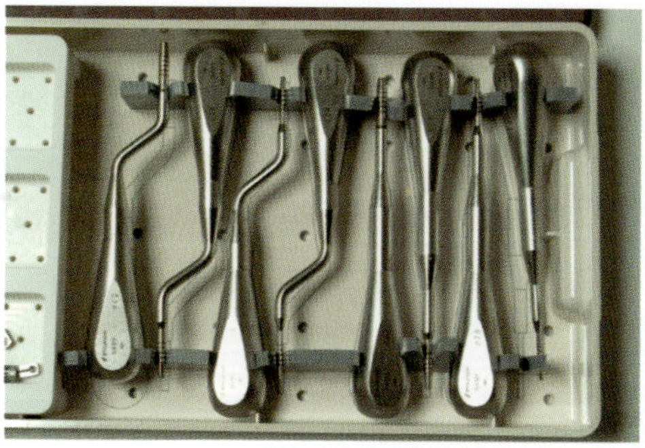

Fig. 15.6c Selection of sinus floor elevation instruments.

(d)

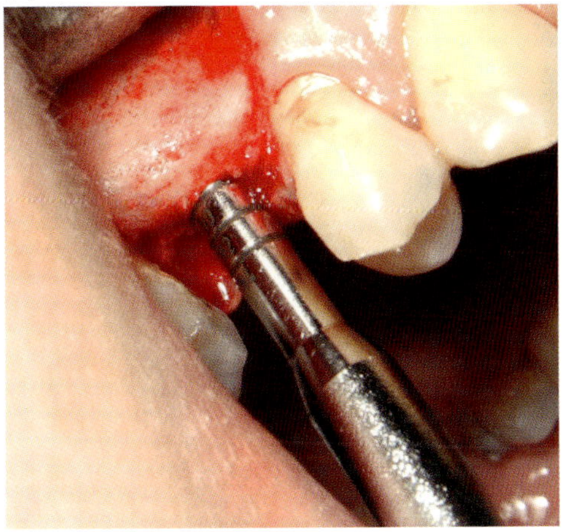

Fig. 15.6d Sinus elevator inserted into implant osteotomy site. Manual pressure or malleting can be used to fracture the maxillary sinus floor.

(e)

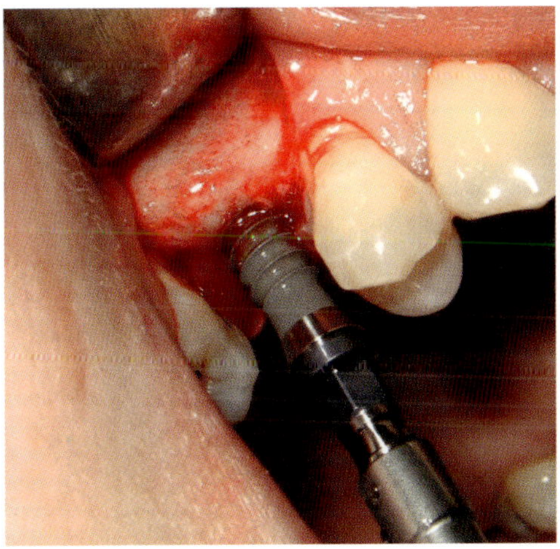

Fig. 15.6e Implant inserted into elevated sinus floor site.

(Summers 1994; Figs. 15.6f–j). Implants can be placed with an osteotome technique if there is at least 5 mm of bone height present (Jensen 1999). If the alveolar ridge has a VBH less than 5 mm, then primary stability of implants may not be achieved. Instead, implants could be placed in a delayed or second-stage surgery after graft remodeling is completed (Summers 1994; Jensen 1999). While these techniques have been used to regenerate lost bone, the factors that contribute to the survival rate of sinus augmentation and dental implant placement are still the subject of discussion. The recent literature concerning sinus grafts showed differing long-term results depending on which type of bone graft material was used (Ewers 2005). Moreover, it has been documented that there are no differences in implant survival

(f)

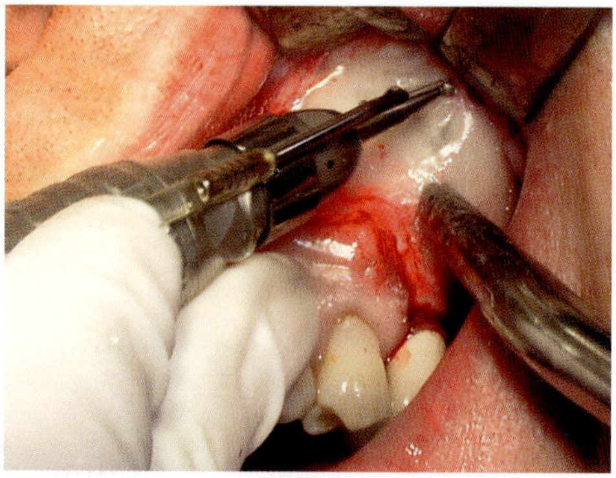

Fig. 15.6f Lateral approach outlining window for open sinus floor augmentation.

(g)

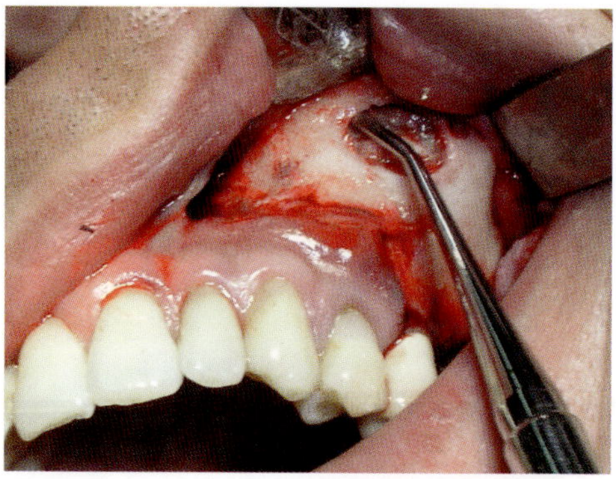

Fig. 15.6g Lateral maxillary infractured to allow access for open sinus floor augmentation.

(h)

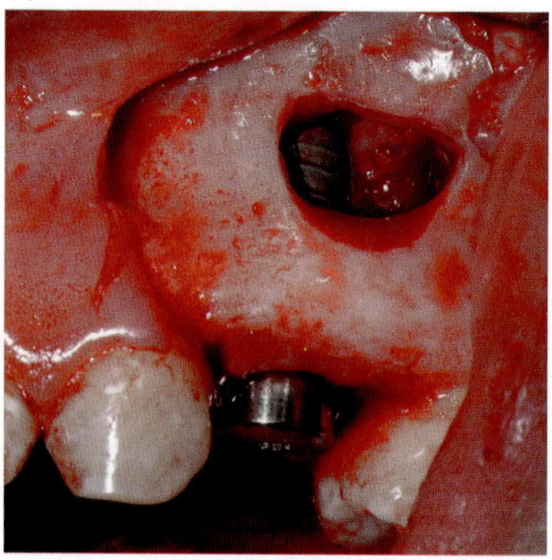

Fig. 15.6h Insertion of a dental implant fixture at same surgery as sinus floor augmentation.

(i)

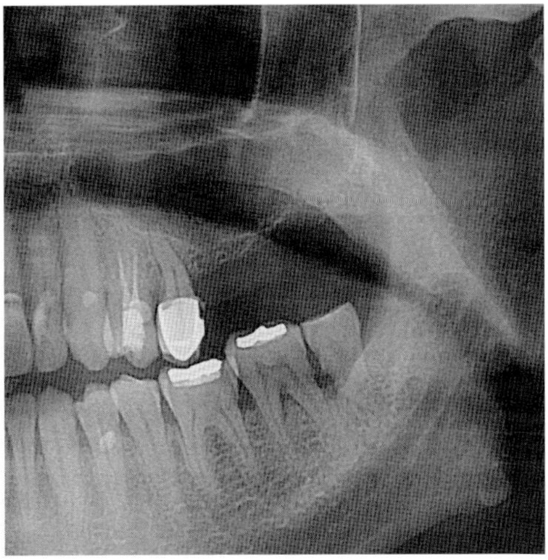

Fig. 15.6i Preoperative orthopantomogram showing well pneumatized sinus where there was too little bone to allow closed sinus floor elevation.

(j)

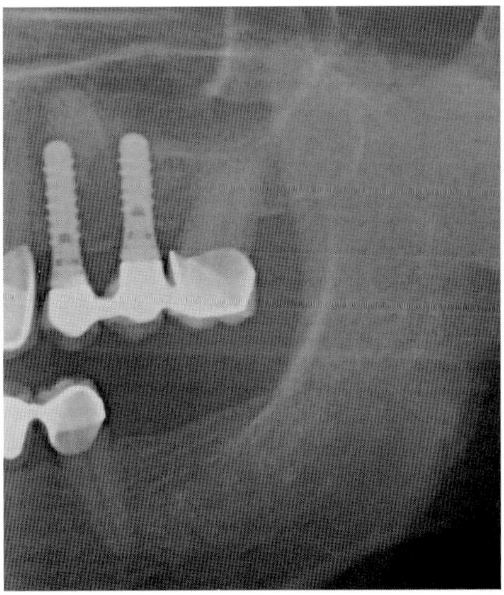

Fig. 15.6j Post-operative orthopantomogram showing two implants inserted with a concurrent open sinus floor elevation and bone grafting.

rates if either osteotome or lateral window technique with synchronous implant placement were performed (Fugazzotto and Vlassis 1998; Kahnberg et al. 2001; Jurisic et al. 2008).

Lateral ridge augmentation is the most commonly used method to augment a deficient mandibular alveolus in preparation for dental implant treatment today (Figs. 15.7a–d). Alveolar ridges in the maxilla which are deficient in the transverse dimension are augmented

(a)

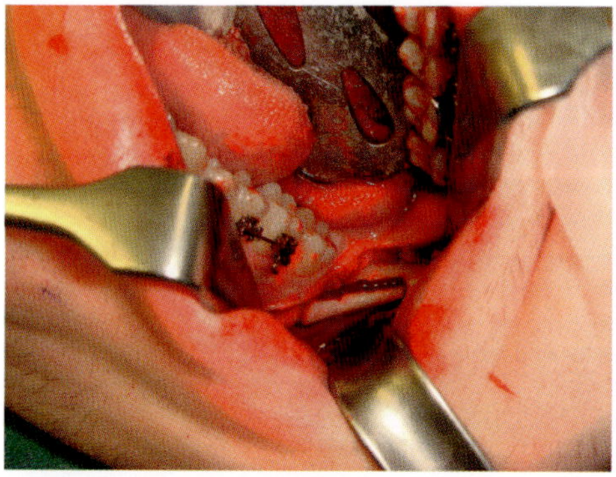

Fig. 15.7a Harvesting of a cortical strut of bone from the left lateral ramus of the mandible.

(b)

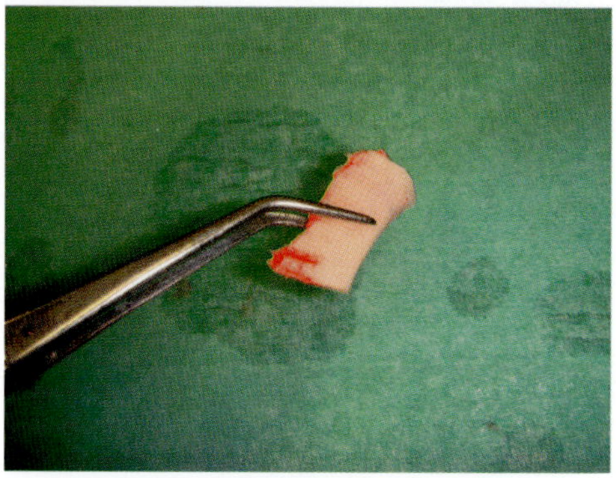

Fig. 15.7b Cortical bone graft perfect for lateral augmentation.

(c)

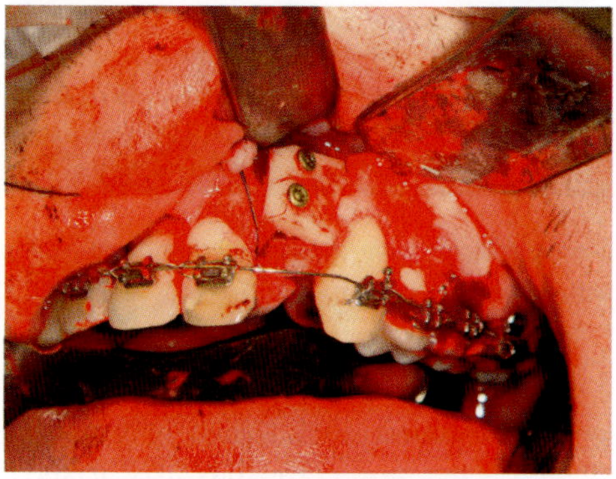

Fig. 15.7c Cortical bone graft secured with two intraosseous screws. The graft will be covered by a resorbable membrane before flap closure.

(d)

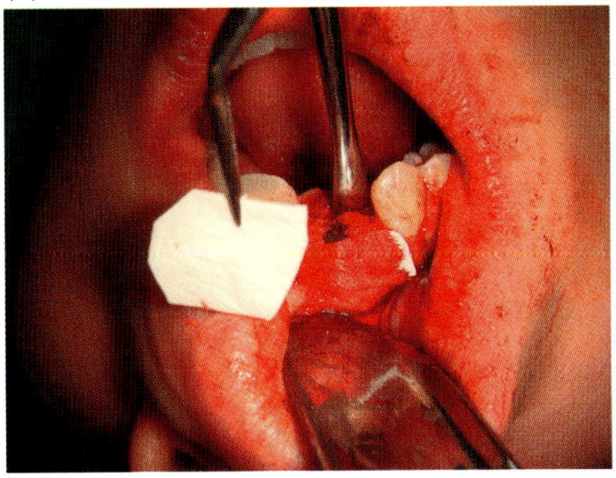

Fig. 15.7d Resorbable membranes placed in two layers to cover particulate bone graft in lateral augmentation procedure.

predictably with the placement of a bone graft and covered laterally with a resorbable membrane (Lindfors et al. 2010). Lateral ridge augmentation is stable with both block cortical and particulate bone grafts, whereas the results of vertical ridge augmentation tend to be unpredictable. Both non-resorbable membranes such as titanium reinforced polytetrafluoroethylene (PTFE) membranes and resorbable collagen membranes have been used (Bornstein et al. 2008).

Hyperbaric oxygen therapy (HBOT)

One maneuver surgeons have learned is to amplify the oxygen tension in a poorly vascularized wound to help promote healing. Some wounds are poorly vascularized due to excessive scarring or from repeated failed surgical attempts (Sándor et al. 2010). Radiation therapy also causes tissues in the irradiated field to become hypovascular. HBO can help in the healing of problem wounds in the dentofacial skeleton (Fok et al. 2008).

HBOT is defined as intermittent exposure to 100% oxygen under pressures greater than 1 absolute atmosphere (ATA). The concentration of oxygen in the atmosphere is 21%. At 1 ATA, the oxygen in blood is almost entirely carried by hemoglobin. Ninety five percent of oxygen carried in the arterial blood is chemically bound to hemoglobin while only 3% is dissolved in plasma. One gram of hemoglobin carries a maximum of 1.34 ml of oxygen. Fully saturated hemoglobin (100%) in 100 ml of blood carries approximately 20 ml of oxygen. Ninety seven percent saturated hemoglobin in 100 ml of blood carries 19.5 ml of oxygen. This amount is reduced to 5 ml of oxygen while passing through capillaries. Increasing the oxygen-carrying capacity of blood by increasing hemoglobin saturation is not possible (Jan et al. 2006).

At sea level, gas pressure is 760 mmHg or 1 ATA. Arterial hemoglobin saturation is 97%, while venous hemoglobin saturation is 70%. Inhalation of HBO increases the quantity of oxygen dissolved in plasma. At 1 ATA, the amount of dissolved oxygen in 100 ml of plasma is 0.449 ml. When inhaling 100% oxygen at 1 ATA, oxygen concentration increases to 1.5 ml/100 ml of plasma. When inhaling 100% oxygen at 3 ATA, the amount of dissolved oxygen in 100 ml of plasma increases to 6.422 ml/100 ml of plasma, which is enough to meet the basic metabolic needs of healing tissues in the human body (Jan et al. 2006, 2009, 2010; Fok et al. 2008).

The driving force for oxygen diffusion from the capillaries to tissues can be estimated by the difference between the partial pressure of oxygen on the arterial side and the venous side of the capillaries. The difference in the partial pressure of oxygen from the arterial side to the venous side of the capillary system is approximately 37 times greater when breathing 100% oxygen at 3 ATA than air at 1 ATA (Jan et al. 2006, 2009, 2010; Fok et al. 2008).

Distraction osteogenesis

Gradual periosteal stretching

Distraction osteogenesis involves osteotomy of a bone with minimal periosteal disruption and slow continuous traction on the ends of the osteotomized bone to produce a lengthening that is unsurpassed by standard osteotomy techniques. There is evidence that during this process bone and other tissues are formed to compensate for this lengthening. Some refer to this process as histiogenesis. Distraction osteogenesis actually recapitulates all the processes of embryonic bone formation to produce new bone without requiring a bone graft. The levels of growth factors such as BMPs, PDGF and VEGF are markedly elevated in the distraction regenerate.

The treatment of alveolar defects includes guided bone regeneration using a variety of membranes, onlay grafting of autogenous bone, connective tissue grafting and alloplastic augmentation. Vertical alveolar defects are difficult to overcome in a predictable manner using autogenous bone grafts and often lead to esthetic shortcomings (Simion et al. 2001; Belser et al. 2004). Distraction osteogenesis of the maxillary alveolus permits correction of alveolar defects oftentimes without the use of a bone graft.

Alveolar distraction osteogenesis (ADO) may offer several advantages over bone grafting alone in the treatment of vertical alveolar defects: no donor site is required; distraction of bone and surrounding soft tissue occurs simultaneously; the transport segment is a form of pedicled graft which is never separated from its blood supply, thus maximizing vitality and minimizing resorption; and it has the potential for better control of vertical height, esthetics and biomechanical loading (Clarizio 2002; Sándor et al. 2005).

Alveolar distraction devices have three basic components: an upper member, a distraction rod and a lower member/base plate supporting the vertical force of distraction. These devices can be classified as intra-osseous or extra-osseous; uni-, bi- or multi-directional; non-resorbable or resorbable (not requiring a second surgery to remove distractor components); and prosthetic (can remain in place to be used to support the dental prosthesis) or non-prosthetic (must be removed following distraction and replaced with a dental implant) (Chin and Toth 1996; Stucki-McCormick et al. 2002).

ADO is indicated for the treatment of alveolar defects where the alveolar processes are atrophic and deficient. ADO can also be used to correct vertical defects caused by ankylosis and submergence of primary teeth retained in the absence of succedaneous teeth (Fig. 15.1). ADO is contraindicated in severe atrophy where there is insufficient bone to allow safe hardware placement between tooth roots and the floor of the nose, the maxillary sinus or the inferior alveolar nerve. It may also be contraindicated in cases of severe osteoporosis where bone quality is poor, or in patients who are unlikely to demonstrate compliance with the rigors of the distraction process. This latter requirement in an adolescent patient may be the most important. ADO is a labor intensive technique with a significant transitional morbidity. Bone grafts may greatly simplify treatment and should always be considered as an alternative in young patients.

The first step in ADO is to plan the vector of distraction. A distractor is chosen that is capable of delivering a force in the direction of the chosen vector. If teeth are available to anchor a distraction device then an external tooth-borne device can be chosen (Figs. 15.8a and 8b); otherwise, an internal bone-borne device must be selected. The effect of the rigid palatal tissues and the lingual tissues on the vector of distraction should be kept in mind when distracting the maxilla or mandible. Palatal tissues tend to exert pull on the distracting segment causing it to tilt lingually away from the desired vector.

An incision is made either in the vestibule or at the crest of the alveolar process, and a mucoperiosteal flap is elevated. Vertical and horizontal osteotomies are performed through the labial or buccal cortical bone of the alveolus using a saw or a fine fissure bur (Figs. 15.8c–e). The device is then attached to the teeth flanking the partially osteotomized segment (Figs. 15.8d and e). The osteotomies are then completed by extending the cuts through the palatal cortical bone using osteotomes, and the segment is mobilized (Fig. 15.8e) to ensure that there are no bony or dental interferences to unrestricted transport along the selected vector of distraction. The wound is then closed.

(a)

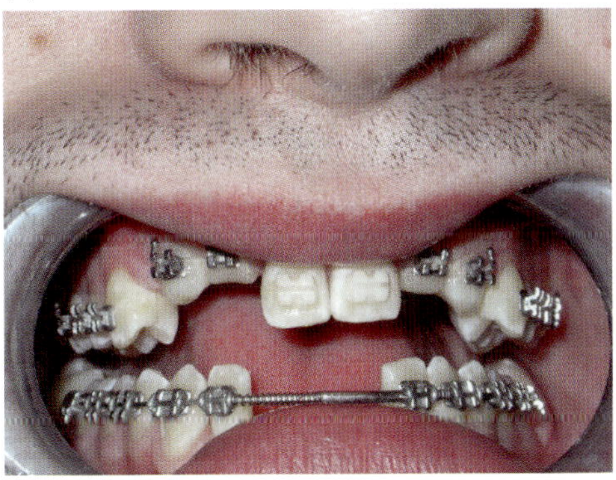

Fig. 15.8a Oligodontia patient with ankylosed deciduous maxillary lateral incisors and canine teeth. Note the vertical hypodevelopment of the maxillary alveolus due to the ankylosed teeth.

(b)

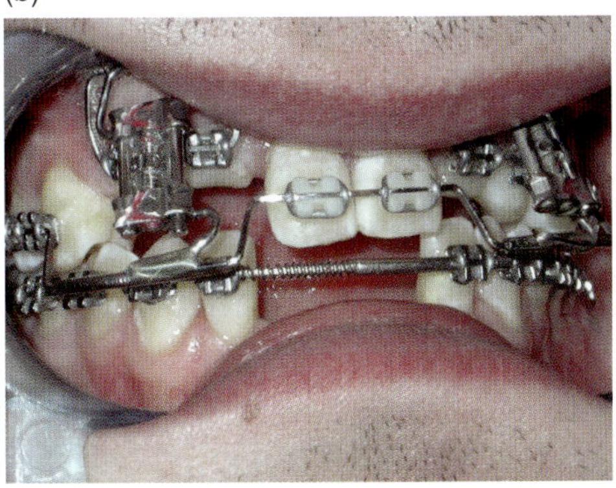

Fig. 15.8b Distraction hardware attached to the ankylosed deciduous teeth bilaterally.

(c)

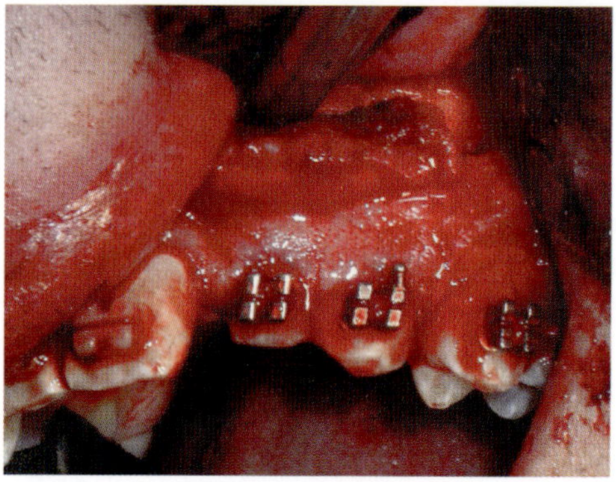

Fig. 15.8c Hardware removed and segmental osteotomy performed bilaterally to enable a two tooth segment with the deciduous teeth to move downwards vertically.

(d)

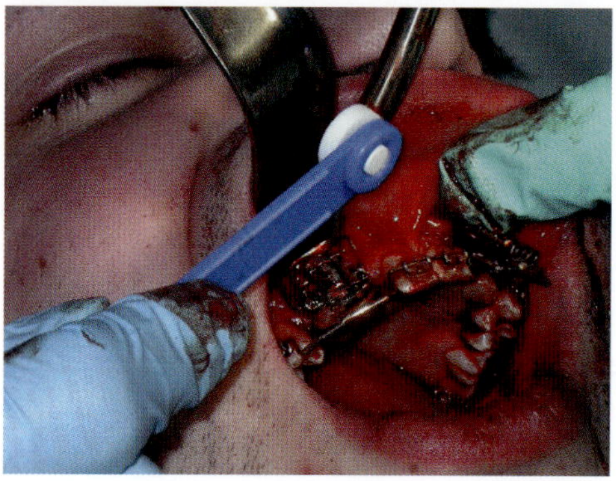

Fig. 15.8d Hardware reattached and device is activated.

(e)

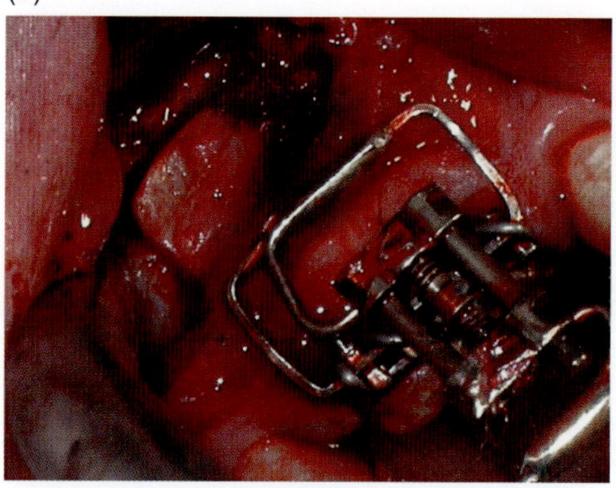

Fig. 15.8e Note the gap between the distracted segment and the superior aspect of the maxilla.

After a 5- to 7-day latency period the segment is distracted once or twice daily at a rate of 0.5–1.0 mm per day until the desired bony position is attained. Overdistraction of the segment by 1–2 mm may minimize relapse. A consolidation phase of 6–12 weeks with the distractor in place allows undisturbed healing of the distracted bone to occur. If teeth are present in a configuration which, when united by fixed orthodontic appliances, can facilitate stabilization of the segment, then the distractor can be removed. Fixed orthodontic appliances should be worn for the duration of the consolidation phase (Figs. 15.8f–h). At some point following the consolidation phase, all metal distractors must be removed, unless they are resorbable. If ankylosed teeth were used for anchorage of the distraction segment, they are extracted following the removal of the distraction hardware (Fig. 15.8h). Dental implants can then be placed into the distracted alveolar segment and restored in their new ideal position (Figs. 15.8i and j).

(f)

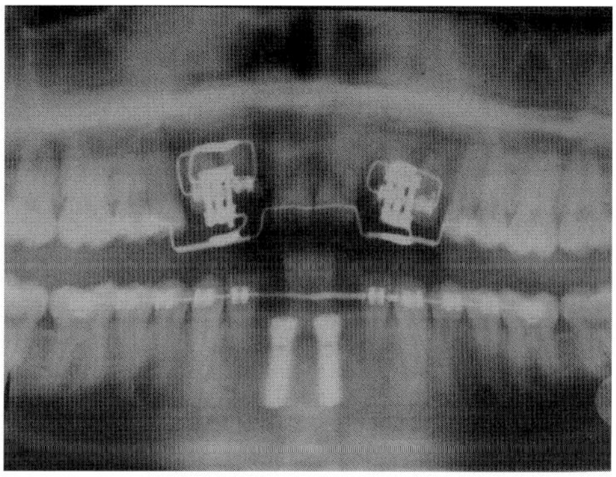

Fig. 15.8f Immediate post-operative orthopantomogram.

(g)

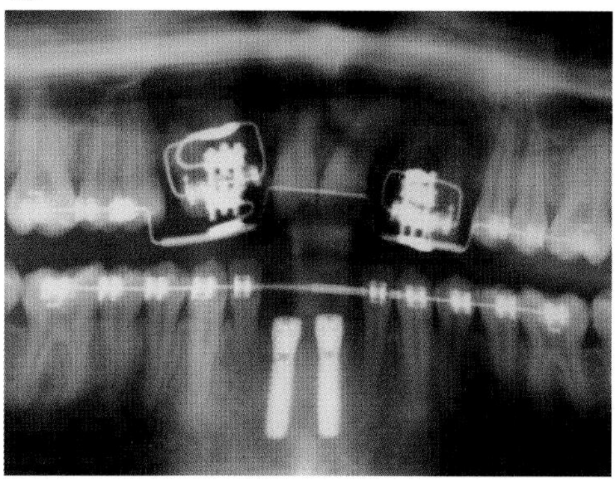

Fig. 15.8g Orthopantomogram at the end of distraction.

(h)

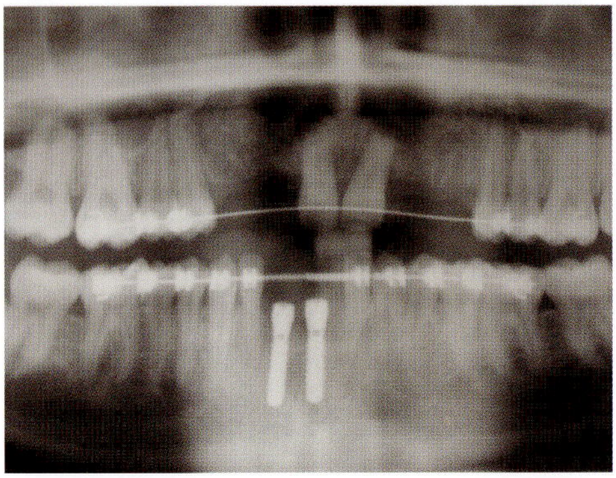

Fig. 15.8h Orthopantomogram in retention phase following extraction of the expendable ankylosed deciduous teeth.

(i)

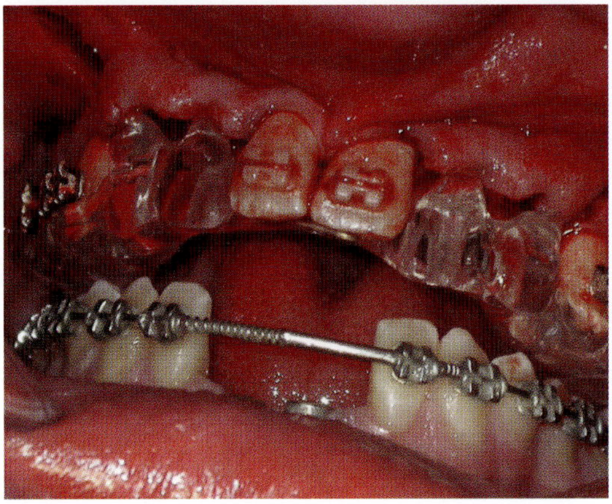

Fig. 15.8i Stent to guide implant placement.

(j)

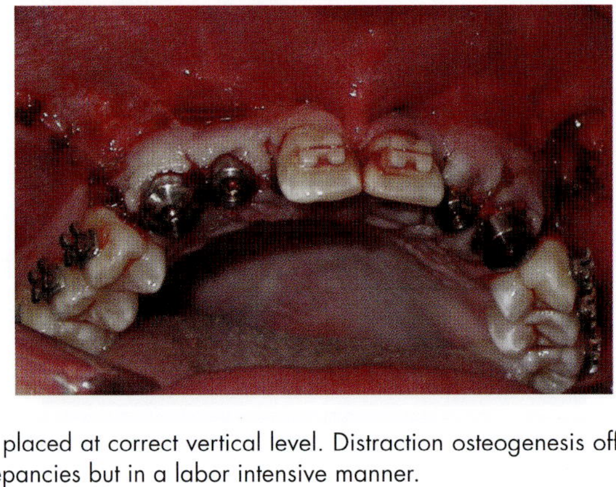

Fig. 15.8j Implants placed at correct vertical level. Distraction osteogenesis offers a method to correct vertical alveolar discrepancies but in a labor intensive manner.

The distracting dental implant

There are clear advantages to having a device that can be used to correct a vertical bony defect by distraction osteogenesis and which can also serve as the anchor for a prosthesis following completion of the distraction. Such an intra-osseous, prosthetic distraction device with completely internalized components is presently in the preclinical stage of development (Figs. 15.8k and l). The distracting implant comprising a fixture connected to a footing by means of a retaining screw is placed within the bone. When the assembly is completely

(k)

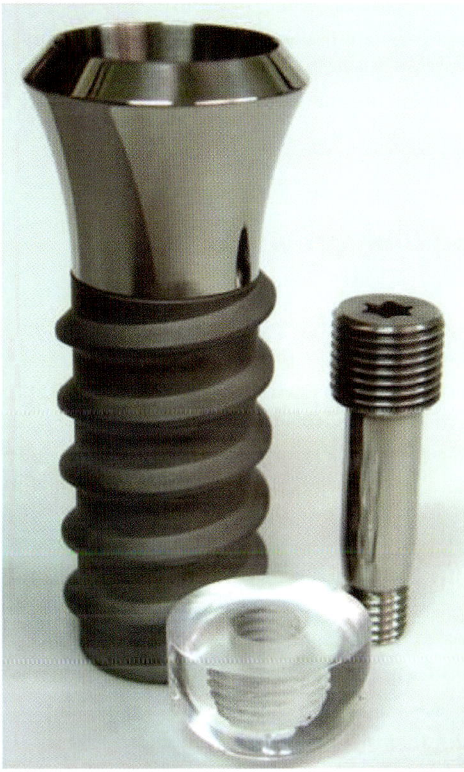

Fig. 15.8k Distracting dental implant.

(l)

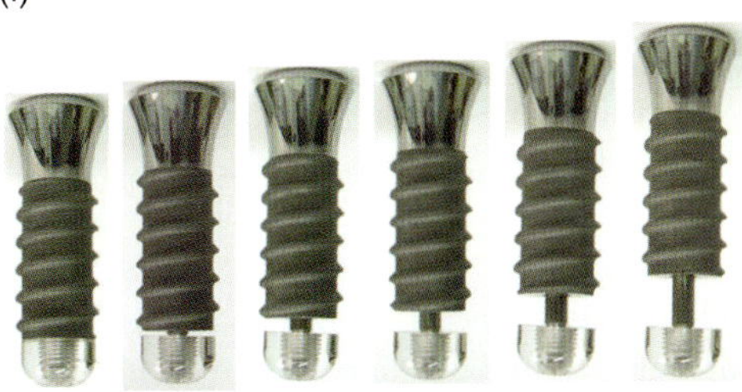

Fig. 15.8l Distracting dental implant in series as it distracts.

installed, the proximal surface of the footing bears against the bottom of the osteotomy. Following the completion of the distraction process, the distracting dental implant is used to support a dental prosthesis.

Guidance of implant placement

Although the distracting dental implant is a unidirectional distraction device, its trajectory can be guided to a certain extent using orthodontic forces or a prosthodontic docking station. A further consequence of the unidirectional nature of the distracting dental implant is that the vector of distraction will be defined primarily by the implant's longitudinal axis. To a certain extent, the geometry of the corticotomy can be designed to counter-pull from the lingual or palatal mucoperiosteum. As the trajectory of the distracting implant depends substantially on the vector of distraction, it is of critical importance to have control over the spatial location and axial inclination of the implant. An implant positioning device with the capability to control spatial location and axial inclination is currently under development.

Tissue engineering with growth factors BMPs and VEGF

With the constraints of both autogenous bone and allogeneic bone, scientists have focused on the fabrication of completely synthetic bioimplants. By the late 1980s the active factor responsible for the induction of bone was identified, bone morphgenetic protein (BMP). BMP is regarded as a morphogen, a protein that replicates the embryonic induction of bone formation (Urist et al. 1983). BMP can induce pluripotent mesenchymal stem cells to differentiate into bone-forming osteoblasts. BMP-2, 4 and 7 have been shown to stimulate *de novo*, *in vitro* and *in vivo* bone formation in various animal models. Currently, there are many BMPs that have been isolated, and with the exception of BMP-1, they are all members of the TGF-β superfamily (Clokie et al. 2002). In the early 1990s the ability to fabricate these proteins synthetically using recombinant technology was developed, and in 2006 this lead finally to the development products OP-1 (BMP-7; Stryker, Allendale, New Jersey, USA) and Infuse (BMP-2; Medtronic, Fridley, Minnesota, USA), both of which are now available for clinical use (Moghadam et al. 2004).

It has become apparent that one of the greatest challenges to the clinical application of BMP has been the identification of an acceptable carrier. Investigations of various delivery agents have identified certain ones as being more effective for the optimal clinical application of BMP. Over the past decade our group has explored the use of a reverse phase block medium as a carrier for BMP, and while others have struggled to achieve acceptable clinical results, our first BMP bioimplant was successfully made in 1999. Since that time our group has reconstructed ten human mandibular defects using bioimplants consisting of OP-1 (BMP-7; Stryker Biotech, Allendale, New Jersey, USA) and DynaGraft Putty (DBM in a reverse phased medium; IsoTis, Irvine, California, USA) (Clokie and Sándor 2008).

The BMP bioimplant was created by manually mixing BMP-7 (OP-1; Stryker Biotech, Allendale, New Jersey, USA) with 10 cc of DBM in a reverse phased medium (DynaGRaft Putty, IsoTis, Irvine, California, USA) and then molding it to form the shape of the resected segment of mandible (Figs. 15.9a–e). This was then inserted into the defect in the mandible

(a)

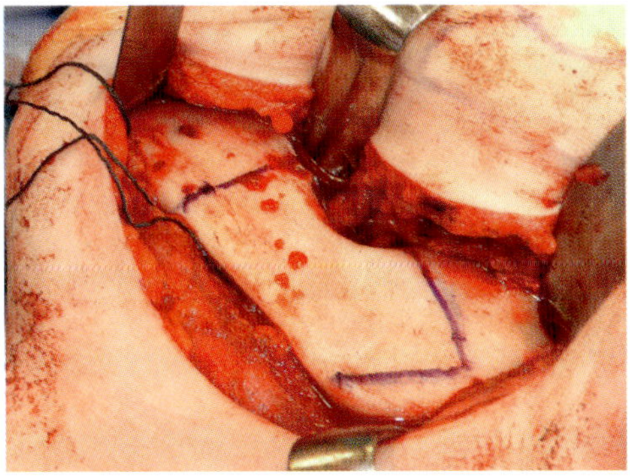

Fig. 15.9a Mandibular resection to treat ameloblastoma.

(b)

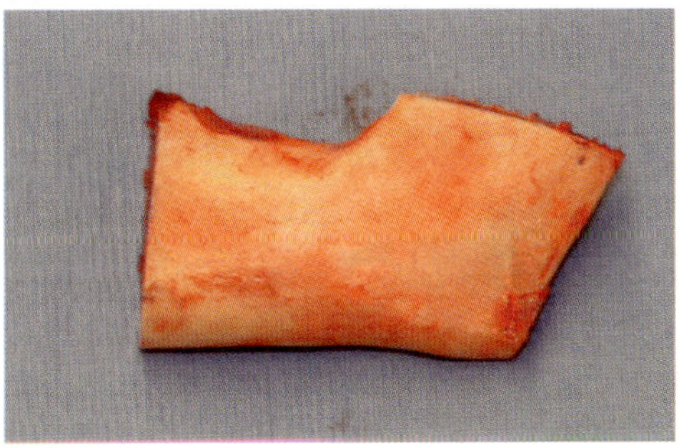

Fig. 15.9b Resected mandibular fragment.

(c)

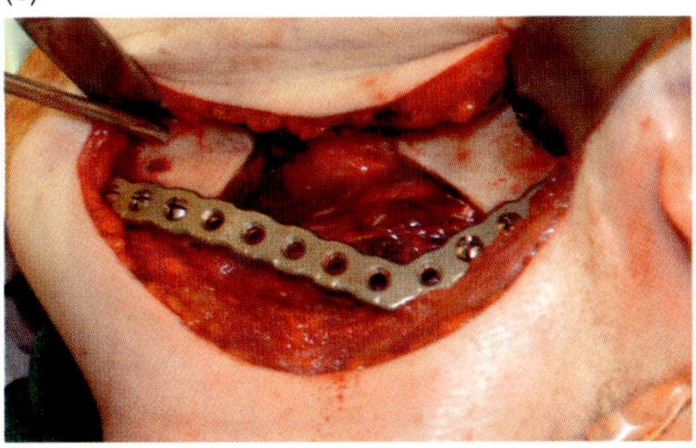

Fig. 15.9c Gap caused by resection is larger than a critical-sized defect and will not heal without some osteogenic intervention.

(d)

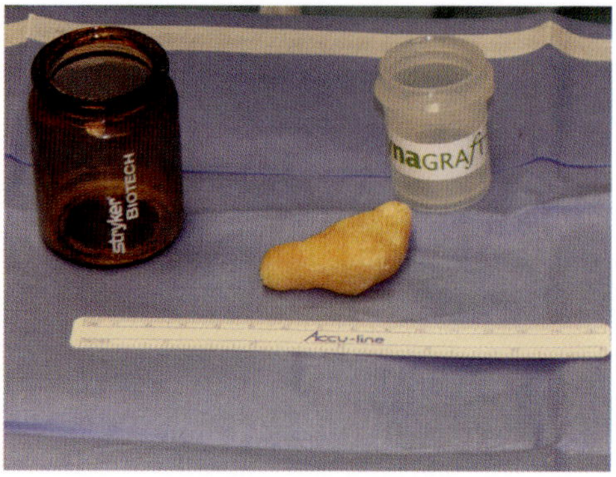

Fig. 15.9d Demineralized bone matrix mixed with BMP-7 to form osteogenic bioimplant.

(e)

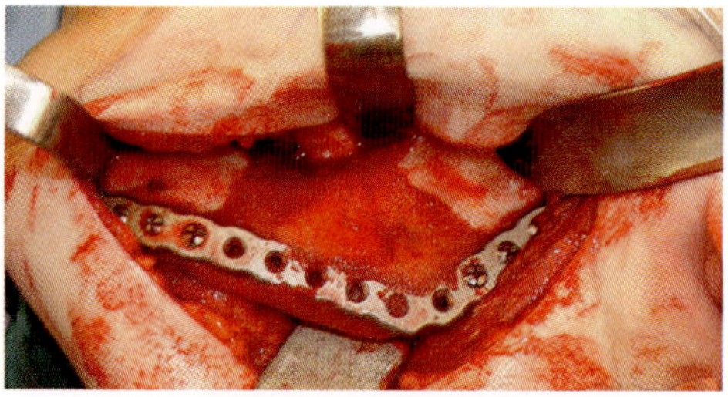

Fig. 15.9e Construct placed into wound and surrounded by muscle tissue in the closure of the wound.

(f)

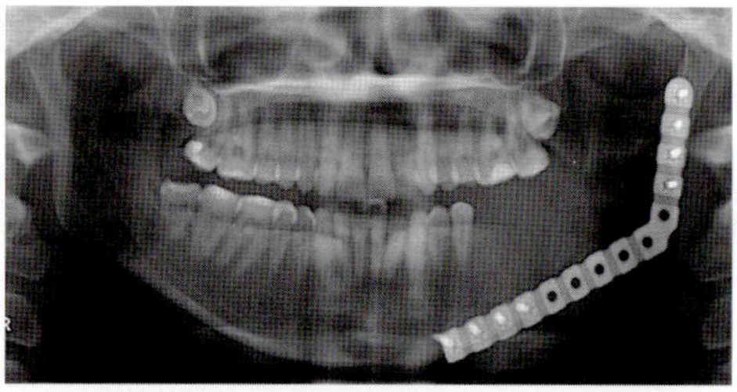

Fig. 15.9f Post resection radiograph.

and the muscular sling surrounding the mandible was re-approximated to ensure complete coverage of the bioimplant (Fig. 15.9e). The superficial tissues were then closed in a traditional fashion. Patients were carefully followed both clinically and radiographically to ensure proper integration of the bioimplant with the mandible (Fig. 15.9f).

Tissue engineering with stem cells and growth factors

Interdependency exists between adipogenesis, the formation of fat tissue from stem cells, and osteogenesis, the formation of bone from its stem cell precursors. Adipose-derived adult mesenchymal stem cells may be useful in future bone regeneration and tissue engineering efforts. We will now discusses possible future relationships between autogenous adipose-derived stem cells, growth factors and resorbable scaffolds in the context of future tissue engineering efforts.

The field of tissue engineering

Tissue engineering efforts include the vital collaboration between cell biologists, biochemists, material scientists, engineers and clinicians. In order to understand the complex role of the various components of tissue engineering, one can consider an equilateral triangle where stem cells, resorbable scaffolds and bioactive molecules such as growth factors continuously interact with each other (Fig. 15.3). It is the understanding of the nature of the interactions between these three key components that tissue engineering is built upon.

Sources of stem cells

The source of cells for tissue engineering depends on the structure that is to be replaced. Human embryonic stem cells (hESC) are pluripotent stem cells isolated from the inner mass of human blastocysts. While these cells have great potential due to their differentiation capacity, there are problems that must be solved prior to their clinical use in tissue engineering. The problems with hESC include culturing hESC without exposure to animal proteins, avoidance of teratoma development and immune rejection by the recipient host (Grinnemo et al. 2008). For the present time it is adult stem cells that are used clinically. Those cells with the lowest morbidity in harvesting and those that still retain a degree of pluripotentiality would be the most advantageous in the tissue engineering of bone, for example.

One source of mesenchymal stem cells (MSC) for bone regeneration is adipose tissue to provide adipose-derived stem cells (ASC). This should not be surprising as there is interdependency between adipogenesis and osteogenesis (Gimble et al. 2006). Certainly the harvesting of adipose tissue is not morbid and may even be advantageous for some if liposuction were used as the harvesting method (Figs. 15.10a and b).

Stimulating stem cells

Using the tissue engineering model, autogenous ASCs could be harvested from a patient having a liposuction procedure and used to seed a resorbable scaffold (Suuronen and Asikainen 2004) which was made using CAD/CAM technology to the precise dimensions of a missing segment of bone, for example. The seeded cells could be stimulated by physical means using vibration (Tirkkonen et al. 2011), magnetic, galvanic, ultrasound or laser stimulation, along with hypoxic or hyperoxic gradients (Sándor et al. 2010) or growth factors such as TGF-β1 (Clokie and Bell 2003) or the BMPs (Hu et al. 2005) to guide the differentiation and growth of the cells. In some cases the surface configuration of a particular scaffold may stimulate stem cells to differentiate in a certain direction. Bioactive glasses, for example, are known to cause mesenchymal stem cells to differentiate into osteoblasts.

(a)

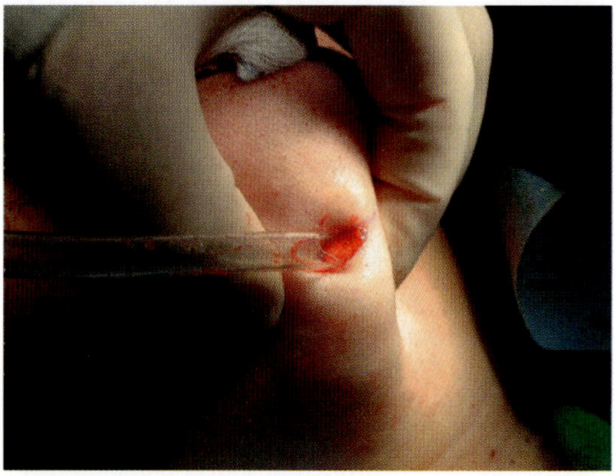

Fig. 15.10a Liposuction is one convenient and minimally morbid way of harvesting adipose-derived stem cells for cell culturing and tissue engineering purposes.

(b)

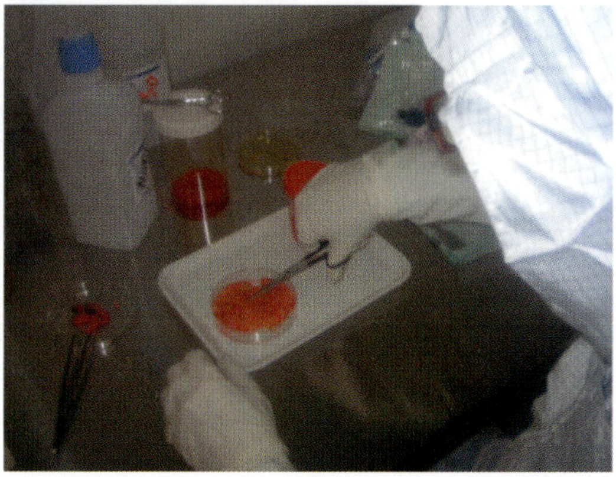

Fig. 15.10b Fat cells are isolated in the laboratory and mesenchymal stem cells are grown out in culture.

Manipulating the construct

Once the cells have populated the scaffold (Figs. 15.10c and d), the resulting bioimplant or construct could be transplanted into the patient to restore the defect. This *ex vivo* derived reconstruction has one major obstacle. The vitality of the bioimplant is entirely dependent upon the vascularity of the recipient bed. To this end, growth factors such as VEGF could be used to stimulate angiogenesis (Marx et al. 1998) to help vascularize the construct.

Future directions

Another source of stem cells could be from suction trap aspirates of bone during mandibular third molar removal (Lindholm et al. 2003; Mesimäki et al. 2009). This technique would allow stem cell harvesting during one of the most common oral surgical procedures

(c)

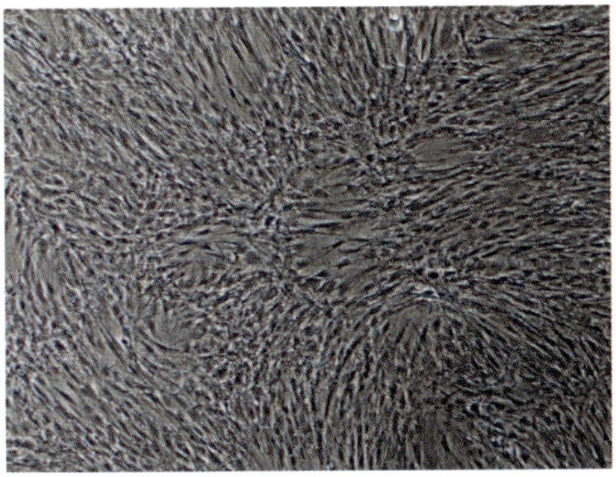

Fig. 15.10c The appearance of adipose-derived stem cells grown in cell culture. These cells can be frozen for storage and later usage.

(d)

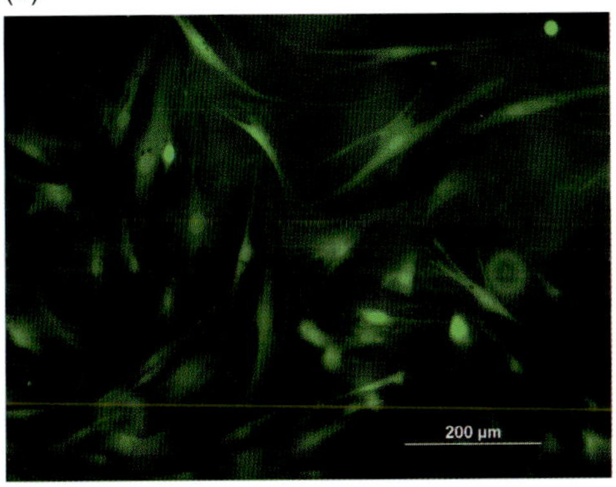

Fig. 15.10d Live/dead staining of adipose stem cells attached onto a scaffold of resorbable biomaterial fibers (3 hour time point). Scale 200 μM. Green cells are viable.

performed today. Third molar removal also presents some new opportunities. The removed developing third molar follicle can yield follicular cells, cementoblast-like cells and dental pulp stem cells which can also be cultured and studied. The receptors of these cells can be characterized and this is an important first step in the understanding of these cells and their possible future utilization.

SPECIFICALLY DIFFICULT WOUNDS

Maxillectomy cavities

The incidence of oral cancer increases with age in all parts of the world. In Western countries 98% of the patients are over 40 years of age (Llewellyn et al. 2001). In high prevalence areas of the world many of the patients are less than 35 years of age owing to heavy usage of various forms of tobacco. There has been an alarming rise in the incidence of oral cancer during the last three decades particularly among younger men, and the trend appears to be continuing (Llewellyn et al. 2001).

Squamous cell carcinoma of the oral cavity is rare in pediatric patients. The tongue and lower lip are the most frequently reported sites (Thompson et al. 1999). In this chapter we illustrate a rare case of a squamous cell carcinoma of the maxillary gingiva in a 10-year-old female who was treated and reconstructed by a multidisciplinary team.

Such malignant tumors require clear surgical margins for survival. Maxillectomy defects often involve multiple missing teeth, alveolar bone, and attached and alveolar mucosa and may have large openings or fistulae connecting the mouth with the nasal cavity or maxillary sinus. Such wounds are challenging to manage.

The management of a maxillectomy defect is illustrated in the following case of a 10-year-old female (Figs. 15.11a–g) who underwent a left partial maxillectomy via an intraoral approach with a left elective supraomohyoid neck dissection. The intraoral defect was packed with iodine-impregnated gauze and immediately reconstructed with a prefabricated obturator which was secured in position using palatal screws. The goal of the obturator was to allow healing of the tissues remaining in the maxillectomy defect by granulation or

(a)

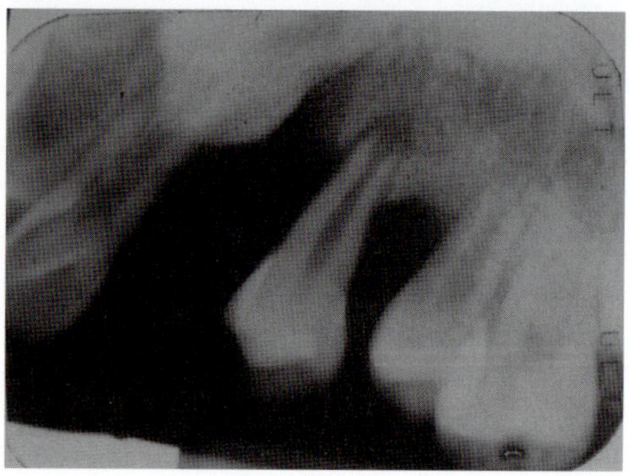

Fig. 15.11a Ten-year-old female with radiographic image of aggressive bone destruction due to a squamous cell carcinoma of the maxillary alveolus.

(b)

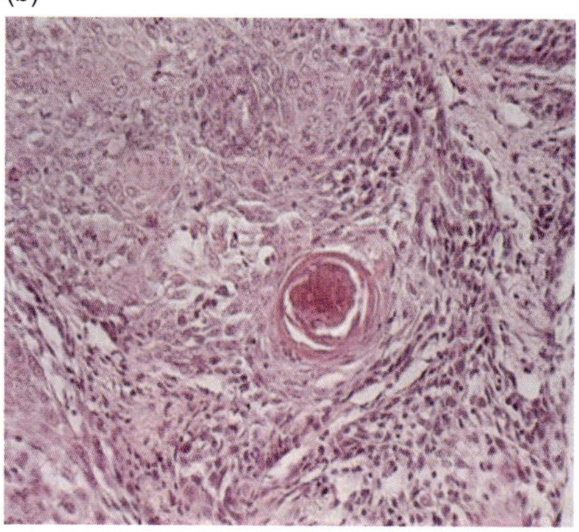

Fig. 15.11b Histologic appearance of well differentiated squamous cell carcinoma.

(c)

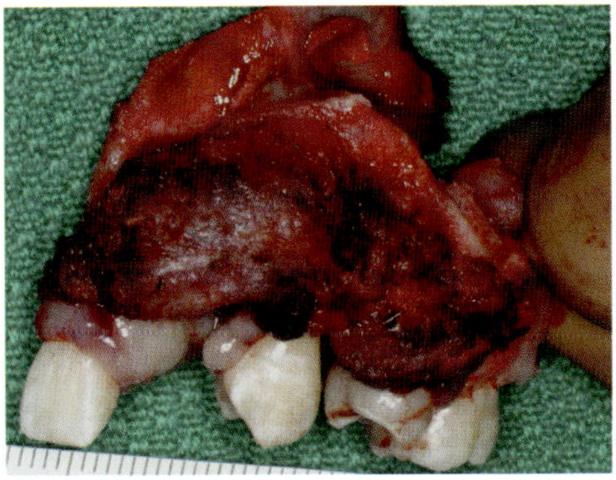

Fig. 15.11c Maxillary resection specimen with clear margins resulting in large dentofacial defect with significant oral antral fistula.

(d)

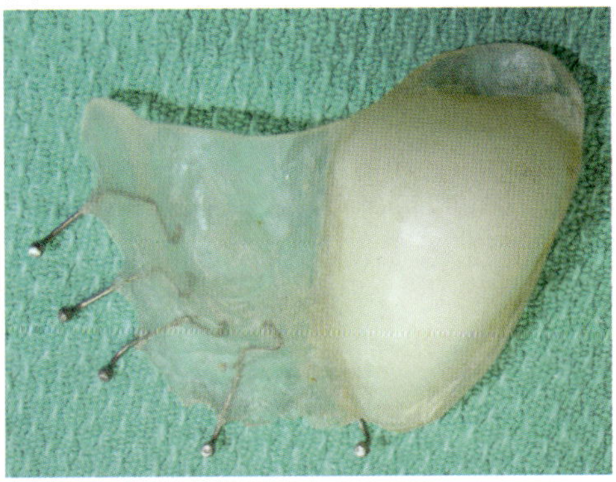

Fig. 15.11d Temporary obturator made pre-operatively.

(e)

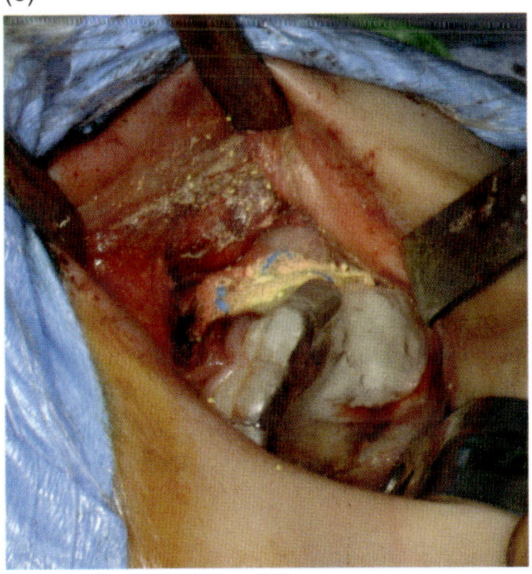

Fig. 15.11e Obturator inserted with iodine-impregnated gauze packing to obdurate oral antral fistula and encourage healing by secondary intention.

(f)

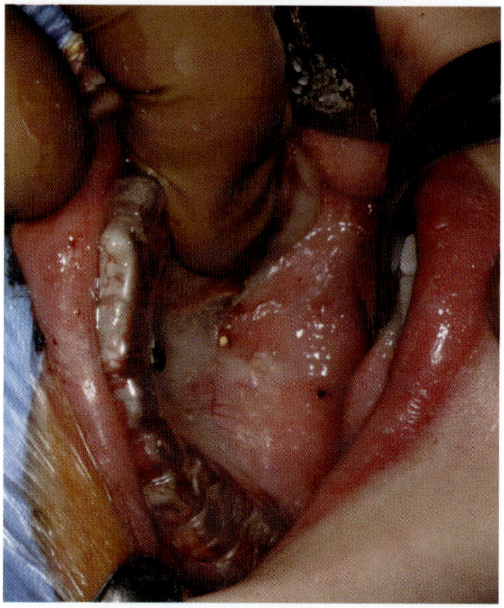

Fig. 15.11f Obturator secured with palatal transosseous screw to retain obturator, facilitating swallowing without nasal regurgitation of food and making speech more intelligible.

(g)

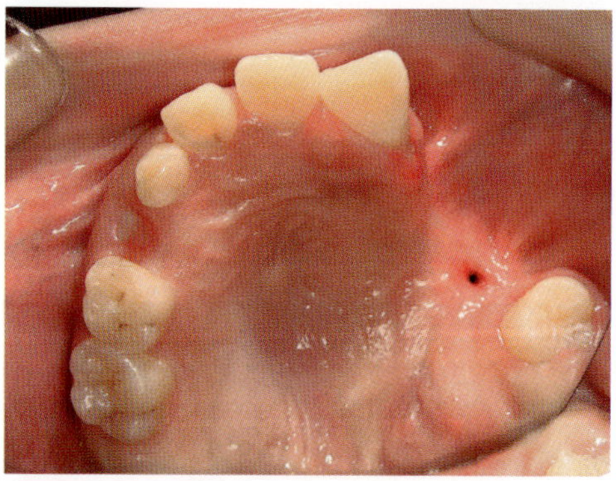

Fig. 15.11g Maxillectomy defect in healed state with pinhole oral antral fistula.

secondary intention. The obturator also minimizes the impact of large oronasal and oral antral fistulae by separating the oral and nasal cavities. This makes speech much more intelligible and aids in swallowing as well.

The surgical specimen demonstrated an invasive squamous cell carcinoma with negative margins. None of the lymph nodes from the neck dissection specimen showed any evidence of metastatic disease. The obturator and packing were removed 2 weeks post surgery and a hollow obturator ultimately bearing prosthetic teeth was inserted. Such obturators form the backbone of prosthetic reconstruction. Future options for the patient include prosthetic reconstruction versus a vascularized tissue transfer with dental implants. In the long term the teeth adjacent to the borders of the resection are prone to periodontal tissue loss and failure.

Wound infections necrotizing fasciitis

Necrotizing fasciitis (NF) is a rapidly spreading-life threatening infection involving the superficial fat and fascial layers with necrosis of the overlying skin. The lesion was first described during the American Civil War (Chattar-Cora et al. 2002) and has been reported extensively in the general surgery literature. It is most common in the perineum, abdominal wall and extremities. It is most often seen in the elderly and immunocompromised patients (Mohammedi et al. 1999). NF is less common in the head and neck, especially in the face. This rare infection (Shindo et al. 1997) can result from dental, (Stoykewych et al. 1992; Dale et al. 1999; Umeda et al. 2003) sinus (Raboso et al. 1998), peritonsillar (Hadfield et al. 1996; Skitarelic et al. 1999) and salivary gland (Marioni et al. 2003) infections or secondary to surgery (Feinerman et al. 1999) or trauma (Shindo et al. 1997). The causative agents have classically been described as group A beta-hemolytic streptococci and staphylococci, and also include obligate anerobic bacteria (Banerjee et al. 1996; Umeda et al. 2003). If not promptly recognized and treated the infection may spread into the deep spaces of the neck and compromise the airway, as well as spreading into the mediastinum, producing life-threatening sepsis. Such wounds require extreme measures.

The management of NF is illustrated by the following case: a 57-year-old female with a moderate right buccal space infection with right submandibular involvement secondary to grossly decayed tooth numbers 46 and 47. The parapharyngeal spaces were clear and there was no airway compromise. The patient was admitted for intravenous antibiotics, observation and analgesia. Unfortunately on the night of her admission, she pulled out her intravenous catheter and discharged herself from the hospital against medical advice (AMA). Multiple attempts at contacting her were unsuccessful.

Five days later, she returned to the emergency department with marked deterioration. She appeared toxic, was febrile and tachycardic. There was a large necrotic region on the right cheek extending from the zygomatic arch superiorly to below the mandible inferiorly (Fig. 15.12a). There was severe right temporal, bilateral submandibular, cervical and floor of the mouth swelling.

The skin appeared grossly abnormal, with a spectrum of findings ranging from erythema, patchy areas of bullae to frank necrosis. There was marked crepitus noted from the zygomatic region to the laryngeal cartilages in the neck. The patient was taken to the operating room for immediate endotracheal intubation which was performed uneventfully. An emergent CT scan was obtained after the airway was secure and revealed the presence of severe subcutaneous gas formation and marked generalized head and neck edema (Fig. 15.12b).

The patient was taken to the operating room where immediate complete debridement of all necrotic tissue was performed until bleeding tissue was encountered. The areas of debridement needed to be extended throughout the operation as the zones of involvement and necrosis were seen to extend and increase during the surgery (Figs. 15.12c and d). Clindamycin 900 mg iv q 8 h was started following an intra-operative infectious disease consultation. Exploration and decompression of all involved fascial spaces was also completed, and tooth numbers 46 and 47 were extracted. Multiple tissue samples were sent for culture, which later revealed the presence of a mixed infection, including *Streptococcus milleri*, coagulase negative *Staphylococcus* and anerobic gram negative bacilli. The wound was packed with iodine gauze (Fig. 15.12e). Intra-operatively, the patient exhibited signs of septic shock with hemodynamic instability requiring inotropic agents to maintain her blood pressure. She was transferred to the intensive care unit (ICU) and remained intubated.

The patient stayed in the ICU for approximately 2 weeks. A total of six sessions of hyperbaric oxygen treatment (HBOT) were administered during the initial period in the ICU.

(a)

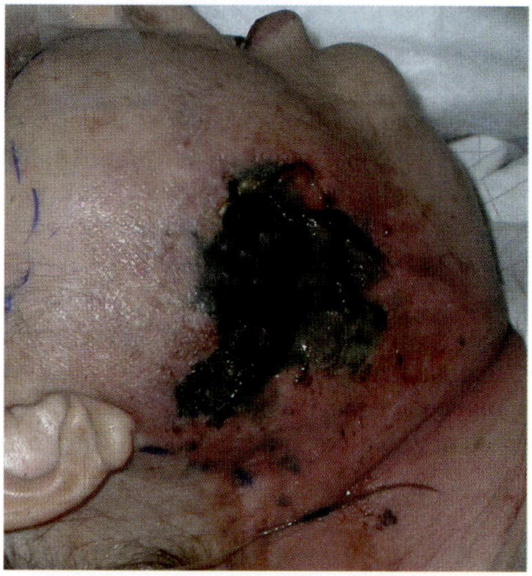

Fig. 15.12a Patient with full-thickness necrosis of the cheek and initial extensive bullae and erythema from the zygomatic arch to the inferior border of the mandible.

(b)

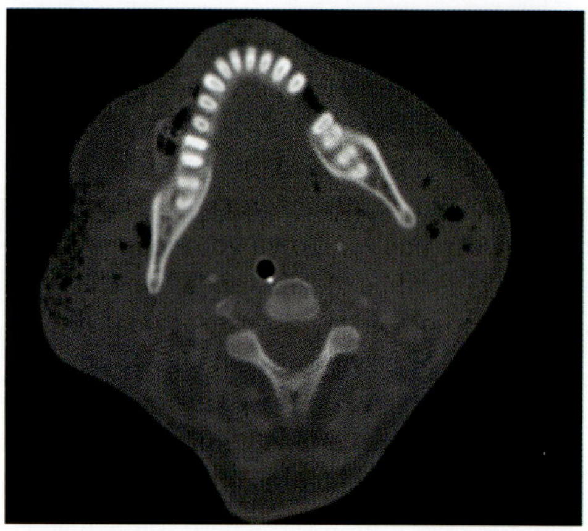

Fig. 15.12b Pre-operative CT scan showing marked edema and extensive subcutaneous gas formation which is also present in the parotid gland bilaterally.

Wound care in the form of frequent poviodine-soaked gauze changes and debridements of further necrotic tissue were performed. The patient was also taken to the operating room on one occasion for further debridement and partial decortication of the now exposed surfaces of the mandible and zygoma. The mandible was covered using a split sternocleidomastoid muscle flap, and all teeth with questionable prognosis were extracted.

At a later date, when the wound bed was judged to be adequate (Fig. 15.12f), multiple strips of split thickness skin grafts were taken from the lateral thigh and grafted to the exposed areas to provide primary cutaneous coverage over the large exposed area left by the surgical debridements (Fig. 15.12g).

(c)

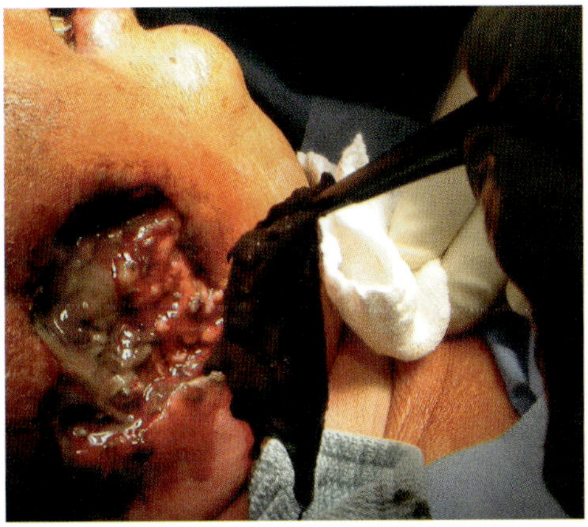

Fig. 15.12c Necrotic tissue excised from the wound. The margins of the excision had to be extended several times at surgery as the lesion continued to spread intra-operatively.

(d)

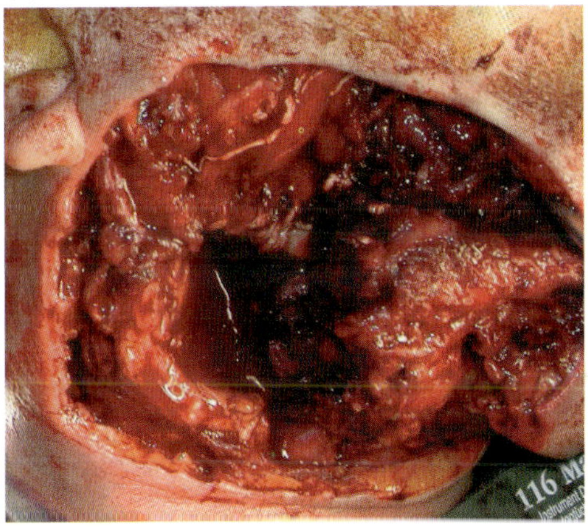

Fig. 15.12d Post-operative defect after extensive resection of all necrotic tissues.

(e)

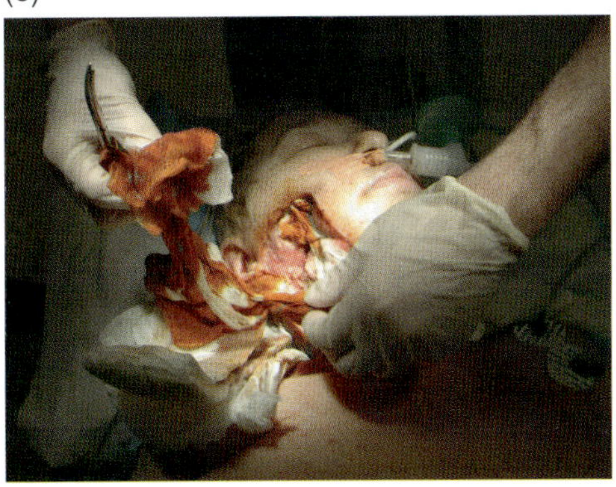

Fig. 15.12e Wound managed using iodine-soaked gauze dressings.

(f)

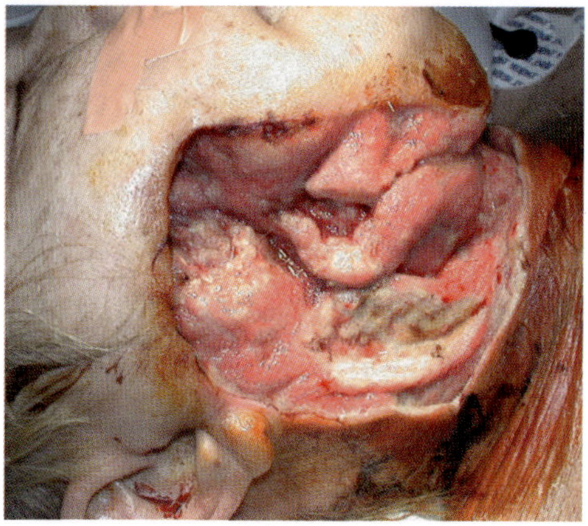

Fig. 15.12f The appearance of fresh granulation tissue signals the improvement of the wound and its readiness for skin grafting.

(g)

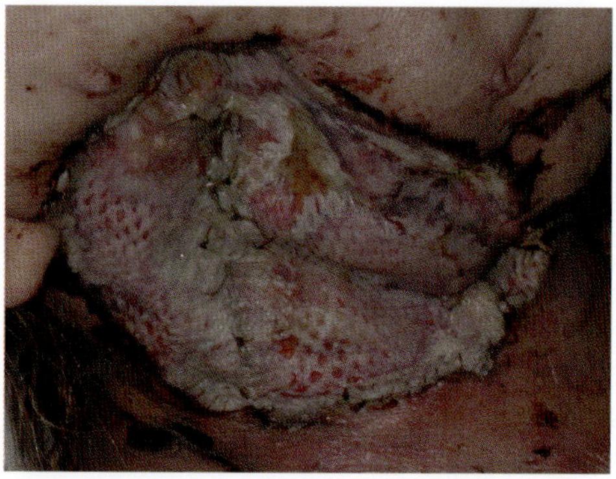

Fig. 15.12g Split thickness skin grafts with perforations placed over the resection defect.

(h)

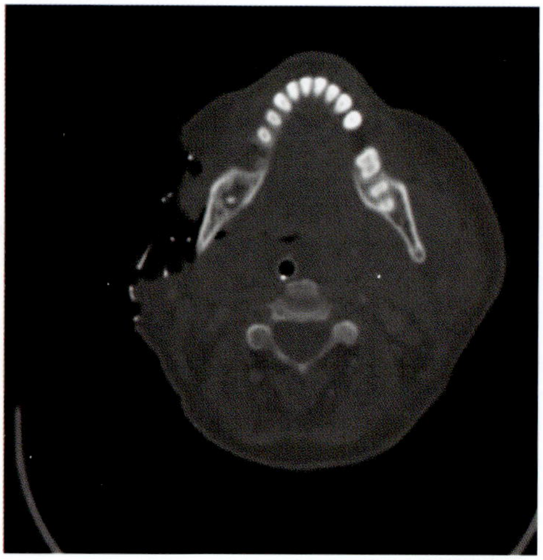

Fig. 15.12h Post-operative CT scan showing resolution of the infection and the defect of the right face due to the resection of the necrotic tissue.

(i)

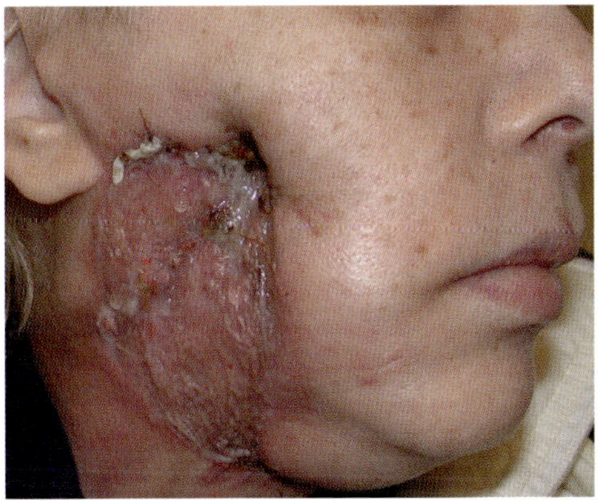

Fig. 15.12i Healed skin grafts 4 weeks after resection.

(j)

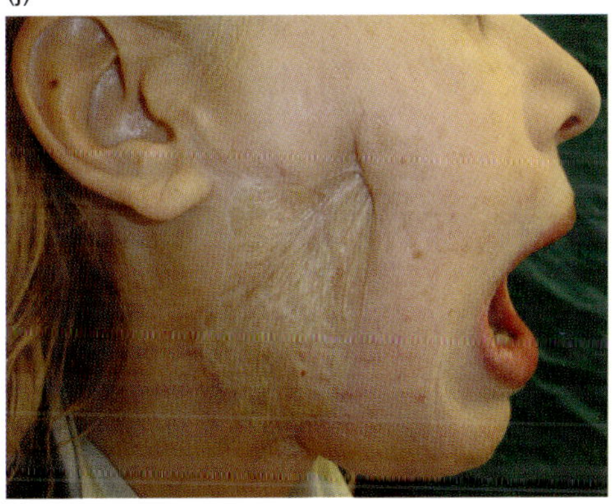

Fig. 15.12j Healed skin grafts 12 months after placement. The loss of a great volume of tissue makes the defect more pronounced though the surrounding soft tissues have healed well despite the life-threatening infection.

At 6 weeks of follow-up, she remained asymptomatic with excellent skin coverage over her large wound (Figs. 15.12h–j) and good oral food intake. Definitive treatment to provide bulk and improved cosmesis in the form of further rotational or free vascularized flaps could be considered in the future.

CONCLUSIONS

Large dentoalveolar wounds can be difficult to manage. Surgeons have a number of reconstructive choices such as autogenous bone grafts, vascularized bone grafts and alloplastic materials which depend on the condition of the wound and surrounding soft tissues. Surgeons can also augment the healing potential of large wounds by acute and chronic periosteal stretching, using growth factors and stem cells and by augmenting angiogenesis indirectly by the use of hyperbaric oxygen therapy.

While all these modalities are of interest, costs, access to the various treatment modalities and practicality are issues. Future surgeons will likely combine the useful features of all these modalities to simplify reconstructive, measures with the goal of making the reconstruction of dentofacial defects more predictable with less morbidity.

REFERENCES

Banerjee AR, Murty GE, Moir AA. (1996). Cervical necrotizing fasciitis: a distinct clinicopathological entity. *J Laryngol Otol* 110(1), 81–86.

Barr T, Carmichael NM, Sándor GKB. (2008). Juvenile idiopathic arthritis: a chronic pediatric musculoskeletal condition with significant dental manifestations. *J Can Dent Assoc* 74(9), 813–821.

Bauer SM, Bauer RJ, Velazquez OC. (2005). Angiogenesis, vasculogenesis, and induction of healing in chronic wounds. *Vasc Endovascular Surg* 39(4), 293–306.

Beaumont M, Du Val MG, Loai Y, Farhat WA, Sándor GKB, Cheng HLM. (2010). Monitoring angiogenesis in soft-tissue engineered constructs for calvarium bone regeneration: an in-vivo longitudinal DCE-MRI study. *Nuclear Med Reson Biomed* 23(1), 48–55.

Belser, U, Buser D, Higgenbottom F. (2004). Consensus statements and recommended clinical procedures regarding esthetics in implant dentistry. Proceedings of Third ITI Consensus Conference, Gstaad, Switzerland. *Int. J Oral Maxillofac Implant* 19(Suppl), 73–74.

Bornstein MM, Chappuis V, von Arx T, Buser D. (2008). Performance of dental implants after staged sinus floor elevation procedures: 5-year results of a prospective study in partially edentulous patients. *Clin Oral Implants Res* 19, 1034–1043.

Bourque WT, Gross M, Hall BK. (1992). A reproducible method for producing and quantifying the stages of fracture repair. *Lab Anim Sci* 42(4), 369–374.

Broussard CL. (2003). Hyperbaric oxygenation and wound healing. *J Wound Ostomy Continence Nurs* 30(4), 210–216.

Burchadt H. (1983). The biology of bone graft repair. *Clin Orthop* 174(1), 28–36.

Byrne AM, Bouchier-Hayes DJ, Harmey JH. (2005). Angiogenic and cell survival functions of vascular endothelial growth factor (VEGF). *J Cell Mol Med* 9(4), 777–794.

Canalis E, McCarthy T, Centrella M. (1988). Growth factors and the regulation of bone remodeling. *J Clin Invest* 81(2), 277–81.

Carmichael RP, Sándor GK. (2008). Use of dental implants in the management of cleft lip and palate. *Atlas Oral Maxillofac Clin N Am*, 16(1), 61–82.

Carmichael RP, Sándor GK, Bilko S, Riquelme C. (2008). Reconstruction of an ablative defect of the mandible in a young man using lateral soft tissue matrix expansion grafting and a novel technique for construction of a retrievable fixed prosthesis. *Forum Implantol* 4(1), 12–25.

Chattar-Cora D, Tulsyan N, Cudjoe EA, Onime GD, Pyo DJ, Weinstein L. (2002). Necrotizing fasciitis of the head and neck: a report of two patients and review. *Head Neck* 24(5), 497–501.

Chin M, Toth BA. (1996). Distraction osteogenesis in maxillofacial surgery using internal devices. Review of five cases. *J Oral Maxillofac Surg* 54, 45–53.

Clarizio LF. (2002).Vertical alveolar distraction versus bone grafting for implant cases: the clinical issues. In: Jensen OT (ed.) *Alveolar Distraction Osteogenesis*. Quintessence, Chicago, pp. 59–68.

Clokie CM, Bell RC. (2003). Human transforming growth factor B-1 and its effects on osseointegration. *J Craniofac Surg* 14(3), 268–277.

Clokie CM, Sándor GK. (2008). Reconstruction of 10 major mandibular defects using bioimplants containing BMP-7. *J Can Dent Assoc* 74(1), 67–72.

Clokie CM, Moghadam H, Jackson MT, Sándor GK. (2002). Closure of critical sized defects with allogenic and alloplastic bone substitutes. *J Craniofac Surg* 13(1), 111–121.

Dale RA, Hoffman DS, Crichton RO, Johnson SB. (1999). Necrotizing fasciitis of the head and neck: review of the literature and report of a case. *Spec Care Dentist*19(6), 267–274.

Danis R. (1949). Theorie et pratique de l'osteosynthese. *Lib Acad Med,* 76, 409–429.

Deckers M, Karperien M. (2000). Expression of vascular endothelial growth factors and their receptors during osteoblast differentiation. *Endocrinology* 141(5), 1667–1674.

Dragoo JL, Choi JY, Lieberman JR, et al. (2003). Bone induction by BMP-2 transduced stem cells derived from human fat. *J Orthop Res* 21(4), 622–629.

Ducy P, Zhang R, Geoffroy V, Ridall AL, Karsenty G. (1997). Osf2/Cbfa1: a transcriptional activator of osteoblast differentiation. *Cell* 89(4), 747–754.

Du Val MG, Davidson S, Ho A, et al. (2007). Albright's hereditary osteodystrophyt with extensive heterotrophic ossification of the oral and maxillofacial region: how fetuin research may help a seemingly impossible condition. *J Can Dent Assoc*, 73(9), 845–850.

Emad B. (2006). Vascular endothelial growth factor augments the healing of demineralized bone matrix grafts. *Int J Surg* 4(3), 160–166.

Engsig MT, Chen QJ, Vu TH, et al. (2000). Matrix metalloproteinase 9 and vascular endothelial growth factor are essential for osteoclast recruitment into developing long bones. *J Cell Biol* 151(4), 879–889.

Ewers R. (2005). Maxilla sinus grafting with marine algae derived bone forming material: a clinical report of long-term results. *J Oral Maxillofac Surg* 63, 1712–1723.

Feinerman IL, Tan HK, Roberson DW, Malley R, Kenna MA. (1999). Necrotizing fasciitis of the pharynx following adenotonsillectomy. *Int J Ped Otorhinolaryngol* 48, 1–7.

Fenton C, Nish IA, Carmichael RP, Sándor GKB. (2007). Metatastatic mandibular retinoblastoma in a child reconstructed with soft tissue matrix expansion grafting. *J Oral Maxillofac Surg* 65(11), 2329–2335.

Ferrara N, Gerber HP, LeCouter J. (2003). The biology of VEGF and its receptors. *Nat Med* 9(6), 669–676.

Fok, TCO, Jan A, Peel SA, Clokie CML, Sándor GK. (2008) Hyperbaric oxygen results in an increase in vascular endothelial growth factor (VEGF) protein expression in rabbit calvarial critical sized defects. *Oral Surg Oral Med Oral Pathol Oral Radiol Endodontol*, 105(4), 417–422.

Fugazzotto PA, Vlassis J. (1998). Long-term success of sinus augmentation using various surgical approaches and grafting materials. *Int J Oral Maxillofac Implants* 13, 52–58.

Gimble JM, Zvonic S, Floyd ZE, Kassem M, Nuttall M. (2006). Playing with bone and fat. *J Cell Biochem* 98(2), 251–266.

Glowacki J. (1998). Angiogenesis in fracture repair. *Clin Orthop Relat Res* 355(Suppl), S82–89.

Grinnemo KH, Syven C, Hovatta O, Dellgren G, Corbascio M. (2008) Immunogenicity of human embryonic stem cells. *Cell Tissue Res* 331(1), 67–68.

Hadfield PJ, Motamed M, Glover GW. (1996). Synergistic necrotizing cellulitis resulting from peri-tonsillar abscess. *J Laryngolol Otol* 110(9), 887–890.

Hu Z, Peel SA, Ho SK, Sándor GK, Clokie CM. (2005). Role of bovine bone morphogenetic proteins in bone matrix protein and osteoblast-related gene expression during rat bone marrow stromal cell differentiation. *J Craniofac Surg* 16(6), 1006–1014.

Hu Z, Peel SA, Ho SK, Sándor GK, Clokie CM. (2009a). Comparison of platelet-rich plasma, bovine BMP, and rhBMP-4 on bone matrix protein expression in vitro. *Growth Factors*, 27(2), 280–289.

Hu Z, Peel SA, Ho SK, Sándor GK, Clokie CM. (2009b). Platelet-rich plasma induces MRNA expression of VEGF and PDGF in rat bone marrow stromal cell differentiation. *Oral Surg Oral Med Oral Pathol Oral Radiol Endodont* 107(1), 43–48.

Humber C, Sándor GK, Davis JM, et al. (2010). Bone healing with an in situ formed bioresorbable PEG membrane in rabbit calvarial defects. *Oral Surg Oral Med Oral Pathol Oral Radiol Endodont* 109(3), 372–384.

Jan A, Sándor GK, Iera D, Mhawi, A, Peel SA, Clokie CM. (2006). Hyperbaric oxygen results in an increase in rabbit calvarial critical-sized defects. *Oral Surg Oral Med, Oral Pathol, Oral Radiol Endodont* 101(2), 144–149.

Jan A, Sándor GK, Brkovic BMB, Peel SA, Evans AW, Clokie CM. (2009). Effects of hyperbaric oxygen on grafted and non-grafted calvarial critical-sized defects. *Oral Surg Oral Med Oral Pathol Oral Radiol Endodont* 107(2), 157–163.

Jan A, Sándor GKB, Brkovic BMB, et al. (2010). Effects of hyperbaric oxygen on demineralized bone matrix and biphasic calcium phosphate bone substitutes. *Oral Surg Oral Med Oral Pathol Oral Radiol Endodont* 109(1), 60–67.

Jensen OT. (1999). Treatment planning for sinus grafts. In: Jensen OT (ed.) *The Sinus Bone Graft*. Quintessence, Carol Stream, Illinois, pp. 49–68.

Jurisic M, Markovic A, Radulovic M, Brkovic BMB, Sándor GKB. (2008). Maxillary sinus floor augmentation: comparing osteotome with lateral window immediate and delayed implant placements. An interim report. *Oral Surg Oral Med Oral Pathol Oral Radiol Endodontol* 106, 820–827.

Kahnberg KE, Ekestubbe A, Grondahl K. (2001). Sinus lifting procedure – I. One-stage surgery with bone and implants. *Clin Oral Implant Res* 12, 479–485.

Kainulainen VT, Lindholm TC, Sándor GKB. (2003). Resorboituneen alaleuan rekonstruktio "telttakeppi" tekniikalla. (Reconstruction of an extremely resorbed mandible by the "tent pole" procedure). *Suomen Hammaslääkärilehti (Finnish Dental Journal)* 12, 591–597.

Kleinheinz J. (2005). VEGF-activated angiogenesis during bone regeneration. *J Oral Maxillofac Surg* 63(9), 1310–1316.

Kudyba PS Jr, Loetscher CA, Perciaccante VJ, Jones CT, Cantrell JH. (2006). The fabrication and use of an extraoral surgical guide for implant placement coincident with soft tissue matrix expansion grafts: a clinical report. *J Prosthet Dent* 96(4), 227–232.

Lindfors LT, Tervonen EA, Sándor GKB, Ylikontiola LP. (2010). Guided bone regeneration using a titanium-reinforced ePTFE-membrane and particulate autogenous bone: the effect of smoking and membrane exposure. *Oral Surg Oral Med Oral Pathol Oral Radiol Endodont* April 8 (Epub).

Lindholm TC, Peel SAF, Clokie CML, Sándor GKB. (2003). Cortical bone grafts used to culture bone cells to be used for increasing efficacy of bone morphogenetic proteins in tissue engineered bone substitutes. *J Oral Maxillofac Surg* 61(8)(Suppl 1), 74.

Llewellyn CD, Johnson NW, Warnakulasuriya KA. (2001). Risk factors for squamous cell carcinoma of the oral cavity in young people – a comprehensive literature review. *Oral Oncol* 37, 401–418.

Mandracchia VJ, Nelson SC, Barp EA. (2001). Current concepts of bone healing. *Clin Podiatr Med Surg* 18(1), 55–77.

Marioni G, Bottin R, Tregnaghi A, Boninsegna M, Staffieri A. (2003). Craniocervical necrotizing fasciitis secondary to parotid gland abscess. *Acta Oto-Laryngol* 123(6), 737–740.

Marx R, Carlson E, Eichstaedt R, Schimmele S, Strauss J, Georgeff K. (1998). Platelet rich plasma growth factor enhancement for bone grafts. *Oral Surg Oral Med Oral Pathol Oral Radiol Endod* 85(6), 638–646.

Marx R, Shellenberger T, Wimsatt J, Correa P. (2002). Severely resorbed mandible: predictable reconstruction with soft tissue matrix expansion (tent pole) grafts. *J Oral Maxillofac Surg* 60, 878–88.

McGuire TP, Sándor GKB, Clokie CML. (2003). Advanced mandibular resorption: reliable reconstruction with autogenous graft tent pole technique. *J Oral Maxillofac Surg* 61(Suppl 1), 74.

Mesimäki k, Lindroos B, Törnwall J, et al. (2009). Novel maxillary reconstruction with ectopic bone formation by GMP adipose stem cells. *Int J Oral Maxillofac Surg* 38(3), 201–209.

Midy V, Plouet J. (1994). Vasculotropin/vascular endothelial growth factor induces differentiation in cultured osteoblasts. *Biochem Biophys Res Commun* 199(1), 380–386.

Moghadam HG, Urist MR, Sándor GK, Clokie CM. (2001). Successful mandibular reconstruction using a BMP bioimplant. *J Craniofacial Surg* 12(2), 119–127.

Moghadam HG, Sándor GK, Holmes HI, Clokie CM. (2004). Histomorphometric evaluation of bone regeneration using allogeneic and alloplastic bone substitutes. *J Oral Maxillofac Surg* 62(2), 202–213.

Mohammedi I, Ceruse P, Duperret S, Vedrinne J-M, Bouletreau P. (1999). Cervical necrotizing fasciitis: 10 years' experience at a single institution. *Intens Care Med* 25, 829–834.

Niida S, Kaku M, Amano H, et al. (1999). Vascular endothelial growth factor can substitute for macrophage colony-stimulating factor in the support of osteoclastic bone resorption. *J Exp Med* 190(2), 293–298.

Raboso E, Llavero MT, Rosell A, Martinez-Vidal A. (1998). Craniofacial necrotizing fasciitis secondary to sinusitis. *J Laryngol Otol* 112(4), 371–372.

Sándor GK, Carmichael RP. (2008). Rehabilitation of trauma using dental implants. *Atlas Oral Maxillofac Clin N Am*, 16(1), 83–105.

Sándor GK, Suuronen R. (2008) Combining adipose-derived stem cells, resorbable scaffolds and growth factors: an overview of tissue engineering. *J Can Dent Assoc,* 74(2), 167–170.

Sándor GK, Ylikontiola LP, Serlo W, Carmichael RP, Nish IA, Daskalogiannakis J. (2005). Midfacial distraction osteogenesis. *Oral Maxillofac Surg Clin N Am* 17, 485–501.

Sándor GK, Carmichael RP, Binahmed A. (2008). Reconstruction of ablative defects using dental implants. Dental implants in children, adolescents and young adults. *Atlas Oral Maxillofac Clin N Am* 16(1): 107–123.

Sándor GK, Carmichael RP, Brkovic BM. (2010). Dental implants placed into alveolar clefts reconstructed with bone grafts and tongue flaps. *Oral Surg Oral Med Oral Pathol Oral Radiol Endodontol,* 109(2), e1–e7.

Sándor GK, Lam DK, Ylikontiola LP, Kainulainen V, Oikarinen K, Clokie CM. (2011). Autogenous bone harvesting techniques. In: Kahnberg KE, Anderson L, Pogrel A (eds) *Oral and Maxillofacial Surgery*. Blackwell Munksgaard, Oxford, pp. 383–403.

Schilephake H. (2002). Bone growth factors in maxillofacial skeletal reconstruction. *Int J Oral Maxillofac Surg* 31(5), 469–484.

Schmitt JM, Hwang K, Winn SR, Hollinger JO. (1999). Bone morphogenetic proteins: an update on basic biology and clinical relevance. *J Orthop Res* 17(3), 269–278.

Sheikh AY, Gibson JJ, Rollins MD, Hopf HW, Hussain Z, Hunt TK. (2000). Effect of hyperoxia on vascular endothelial growth factor levels in a wound model. *Arch Surg* 135(11), 1293–1297.

Shindo ML, Nalbone VP, Dougherty WR. (1997). Necrotizing fasciitis of the face. *Laryngoscope* 107(8), 1071–1079.

Simion M, Jovanovic SA, Tinti C, Benfenati SP. (2001). Long-term evaluation of osseointegrated implants inserted at the time or after vertical ridge augmentation. A retrospective study on 123 implants with 1–5 year follow-up. *Clin Oral Implant Res* 12, 35–45.

Simmons D. (1980). Fracture healing. In: Urist MR (ed.) *Fundamental and Clinical Bone Physiology*. JB Lippincott, Philadelphia, pp. 283–330.

Sipola A, Ilvesaro J, Birr E, et al. (2007). Endostatin inhibits endochondral ossification. *J Gene Med* 9(2), 1057–1064.

Skitarelic N, Mladina R, Matulic Z, Kovacic M. (1999). Necrotizing fasciitis after peritonsillar abscess in an immunocompetent patient. *J Laryngol Otol* 113(8), 759–761.

Stoykewych AA, Beecroft WA, Cogan AG. (1992). Fatal necrotizing fasciitis of dental origin. *J Can Dent Assoc* 58, 59–62.

Street J, Winter D, Wang JH, Wakai A, McGuinness A, Redmond HP. (2000). Is human fracture hematoma inherently angiogenic? *Clin Orthop Relat Res* 378(9), 224–237.

Stucki-McCormick S, Moses JL, Robinson R, Laster Z, Mommaerts MY, Jensen OT. (2002). Alveolar distraction devices. In: Jensen OT (ed.) *Alveolar Distraction Osteogenesis*. Quintessence, Chicago, pp. 41–58.

Summers RB. (1994). A new concept in maxillary implant surgery: the osteotome technique. *Compend Cont Educ Dent* 15, 152–160.

Suuronen R, Asikainen A. (2004). Biodegradable materials as tools to fasten bone in face and jaw surgery. *Duodecim* 120(16), 2002–2007.

Tarkka T, Sipola A, Jämsä T, et al. (2003). Adenoviral VEGF-A gene transfer induces angiogenesis and promotes bone formation in healing osseous tissue. *J Gene Med* 5(4), 560–566.

Tatsuyama K, Maezawa Y, Baba H, Imamura Y, Fukuda M. (2000). Expression of various growth factors for cell proliferation and cytodifferentiation during fracture repair of bone. *Eur J Histochem* 44(3), 269–278.

Thompson L, Castle J, Heffner DK. (1999). Oral squamous cell carcinoma in pediatric patients: a clinicopathologic study of 20 cases. *Oral Surg Oral Med Oral Pathol Oral Radiol Endodontol* 88, 204.

Tirkkonen L, Halonen H, Hyttinen J, Kuokkanen H, Sievänen H, Koivisto A-M, Mannerström B, Sándor GK, Suuronen R, Miettinen S, Haimi S (2011). The effects of vibration loading on adipose stem cell number, viability and differentiation towards bone-forming cells. *J Royal Society Interface* 8(65),1736–1747.

Umeda M, Minamikawa T, Komatsubara H, Shibuya Y, Yokoo S, Komori T. (2003). Necrotizing fasciitis caused by dental infection: a retrospective analysis of 9 cases and a review of the literature. *Oral Surg Oral Med Oral Pathol Oral Radiol andEndodontol* 95(3), 283–290.

Urist MR, DeLange RJ, Finerman GA. (1983). Bone cell differentiation and growth factors. *Science* 220(4598), 680–686.

Warnke PH, Coren AJ. (2003). First experiences with recombinant human bone morphogenetic protein 7 (osteogenic protein 1) in a human case in maxillofacial surgery. *Plast Reconstr Surg* 111(10), 2471–2472.

Wozney JM, Lynch SE, Genco RJ, Marx RE. (1999). *Biology and Clinical Application of rhBMP-2: Tissue Engineering: Applications for Maxillofacial Surgery and Periodontics*. Quintessence, Chicago, pp. 103–123.

Yeh LC, Lee JC. (1999). Osteogenic protein-1 increases gene expression of vascular endothelial growth factor in primary cultures of fetal rat calvaria cells. *Mol Cell Endocrinol* 153(1–2), 113–124.

Index

Oral Wound Healing: Cell Biology and Clinical Management, First Edition. Edited by Hannu Larjava.